Fungal Eye Infections

Max Carlos Ramírez-Soto
Editor

Fungal Eye Infections

Epidemiology, Diagnosis and Treatment

Springer

Editor
Max Carlos Ramírez-Soto
Centro de Investigación en Salud Pública,
Facultad de Medicina Humana
Universidad de San Martín de Porres
Lima, Peru

ISBN 978-3-032-19922-5 ISBN 978-3-032-19923-2 (eBook)
https://doi.org/10.1007/978-3-032-19923-2

This Springer imprint is published by the registered company Springer Nature Switzerland AG
The registered company address is: Gewerbestrasse 11, 6330 Cham, Switzerland

Preface

Ocular fungal infections remain an important cause of ocular morbidity and irreversible vision loss, particularly in developing regions. Their incidence has increased markedly over the past decades, largely due to the widespread use of broad-spectrum antibiotics, immunosuppressive therapies, corticosteroids, ocular trauma, and post-operative complications. Unlike bacterial or viral ocular infections, which may be prevented or controlled through vaccines and public health strategies, fungal infections persist owing to their environmental reservoirs, adaptability, and ability to affect both immunocompetent and immunocompromised hosts. These infections may involve the ocular adnexa as well as intraocular structures, with clinical manifestations in both the anterior and posterior segments of the eye.

A wide range of fungal pathogens has been implicated in ocular disease. Among the most important are *Candida* spp., *Aspergillus*, *Fusarium*, *Curvularia* sp., *Alternaria* sp. and *Cryptococcus* spp., mucorales, along with *Penicillium*, and several dimorphic fungi, including *Histoplasma capsulatum*, *Paracoccidioides brasiliensis*, *Blastomyces dermatitidis*, *Sporothrix* spp., and *Coccidioides* spp. While certain species represent classical endemic mycoses, others are emerging opportunistic agents whose clinical significance is increasing in diverse geographic and epidemiological contexts. Over the past decades, several new fungal species have also been recognized as ocular pathogens, expanding the spectrum of organisms of concern.

The diagnosis of ocular fungal infections remains particularly challenging, as their clinical manifestations are often nonspecific and may mimic other ocular disorders, leading to delays in recognition and treatment. Over the past decade, remarkable progress has been made in ocular imaging technologies, microbiological diagnostic techniques—such as polymerase chain reaction and nucleic acid sequencing—and the development of novel antifungal agents. These advances, arising from multiple scientific and clinical disciplines, have substantially improved our understanding of ocular mycoses, yet keeping abreast of them continues to pose a challenge for clinicians and researchers alike.

As a result, the identification of characteristic clinical signs has enhanced early detection and management, contributing to better patient outcomes. Fungal infections of the eye may produce disease either through direct tissue invasion and destruction of essential ocular structures or indirectly through immune-mediated inflammatory responses. Despite their often-insidious onset, these infections can progress rapidly and cause devastating consequences, including irreversible vision loss, if not promptly recognized and treated.

As scientists, clinicians, and medical mycologists, we share the responsibility to dispel uncertainties surrounding ocular fungal infections by replacing speculation with evidence and providing accurate, science-based knowledge. This book was conceived to address these challenges by integrating current evidence and multidisciplinary expertise to present an updated and comprehensive overview of ocular and adnexal fungal infections. It offers concise and practical information designed to help ophthalmologists and eye care practitioners remain abreast of recent advances in diagnostic techniques, antifungal therapies, and surgical approaches, while also serving as a valuable reference for infectious disease specialists, microbiologists, and researchers dedicated to understanding, diagnosing, and managing these complex conditions.

Finally, I am deeply grateful to the contributing authors for their dedication, expertise, and unwavering commitment to advancing the field of ocular infectious diseases. Their collective efforts have enriched this book with current knowledge and valuable clinical insight. I also extend my sincere appreciation to the editorial team at Springer Nature for their guidance and support throughout the development of this work. I hope this book serves both as a practical reference and as an inspiration for continued research and innovation in the prevention, diagnosis, and treatment of ocular fungal infections.

Lima, Peru Max Carlos Ramírez-Soto

About This book

Fungal Eye Infections: Epidemiology, Diagnosis, and Treatment offers an in-depth and forward-looking exploration of one of the most challenging areas in ocular infectious disease. Bringing together the expertise of ophthalmologists, scientists, and medical mycologists, this volume offers a multidisciplinary perspective on the epidemiology, clinical manifestations, diagnosis, and management of both established and emerging fungal infections of the eye.

Each chapter follows a structured format, beginning with an overview and discussion of epidemiology, followed by sections on diagnosis, treatment, and concluding remarks. The content covers fungal infections involving the eyelids, conjunctiva, lacrimal sac, cornea (keratitis), intraocular structures (endophthalmitis and choroiditis), as well as orbital and neuro-ophthalmic fungal infections. The book also addresses the growing challenge of antifungal resistance and highlights the expanding role of artificial intelligence in enhancing diagnostic accuracy and patient management.

Written in a clear, concise, and clinically oriented style, this book is designed to serve as an essential reference for ophthalmologists, infectious disease specialists, microbiologists, and medical mycologists. Its unique integration of clinical and research insights makes it an indispensable resource for understanding, diagnosing, and managing the full spectrum of fungal eye infections.

Contents

About the Editor and Contributors

Editor

Max Carlos Ramírez-Soto, BSc, MPH, PhD, FECMM (https://orcid.org/0000-0003-0471-6746), is a professor and researcher at the Centre for Public Health Research, Department of Medicine, Universidad de San Martín de Porres, Lima, Peru. He graduated in Biological Sciences (BSc) from the Universidad de San Antonio Abad del Cusco, Peru, obtained his Master of Public Health (MPH) from the Universidad Nacional Mayor de San Marcos, Peru, and earned his PhD in Public Health from the Universidad Peruana Cayetano Heredia, Peru. He is a Fellow of the European Confederation of Medical Mycology (FECMM), an active member of numerous professional and academic societies, and a Global Assessor at the Royal Society of Tropical Medicine and Hygiene (UK). His research expertise includes evidence synthesis and the clinical and epidemiological aspects of fungal infections and infectious diseases, with a primary focus on sporotrichosis for more than 15 years. He serves on the Editorial Board of *BMC Medicine*, *BMC Infectious Diseases*, *Scientific Reports*, *Journal of Infection and Public Health*, *Frontiers in Public Health*, *Heliyon*, and *Current Fungal Infection Reports*. He is also an Academic Editor for *PLOS Neglected Tropical Diseases* and *PLOS Global Public Health*, and a Top Peer Reviewer for Web of Science. He has been recognized as an Expertscape World Expert in sporotrichosis, ranked No. 2 worldwide in 2021, and is one of the most highly cited researchers in Peru.

Contributors

Rupesh Agrawal Programme for Ocular Inflammation & Infection Translational Research, Department of Ophthalmology, National Healthcare Group Eye Institute, Tan Tock Seng Hospital, Singapore, Singapore
Lee Kong Chian School of Medicine, Nanyang Technological University, Singapore, Singapore
National Healthcare Group Eye Institute, Tan Tock Seng Hospital, Singapore, Singapore

Guillermo Amescua Bascom Palmer Eye Institute, University of Miami, Miami, FL, USA

Anjali Anil Department of Medical Microbiology, Post Graduate Institute of Medical Education and Research, Chandigarh, India

Alexandro Bonifaz Dermatology Service & Mycology Department, Hospital General de México "Dr. Eduardo Liceaga", Ciudad de México, Mexico

Carlos Cifuentes-González Programme for Ocular Inflammation & Infection Translational Research, Department of Ophthalmology, National Healthcare Group Eye Institute, Tan Tock Seng Hospital, Singapore, Singapore
Lee Kong Chian School of Medicine, Nanyang Technological University, Singapore, Singapore
Ocular Immunology Department, Ophthalmology Research Center, SIGMA Clinic, Cali, Colombia

Oindrilla Dasgupta Translational Pharmaceutics Research Laboratory (TPRL), Department of Pharmacy, Birla Institute of Technology and Sciences (BITS), Pilani, Hyderabad, Telangana, India
Centre for Ocular Drug Delivery Devices, Department of Pharmacy, Birla Institute of Technology and Sciences (BITS), Pilani, Hyderabad, Telangana, India

Jesús Heriberto Dávila-Alquisiras Oftalmology Service, Hospital General de México "Dr. Eduardo Liceaga", Ciudad de México, Mexico

Alejandra de-la-Torre Neuroscience (NEUROS) Research Group, Neurovitae Research Center, Institute of Translational Medicine (IMT). Escuela de Medicina y Ciencias de la Salud, Universidad del Rosario, Bogotá, Colombia

Haroldo Cesar de Oliveira Department of Microbiology, Immunology, and Parasitology, Discipline of Cellular Biology, Federal University of São Paulo (UNIFESP), São Paulo, Brazil

Prashant Garg Shantilal Shanghvi Cornea Institute and Brian Holden Eye Research Centre, KAR Campus, LV Prasad Eye Institute, Hyderabad, Telangana, India

Ana Luisa Hofling-Lima Department of Ophthalmology and Visual Sciences, Escola Paulista de Medicina (EPM), Federal University of São Paulo (UNIFESP), Sao Paulo, Brazil

Jiaxu Hong Department of Ophthalmology, Eye and ENT Hospital, Fudan University, Shanghai, China

Velmurugan Kailasam Translational Pharmaceutics Research Laboratory (TPRL), Department of Pharmacy, Birla Institute of Technology and Sciences (BITS), Pilani, Hyderabad, Telangana, India
Centre for Ocular Drug Delivery Devices, Department of Pharmacy, Birla Institute of Technology and Sciences (BITS), Pilani, Hyderabad, Telangana, India

Nitin Khandagale Translational Pharmaceutics Research Laboratory (TPRL), Department of Pharmacy, Birla Institute of Technology and Sciences (BITS), Pilani, Hyderabad, Telangana, India
Centre for Ocular Drug Delivery Devices, Department of Pharmacy, Birla Institute of Technology and Sciences (BITS), Pilani, Hyderabad, Telangana, India

Jaeryung Kim Subdivision of Neuro-ophthalmology, Department of Ophthalmology, Samsung Medical Center, Sungkyunkwan University School of Medicine, Seoul, South Korea

Wijak Kongwattananon Department of Ophthalmology, King Chulalongkorn Memorial Hospital, Thai Red Cross Society, Bangkok, Thailand
Center of Excellence in Retina, Department of Ophthalmology, Faculty of Medicine Chulalongkorn University and King Chulalongkorn Memorial Hospital, Thai Red Cross Society, Bangkok, Thailand

Esaú López-Jácome Laboratorio de Infectología, Instituto Nacional de Rehabilitación Luis Guillermo Ibarra Ibarra, CDMX, Mexico City, Mexico

Manisha Malani Translational Pharmaceutics Research Laboratory (TPRL), Department of Pharmacy, Birla Institute of Technology and Sciences (BITS), Pilani, Hyderabad, Telangana, India

Tamizhmathy Mannangatty Translational Pharmaceutics Research Laboratory (TPRL), Department of Pharmacy, Birla Institute of Technology and Sciences (BITS), Pilani, Hyderabad, Telangana, India
Centre for Ocular Drug Delivery Devices, Department of Pharmacy, Birla Institute of Technology and Sciences (BITS), Pilani, Hyderabad, Telangana, India

Jayabalan Nirmal Translational Pharmaceutics Research Laboratory (TPRL), Department of Pharmacy, Birla Institute of Technology and Sciences (BITS), Pilani, Hyderabad, Telangana, India
Centre for Ocular Drug Delivery Devices, Department of Pharmacy, Birla Institute of Technology and Sciences (BITS), Pilani, Hyderabad, Telangana, India

Kyung-Ah Park Subdivision of Neuro-ophthalmology, Department of Ophthalmology, Samsung Medical Center, Sungkyunkwan University School of Medicine, Seoul, South Korea

Max Carlos Ramírez-Soto Centro de Investigación en Salud Pública, Facultad de Medicina Humana, Universidad de San Martín de Porres, Lima, Peru

Anderson Messias Rodrigues Department of Microbiology, Immunology, and Parasitology, Discipline of Cellular Biology, Federal University of São Paulo (UNIFESP), São Paulo, Brazil
National Institute of Science and Technology in Human Pathogenic Fungi, São Paulo, Brazil

Alejandro Rodriguez-Garcia Institute of Ophthalmology and Visual Sciences, School of Medicine and Health Sciences, Tecnologico de Monterrey, Monterrey, Mexico

William Rojas-Carabali Colombian Visual Science and Translational Eye Research Institute (CERI), Centre of Excellence in Ocular Inflammation, Bogotá, Colombia
Programme for Ocular Inflammation & Infection Translational Research, Department of Ophthalmology, National Healthcare Group Eye Institute, Tan Tock Seng Hospital, Singapore, Singapore

Shivaprakash M. Rudramurthy Department of Medical Microbiology, Post Graduate Institute of Medical Education and Research, Chandigarh, India

Shridula Sankar Translational Pharmaceutics Research Laboratory (TPRL), Department of Pharmacy, Birla Institute of Technology and Sciences (BITS), Pilani, Hyderabad, Telangana, India

Kun Shan Department of Ophthalmology, Eye and ENT Hospital, Fudan University, Shanghai, China

Aileen Miwa Tabuse Department of Ophthalmology and Visual Sciences, Escola Paulista de Medicina (EPM), Federal University of São Paulo (UNIFESP), Sao Paulo, Brazil

Jazmín Tejeda-Olán Dermatology Service & Mycology Department, Hospital General de México "Dr. Eduardo Liceaga", Ciudad de México, Mexico

Andrés Tirado-Sánchez Dermatology Service & Mycology Department, Hospital General de México "Dr. Eduardo Liceaga", Ciudad de México, Mexico
Internal Medicine Department, Hospital General de Zona 30, Instituto Mexicano del Seguro Social, Ciudad de México, Mexico

Ayush Vasisth Department of Medical Microbiology, Post Graduate Institute of Medical Education and Research, Chandigarh, India

Lucy H. Young Department of Ophthalmology, Mass Eye and Ear, Harvard Medical School, Boston, MA, USA

Henry W. Zhou Department of Ophthalmology, Mass Eye and Ear, Harvard Medical School, Boston, MA, USA

Diagnosis Methods of Ocular Fungal Infections

1

Alexandro Bonifaz, Andrés Tirado-Sánchez,
Jesús Heriberto Dávila-Alquisiras, Jazmín Tejeda-Olán,
Esaú López-Jácome, and Max Carlos Ramírez-Soto

1.1 Introduction

The diagnosis of ocular fungal infections (OFIs) presents a significant clinical and laboratory challenge due to their nonspecific clinical features, which often mimic bacterial, viral, or parasitic infections. Conventional diagnostic methods, such as direct microscopy and fungal culture, are the diagnostic cornerstone for OFIs. However, in recent years, the advent of molecular methods has significantly improved the detection of fungal pathogens, even in culture-negative cases, and this offers the potential for earlier and more accurate diagnosis. Given the global burden of OFIs, particularly in tropical and subtropical regions, a timely and precise diagnosis is crucial to avoid serious complications such as corneal perforation, vision

A. Bonifaz (✉) · J. Tejeda-Olán
Dermatology Service & Mycology Department, Hospital General de México "Dr. Eduardo Liceaga", Ciudad de México, Mexico

A. Tirado-Sánchez
Dermatology Service & Mycology Department, Hospital General de México "Dr. Eduardo Liceaga", Ciudad de México, Mexico

Internal Medicine Department, Hospital General de Zona 30, Instituto Mexicano del Seguro Social, Ciudad de México, Mexico

J. H. Dávila-Alquisiras
Oftalmology Service, Hospital General de México "Dr. Eduardo Liceaga", Ciudad de México, Mexico

E. López-Jácome
Laboratorio de Infectología, Instituto Nacional de Rehabilitación Luis Guillermo Ibarra Ibarra, CDMX, Mexico City, Mexico

M. C. Ramírez-Soto
Centro de Investigación en Salud Pública, Facultad de Medicina Humana, Universidad de San Martín de Porres, Lima, Peru

M. C. Ramírez-Soto (ed.), *Fungal Eye Infections*,
https://doi.org/10.1007/978-3-032-19923-2_1

loss, or even loss of the eye through evisceration or enucleation. Diagnosis is often initiated clinically through slit-lamp examination, followed by the careful collection of ocular specimens prior to treatment. These specimens must be correctly inoculated or transferred to the microbiology laboratory, where clear communication between laboratory staff and medical practitioners is vital. In this context, the laboratory should provide clear guidance on the appropriate specimens required and the most accurate diagnostic approaches for OFIs.

This chapter reviews the current methodologies employed in the laboratory diagnosis of OFIs. We begin with a brief summary of ocular anatomy relevant to specimen collection. This is followed by an overview of the major clinical pathogens associated with fungal infections of the eye and the most commonly implicated pathogens. Finally, we discuss the various diagnostic tools available, including conventional and advanced molecular methods, and examine the role of antifungal susceptibility testing in guiding therapeutic decision-making.

1.2 Anatomy of the Eye

The eye is a specialized sensory organ composed of three concentric layers: the fibrous tunic (sclera and cornea), the vascular tunic or uvea (iris, ciliary body, and choroid), and the inner neural tunic (retina). The anterior segment comprises the cornea,

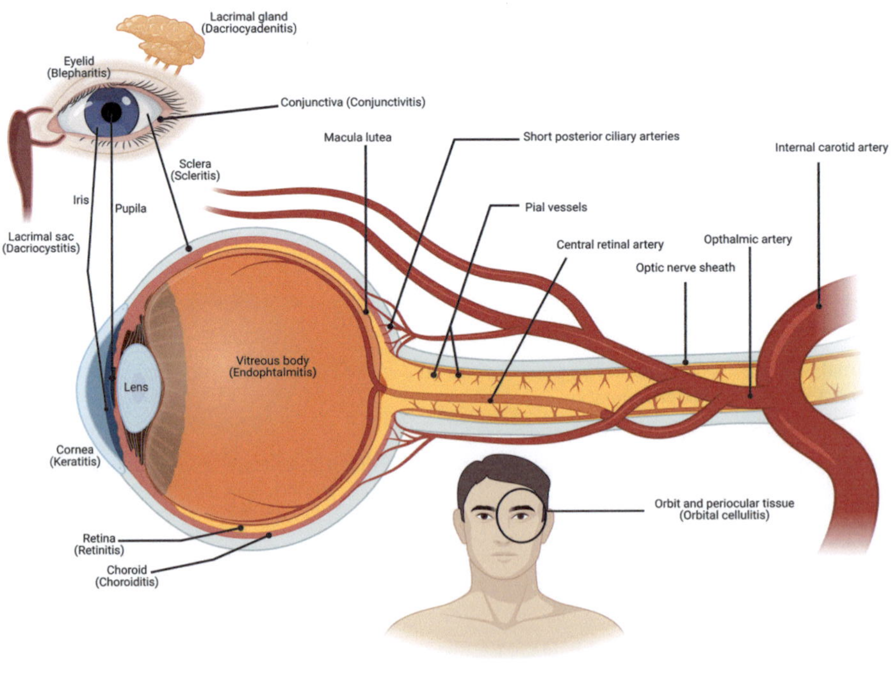

Fig. 1.1 Diagram of the eye and the various types of ocular fungal infections

anterior chamber, iris, posterior chamber, and lens, while the posterior segment includes the vitreous humor, retina, choroid, and optic nerve head (Fig. 1.1). Surrounding the globe are the ocular adnexa, which include the eyelids (palpebrae), conjunctiva, lacrimal apparatus (lacrimal gland, canaliculi, lacrimal sac, and nasolacrimal duct), extraocular muscles, and the bony orbit (Fig. 1.1). These structures are essential for ocular motility, protection, tear production and drainage, and the maintenance of a stable ocular surface environment. Understanding the anatomy of the eye and its adnexa is critical for recognizing the potential sites of infection, particularly in the context of OFIs, which may involve both intraocular and periocular structures [1].

1.3 Classification of Ocular Fungal Infections

OFIs comprise a diverse group of clinical entities that affect both the ocular globe and its adnexal structures [1, 2]. These infections can be broadly categorized into infections of the ocular adnexa and intraocular fungal infections, each presenting distinct etiologies, risk factors, and clinical manifestations [1, 2] (Table 1.1).

1.3.1 Infections of the Ocular Adnexa

Eyelid infections represent a heterogeneous group, ranging from superficial dermatophytosis to subcutaneous (e.g., *Sporothrix* spp.), systemic (e.g., *Paracoccidioides*, *Histoplasma*, *Cryptococcus* spp.), and opportunistic mycoses (e.g., *Candida*, *Aspergillus*, *Mucor* spp.) [3–6]. These infections frequently mimic other dermatologic or inflammatory conditions and often lack pathognomonic signs, leading to diagnostic delays. Fungal blepharitis, although rare in immunocompetent individuals, is typically endogenous due to organisms such as *Malassezia* spp., part of the normal skin microbiota. Clinically, it presents with eyelid erythema, pruritus, and inflammation, occasionally extending to the eyelashes [1, 2, 4].

Fungal conjunctivitis is an uncommon clinical entity that often presents as chronic conjunctival inflammation. It may be associated with trauma, adjacent blepharitis, or inoculation from contaminated fomites. Patients may experience redness, discharge, conjunctival hyperemia, and a foreign body sensation. Common causative organisms include *Candida*, *Aspergillus*, and *Fusarium* spp., though cases due to *Sporothrix* and other endemic fungi have been reported.

Fungal dacryocystitis is an uncommon infection of the lacrimal sac that may result in nasolacrimal duct obstruction. It usually affects immunocompetent individuals and can be associated with chronic blepharitis or introduced by exogenous pathogens such as *Candida*, *Sporothrix*, or *Blastomyces* spp. [1, 2, 5, 6].

Orbital cellulitis due to fungi involves infection of the soft tissues within the orbit and is clinically characterized by proptosis, impaired ocular motility, orbital pain, erythema, and, in severe cases, palpebral necrosis. Rhino-orbito-cerebral mucormycosis is the most common form and is strongly associated with uncontrolled diabetes mellitus, diabetic ketoacidosis, and profound neutropenia. *Aspergillus* spp. may also cause orbital involvement, although less frequently than *Mucor* spp. [1, 2, 4–6].

Table 1.1 Site and type of infection, predisposing factors, and main etiological agents

Site of infection	Type of infection	Frequency/patient type	Etiologic agents (more frequent)
Outer eye: Eyelid, lid margin, conjunctiva, lacrimal system, and periorbital tissue	Subcutaneous infections of eyelid	Immunocompetent	Dimorphic: *Sporothrix* spp., *Paracoccidioides* spp., *Coccidioides immitis*, and *Blastomyces dermatitidis*
	Blepharitis	Immunocompetent	Dermatophytes: *Trichophyton* spp., *Microsporum* spp., and *Arthroderma benhamiae* *Malassezia* sp.
	Dacryocystitis	Rare Immunocompetent	*Malassezia* sp., *Candida* sp., *Sporothrix* sp. *Blastomyces* sp.
	Conjunctivitis (rare)	Immunocompetent	Dimorphic fungi: *Sporothrix schenckii* and *S. brasiliensis* Opportunists: *Candida albicans* and *Fusarium* spp.
	Preseptal cellulitis	Immunocompetent	

Inner eye: Orbital cavity, cornea, anterior chamber, vitreous Humor, iris, uvea, sclera and lens	Fungal keratitis	Common/ immunocompetent trauma from plants contact lens wear post-surgery	**White filamentous fungi** *Fusarium solani* (50%), *F. oxysporum*, *F. verticillioides*, *F. dimerum*, *F. moniliforme*, *F. chlamydosporum* *Aspergillus fumigatus* (20%), *A. niger*, *A. flavus*, *A. glaucus*, *A. terreus*, *A. nidulans*, *A. nomius, A. tamari, A. protuberus* *Acremonium* sp. (formerly *Cephalosporium* sp.), *Aureobasidium pullulans, Colletotrichum* sp., *Cylindrocarpon lichenicola, Geotrichum* sp., *Lecythophora* sp., *Monosporium* sp., *Paecilomyces* sp., *Penicillium* sp., and *Scedosporium apiospermum complex*, *Scopulariopsis* sp., and *Verticillium* sp. **Dematiaceous filamentous fungi (melanized):** *Alternaria* sp., *Bipolaris* sp. (formerly reported, the species are now within the genus *Curvularia), Cladosporium* sp., *Curvularia* sp. (the most frequent), *Drechslera* sp., *Exophiala* sp., *Exserohilum* sp., *Macrophoma* sp., *Phialophora* sp., Bipolaris *Phoma* sp., *Pyrenochaeta keratinophila, Neoscytalidium* sp., *Chaetomium atrobrunneum, Colletotrichum truncatum, Fonsecaea pedrosoi, Papulaspora equi, and Ulocladium* sp. **Yeasts:** *Candida albicans, C. Parapsilosis, C. Dubliniensis, Trichosporon asahii, Dipodascus capitatus (Saprochaete capitata)* and *Rhodotorula mucilaginosa*
	Exogenous endophthalmitis	Rare Immunosuppression Trauma Surgical complications Intravenous drug use	*Candida albicans* infection, *Candida* spp. Other yeasts: *Rhodotorula* spp., *Cryptococcus* spp., *Geotrichum* spp., *Trichosporon* spp., *Malassezia* spp., and *saccharomyces* spp. Achloric algae (due to their yeast-like behavior such as *Prototheca* spp.)
	Endogenous endophthalmitis	Rare Immunosuppressed	Filamentous fungal infections Disseminated infections caused by *Aspergillus* spp., *Fusarium* spp., *and Scedosporium* spp. Dimorphic fungi: *Histoplasma capsulatum, Coccidioides* spp., *Blastomyces dermatitidis, Paracoccidioides brasiliensis, and Sporothrix schenckii complex*
	Choroiditis	Rare immunosuppressed	Opportunists: *Candida albicans, Cryptococcus neoformans*, and *Fusarium* sp. Dimorphic: *Blastomyces dermatitidis, Histoplasma capsulatum*
	Orbital cellulitis	Decompensated diabetes mellitus Immunocompromised (neutropenia)	Mucorales (*Rhizopus)* and *Aspergillus*

1.3.2 Intraocular Fungal Infections

Intraocular fungal infections include keratitis, endophthalmitis (exogenous and endogenous), and choroiditis. These entities represent serious, vision-threatening conditions that require prompt recognition and management.

Fungal keratitis, also known as fungal corneal ulcer, is the most common form of ocular fungal infection (OFI). It is an exogenous opportunistic infection, typically associated with corneal trauma—either accidental (e.g., from plant material) or iatrogenic (e.g., post-surgical)—and is often worsened by the inappropriate use of topical corticosteroids or antibiotics. Most cases occur in individuals with compromised immunity [1, 2]. Its global incidence remains unknown and varies significantly depending on geographic, socioeconomic, and environmental factors. It is considered a neglected disease, with a particularly high burden in low-income regions such as South Asia and Africa [3–7]. The causative agents of keratitis are generally classified into four main groups: hyaline filamentous fungi (hyalohyphomycetes), dematiaceous or melanized fungi (phaeohyphomycetes), yeasts, and, less commonly, actinomycetes—bacterial organisms capable of mimicking fungal infections (pseudomycoses). The condition is most commonly associated with environmental fungi such as *Fusarium* spp. (50–65%) and *Aspergillus* spp. (around 25%), though the distribution varies by geographic region [1, 4, 8–10, 15]. Major risk factors include ocular trauma involving plant material, contact lens use, and poor hygiene [4, 5, 22–25]. Other etiologic agents include a broad range of hyaline fungi such as *Acremonium*, *Paecilomyces*, *Penicillium*, and *Scedosporium* spp. [1, 4, 14], as well as melanized fungi like *Curvularia*, *Alternaria*, *and Cladosporium* spp. [16, 17], which are more prevalent in tropical and subtropical climates. Yeasts such as *Candida*, *Trichosporon*, and *Rhodotorula*, as well as actinomycetes like *Nocardia asteroides*, *N. brasiliensis*, and *N. farcinica*, have also been identified in a smaller proportion of cases [1, 4, 18–21].

Fungal endophthalmitis is a severe intraocular infection caused by filamentous fungi or yeasts and presents with symptoms such as conjunctival hyperemia, ocular pain, floaters, and progressive vision loss [6, 9]. *Exogenous* cases are typically associated with trauma, ocular surgery, or intravenous drug use and involve organisms such as *Candida* spp., *Rhodotorula*, *Trichosporon*, and *Saccharomyces* spp. [9]. *Endogenous* forms result from hematogenous dissemination of systemic mycoses, particularly in immunocompromised patients. The most frequently implicated pathogens include *Aspergillus*, *Fusarium*, *Scedosporium*, and dimorphic fungi such as *Blastomyces*, *Histoplasma*, *Paracoccidioides*, and *Sporothrix* spp. [1–6].

Fungal choroiditis is generally caused by opportunistic pathogens like *Candida* and *Cryptococcus*, particularly in individuals with impaired immunity. It may also manifest secondarily in the context of disseminated systemic fungal infections such as blastomycosis or histoplasmosis, leading to inflammation of the choroidal vasculature and potential extension to adjacent ocular tissues [1, 2, 6].

1.4 Laboratory Diagnosis

1.4.1 Sample Collection Protocol

In cases of fungal keratitis, it is recommended that the patient be seated in a fixed ophthalmic examination chair (with forehead and chin support) to ensure greater head stability. Ideally, the patient should be advised to wear an eye patch to keep the eye open and prevent sudden movements of the eyelids. (Fig. 1.2) The following protocol is recommended for sample collection:

(a) The eye should be anesthetized with 0.5% proparacaine or tetracaine hydrochloride (0.5%) drops. The recommended application is one or two drops of the solution in the eye, which will provide local anesthesia for 5–10 min.
(b) To ascertain the extent of corneal damage, it is recommended to add fluorescein or acridine orange, which emit an orange color under blue light. A number of solutions have been developed that incorporate this substance in conjunction with analgesics. (Fig. 1.3).
(c) Following the administration of ophthalmic anesthetics and the observation of the ulcer's periphery, the base and edges are meticulously scraped using a scalpel blade or Kimura spatula (sterile), employing gentle pressure to avoid injury to the underlying tissue. Given the delicacy of the procedure, it is strongly recommended that the sample be obtained by a specialist, such as ophthalmologist or qualified technical personnel.
(d) In the case of other types of ophthalmological infections as blepharitis, conjunctivitis, dacryocystitis, endophthalmitis, and uveitis, the secretions should be collected in a syringe and placed in a sterile container for subsequent fresh examination, staining, and culture. Similarly, in cases of orbital cellulitis (mucormycosis, aspergillosis), it is recommended to obtain tissue samples for further evaluation and management [1, 4, 7, 12, 13, 14, 22, 26–28].
(e) Specimens must be transported to the testing lab immediately. If delays occur, contact the lab for storage guidance. Swabs go in transport media at room

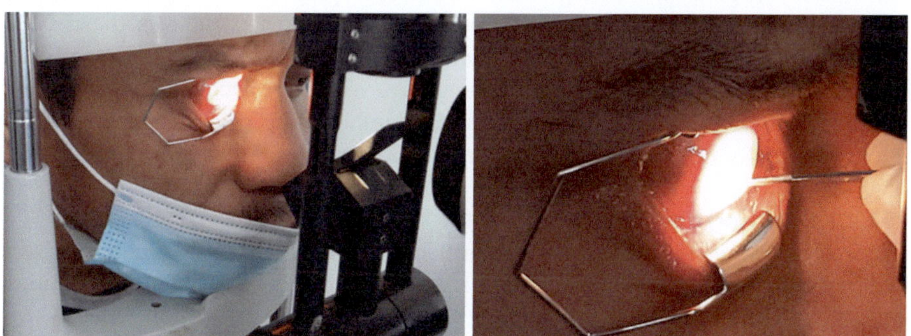

Fig. 1.2 Sampling of fungal keratitis

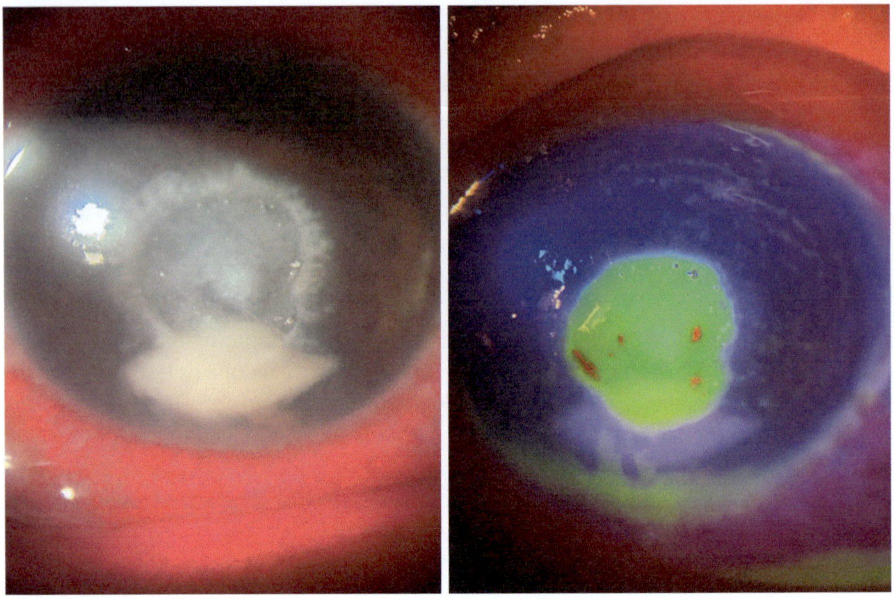

Fig. 1.3 Fungal keratitis due to *Fusarium* sp. with hypopyon. Fluorescein demarcation

temperature; fluids stay in original containers (syringe with needles removed) or sterile specimen containers. Tissues should remain intact, moistened with sterile saline, and treated like tissue if they include foreign objects or are collected on filter paper [1]. (Table 1.2).

1.4.2 Organism Identification and Reporting

The source, type, and suspected infection of the specimen are critical for its appropriate triage to ensure clinically actionable results. This information enables optimal microbiological processing, including proper preparation, examination, and culture—particularly important for irreplaceable specimens, such as those from ocular sources. This ensures optimal microbiological processing, including proper specimen preparation, examination, and culture, which is especially important for often irreplaceable specimens such as ocular samples. The sample is then divided into two parts for observation: fresh examination and/or staining and for cultures.

1.4.2.1 Staining and Fresh Examination

Generally, fresh examinations are performed using KOH (10%), a diagnostic test that has proven useful in analyzing material collected from cases of fungal keratitis and other forms of ocular pathology. A rapid observation reveals the presence of two distinct types of images in cases of corneal ulcers. In infections caused by filamentous fungi, the most common findings include broad, tortuous, and irregular hyphae

Table 1.2 Ocular sample collection for laboratory diagnosis of fungal infections

Sample type	Collection method	Indications	Laboratory tests	Remarks
Corneal scraping	Scraped from ulcer margins and base using sterile blade/spatula under anesthesia	Fungal keratitis	KOH mount, calcofluor white stain, fungal culture, PCR	Most common sample for fungal keratitis diagnosis
Conjunctival swab	Sterile swab from lower fornix	Suspected fungal conjunctivitis	KOH mount, gram stain, fungal culture	Less sensitive than scraping for fungal diagnosis
Aqueous humor	Paracentesis with fine needle under aseptic conditions	Fungal endophthalmitis and uveitis	KOH mount, fungal culture, PCR	Limited yield, used when corneal or vitreous samples unavailable
Vitreous humor	Vitreous tap or biopsy via pars plana	Fungal endophthalmitis	KOH mount, fungal culture, PCR, cytology	High diagnostic value in intraocular fungal infections
Lens material	Removed during cataract or vitrectomy surgery	Suspected lens-induced infection	Culture, histopathology, PCR	Especially for delayed-onset fungal endophthalmitis
Intraocular membranes	Obtained during vitrectomy	Fungal Endophthalmitis	Histopathology, fungal culture, PCR	Useful in chronic or unresponsive cases
Tear film / lacrimal secretions	Schirmer strip or swab	Chronic dacryocystitis Canaliculitis	Fungal culture, KOH stain	Rare, used for superficial or nasolacrimal infections
Contact lens & case	Collected directly	Contact lens-related fungal keratitis	Fungal culture	Should be examined alongside corneal scrapings
Eyelid margin scraping/ periorbital tissue	Scraping with sterile blade	Blepharitis, meibomianitis and periocular tinea	Fungal culture, KOH stain	Collect samples from the active lesion margin
Orbital cavity	Collect tissue and/or discharge/ purulent material	Orbital cellulitis	Fungal culture, histopathology	Whenever possible, obtain deep tissue samples and ensure measures are taken to prevent secondary contamination

that are septate and poorly branched, typically seen in species such as *Fusarium*, *Scedosporium*, and *Acremonium*. Infections caused by *Aspergillus* species present with hyaline, septate, and regularly branching hyphae, often exhibiting a characteristic 45° angle of bifurcation. On rare occasions, dark, septate, and branched hyphae emerge for black or melanized fungi (*Curvularia, and Alternaria*) [27]. In case of infection by *Candida* spp., blastoconidia and pseudohyphae are observed. In cases associated with *Nocardia* sp., Gram staining is the preferred method due to its ability to reveal multiple thin (1 μm) Gram-positive filaments [27].

As indicated by the literature, direct examinations with calcofluor white plus KOH (10–20%) are also useful for the diagnosis of ocular fungal infections—especially fungal keratitis and endophthalmitis; a direct fluorescence microscope is required for this procedure. In general, a small sample volume is added and subsequently observed after 2 min. calcofluor white is a fluorescent dye that binds specifically to chitin and cellulose in fungal cell walls. For corneal scrapings from suspected infectious ulcers, the sample is smeared onto a clean slide, and a drop of 10% KOH mixed with calcofluor white stain is added. The slide is then covered with a coverslip and examined under a fluorescence microscope. Fungal hyphae—such as those of *Fusarium* or *Aspergillus*—appear as bright fluorescent filaments. In intraocular samples, such as vitreous aspirates, aqueous humor, or lens material from suspected cases of endophthalmitis, direct microscopy using calcofluor white can rapidly detect fungal filaments. This technique has been demonstrated to be more effective and sensitive than the traditional KOH technique. The fungal elements manifest as yellow-green coloration [1, 4, 22, 27].

Additionally, smears can be prepared from the samples and stained using various techniques, including Giemsa and Periodic Acid-Schiff (PAS). Giemsa stain may weakly stain hyphae or yeast in a blue-violet color. PAS highlights fungal cell walls in magenta due to their polysaccharide content and is particularly effective for detecting yeasts and hyphae in tissues or scrapings. Other stains such as acridine orange, Grocott's methenamine silver, and Papanicolaou can also be employed for fungal detection [1, 22, 27].

Direct examinations and stains are regarded as rapid tests. However, the available evidence suggests that these tests have low sensitivity (60% to 70%) and specificity (40% to 66%), leading to the possibility of false negative interpretations [1, 14, 22, 27]. (Figs. 1.4 and 1.5).

1.4.3 Culture

Cultures are widely regarded as the gold standard for diagnosis; in specialized laboratory settings, the proportion of cultures yielding positive results can reach up to 70%, a finding contingent on the method of sample collection and the patient's antifungal therapy status. The recommended protocol entails repeated execution of the process, spanning several days, in standard media formulations devoid of antibiotics such as Sabouraud dextrose agar, Sabouraud dextrose agar containing antibiotics, potato dextrose agar (PDA), yeast extract, and brain heart infusion (BHI) agar.

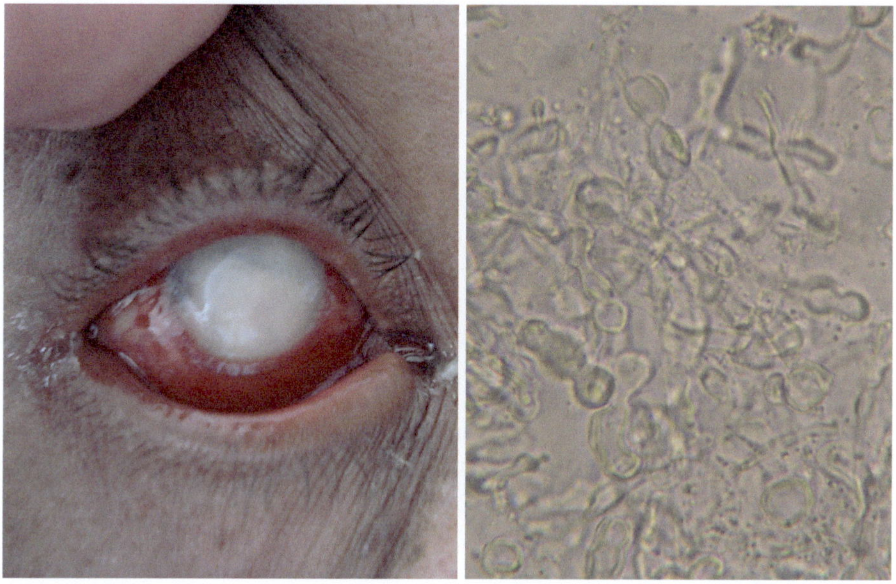

Fig. 1.4 *Fusarium* keratitis. Direct examination with multiple irregular hyphae (KOH, 40x)

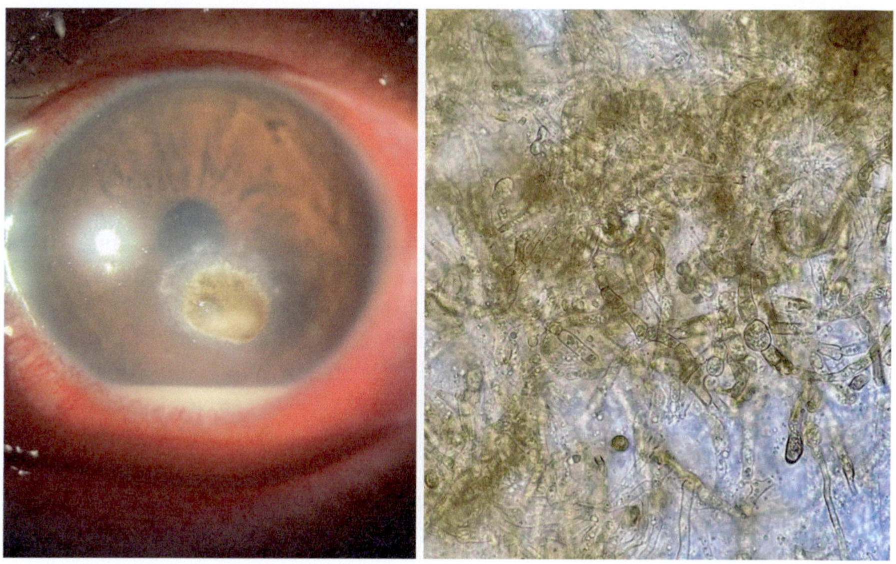

Fig. 1.5 *Curvularia* keratitis. Direct examination with dark, septate hyphae (KOH, 40x)

In most cases, fungal keratitis results in the rapid development of fungal colonies. This development occurs within a time span of 3–5 days at temperatures ranging from 25 to 28 °C. The characteristics that these colonies exhibit are determined by the specific fungal strain identified. Table 1.3 lists the fungal pathogens that infect ocular tissues.

The incubation period is extended to a maximum of 30 days in cases of primary pathogenic mycoses, including sporotrichosis, paracoccidioidomycosis, and blastomycosis. In cases of fungal keratitis and other infections caused by contaminating filamentous fungi, the criterion for determining etiology involves the retrieval of at least two or three positive cultures at different times. However, in cases where the etiological agent is a primary pathogenic fungus, the presence of pure isolation and correlation with parasitic observation serves as a diagnostic indicator [1, 4, 22, 27–31].

As observed in direct examinations and stains, cultures are obtained in approximately 60–70% of cases and require more time to develop and allow for subsequent identification; nevertheless, these tests prove useful not only for species identification but also in the processing of in vitro susceptibility testing [1, 22, 31–34] (Fig. 1.6). (Table 1.2).

1.4.4 Polymerase Chain Reaction (PCR)

PCR tests are performed on various regions of nucleic acids to obtain specific probes or primers. The most commonly used are the ITS-5.8S rRNA, 18S rRNA, 28S rRNA, and ITS2 regions. The results of this test are then compared with genetic information databases, such as GenBank, with a particular emphasis on the Basic Local Alignment Search Tool (BLAST) system. The use of these techniques has been reported sensitivity and specificity rates ranging from 70% to 93% and 89% to 100%, respectively [1, 22, 27, 35, 36]. Consequently, the PCR techniques are regarded as the gold standard for the identification of the most prevalent fungi. This is because these are rapid tests that exhibit high reliability and can be performed either directly on the specimen or the isolated culture (Table 1.4). In the research conducted by Thomas et al., the combination of direct examination with culture yielded a 78% positive outcome, in contrast to the 93% positive results obtained through PCR [37]. It has been observed that the results of PCR and microbiological studies frequently exhibit a high degree of concordance. Nevertheless, the primary function of PCR is as a diagnostic adjunct, especially in cases where cultures yield negative results or when the disease is in early stages [38].

Table 1.3 Type of ocular fungal infection, main mycological data for diagnosis

Types of fungi	Most frequent etiological agents	Direct examination and staining observations	Cultures (Sabouraud dextrose agar medium)	Reproductive forms	Associated ocular infections
Hyaline fungi	*Fusarium complex* *Scedosporium* sp.	Hyaline, irregular, septate, and bifurcated hyphae	Fast-growing white colonies with various pigments diffusible to the medium	*Fusarium:* Conidiophores with spindle-shaped macroconidia and microconidia *Scedosporium:* Conidiophores with pyriform microconidia	Keratitis
Dematiaceous fungi (melanized)	*Curvularia* sp. *Alternaria* sp.	Dark, regular, septate, and bifurcated hyphae	Fast-growing black or dark-green colonies with dark pigment	*Curvularia:* Macroconidia with transverse and curved septa *Alternaria:* Dictyoconidia with transverse and longitudinal septa arising from the hyphae	Keratitis
Yeasts	*Candida albicans*	Pseudohyphae and blastoconidia	Fast-growing creamy-white colonies	Round and oval blastoconidia	Blepharitis Endophthalmitis, conjunctivitis, chorioretinitis and keratitis
Actinomycetes	*Nocardia* spp.	Thin filaments (<1 mm) gram-positive and acid-fast	Slow growing, limited rocky colonies	Thin filaments less than 1 mm long with coccoid and rod-shaped gram-positive bacteria	Keratitis, scleritis and orbital cellulitis
Dimorphic fungi	*Paracoccidioides brasiliensis,* *Blastomyces dermatitidis,* *Sporothrix schenckii*	Yeast-like cells or budding forms observed in tissue; may show oval or cigar-shaped yeasts in stained smears	Yeast-like or budding cells observed in tissue; oval or cigar-shaped yeasts may be seen in stained smears	Slow-growing colonies; yeast form at 37 °C and mycelial form at room temperature	Palpebral infections, endophthalmitis, choroiditis and conjunctivitis (rare)

(continued)

Table 1.3 (continued)

Types of fungi	Most frequent etiological agents	Direct examination and staining observations	Cultures (Sabouraud dextrose agar medium)	Reproductive forms	Associated ocular infections
Mucorales (Zygomycetes)	*Rhizopus* spp., *Mucor* spp., *Lichtheimia* spp.	Broad, non-septate hyphae with right-angle branching	Rapid growth; fluffy gray-white colonies	Sporangiospores inside sporangia	Orbital cellulitis and rhino-orbital-cerebral mucormycosis
Dermatophytes	*Trichophyton* spp. and *Microsporum* spp.	Septate hyphae and arthroconidia observed in KOH preparation or stained smears	Cottony or powdery colonies; the pigment may vary depending on the species	Yeast and mycelial forms (temperature-dependent dimorphism)	Periocular tinea

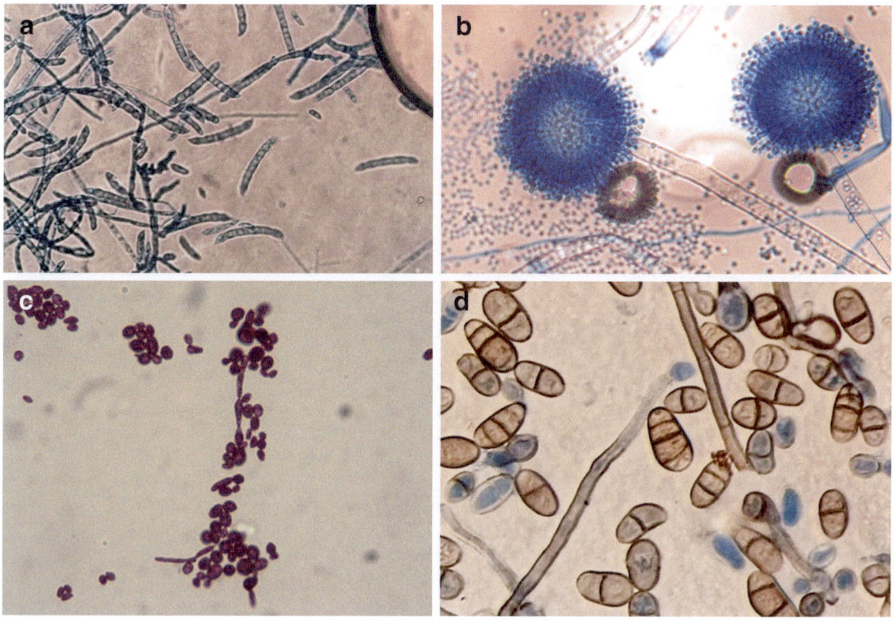

Fig. 1.6 Microscopy of the 4 main etiologic agents. (**a**) *Fusarium solani*. (**b**) *Aspergillus flavus*. (**c**) *Candida albicans*. (**d**) *Curvularia lunata*

1.4.5 Proteomics

The majority of the etiological agents isolated from fungal keratitis can be identified with high accuracy using matrix-assisted laser desorption/ionization-time of fly (MALDI-TOF) mass spectrometry (MS). This method entails extensive extraction for filamentous fungi and merely requires the maintenance of a current equipment database [1, 22, 39, 40].

1.4.6 Histopathology

It is particularly useful when direct examination yields negative results; histopathology reveals an acute and suppurative inflammatory process with areas of coagulative necrosis. To adequately highlight the fungal elements (hyphae), it is necessary to employ staining techniques such as PAS or Gomori-Grocott staining. The arrangement of hyphae in fungal keratitis is typically observed to be parallel aligned to the corneal lamellae and Descemet's membrane. In certain cases, hyphae may even be found traversing these structures, a phenomenon that is particularly evident following corticosteroid therapy [1, 4, 41].

Table 1.4 Molecular methods for the diagnosis of ocular fungal infections

Molecular technique	Genetic target	Advantages	Limitations	Clinical application	Reference
Conventional PCR	ITS, 18S rRNA, 28S rRNA	High sensitivity and specificity; rapid	Risk of contamination; requires primer design	General detection of fungi in ocular specimens	[35–37]
Real-time PCR (qPCR)	Species- or genus-specific fungal DNA	Quantitative; high sensitivity; reduced contamination risk	Requires specialized equipment and standardization	Early and specific diagnosis of *Fusarium*, *aspergillus*, etc.	[41, 42]
Multiplex PCR	Multiple fungal genes	Detects multiple pathogens simultaneously	Complex primer design; cross-reactivity risk	Differential diagnosis when multiple fungi are suspected	[35, 62–65]
Nested PCR	ITS, 18S rRNA	Highly sensitive, suitable for low DNA load samples	Time-consuming; higher contamination risk	Detection in paucibacillary ocular samples	63–66]
Sanger sequencing	PCR amplicons (ITS, D1/D2, 28S rRNA)	Precise species-level identification	Costly; cannot resolve mixed infections	Confirmation of rare or unusual fungi	[38]
Next-generation sequencing (NGS)	Total fungal and host DNA	Detects unculturable and unexpected fungi; metagenomic profiling	High cost; requires bioinformatics expertise	Atypical, recurrent, or polymicrobial infections	[62–65]

The efficacy of the histopathology is approximately 85%, yet its specificity is low, due to the inability to identify the type of etiological agent involved, a limitation that is similar to that of staining. It is important to acknowledge that this technique is considered to be invasive and is preferred when microbiological tests yield negative results [1, 42].

1.4.7 In Vivo Confocal Microscopy

This noninvasive diagnostic technique is performed directly on the subject, providing high-contrast, three-dimensional images. This system is used in ophthalmological applications for the corneal analysis. It facilitates the visualization of all corneal layers, thereby enabling the detection of microbes, with a particular emphasis on fungi and amoebae. The primary benefit of this technique is that it enables precise assessment of the ulcer's depth and extent. However, its efficacy as a sole diagnostic tool is considered limited, thereby requiring its integration with additional diagnostic techniques, such as microbiological studies, to increase diagnostic precision [42, 43].

In the study conducted by Vaddavalli et al. [44], a sample of approximately 150 cases was examined, resulting in sensitivity and specificity rates of 89% and 93%, respectively. Considering the aforementioned discussion and in accordance with the findings of recent studies [42–44], this technique has been deemed noninvasive and of significant utility, as it yields immediate results.

1.5 Antifungals and Susceptibility Testing

The treatment of OFIs, particularly fungal keratitis, poses a significant challenge due to the limited availability of ophthalmic antifungal agents [45]. Natamycin (pimaricin) is a commonly used and effective option. It is available as a 5% ophthalmic suspension or cream and is typically administered every hour during the day and every 2 h at night [46]. This polyene antifungal has broad-spectrum activity against several fungal pathogens, including *Fusarium*, *Aspergillus*, and dematiaceous (melanized) fungi [11]. However, certain *Fusarium* strains have shown resistance to antifungal therapy. In vitro studies have indicated that natamycin exhibits lower minimum inhibitory concentrations (MICs) against *Fusarium* spp. compared to voriconazole, suggesting superior potency in this context [47]. An amphotericin B suspension at a concentration of 1 mg/mL is also employed; nevertheless, this antifungal agent is associated with a considerable toxicity profile despite its broad therapeutic index. Ocular toxicity, particularly corneal epithelial irritation, is a well-documented adverse effect. In selected cases, intravitreal injection of amphotericin B has been employed as a therapeutic approach for fungal endophthalmitis [11, 46, 47].

Voriconazole has proven effective in treating fungal keratitis, as supported by multiple clinical studies. It is administered in a 1% solution, once-hourly during daytime and twice-hourly during nighttime. This agent has rapidly emerged as the treatment of choice in many cases of fungal keratitis due to its broad spectrum of antifungal activity and excellent penetration into the corneal stroma [11]. In comparative studies with natamycin [47, 48], voriconazole demonstrated greater efficacy, particularly in cases caused by *Aspergillus* and *Candida* species [48, 49]. These findings suggest that voriconazole may offer comparable or even statistically superior clinical outcomes. However, this contrasts with the results reported by Prajna et al. [48], in which natamycin was associated with significantly better clinical and microbiological outcomes in filamentous fungal keratitis compared to voriconazole. Notably, natamycin's efficacy is especially evident in keratitis caused by *Fusarium* species [48]. The combination of natamycin and voriconazole has also been identified as effective and may be considered for regular use in the future, particularly in cases of refractory or recurrent OFIs [50].

Antifungal susceptibility testing is crucial for guiding antifungal therapy, particularly due to rising rates of antifungal resistance and the growing diversity of fungal pathogens. Their objective is to determine the MICs of antifungal agents against clinical fungal isolates, thereby informing treatment choices and supporting surveillance of resistance trends. The Clinical and Laboratory Standards Institute (CLSI) and the European Committee on Antimicrobial Susceptibility Testing (EUCAST) establish protocols for broth microdilution, which is the reference method for MIC determination. The performance of susceptibility testing should be guided by the CLSI documents M27 (for yeasts) and M38 (for filamentous fungi), in conjunction with the EUCAST system [51, 52]. This testing should be conducted using both broth microdilution and disk diffusion methods. The cut-off points for each fungus can be found in the corresponding documents for the methods used. CLSI document M60 contains multiple clinical breakpoints for *Candida* species, while document M61 provides clinical breakpoints for *A. fumigatus* specifically against voriconazole [53]. Epidemiological cutoff values (ECVs) for both yeasts and molds are reported in CLSI document M59 [54]. There are also commercial alternative methods, such as gradient diffusion methods (Etest™) and colorimetric assays (e.g., Sensititre™ YeastOne™), which offer more practical workflows in routine settings, though with some limitations in terms of accuracy or cost [57]. Emerging technologies like MALDI-TOF MS-based susceptibility approaches show promise for rapid detection but remain under investigation and lack standardization [58] (Table 1.5). Both CLSI and EUCAST periodically publish clinical breakpoints derived from pharmacokinetic/pharmacodynamic data and clinical outcome studies. However, for many uncommon or emerging fungal pathogens, only ECVs are available. As ECVs do not predict clinical outcomes, it is essential to acknowledge the limitations of MIC-based testing and to interpret susceptibility results within a context clinical, pharmacological, and mycological framework to guide effective antifungal therapy [59].

It is imperative to acknowledge that the values reported for yeasts are typically associated with blood levels and may not necessarily reflect the levels present in the

Table 1.5 Methods for antifungal susceptibility testing

Method	Target organisms	Brief description	Advantages	Limitations	Reference
Broth microdilution (CLSI M27/M38)	Yeasts (M27), filamentous fungi (M38)	Reference method to determine minimum inhibitory concentration (MIC) using RPMI medium	Standardized, reproducible MIC values; widely accepted	Labor-intensive, requires trained personnel, slow turnaround time	[51–53]
EUCAST broth microdilution	Yeasts, molds	Similar to CLSI; differs in media composition and breakpoints	Harmonized within Europe; regularly updated breakpoints	Limited data for some molds and rare fungi	[55]
Disk diffusion (CLSI M44)	Yeasts	Disks with antifungal agents on agar; measures inhibition zones	Simple, low cost, useful for initial screening	Not quantitative; not suitable for filamentous fungi	[56]
Etest (gradient diffusion strip)	Yeasts, filamentous fungi	Plastic strips with antifungal gradient placed on agar; MIC read at inhibition ellipse	Easy to use, direct MIC estimation, suitable for routine labs	Costly; affected by medium composition and incubation conditions	[57]
Commercial colorimetric assays (e.g., Sensititre™, YeastOne™)	Yeasts, some molds	Pre-prepared panels with colorimetric indicators to determine MIC	Rapid, user-friendly, compatible with automated systems	Expensive; limited mold panel coverage; interpretation may vary	[57]
MALDI-TOF MS-based AFST *(experimental)*	Yeasts, molds (under study)	Uses spectral changes after antifungal exposure to infer susceptibility	Potentially rapid; culture-independent variants under development	Still experimental; no validated standards; high cost of equipment	[58]

eye. A high prevalence of drug resistance has been documented in fungal species associated with fungal keratitis, including *Fusarium* and *Aspergillus*, particularly in cases resulting from traumatic injury with vegetables. This increased resistance may be partly explained to the widespread use of antifungal medications, particularly triazoles, which can result in the development of voriconazole resistance [60, 61]. Certain fungi, such as *Aspergillus terreus*, *Lomentospora prolificans*, and *Purpureocillium lilacinum*, demonstrate intrinsic resistance to amphotericin B. These organisms may exhibit augmented MICs against natamycin and, in certain instances, exhibit resistance. Infections caused by *F. solani* complex are associated with poorer clinical outcomes and higher voriconazole resistance than other *Fusarium* spp. Importantly, detection of intrinsically voriconazole-resistant fungi, such as Mucorales, should prompt alerts to inform ophthalmologists [1].

Antifungal susceptibility testing should be routinely available in clinical laboratories, and MIC results should be reported even in the absence of established clinical breakpoints. In practice, fungal identification to the genus and species level, combined with isolate-specific susceptibility data, often provides clinically relevant and actionable information.

1.6 Conclusions

OFIs are a heterogeneous group of conditions, ranging from superficial adnexal involvement to deep intraocular infections such as keratitis, endophthalmitis, and choroiditis. Diagnosis typically involves direct examination, staining, biopsy, and fungal culture—the current gold standard—which also enables antifungal susceptibility testing using CLSI and EUCAST methodologies such as broth microdilution and disk diffusion. In cases of common contaminants, multiple isolates may be needed and definitive identification is confirmed by molecular or proteomic methods. Here highlights the critical role of the mycology laboratory in supporting diagnosis and treatment of OFIs, while emphasizing the need for further advances, including standardizing molecular diagnostics and expanding susceptibility testing for molds.

References

1. Leal SM Jr, Rodino KG, Fowler WC, Gilligan PH. Practical guidance for clinical microbiology laboratories: diagnosis of ocular infections. Clin Microbiol Rev. 2021;34(3):e0007019. https://doi.org/10.1128/CMR.00070-19.
2. Ramírez-Soto MC, Bonifaz A. Ocular fungal infections. J Fungi (Basel). 2022;8(10):1078. https://doi.org/10.3390/jof8101078.
3. Reginatto P, Agostinetto GJ, Fuentefria RDN, Marinho DR, Pizzol MD, Fuentefria AM. Eye fungal infections: a mini review. Arch Microbiol. 2023;205(6):236. https://doi.org/10.1007/s00203-023-03536-6.
4. Clare G, Kempen JH, Pavésio C. Infectious eye disease in the 21st century-an overview. Eye (Lond). 2024;38(11):2014–27. https://doi.org/10.1038/s41433-024-02966-w.

5. Bonifaz A. Queratitis micótica. In: Micología médica básica. 6th ed. McGraw-Hill; 2020. p. 683–96. ISBN: 978-607-15-1438-7.
6. Klotz SA, Penn CC, Negvesky GJ, Butrus SI. Fungal and parasitic infections of the eye. Clin Microbiol Rev. 2000;13(4):662–85. https://doi.org/10.1128/CMR.13.4.662.
7. Gaffi Reports. https://gaffi.org/call-to-action-fungal-keratitis-should-be-accepted-as-a-neglected-tropical-disease-ntd-by-the-world-health-organization-who. (Oct 10, 2022).
8. Brown L, Kamwiziku G, Oladele RO, Burton MJ, Prajna NV, Leitman TM, Denning DW. The case for fungal keratitis to be accepted as a neglected tropical disease. J Fungi (Basel). 2022;8(10):1047. https://doi.org/10.3390/jof8101047.
9. Bihaniya H, Rudraprasad D, Joseph J. Pathobiology of fungal Endophthalmitis: a major review. ACS Infect Dis. 2024;10(9):3126–37. https://doi.org/10.1021/acsinfecdis.4c00442.
10. Cintra MEC, da Silva DM, Al-Hatmi AMS, Bastos RW, Rossato L. Fusarium keratitis: a systematic review (1969 to 2023). Mycopathologia. 2024;189(5):74. https://doi.org/10.1007/s11046-024-00874-x.
11. Arboleda A, Ta CN. Overview of Mycotic keratitis. Cornea. 2024;43(9):1065–71. https://doi.org/10.1097/ICO.0000000000003559.
12. Bonifaz A, Gordillo-García L, Fest-Parra S, Tirado-Sánchez A, García-Carmona K. Mycotic keratitis. Keratitis due to Fusarium (Chap. 2). In: Mahendra RM, Occhiuto ML, editors. . London: CRC Press (Taylor & Francis); 2019. p. 18–32.
13. Vanzzini Zago V, Manzano-Gayosso P, Hernández-Hernández F, Méndez-Tovar LJ, Gómez-Leal A, López MR. Mycotic keratitis in an eye care hospital in Mexico City. Rev Iberoam Micol. 2010;27:57–61.
14. Bisen AC, Sanap SN, Agrawal S, Biswas A, Mishra A, Verma SK, et al. Etiopathology, epidemiology, diagnosis, and treatment of fungal keratitis. ACS Infect Dis. 2024;10(7):2356–80. https://doi.org/10.1021/acsinfecdis.4c00203.
15. Al-Hatmi AMS, Castro MA, de Hoog GS, Badali H, Alvarado VF, Verweij PE, et al. Epidemiology of aspergillus species causing keratitis in Mexico. Mycoses. 2019;62:144–51.
16. Araiza J, Tirado-Sánchez A, Bonifaz A. Mycotic keratitis caused by dematiaceous fungi (chap 3). In: Mahendra RM, Occhiuto ML, editors. Mycotic keratitis. London: CRC Press (Taylor & Francis); 2019. p. 33–44.
17. Rai M, Ingle AP, Ingle P, Gupta I, Mobin M, Bonifaz A, Alves M. Recent advances on mycotic keratitis caused by dematiaceous hyphomycetes. J Appl Microbiol. 2021 Oct;131(4):1652–67. https://doi.org/10.1111/jam.15008.
18. Durand ML. Bacterial and fungal endophthalmitis. Clin Microbiol Rev. 2017;30:597–613.
19. Chaidaroon W, Tantayakom T. Nocardia keratitis in a human immunodeficiency virus patient. Jpn J Ophthalmol. 2004;48:272–5.
20. Rao SK, Madhavan HN, Sitalakshmi G, Padmanabhan P. Nocardia asteroides keratitis: report of seven patients and literature review. Indian J Ophthalmol. 2000;48:217–21.
21. Kalavathy CM, Parmar P, Ramalingam K, et al. Trimethoprim-sulphamethoxazole therapy in Nocardia keratitis. Clin Experiment Ophthalmol. 2004;32:424–8.
22. Miller JM, Binnicker MJ, Campbell S, Carroll KC, Chapin KC, Gilligan PH, et al. A guide to utilization of the microbiology Laboratory for Diagnosis of infectious diseases: 2018 update by the Infectious Diseases Society of America and the American Society for Microbiology. Clin Infect Dis. 2018;67(6):e1–e94. https://doi.org/10.1093/cid/ciy381.
23. Ahearn DG, Zhang S, Stulting RD, Schwam BL, Simmons RB, Ward MA, et al. Fusarium keratitis and contact lens wear: facts and speculations. Med Mycol. 2008;46:397–410.
24. Chang DC, Grant GB, O'Donnell K, Wannemuehler KA, Noble-Wang J, Rao CY, et al. Multistate outbreak of Fusarium keratitis associated with use of a contact lens solution. JAMA. 2006;23:953–63.
25. Yi J, Sun Y, Zeng C, Kostoulias X, Qu Y. The role of biofilms in contact lens associated fungal keratitis. Antibiotics (Basel). 2023;12(10):1533. https://doi.org/10.3390/antibiotics12101533.
26. Kaliamurthy J, Thomas PA. Is inclusion of Sabouraud dextrose agar essential for the laboratory diagnosis of fungal keratitis? Indian J Ophthalmol. 2011;59:263–4.

27. Gray LD, Gilligan PH, Fowler WC. Cumitech 13B. Laboratory diagnosis of ocular infections. Washington, DC: ASM Press; 2010.
28. Kanungo R, Srinivasan R, Rao R. Acridine orange staining in early diagnosis of mycotic keratitis. Acta Ophthalmol. 1991;69:750–3.
29. Sharma S, Silverberg M, Metha PE, et al. Early diagnosis of keratitis mycotic. Predictive value of potassium hydroxide preparation. Indian J Ophthalmol. 1998;46:31–5.
30. Thomas PA, Kuriakose T. Use of lactophenol cotton blue mounts of corneal scrapings as an aid in the diagnosis of mycotic keratitis. Diag Microbiol Infect Dis. 1991;14:219–24.
31. Bharathi MJ, Ramakrishnan R, Vasu S, et al. Epidemiological characteristics and laboratory diagnosis of fungal keratitis. A three-year study. Indian J Ophthalmol. 2003;51:315–21.
32. Mahmoudi S, Masoomi A, Ahmadikia K, Tabatabaei SA, Soleimani M, Rezaie S, et al. Fungal keratitis: an overview of clinical and laboratory aspects. Mycoses. 2018;61:916–30.
33. Sharma S, Kunimoto DY, Gopinathan U, et al. Evaluation of corneal scraping smear examination methods in the diagnosis of bacterial and fungal keratitis: a survey of eight years of laboratory experience. Cornea. 2002;21:643–7.
34. Iqbal NJ, Boey A, Park BJ, Brandt ME. Determination of in vitro susceptibility of ocular Fusarium spp. isolates from keratitis cases and comparison of clinical and laboratory standards institute M38-A2 and E test methods. Diagn Microbiol Infect Dis. 2008;62:348–50.
35. Thomas PA, A Teresa P, Theodore J, Geraldine P. PCR for the molecular diagnosis of mycotic keratitis. Expert Rev Mol Diagn. 2012;12:703–18.
36. Vengayil S, Panda A, Satpathy G, Nayak N, Ghose S, Patanaik D, Khokhar S. Polymerase chain reaction-guided diagnosis of mycotic keratitis: a prospective evaluation of its efficacy and limitations. Invest Ophthalmol Vis Sci. 2009;50:152–6.
37. Thomas PA, Kaliamurthy J. Mycotic keratitis: epidemiology, diagnosis and management. Clin Microbiol Infect. 2013;19:210–20. https://doi.org/10.1111/1469-0691.12126.
38. Hammoudeh Y, Suresh L, Ong ZZ, Lister MM, Mohammed I, Thomas DJI, et al. Microbiological culture versus 16S/18S rRNA gene PCR-sanger sequencing for infectious keratitis: a three-arm, diagnostic cross-sectional study. Front Med (Lausanne). 2024;11:1393832. https://doi.org/10.3389/fmed.2024.1393832.
39. Rohilla R, Meena S, Mohanty A, Gupta N, Kaistha N, Gupta P, et al. Etiological spectrum of infectious keratitis in the era of MALDI-TOF-MS at a tertiary care hospital. J Family Med Prim Care. 2020;9(9):4576–81. https://doi.org/10.4103/jfmpc.jfmpc_630_20.
40. Bagga B, Das S, Tawde Y, Singh S, Shaw T, Sharma S, Ghosh A. Fusarium keratitis from a comprehensive eye health Care Facility in South India: molecular characterization by MALDI-TOF versus polymerase chain reaction sequencing, species complex distribution, and clinical correlation. Cornea. 2023;42(9):1150–62. https://doi.org/10.1097/ICO.0000000000003315.
41. Dutta A, Sahu SK, Das S, Mohanty A, Priyadarshini SR. The role of corneal biopsy in the management of microbial keratitis. Indian J Ophthalmol. 2024;72(4):571–7. https://doi.org/10.4103/IJO.IJO_1263_23.
42. Ghenciu LA, Faur AC, Bolintineanu SL, Salavat MC, Maghiari AL. Recent advances in diagnosis and treatment approaches in fungal keratitis: a narrative review. Microorganisms. 2024;12(1):161. https://doi.org/10.3390/microorganisms12010161.
43. Nielsen E, Heegaard S, Prause JU, Ivarsen A, Mortensen KL, Hjortdal J. Fungal keratitis—improving diagnostics by confocal microscopy. Case Rep Ophthalmol. 2013;193:303–10.
44. Vaddavalli PK, Garg P, Sharma S, Sangwan VS, Rao GN, Thomas R. Role of confocal microscopy in the diagnosis of fungal and acanthamoeba keratitis. Ophthalmology. 2011;118:29–35.
45. Austin A, Lietman T, Rose-Nussbaumer J. Update on the management of infectious keratitis. Ophthalmology. 2017;124:1678–89.
46. Mascarenhas M, Chaudhari P, Lewis SA. Natamycin ocular delivery: challenges and advancements in ocular therapeutics. Adv Ther. 2023;40(8):3332–59. https://doi.org/10.1007/s12325-023-02541-x.
47. Arora R, Gupta D, Goyal J, Kaur R. Voriconazole versus natamycin as primary treatment in fungal corneal ulcers. Clin Experiment Ophthalmol. 2010;24:125–8.

48. Prajna NV, Krishnan T, Mascarenhas J, Rajaraman R, Prajna L, Srinivasan M, et al. The mycotic ulcer treatment trial: a randomized trial comparing natamycin vs voriconazole. JAMA Ophthalmol. 2013;131:422–9.
49. Al-Hatmi AM, Bonifaz A, de Hoog G, Vázquez-Maya L, García-Carmona K, Meis JF, et al. Keratitis by Fusarium temperatum, a novel opportunist. BMC Infect Dis. 2014;14:588.
50. Lalitha P, Sun CQ, Prajna NV, Karpagam R, Geetha M, O'Brien KS, et al. In vitro susceptibility of filamentous fungal isolates from a corneal ulcer clinical trial. Mycotic ulcer treatment trial group. Am J Ophthalmol. 2014;157:318–26.
51. CLSI. CLSI standard M38—reference method for broth dilution antifungal susceptibility testing of filamentous fungi. 3rd ed. Wayne: CLSI; 2017.
52. CLSI. CLSI standard M27—reference method for broth dilution antifungal susceptibility testing of yeasts. 4th ed. Wayne: CLSI; 2017.
53. CLSI. CLSI standard M59—epidemiologic cutoff values for antifungal susceptibility testing. 2nd ed. Wayne: CLSI; 2018.
54. Clinical and Laboratory Standards Institute (CLSI). Epidemiological cutoff values for antifungal susceptibility testing. CLSI supplement M59. 2nd ed. Wayne: CLSI; 2018.
55. Anonymous. EUCAST definitive document EDef 7.1: method for the determination of broth dilution MICs of antifungal agents for fermentative yeasts. Clin Microbiol Infect. 2008;14:398–405.
56. CLSI. Method for antifungal disk diffusion susceptibility testing of yeasts; approved guideline—second edition (M44-A2). Wayne: CLSI; 2009.
57. Paranos P, Espinel-Ingroff A, Meletiadis J. Commercial methods for antifungal susceptibility testing of saprophytic molds: can they be used to detect resistance? J Fungi (Basel). 2024;10(3):214.
58. Grizante Barião PH, Cayún Y, Sepúlveda M, Tonani L, Gonçalves de Almeida OG, Cornejo P, et al. MALDI-TOF MS: a quick method to detect the susceptibility of Fusarium spp. Clinical Isolates to Amphotericin B Microorganisms. 2023;11(7):1834.
59. Arendrup MC, Meletiadis J, Mouton JW, Guinea J, Cuenca-Estrella M, Lagrou K, Howard SJ, Subcommittee on antifungal susceptibility testing (AFST) of the ESCMID European Committee for Antimicrobial Susceptibility Testing (EUCAST). EUCAST technical note on isavuconazole breakpoints for aspergillus, itraconazole breakpoints for Candida and updates for the antifungal susceptibility testing method documents. Clin Microbiol Infect. 2016;22(6):571.e1.
60. Dallé da Rosa P, Nunes A, Borges R, Batista B, Meneghello Fuentefria A, Goldani LZ. In vitro susceptibility and multilocus sequence typing of Fusarium isolates causing keratitis. J Mycol Med. 2018;28(3):482–5. https://doi.org/10.1016/j.mycmed.2018.05.001.
61. Manzi S, de Souza PF, Milanez EPR, de Andrade ARC, Silva L, Silva ML, Monteiro RC, et al. Antifungal susceptibility, clinical findings, and biofilm resistance of Fusarium species causing keratitis: a challenge for disease control. Braz. J Microbiol. 2025 Mar;56(1):341–52. https://doi.org/10.1007/s42770-024-01611-8.
62. Krichevskaya GI, Kovaleva LA, Zyurnyayeva ID, Makarov PV, Andryushin AE. The effectiveness of PCR in diagnosis of fungal keratitis. Oftalmologia. 2020;17(4):824–9. https://doi.org/10.18008/1816-5095-2020-4-824-829.
63. Behera HS, Srigyan D. Evaluation of polymerase chain reaction over routine microbial diagnosis for the diagnosis of fungal keratitis. Optom Vis Sci. 2021;98(3):280–4. https://doi.org/10.1097/opx.0000000000001652.
64. Hoffman JJ, Dart JKG, De SK, Carnt N, Cleary G, Hau S. Comparison of culture, confocal microscopy and PCR in routine hospital use for microbial keratitis diagnosis. Eye (Lond). 2022;36(11):2172–8. https://doi.org/10.1038/s41433-021-01812-7.
65. Toumasis P, Tsantes AG, Tsiogka A, Samonis G, Vrioni G. From clinical suspicion to diagnosis: a review of diagnostic approaches and challenges in fungal keratitis. Clin Med. 2024;13(1):286. https://doi.org/10.3390/jcm13010286.

Ocular Drug Delivery of Antifungal Agents

2

Oindrilla Dasgupta, Tamizhmathy Mannangatty, Shridula Sankar, Nitin Khandagale, Velmurugan Kailasam, Manisha Malani, Prashant Garg, and Jayabalan Nirmal

2.1 Introduction

Invading fungal strains can incite different reactions in the host even if they may belong to the same species. The treatment strategy for each infection must be approached rationally and with careful consideration of the susceptibility of fungal strains to different antifungal agents [1]. Of the more than 100 identified fungal species, *Aspergillus, Fusarium,* and *Candida* are the most prevalent species that cause ocular fungal diseases [2]. The choice of antifungal agent thus depends on its spectrum of activity and potency against the isolated fungal strain and its bioavailability [3]. On the other hand, the severity and location of the fungal infection determine the dosage regimen and the route of administration [3, 4].

Corneal infections like fungal keratitis and other anterior segment diseases are typically treated using eye drops. Eye drops are the most widely used delivery system for topical administration of drugs to the eye, due to their lack of invasiveness, systemic side effects, and ease of handling. However, the delivery of antifungal agents through eye drops possesses several limitations [5]. Most antifungal drugs that have been developed are hydrophobic in nature with poor water solubility. This

O. Dasgupta · T. Mannangatty · N. Khandagale · V. Kailasam · J. Nirmal (✉)
Translational Pharmaceutics Research Laboratory (TPRL), Department of Pharmacy, Birla Institute of Technology and Sciences (BITS), Pilani, Hyderabad, Telangana, India

Centre for Ocular Drug Delivery Devices, Department of Pharmacy, Birla Institute of Technology and Sciences (BITS), Pilani, Hyderabad, Telangana, India
e-mail: nirmalj@hyderabad.bits-pilani.ac.in

S. Sankar · M. Malani
Translational Pharmaceutics Research Laboratory (TPRL), Department of Pharmacy, Birla Institute of Technology and Sciences (BITS), Pilani, Hyderabad, Telangana, India

P. Garg
Shantilal Shanghvi Cornea Institute and Brian Holden Eye Research Centre, KAR Campus, LV Prasad Eye Institute, Hyderabad, Telangana, India

M. C. Ramírez-Soto (ed.), *Fungal Eye Infections*,
https://doi.org/10.1007/978-3-032-19923-2_2

makes them highly challenging to formulate, leading to development of suspensions or emulsions to prepare eye drops. Drugs with higher molecular weight (such as amphotericin B, natamycin, or ketoconazole) have poor permeation through the corneal epithelium [4, 5]. Natamycin suspension eye drops is the only FDA-approved treatment currently available for fungal keratitis [6]. Among the polyene therapeutics, amphotericin B is widely repurposed for the treatment of fungal keratitis, due to its broad-spectrum activity, rare fungal strain resistance, and cross-resistance cases [7], although it has not yet been approved by the US Food and Drug Administration (FDA) for the treatment of fungal keratitis. Azoles such as ketoconazole, fluconazole, and voriconazole are also reconstituted as eye drops when the requirement arises [8].

The antifungal agent used to treat mycotic keratitis should be readily accessible. If the direct microscopy results are clear and in line with the clinical evaluation, treatment can be started; if not, therapy should be paused until culture results are obtained. Regardless of whether direct microscopy shows septate hyphae or yeast cells, topical natamycin (5%) is typically used as the first line of treatment for superficial keratomycoses. For deep corneal infections, additional antifungal medications (such as amphotericin B, ketoconazole, or itraconazole) are added [1].

Subconjunctival, intracameral, and intrastromal injections are used in cases of deeper recalcitrant infections. Patients with scleral or limbal involvement, endophthalmitis, an imminent perforation, or a perforated corneal ulcer, juvenile patients, resistant patients, and postkeratoplasty patients are treated systemically with oral antifungal drugs [9]. The route of administration is based on achieving sufficient drug concentration to the infected site; thus, the site of administration is kept as close to the site of action as possible. The route of administration and the antifungal drug is ultimately chosen to provide the most efficient treatment while minimizing the potential side effects.

2.2 Antifungal Agents in Ocular Therapy

2.2.1 General Classification of Antifungal Agents

Antifungal agents can be broadly categorized into several classes (Table 2.1), including polyenes, azoles, pyrimidines, allylamines, echinocandins, and heterocyclic benzofurans. Among these, polyenes and azoles are the most frequently used in clinical practice.

2.2.1.1 Polyenes

Polyenes represent the earliest class of antifungal drugs and still play a crucial role in the management of ocular fungal infections. Polyenes act by affecting the integrity of fungal cell walls by binding to ergosterol, a sterol found exclusively in fungal cell membranes, which leads to membrane disruption and subsequent leakage of vital cellular contents. Natamycin, amphotericin B, and nystatin are the key drugs in this category used for managing ocular fungal infections. However, nystatin is no

Table 2.1 Summary of clinical usage of antifungal agents for ocular diseases

Antifungal agent	Route of administration	Concentration	Formulation used	Ref.
Natamycin	Topical	5% w/v	Suspension	[13]
	Intrastromal injection	10 μg/0.1 ml	Diluted natamycin suspension	[84]
Amphotericin B	Topical	0.15% w/v	Liposomal solution	[85]
	Intrastromal + intravitreal injection	5 to 10 μg per 0.1 ml	Fungizone (powder for injection)	[24]
	Intracameral injection	10 μg per 0.1 ml	Fungizone® (powder for injection) reconstituted using balanced salt solution	[25]
	Subconjunctival injection	1.5 mg per 0.3 ml	Amphotericin B reconstituted using 5% dextrose	[86]
Voriconazole	Topical + Oral	1% w/v	–	[29, 30]
	Oral	200 mg	Powder	[29, 30]
	Intrastromal injection	50 μg/0.1 mL	VFEND® (powder for injection) reconstituted with distilled water	[39]
	Intrastromal injection	0.5 mg/ml (50 μg/0.1 ml)	VFEND® (powder for injection) reconstituted with lactated ringer (LR) solution	[40], [41]
	Intracameral + intrastromal injection	50 μg/0.1 ml	VFEND® (powder for injection) reconstituted with lactated ringer (LR) solution	[87]
Miconazole	Topical + subconjunctival injection	10 mg/ml	–	[88]
Fluconazole	Topical + Oral	2% w/v (2 mg/ml) + 37.5 mg/kg	Diflucan for injection reconstituted with 0.9% NaCl + Diflucan oral tablets	[47]
	Oral	200 mg		[46]
	Subconjunctival injection	2% w/v (2 mg/ml)	–	[50]
	Subconjunctival injection	2% w/v (2 mg/ml)	Intravenous powder for injection reconstituted	[89]
Posaconazole	Oral + topical	200 mg (qid) + 4 mg / 0.1 ml (hourly)	Noxafil® oral suspension	[60], [62]
	Oral + topical	200 mg (qid) + 100 mg/ml	Noxafil® oral suspension	[63]
Itraconazole	Topical	0.1% w/v (1 mg/ml)	Itraconazole powder reconstituted in artificial tear solution	[67]
	Topical + Oral	0.1% w/v (1 mg/ml) + 100 mg (twice daily)	Itraconazole powder reconstituted in artificial tear solution	[67]
	Oral	200 mg daily	Itraconazole 50 mg capsules	[65]

(continued)

Table 2.1 (continued)

Antifungal agent	Route of administration	Concentration	Formulation used	Ref.
Caspofungin	Topical	0.5% w/v	–	[90]
	Intravitreal injection	250 μg/0.1 ml	–	[91]
	Intravitreal injection	100 μg/0.1 ml	Cancidas® powder for injection	[92]
	Intravitreal injection + intravenous injection	50 μg/0.1 ml	–	[93]
	Topical + intrastromal injection	0.5% w/v	Cancidas® powder for injection reconstituted with water for injection	[72]
	Topical + Intracameral injection	50 μg/0.1 ml	–	[94]
Micafungin	Topical	0.1% w/v	Powder for injection reconstituted with sterile saline solution	[76], [77]

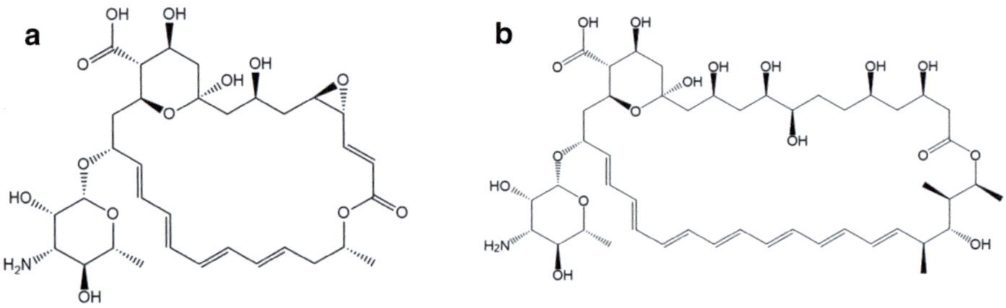

Fig. 2.1 Structure of natamycin (**a**) and amphotericin B (**b**)

longer commonly used for eye infections due to its limited tissue penetration, potential toxicity, and documented resistance [10]. Natamycin and amphotericin B, on the other hand, continue to be the primary choices in the polyene class of drugs for treating fungal infections of the eye (Fig. 2.1) [11].

Natamycin

Natamycin is the most widely used topical antifungal drug and is currently the only antifungal agent approved by the USFDA in 1978 specifically for the treatment of fungal keratitis. It is derived from *Streptomyces natalensis* and is commercially available as a 5% suspension (50 mg/ml) [12]. Natamycin exhibits a broad spectrum of action and is effective against numerous fungal pathogens, including *Fusarium*, *Aspergillus*, *Alternaria*, *Candida*, *Cephalosporium*, *Colletotrichum*, *Curvularia*, *Lasiodiplodia*, *Scedosporium*, *Trichophyton*, and *Penicillium* species [13].

Treatment typically begins with one drop administered every 1 to 2 hours, depending on the severity of the infection. As clinical improvement occurs, the frequency is gradually tapered. Once the infection is resolved, a maintenance dose of four times daily is generally continued for at least 4 weeks [14]. The effectiveness of natamycin has been strongly supported by clinical evidence. The Mycotic Ulcer Treatment Trial-1 (MUTT-1), a multicenter randomized trial, compared natamycin with voriconazole in 368 patients with smear-positive filamentous fungal ulcers and best corrected visual acuity (BCVA) between 20/40 and 20/400. At the 3-month follow-up, those treated with natamycin showed better visual outcomes and a reduced rate of corneal perforation compared to the voriconazole group [15]. The benefits were particularly notable in patients with *Fusarium* infections, which comprised 40% of the study population. In contrast, patients with non-*Fusarium* infections (*Aspergillus*—17%, others—43%) responded similarly to both treatments [15].

Common adverse effects include ocular redness, stinging or burning, and excessive tearing. Additionally, undissolved drug particles in suspension formulation may accumulate on the corneal surface, in the conjunctival fornices, and along the eyelid margins [16].

Amphotericin B

Amphotericin B is produced by the actinomycete *Streptomyces nodosus.* It was approved by the FDA in the 1960s due to its great efficiency in controlling disseminated fungal infections.

[17]. Amphotericin B acts by increasing cell permeability through the formation of pores or channels in the fungal cell membrane upon binding to ergosterol and by promoting oxidative action on cells, thus altering their metabolic functions. It also binds nonspecifically to cholesterol in human cells, which is the main reason for its side effects [18]. Its primary effect is to inhibit fungal growth, though it can kill fungi at higher concentrations within the affected tissue [19].

Amphotericin B is among the few drugs reported in the literature to be administered via multiple ocular routes—including subconjunctival, intrastromal, intracameral, intravitreal, and topical applications. Topical treatment, typically the first-line approach for fungal keratitis, involves using concentrations of 1.5–5 mg/ml applied hourly during the initial phase and then reduced to every 4 hours once a clinical response is achieved. The commercially available powder for injection is reconstituted in distilled water to prepare a 0.15% (1.5 mg/mL) solution of amphotericin B suitable for ocular administration [7]. To enhance corneal drug penetration, periodic removal of the corneal epithelium is often recommended [20]. Clinical studies have shown that the drug is well tolerated and effective when administered in both drop and ointment forms [21]. Additionally, intrastromal injection has been found to yield better therapeutic outcomes than subconjunctival administration, particularly in patients with poor treatment adherence, due to fewer side effects and more sustained drug levels in the cornea compared to topical or intracameral routes [22]. Amphotericin B when administered intravenously 0.7–1 mg/kg/day has a $t_{1/2}$ of 15 days and mainly accumulates in the liver and the spleen. Approximately 10% of the drug gets eliminated through urine when administered as liposomal formulation, whereas in some cases the drug is excreted unchanged. There are no oral formulations of amphotericin B due to its poor solubility [23].

In several reported cases, keratitis that did not respond to topical therapy was successfully treated with intrastromal injections of amphotericin B at concentrations ranging from 5 to 10 μg per 0.1 ml [24]. However, additional controlled studies are necessary to confirm these outcomes. Intracameral injection is typically reserved for severe infections that extend beyond Descemet's membrane and involve the anterior chamber and lens. Despite its effectiveness, this route has been associated with adverse effects such as cataract formation, temporary inflammation in the anterior chamber within 24 hours due to amphotericin B's immune-enhancing properties, iritis, and corneal edema, though these effects are generally reversible [25, 26]. For fungal endophthalmitis, intravitreal administration of amphotericin B remains the preferred treatment. While it exhibits broad-spectrum antifungal activity, its effectiveness in intraocular infections is constrained by limited ocular penetration and the risk of toxicity within the eye.

2.2.1.2 Azoles

First introduced into clinical use during the 1970s, azoles marked a significant breakthrough in antifungal treatment. Compared to polyenes, they offer a broader antifungal spectrum and are associated with fewer side effects. Azoles exert their effect by targeting a fungal cytochrome P-450 enzyme that plays a role in the 14α-demethylation of lanosterol or 25-methylenedihydrolanosterol. This inhibition disrupts ergosterol synthesis, leading to the buildup of 14α-methylated sterols, which compromises fungal cell membrane integrity. The resulting increase in membrane permeability, along with the disruption of membrane-bound enzymes, halts fungal growth and eventually causes cell death [27]. In ophthalmology, commonly used imidazoles include miconazole and ketoconazole. Among the first-generation triazoles, itraconazole and fluconazole are frequently prescribed. The more recent second-generation triazoles, such as voriconazole and posaconazole, have been introduced into clinical practice over the past decade [28].

Voriconazole

Voriconazole is considered the second most effective topical agent for treating fungal keratitis (Fig. 2.2a). Although it is approved by the USFDA for oral and intravenous use in managing invasive aspergillosis and recalcitrant infections caused by *Fusarium* species and *Scedosporium apiospermum*, its application in ophthalmology is off-label. For ocular use, the injectable formulation is reconstituted to prepare a 1% (10 mg/ml) solution suitable for topical administration [29, 30].

Voriconazole possesses a broad antifungal spectrum, showing effectiveness against a range of pathogens including *Aspergillus*, *Candida*, *Cryptococcus*, *Fusarium*, and *Scedosporium* species. However, its efficacy against fungi belonging to the *Mucorales* order is limited [31, 32]. Voriconazole can be delivered through various routes, including oral capsules, intracameral and intrastromal injections, as well as intravitreal administration. The oral capsule formulation is quickly absorbed, with the average time to reach peak plasma levels (T_{max}) ranging from approximately 1.43 to 1.81 h for 200 mg and 400 mg doses, respectively [33, 34]. Since voriconazole is metabolized in the liver, regular monitoring of liver enzyme levels is recommended during treatment. The common side effects of oral voriconazole

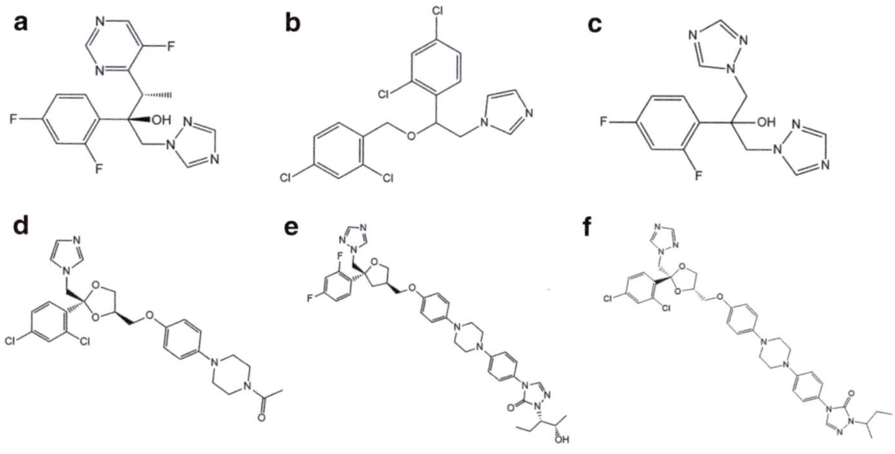

Fig. 2.2 Structures of azoles. (**a**) Voriconazole, (**b**) miconazole, (**c**) fluconazole, (**d**) ketoconazole, (**e**) posaconazole, and (**f**) itraconazole

include visual disturbances, color vision changes, and photophobia occurring in approximately 30% of patients; however, these effects are typically temporary. Like fluconazole, voriconazole demonstrates excellent gastrointestinal absorption and bioavailability [35].

Compared to polyenes, voriconazole offers greater stability when exposed to light and temperature, maintaining its effectiveness for up to 30 days [36, 37]. Research conducted in horses demonstrated that the drug can penetrate the cornea even when the epithelium remains intact [38]. Intrastromal administration of voriconazole has been recommended in cases of deep keratitis that do not respond to topical or oral treatment. Studies have reported successful outcomes in three patients with keratitis resistant to topical natamycin, following intrastromal injection of voriconazole at a dose of 50 μg/0.1 ml [39]. Similarly, Siatiri et al. documented the resolution of three *Fusarium* keratitis cases that had not improved with topical therapy but responded to intrastromal voriconazole [40]. Additionally, a study involving 13 patients also supported the use of intrastromal voriconazole for treating refractory keratitis [41].

Miconazole

Miconazole was originally formulated as a topical treatment for superficial fungal infections. Although systemic administration has shown effectiveness, its use has declined due to adverse cardiovascular and liver-related side effects [42]. Like other azole antifungals, Miconazole disrupts ergosterol synthesis in fungal cell membranes. Additionally, it inhibits peroxidase enzymes, leading to the buildup of free radicals within the fungal cytoplasm, ultimately causing cell death (Fig. 2.2b)) [43]. Miconazole is available in a 10 mg/ml solution, which is used both topically and intravenously. When the epithelium is removed, this concentration shows effective tissue penetration. It may also be administered subconjunctivally in doses of

5–10 mg to treat ocular infections caused by fungi such as *Candida*, *Fusarium*, *Curvularia*, and *Aspergillus [44]*. Laboratory studies have shown miconazole to be more potent than ketoconazole and itraconazole against *Aspergillus* species, *Candida albicans*, and other non-*albicans* strains [44].

Fluconazole

Fluconazole (Fig. 2.2c) is well absorbed through the gastrointestinal tract and remains stable under the acidic conditions of the stomach. Peak plasma concentrations (C_{max}) are comparable following both oral and intravenous administration. It demonstrates effective ocular tissue penetration, with aqueous humor concentrations approaching those found in plasma [45]. Oral dosing at 200–400 mg per day has proven beneficial in managing ocular fungal infections, either alone or in combination with topical natamycin [46]. A study comparing the efficacy of topical and oral administration of fluconazole showed no significant difference between the treatment efficacy of 2% w/v topical fluconazole eye drops (8 times daily) and orally administered fluconazole (37.5 mg/kg twice daily) [47]. When combined with topical amphotericin B and administered via subconjunctival injection, fluconazole provides a broader antifungal spectrum while reducing amphotericin B-associated toxicity [48, 49]. Yilmaz et al. demonstrated that daily subconjunctival injections of 2 mg/ml fluconazole for 10 days successfully treated approximately 60% of fungal keratitis cases [50].

Topically applied fluconazole eye drops (2 mg/ml) were found to achieve therapeutic concentrations within the corneal tissue in rabbit models infected with *Aspergillus fumigatus* [51]. Despite its ability to penetrate the vitreous humor when taken orally, fluconazole shows limited efficacy against filamentous fungi such as *Aspergillus* and *Fusarium* species due to their inherent resistance [47], making it less suitable for treating fungal endophthalmitis caused by these pathogens. Nonetheless, fluconazole has been used successfully in cases of endogenous endophthalmitis caused by *Candida* species [52].

Ketoconazole

Ketoconazole is a synthetic imidazole derivative with lipophilic properties (Fig. 2.2d). It acts as a 14α-sterol demethylase inhibitor, disrupting ergosterol synthesis and altering fungal cell membrane integrity, leading to cell lysis [53]. It exhibits broad in vitro activity against *dermatophytes, Candida* species, dimorphic fungi, and some molds and bacteria, though its effect on filamentous fungi is limited [54, 55].

It demonstrates good oral absorption and tissue distribution, achieving peak serum levels (2–3 μg/mL) within 2–3 h of a 200 mg dose [53, 56]. It exhibits high plasma protein binding (~99%) and undergoes hepatic metabolism primarily via CYP3A4, with negligible central nervous system (CNS) penetration. Elimination is biphasic, with initial and terminal half-lives of approximately 2 and 8 h, respectively. Around 13% is excreted in urine (2–4% unchanged), and 57% via feces [56]. Animal studies showed high corneal concentrations of ketoconazole postoral administration, with sustained levels even 24 hours later [57].

Shibashi documented complete resolution of fungal corneal ulcers in two culture-confirmed cases of *Fusarium* keratitis when oral ketoconazole was used as an adjunct to topical natamycin [55]. In another study, Thomas et al. observed full healing in 67% of patients (20 out of 30) with mycotic keratitis who received oral ketoconazole [53]. A randomized controlled trial by Rajaraman and colleagues involving 115 patients compared the efficacy of topical 5% natamycin with and without oral ketoconazole. The results showed no significant difference in healing rates (72% in the oral ketoconazole group vs. 68% in the non-ketoconazole group) or in final visual outcomes. These findings suggest that the addition of oral ketoconazole to topical natamycin therapy offers no substantial advantage [58]. The most important adverse effect is hepatotoxicity (3.6%–4.2%), necessitating regular liver and renal function monitoring; other potential side effects include endocrine and gastrointestinal problems [59].

Posaconazole

Posaconazole, a second-generation triazole and synthetic analogue of itraconazole, has effectively treated mycotic keratitis (Fig. 2.2e). It has been used alone and in combination with other antifungal agents with successful outcomes [60]. It is a broad-spectrum antifungal agent with similarities to voriconazole. It is effective against a wide range of *Candida* species, including strains resistant to fluconazole. Also, it exhibits potent activity against filamentous fungi like *Aspergillus*, *Fusarium*, and members of the *Mucorales* order [59]. Posaconazole demonstrates good oral absorption and binds extensively to plasma proteins (about 98%) and shows limited distribution to the cerebrospinal fluid and ocular tissues. It undergoes hepatic metabolism and is primarily eliminated via the bile and feces. The drug has a long elimination half-life, ranging from 25 to 35 hours [59].

Posaconazole has demonstrated efficacy in treating fungal keratitis, which is resistant to commonly used antifungals such as ketoconazole, fluconazole, and voriconazole. Altun and colleagues reported successfully managing two refractory keratitis cases using topical (0.1 mg/mL) and oral posaconazole (200 mg four times daily). These cases had previously failed to respond to standard antifungal agents, including natamycin, voriconazole, fluconazole, and amphotericin B [60]. Cuenca-Estrella et al. also found posaconazole effective against fungal isolates resistant to fluconazole and itraconazole [61]. Tu and co-authors detailed three cases of persistent *Fusarium* keratitis that were successfully treated with posaconazole [62]. Similarly, Sponsel and colleagues reported complete resolution of a *Fusarium* infection resistant to amphotericin B and natamycin using oral posaconazole (200 mg four times daily) in conjunction with a 10% topical solution (100 mg/mL, prepared from the oral formulation) [63]. Posaconazole is generally well tolerated, even with extended use. Common side effects include gastrointestinal symptoms such as nausea, vomiting, diarrhea, abdominal discomfort, fever, and headache. Other adverse reactions may involve hypokalemia, skin rashes, low platelet counts, and elevated liver enzymes [64].

Itraconazole

Itraconazole is a synthetic dioxolane triazole antifungal agent, and its mechanism of action is comparable to that of other triazoles, acting as a 14α-sterol demethylase inhibitor (Fig. 2.2f). By blocking ergosterol synthesis, itraconazole disrupts cell membrane integrity, ultimately leading to increased permeability and fungal cell lysis [65]. It is effective against *Candida* and *Aspergillus* species [31, 66]. Itraconazole is marketed in both systemic and topical dosage forms, with the topical formulation commonly available as a 1% solution (10 mg/ml) [67].

Despite its therapeutic potential, itraconazole demonstrates relatively poor bioavailability, solubility, and ocular tissue penetration following oral administration when compared with other azole antifungals [59]. Similar to ketoconazole, its gastric absorption is dependent on an acidic environment. However, the oral solution formulation achieves higher absorption (~80%) and is not influenced by gastric pH or food intake [68]. Serum levels are generally higher with the oral solution than with tablets. Owing to its strong plasma protein binding (~99%), ocular concentrations of itraconazole are considerably lower than those achieved with fluconazole or voriconazole [69].

Clinical evidence highlights the role of itraconazole in fungal keratitis. Thomas et al. reported that 22 of 40 patients (55%) with mycotic keratitis responded to oral itraconazole (200 mg daily for 17 days), with more favorable outcomes in cases caused by *Aspergillus* species [65]. Similarly, in a randomized controlled trial, Agrawal et al. evaluated oral itraconazole in combination with topical itraconazole. Complete resolution was achieved in 42 eyes (77%), while 12 eyes (22.2%) showed poor response. Of these, four cases involved *Fusarium* spp., suggesting limited effectiveness of Itraconazole against this pathogen [67].

The most frequent side effects of itraconazole include rash, headache, and gastrointestinal discomfort. More severe toxicities, such as hepatotoxicity and liver failure, represent the most significant risks associated with Itraconazole therapy [59].

2.2.1.3 Echinocandins

Echinocandins are a class of semisynthetic lipopeptide antifungal agents that exert their effect by inhibiting the synthesis of β-1,3-D-glucan, an essential component of the fungal cell wall. This mechanism compromises cell wall integrity and leads to fungal cell death. Notable members of this group include Micafungin, Anidulafungin, and Caspofungin, all of which show strong activity against a variety of *Candida* species and *Aspergillus* species (Fig. 2.3). These agents are not effectively absorbed when administered orally and are therefore available only in parenteral formulations. They exhibit relatively long elimination half-lives, ranging from approximately 10 to 26 h, enabling once-daily dosing. Echinocandins when given through the intravenous route (Capsofungin: 70 mg for 1 dose and 50 mg/day; Micafungin: 100 to 150 mg / day and 50 mg/day later on) have limited penetration into the central nervous system and ocular tissues, resulting in low concentrations at these sites [59]; thus the ocular bioavailability of these drugs through intravenous route is comparatively lower.

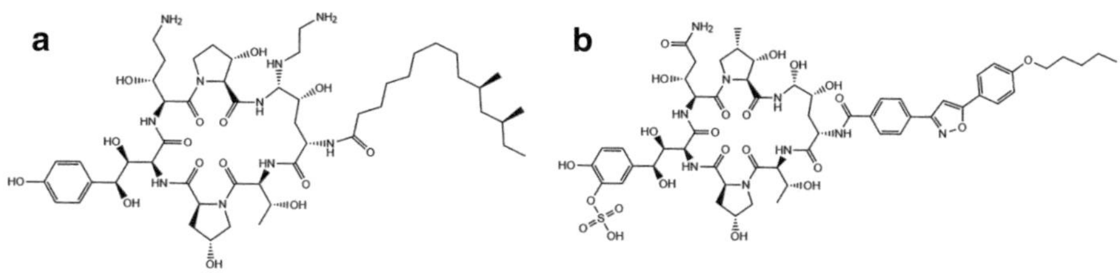

Fig. 2.3 Structures of echinocandins. (**a**) Caspofungin and (**b**) Micafungin

Caspofungin

The first approved echinocandin has shown promise in treating refractory fungal eye infections. Topical Caspofungin formulations (0.5% and 1%) have demonstrated effectiveness in managing cases of resistant mycotic keratitis. Intravenous Caspofungin has also been used with success in the treatment of fungal endophthalmitis [70]. A study by Neoh et al. reported that a 0.5% Caspofungin solution remained stable for up to 28 days when stored at 4 °C, but its stability reduced to just 3 days at room temperature, 25 °C [71]. Additionally, its use was effective in treating *Alternaria* keratitis [72]. In rabbit models of *Candida* keratitis, topical Caspofungin (0.5%) was found to be as effective as amphotericin B (0.15%), with no significant ocular toxicity [73]. Similar efficacy was observed with 1% Caspofungin in treating *Fusarium solani* keratitis in experimental settings [74].

Micafungin

Another echinocandin shares a similar mode of action with Caspofungin. It is FDA-approved for systemic treatment of esophageal candidiasis, but its ophthalmic use remains off-label [75]. In clinical studies, topical Micafungin 0.1% (1 mg/mL) demonstrated beneficial effects in cases of *Candida* keratitis that did not respond to conventional antifungals. Matsumoto et al. observed outcomes comparable to fluconazole 0.2% in such cases [76]. Moreover, a study by Trujillo et al. indicated that Micafungin had similar therapeutic efficacy to natamycin in treating *Alternaria* keratitis in animal models [77, 78]. Overall, echinocandins are well tolerated, with minimal side effects. Reported adverse events include mild infusion-related reactions, gastrointestinal discomfort, headache, and elevated liver enzyme levels, such as aminotransferases [59].

2.2.1.4 Pyrimidines

The pyrimidine class of antifungal agents is represented by 5-fluorocytosine (5-FC), also known as flucytosine, which is unique among antifungals for its intracellular mode of action. Once taken up by fungal cells, flucytosine is enzymatically converted into 5-fluorouracil (5-FU)—a potent antimetabolite that disrupts fungal DNA synthesis [79].

Flucytosine can be administered topically as a 1% solution, orally at a dose of 150 mg/kg/day, or intravenously. It exhibits antifungal activity primarily against *Candida* and *Cryptococcus* species and has inconsistent activity against certain *Aspergillus* strains. Its therapeutic role is mainly adjunctive, especially in the treatment of yeast keratitis, because resistance can develop quickly when used as monotherapy for *Candida* or *Cryptococcus* keratitis. Its effectiveness against *Fusarium* species is limited [80].

Flucytosine is often used in combination with amphotericin B, especially for treating *Candida* endophthalmitis, due to their synergistic effect [81]. Studies in both animals and humans have shown that this combination achieves high intraocular drug levels [82]. However, flucytosine's clinical utility in ocular infections is constrained by its narrow antifungal spectrum and poor ocular penetration [83]. Potential side effects include bone marrow suppression, alopecia, and other systemic toxicities.

2.2.2 Considerations for Pediatric and At-Risk Patients

Specific criteria are considered before prescribing the antifungals to neonates, children, pregnant women, and immunocompromised patients [95]. The ocular fungal infections in children have become a rising concern due to immunodeficiencies. In mild to moderate cases of fungal infections, a natamycin suspension (5 mg/mL) and amphotericin B drops (1.5 mg/mL) are prescribed for the treatment of fungal keratitis for children >2 years [96]. A voriconazole treatment is warranted for *Aspergillus* spp. which when rendered ineffective is given along with oral posaconazole (200 mg for 4 times a day) [62]. For severe fungal infections, systemic antifungal therapies are recommended along with surgical removal of the infected area. The dosage regimen varies for children and normal adults because of the body mass ratio [97]. Choosing an appropriate therapy for children is a serious concern, as it may cause an adverse reaction or resistance to the given drug. The predominant prevalence occurs in the neonatal intensive care unit in premature infants. The isolated species among the NICU are *Candida albicans* and *Candida parapsilosis* [95]. A 3–6 mg/kg orally twice weekly for 6 weeks of fluconazole is given as a treatment initially. Later, the clinical trials showed an increase in morbidity and mortality. The Society of Pediatric Infectious Disease and Management has regulated fluconazole as 3 mg/kg/day in neonates with a weight < 1.5 grams, for a period at risk. The indications and symptoms are also managed by oral nystatin suspension (100,000 IU/mL) when there is resistance against the azole antibiotics.

Continuous therapeutic drug monitoring is recommended for immunocompromised patients. The patients undergoing chemotherapy or organ transplantation are at a high risk of infectious diseases. While the antifungal therapy has been proven to be safe during the process in clinical trials, an effective treatment is achieved when used in conjunction [98]. For the pediatric population undergoing Hematopoietic Stem Cell Transplant (HSCT), a maximum dose of 400 mg/day of fluconazole is given through i.v [99]. The treatment of voriconazole is recommended for HSCT patients. The ages between 2 and 12 receive 16 mg/kg/day twice a day i.v. with an initial dose of 18 mg/kg/day. The population above 15 receives 8 mg/kg/day twice a day i.v. with an initial dose of 12 mg/kg/day [100]. Patients undergoing cancer treatment are generally treated with the same doses as the general population, but daily follow-up of the treatment is done [101].

Table 2.2 Oral and topical agents prescribed for the FDA categories of pregnant patients

FDA categories	Indications	Oral agents	Topical agents
A	Controlled studies of women failed to demonstrate a risk to the fetus in the first trimester, and the possibility of fetal harm appears remote	–	Amphotericin B
B	Either animal studies do not indicate a risk to the fetus and there have been no controlled studies in pregnant women or animal studies have indicated fetal risk but controlled studies of pregnant women failed to demonstrate a risk	Terbinafine Ciclopirox Clotrimazole Naftifine Oxiconazole	–
C	Either animal studies indicate a fetal risk and there have been no controlled studies of women or there are no available reports of studies of women or animals	Ketoconazole Fluconazole (150 mg/day) Itraconazole Econazole Miconazole Griseofulvin Butenafine Nystatin	Natamycin
D	There is positive evidence of fetal risk, but there may be certain situations where the benefit may outweigh the risk (e.g., life-threatening or serious diseases for which other drugs are ineffective or carry a greater risk)	Fluconazole (400–600 mg/day) Voriconazole 5-Fluorocytosine	Voriconazole 5-Fluorocytosine
X	There is definite fetal risk, according to studies of animals or humans or on the basis of human experience, and the risk clearly outweighs any benefit in pregnant women	–	–

The USFDA has given specific pregnancy risk categories (A, B, C, D, and X) and pregnancy lactation and labeling rule guidance for pregnant women [102]. A few of the drugs on the list, when taken orally, show little toxicity when taken orally, but are regarded safe topically. So far, amphotericin B is considered as the safest treatment for pregnant women (Table 2.2) [103]. However, the clinician's prescription always outweighs the benefit-to-risk ratio [104].

2.2.3 Combination Therapy of Antifungal Agents

Over the last few decades, there has been a substantial amount of research on the development of new antifungal agents. Thus, there eventually comes a scenario where a combination of different agents can be used in the treatment of fungal diseases. Combination therapy is used to broaden the spectrum of activity, lower the toxicity produced by certain drugs, produce a synergistic effect, and enhance the efficacy of the treatment [105]. The increased activity with a lower dose could also reduce the potential of development of antifungal resistance. Natamycin is commonly administered alongside intraocular injections of other antifungal agents. However, recently, the combination of natamycin and voriconazole has received a considerable amount of attention due to their synergistic effect [106, 107]. However, combination therapy of ocular infections can include multiple routes of administration for different drugs in the same treatment. In a treatment trial for fungal keratitis, amphotericin B eye drops were administered alongside fluconazole subconjunctival injections for treatment [49]. A few examples of successful combination therapy for antifungal ocular infections are given in Table 2.3.

2.2.4 Adverse Events and Ocular Toxicity of Antifungal Agents

Ocular administration of antifungal agents can result in a range of adverse events and toxicities, which vary depending on the specific drug, route of administration, and patient-related factors [113].

Both topical and systemic antifungal therapies are associated with ocular side effects. Topical agents, such as natamycin and amphotericin B, generally cause milder, surface-level adverse reactions, including eyelid and periorbital edema, conjunctival irritation, foreign body sensation, burning, tearing, stinging, and redness. Amphotericin B is notably cytotoxic to corneal epithelial cells, potentially leading to corneal edema, neovascularization, iritis, cataract, and even retinal toxicity when administered intravitreally or at high concentrations. Natamycin is mostly associated with local discomfort and occasional adherence of drug particles to ulcerated epithelium but otherwise exhibits a favorable safety profile for ocular use [114].

Systemic antifungals, including voriconazole and other azoles, can cause more severe and occasionally vision-threatening complications, such as toxic optic neuropathy, macular opacity, disturbances in color vision, photophobia, and, in rare cases, visual hallucinations. Voriconazole, for example, is linked to a high incidence (15–33%) of reversible visual disturbances, b-wave attenuation on ERG, and, rarely, optic nerve dysfunction. Some antifungals may also induce intraocular inflammation, lenticular damage, and glaucoma if delivered by intraocular injection [115].

Gene-association and pharmacovigilance studies have implicated molecular pathways such as PI3K-Akt and CES1-associated metabolism in mediating or modulating these toxicities, highlighting the complexity of antifungal ocular safety profiles [113].

These findings emphasize the need for close monitoring of ocular status during antifungal therapy, careful selection and dosing of agents based on toxicity profiles, and further studies to elucidate underlying mechanisms and risk factors of antifungal-induced ocular adverse events [114]. A summary of the ocular toxicity caused by antifungal agents is given in Table 2.4.

Table 2.3 Combination antifungal therapy for ocular fungal diseases

Combination therapy	Dose	Mode of administration	Study observations	Reference
Voriconazole and Caspofungin	2% and 0.5%	Intrastromal, topical, oral Voriconazole and topical & intrastromal Caspofungin	Administered to a single patient with *Alternaria keratitis*. Findings show that voriconazole and Caspofungin have synergistic effect in the treatment of yeasts or filamentous fungi	[72]
Fluconazole, amphotericin B and 5-fluorocytosine	1.0% w/v, 0.05% w/v and 0.8% w/v	–	Synergistic effect was observed between fluconazole and amphotericin B and between fluconazole and 5-FU in the treatment of fungal endophthalmitis induced in rat model	[81]
Amphotericin B and fluconazole	0.02% w/v and 0.2% w/v	Amphotericin B eye drops and fluconazole subconjunctival injection	Administered in humans with fungal keratitis. Showed successful healing of fungal keratitis and reduced side effects from local administration	[49]
Ketoconazole and ketorolac	2.0% w/v and 0.5% w/v	Topical polymeric gel	Combination effect observed in vivo in a rabbit model. Ketorolac reduced the inflammatory cells compared to plain ketoconazole administration	[108]
Moxifloxacin and liposomal amphotericin B	0.1% w/v and 0.01% w/v	Intravitreal injection	Administered in fungal endophthalmitis-induced rabbit model. Synergistic effect observed in vitro but not in vivo. Two–eightfold increase in antifungal activity seen in in vitro with the addition of moxifloxacin	[109]
Natamycin and azithromycin	0.06% w/v and 0.05% w/v	–	Natamycin and azithromycin showed synergistic effect against *Aspergillus flavus* species complex and *Fusarium solani* in vitro	[110]
Amphotericin B and voriconazole	0.005% w/v and 0.1% w/v	Intravitreal injection	Administered in humans with fungal endophthalmitis with filamentous fungal infection. There was an improvement in the visual acuity of 58.33% of the cases	[111]
Ketoconazole and miconazole	5 mg and 200 mg	Miconazole eye drop and subconjunctival injection and ketoconazole oral tablets	Administered in 20 patients with fungal keratitis. Treatment was successful in 13 out of the 20 patients	[112]

Table 2.4 Comparative ocular and systemic adverse events of key antifungal agents

Antifungal agent	Class	Route of administration	Ocular adverse events	Systemic adverse events	Key toxicity mechanism	References
Natamycin	Polyene	Topical	Minor irritation and discomfort, blurred vision	Low systemic absorption; high LD_{50}	Binds ergosterol; forms membrane "blisters," not pores; low affinity for cholesterol	[116–118]
Amphotericin B	Polyene	Topical	Dose-dependent ocular toxicity, low cell viability, impaired membrane integrity	Nephrotoxicity, hypokalemia, chills	Binds ergosterol and, secondarily, mammalian cholesterol; forms transmembrane channels, causing ion leakage	[119]
		Intravitreal	Retinal toxicity, acute visual loss, focal retinal damage	Limited due to local administration	Direct cytotoxicity due to binding to cholesterol in retinal cell membranes	
		Systemic	Poor ocular penetration	Severe nephrotoxicity, hypokalemia, hypomagnesemia, chills, fever, anemia	High affinity for cholesterol in mammalian cells; systemic distribution causes widespread off-target damage	
Voriconazole	Azole	Topical, systemic, intravitreal	Photophobia, blurred vision, color vision changes, visual hallucinations	Nausea, vomiting, abnormal liver function, rash, fever, chills	Inhibits fungal cytochrome P450-dependent enzyme 14α-sterol demethylase; visual effects are likely tied to drug-specific off-target effects on the retina and optic nerve	[120]
Miconazole	Azole	Topical, subconjunctival	No visible ocular toxicity in rabbit studies with topical use	Blurred vision, nausea, vomiting, diarrhea, anorexia, phlebitis, tachycardia, arrhythmias, fever, chills	Inhibits ergosterol synthesis; may also inhibit endogenous respiration	[121]

Fluconazole	Azole	Topical, oral	Xerosis (dry eyes) as a systemic side effect	Headache, dizziness, nausea, vomiting, diarrhea, stomach pain, visual field defects, seizures, hallucinations	Inhibits ergosterol synthesis	[122, 123]
Posaconazole	Azole	Topical (off-label), oral	Blurred vision, photophobia, reduced visual acuity, scotoma, diplopia	Nausea, vomiting, diarrhea, hypokalemia, hypomagnesemia, QT prolongation, liver damage, neurotoxicity, hallucinations	Inhibits ergosterol synthesis; broadest spectrum triazole	[124, 125]
Itraconazole	Triazole	Topical, oral, subconjunctival	Blurred/double vision, irritation, burning sensation, eye defects in babies of exposed mothers	Cardiotoxicity (decreased heart contractility, fast heartbeat), hepatotoxicity, nausea, vomiting, diarrhea, abdominal pain, headache, dizziness, runny nose, hair loss	Inhibits ergosterol synthesis via cytochrome P450-dependent enzyme 14α-sterol demethylase; cardiotoxicity is a rare but noted side effect.	[126, 127]
Micafungin	Echinocandin	Topical, intravenous	No apparent ocular toxicity to the cornea in preclinical studies	Blurred vision, headaches, confusion, seizures, nausea, vomiting, fever, rash, phlebitis	Inhibits β-(1,3)-D-glucan synthesis in the fungal cell wall	[128]
Caspofungin	Echinocandin	Intravitreal, intravenous	Low toxicity at therapeutic intravitreal doses in mice	Fever, rash, nausea, phlebitis, septic shock, hypokalemia	Inhibits β-(1,3)-D-glucan synthesis in the fungal cell wall	[129]

2.3 Limitations to Effective Ocular Drug Delivery

Despite the extensive research on the development of new antifungal agents, administration of these drugs to the eye is highly challenging. The eye's complex anatomical framework affects drug transport to the site of action. Understanding these aspects is essential for rationalizing the design for the delivery of drugs using novel delivery systems. The anatomical and physiological ocular barriers significantly affect drug stability, distribution, and overall therapeutic efficacy (Fig. 2.4) [130, 131].

2.3.1 Static Barriers to Ocular Drug Delivery

The cornea and blood-ocular barriers are static barriers that must be addressed to design effective ocular drug delivery systems [133]. Due to their unique physicochemical properties and multilayered composition, these barriers inherently restrict drug absorption and distribution.

2.3.1.1 Cornea

The cornea, a transparent and avascular anterior tissue, serves as a major static barrier to topically administered drugs. The alternating lipophilic and hydrophilic layers impose distinct permeability challenges for different drug classes. The corneal

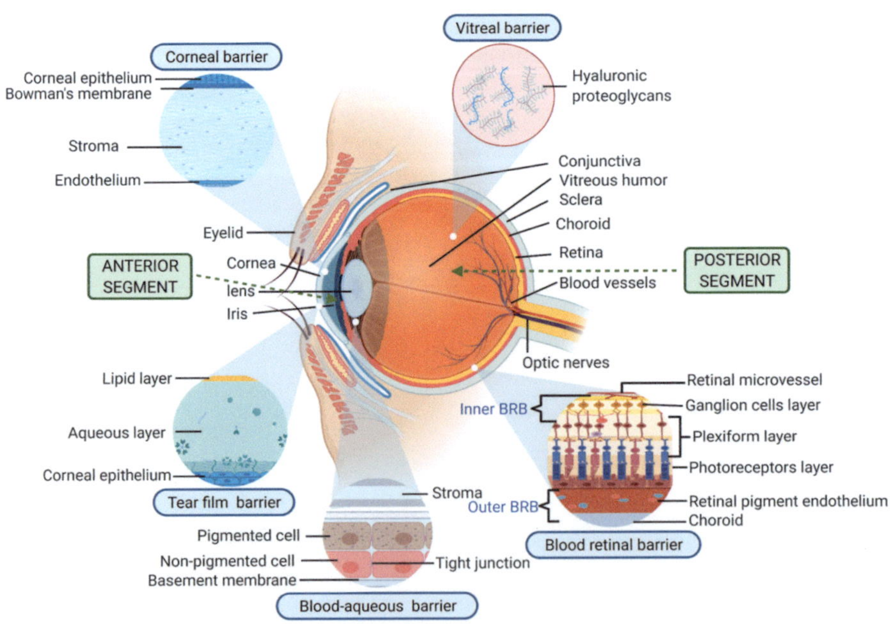

Fig. 2.4 Physiological and anatomical barriers to ocular drug delivery [132]

epithelium is lipophilic, facilitating the diffusion of small, nonpolar molecules, thereby necessitating the consideration of drug physicochemical properties and formulation strategies for large molecules [134, 135]. The stroma is a hydrophilic matrix that exhibits low resistance to polar molecules [136]; however, it imposes a significant barrier to nonpolar drugs and may serve as a reservoir for sustained release [137].

2.3.1.2 Blood-Ocular Barrier

The blood-ocular barrier comprises two selective systems: the blood-aqueous barrier (BAB) and the blood-retinal barrier (BRB) [138, 139]. The BAB is formed by the ciliary body's non-pigmented epithelial cells and the iris vasculature's endothelial cells [140], whereas the BRB is composed of the tight junctions in the retinal pigment epithelium (RPE) and retinal vascular endothelium. These highly selective barriers limit the ocular bioavailability of topically administered drugs, thereby necessitating alternative delivery approaches for anterior, like fungal keratitis, and posterior segment diseases, such as fungal endophthalmitis.

2.3.2 Dynamic Barriers in Ocular Drug Delivery

While static barriers constitute the anatomical framework of the eye's defense system, dynamic barriers rely on physiological mechanisms that actively dilute, remove, or redistribute drug formulations. These dynamic processes pose significant challenges in maintaining therapeutic drug concentrations at the target site.

2.3.2.1 Tear Film

The tear film plays a pivotal role in ocular protection and providing optical clarity [141]. Despite its minimal thickness (~6 μm), the tear film is a trilaminar structure consisting of a superficial lipid layer, a middle aqueous layer, and an innermost mucin layer. Each component plays distinct roles in drug solubility, retention, and potential degradation [142].

Tear turnover is rapid, with an estimated flow rate of ~1 μL/min and a total volume of 7–9 μL. Complete turnover can occur within minutes, significantly limiting drug contact time on the ocular surface [143]. The average blink rate—ranging from 2 to 50 times per minute—further contributes to drug washout and reduces bioavailability [144].

2.3.2.2 Nasolacrimal Drainage

The nasolacrimal drainage system is a critical dynamic mechanism that removes tear fluid and drug residues from the ocular surface. Following topical administration, a substantial fraction (up to 80%) of the drug dose may be lost via nasolacrimal drainage within 15 to 30 seconds, severely reducing drug residence time and ocular bioavailability [137, 145]. Improving the drug residence on the cornea using mucoadhesive polymers, viscosity enhancers, and punctal plugs has been explored to prolong residence time and mitigate rapid clearance [146, 147].

2.3.2.3 Conjunctival Blood Flow

The conjunctiva is a vascularized mucous membrane that lines the inner eyelids and covers the sclera [148, 149]. Drugs absorbed through the conjunctival epithelium may undergo rapid clearance via conjunctival capillaries into the systemic circulation, reducing their local ocular bioavailability. Formulating drugs that could restrict their flow towards the conjunctiva can reduce the efflux of the drug.

Dynamic barriers such as tear turnover, blinking, nasolacrimal drainage, and conjunctival blood flow substantially hinder ocular drug delivery. These barriers not only reduce drug residence time but also contribute to drug loss and systemic exposure. Overcoming these challenges requires an integrated approach considering drug physicochemical properties, formulation strategies, and ocular physiological processes. Novel delivery systems are being developed to counteract these dynamic mechanisms and improve therapeutic outcomes [150].

2.4 Advanced Ocular Drug Delivery Systems

As discussed in the previous section, drug delivery to the eye is complex and highly challenging due to the various anatomical and physiological barriers and the high clearance rate of topical eye drops. The chemical characteristics of many of the antifungal drugs also make them difficult to formulate. Polyenes like amphotericin B and natamycin have poor solubility and permeability [7, 151]. Certain azoles such as ketoconazole and itraconazole have also shown poor corneal permeability [4]. Due to this, the prescribed eye drops need to be administered quite frequently leading to poor patient compliance. The higher dosing concentration also gradually leads to the development of antifungal resistance. Therefore, extensive research is being conducted to develop novel drug delivery systems to improve the delivery of these antifungal drugs to the eye and thereby improve the efficacy of the treatment (Fig. 2.5).

2.4.1 Nano-formulations

2.4.1.1 Nanoparticles

Polymeric nanoparticles have been widely used in the field of drug delivery to increase the solubility of large and hydrophobic molecules [152]. The size range of nanoparticles could also help crossing the corneal barriers and thus improving their bioavailability. Polymeric nanoparticles have also been used to stabilize drugs that may undergo degradation in aqueous solutions [153]. Eudrajit RL 100 was used to prepare amphotericin B nanoparticles using nanoprecipitation method. Not only did it help sustain the release for over 24 hours, the nanoparticle solution was stable at room temperature and refrigerated conditions for up to 2 months [153]. Chitosan/lecithin nanoparticles loaded with amphotericin B for the treatment of fungal keratitis showed more than threefold increase in corneal residence due to its high mucoadhesion and more than twofold increase in bioavailability compared to marketed

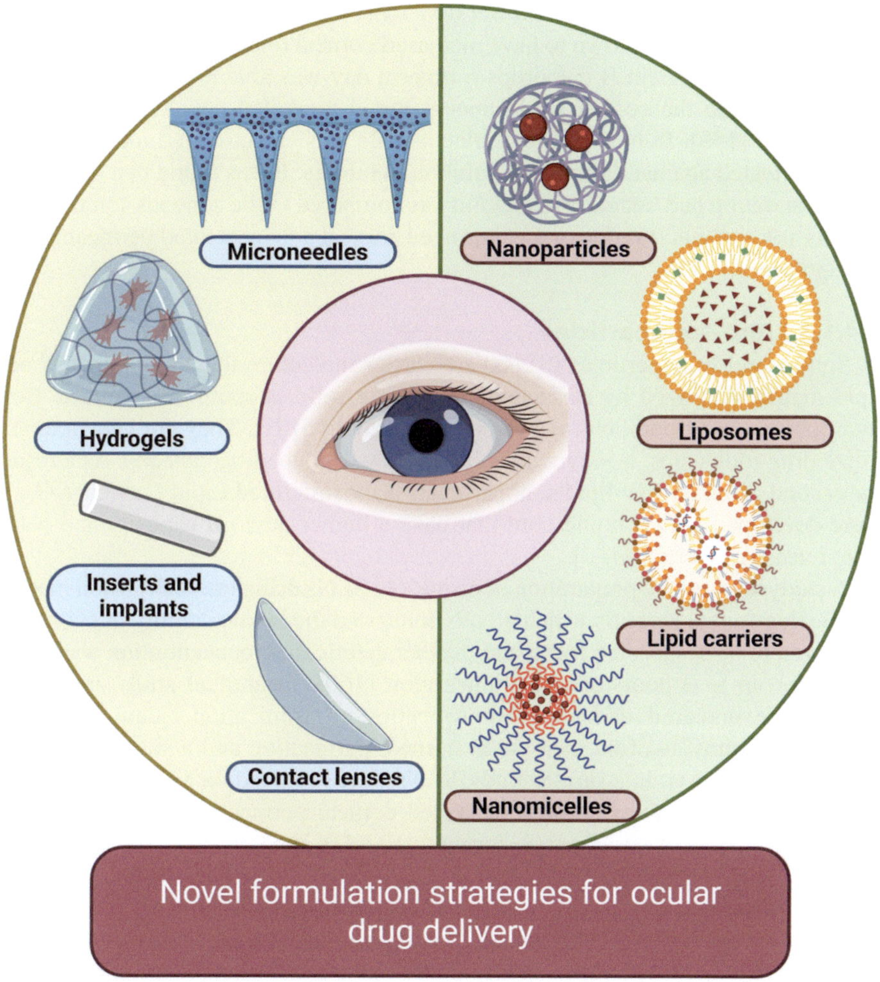

Fig. 2.5 Novel strategies for ocular drug delivery (Created with BioRender.com)

solution [154]. In another study, terconazole-loaded nanoparticles were prepared using Eudrajit RLPO® which showed sustained release for up to 24 h and better antifungal activity compared to plain terconazole [155].

2.4.1.2 Liposomes

Liposomes are bilayered vesicular structures made up of phospholipids with an aqueous core that can act as carriers for both hydrophilic and lipophilic compounds [156]. The encapsulated drug can reach the outer surface either through passive diffusion or vesicular erosion. The rate of drug release is usually dependent on the size of the liposomal structure, lipid property, and the hydrophilicity of the drug [156, 157]. AmBisome® is a liposomal powder of amphotericin B that was developed as an alternative to Fungizone, with lower toxicity [7]. Topical liposomal amphotericin B eye drops were also shown to have increased corneal retention. Administration of liposomal amphotericin B eye drops 6 times a day was able to maintain the same concentration in the cornea as the reconstituted marketed powder eye drops 24 times a day [158]. In another study, fluconazole was encapsulated into liposomes and were tested against fluconazole solution in rabbits. It was found that the liposomal formulation had better bioavailability as compared to the aqueous solution. The authors suggest that it is due to the improved corneal adherence and permeability of the liposomes [159].

2.4.1.3 Lipid Nanoparticles

Solid Lipid Nanoparticles (SLNs) are carrier molecules that are composed of a lipid matrix stabilized by surfactants which are solid at room temperature. Both hydrophilic and lipophilic drugs can be loaded onto SLNs. They are known to stabilize drug molecules; however, they have a low drug loading capacity. As a result, the second generation of lipid nanoparticles, Nanostructured Lipid Carriers (NLCs) were developed with a liquid core that have a higher payload capacity and better drug release properties [140].

A study showed the preparation of econazole SLNs using microemulsion method for treating fungal keratitis which greatly improved the bioavailability of econazole compared to its suspension form, and the therapeutic drug concentration was maintained for up to 3 hours after administration [160]. In another study, natamycin SLNs were prepared using the emulsification-ultrasonication technique, which showed an almost twofold increase in corneal permeation and a sustained release for about 10 h [161]. In a similar study, SLNs were prepared for voriconazole using hot-melt extrusion. They showed enhanced corneal permeation and were able to sustain the release of voriconazole for up to 10 h [162].

2.4.1.4 Micelles

Micelles are molecules of surfactants that self-aggregate in aqueous solution, with a hydrophobic core and a hydrophilic shell. These features make micelles particularly useful for solubilizing hydrophobic drugs [163]. Natamycin-encapsulated polymeric nanomicelles using tocopherol polyethylene glycol 1000 succinate (TPGS) showed better antifungal activity after administration 4 times a day compared to 12 times a day administration of 5% natamycin suspension. The nanomicelles were also able to improve the corneal permeability of natamycin [6]. TPGS was also used to formulate posaconazole-loaded nanomicelles. The nanomicelles showed higher corneal and scleral permeation than the marketed suspension in an ex vivo study [164]. In another study, amphotericin B-loaded PEG-PPG micelles were prepared by modifying it using polyhedral oligomeric silsesquioxane (POSS) to improve its mucoadhesion. The micelles showed corneal retention for up to 4 h after administration. It also showed improved antifungal activity [165].

2.4.2 Hydrogels

Hydrogels have been explored for anterior as well as posterior drug delivery, while contact lenses are better suited for corneal diseases such as fungal keratitis. Due to the increased adhesion of hydrogels, they are not affected by blinking or tear secretion, thus prolonging the residence time of drug on the ocular surface [166]. An amphotericin B nanohydrogel system developed using hyaluronic acid was expected to not only increase corneal retention but also shown to have lower toxicity than the available amphotericin B eye drops [167]. Another study developed a hydrogel system loaded with econazole-cyclodextrin complexes for the treatment of fungal keratitis. The hydrogel was able to sustain the release and increase the corneal residence of the drug [168].

In situ gelling systems are more commonly used for posterior segment diseases but have been explored for anterior infections as well. In situ gelling systems are in liquid state when injected and then subsequently undergo gelation after exposure to specific stimuli, such as temperature, pH, ion, UV light etc. [166]. A study showed the preparation of a thermos-responsive hydrogel system made of Poloxamer 407, loaded with fluconazole nanoparticles which showed prolonged drug release with penetration into the deeper tissues [169]. Hydrogels have not much been explored for deeper fungal infections; however, it has been demonstrated that hydrogels can stabilize proteins by reducing their mobility within the network structure and thus has a lot of scope as a sustained delivery system [170].

2.4.3 Contact Lenses and Microneedle Patches

Contact lenses and microneedles are better suited for anterior diseases as they are able to maintain consistent contact with the site of action. Contact lens-based drug delivery has a bioavailability of about 50%, compared to the 5% of eye drops [171]. This allows us to reduce the drug loading concentration, thus lowering the risk of antifungal resistance. The most commonly used method of developing antifungal contact lenses is by soaking commercially available contact lenses in drug solution to load the drug onto the lens [172]. A study compared the loading and release of natamycin of five different commercially available contact lenses [173]. It was found that after soaking for 24 hours, the drug loading was similar among the five contact lenses; however, sustained release was not obtained. All five contact lenses showed burst release in the first 30 minutes, and the remaining drug was released within the hour [173]. They concluded that the material of the contact lens plays a major role in the ability of the contact lens to sustain the release. On the other hand, hydrophilic drugs also tend to release from the contact lenses faster. A study used vitamin E to slow down the release of drug from the contact lens [174]. Fluconazole was loaded onto three different commercial lenses (NIGHT&DAY™, ACUVUE® OASYS™, and O_2OPTIX™) by soaking method. The increase in concentration of vitamin E proportionally slowed down the release of fluconazole from the contact lenses for more than 9 days with 66% of vitamin E loading [174].

Another study prepared a prototype contact lens by encapsulating econazole-loaded PLGA (poly(lactic-co-glycolic acid)) films with pHEMA [175]. These drug-eluting contact lenses were found to retain their fungicidal activity for up to 3 weeks. Aside from contact lenses, biodegradable corneal patches have also been explored for fungal keratitis. An amphotericin B-loaded corneal patch was developed that can provide sustained release for up to 12 hours [176]. Loading the drug onto the polymeric patch was also able to stabilize amphotericin B for up to 60 days at room temperature [176].

Microneedles are a minimally invasive alternative to intraocular injections that can increase the permeability of drugs across the corneal barrier [177]. Dissolvable microneedles are made of water-soluble biocompatible polymers that release the drug into the target site through erosion. Other types such as coated and hollow microneedles have also been used for ocular drug delivery [178, 179]. In a study, an amphotericin B-loaded microneedle ocular patch was developed for the treatment of fungal keratitis. The liposomal amphotericin B-loaded microneedle patches were shown to improve the efficacy of the treatment at lower concentrations of amphotericin B, thus lowering the potential for systemic toxicity [180]. Another study also attempted to prepare amphotericin B-loaded microneedles using polyvinyl pyrrolidone (PVP) and hyaluronic acid for the fabrication of the microneedle patch. Drug loading was increased by using a plain drug instead of liposomal amphotericin B. It showed increased corneal penetration and high antifungal activity compared to amphotericin B solution [181]. In another study, voriconazole was formulated into micelles and loaded onto PVP microneedles. The microneedles were able to sustain the release for up to 12 hours and significantly increased the corneal permeation compared to eye drops [182].

2.4.4 Intraocular Inserts and Implants

Ocular inserts are another mode of extended drug delivery. They hold an advantage over contact lenses and hydrogels as they do not compromise visual acuity. Ocular inserts are placed in the conjunctival sac and are able to provide a sustained release of drug in the anterior region [183]. In a study, voriconazole was formulated in a sponge-like biodegradable ocular insert using carboxymethyl cellulose, gellan gum, sodium alginate, xanthan gum, and chitosan. The insert showed high mucoadhesion and sustained antifungal activity after administration in the conjunctival sac. The sponge-like nature was expected to reduce the foreign body sensation [184]. Another study aimed to develop fluconazole-loaded ocular inserts made of chitosan. The fibrous inserts prepared using freeze-drying technique showed sustained release of the drug as compared to the fluconazole solution and had better permeation across bovine cornea [185].

Injectable implants have been extensively studied for their application in posterior segment ocular diseases. Many intravitreal implants are available commercially for inflammatory diseases [186]. An intravitreal implant for the delivery of voriconazole was prepared using different concentrations of PLGA for the treatment of fungal endophthalmitis. The PLGA-voriconazole implants were observed to have a sustained therapeutic effect for up to 8 weeks [187].

2.5 Future Directions in Ocular Antifungal Drug Delivery

The treatment for fungal infections primarily relies on the topical eye drops such as voriconazole, natamycin, and amphotericin B. Though these drugs can reduce the incidence of fungal keratitis, the emergence of resistant fungal strains, particularly of *Fusarium*, *Aspergillus*, and *Candida,* has compromised the effectiveness of these therapies. To tackle the antifungal resistance, more vigorous treatment protocols are needed for the management of diseases [188].

Though these drugs can improve the vision, challenges still pertain to the antifungal resistance that is significantly emerging in the clinics, requiring a change in the prescription doses. This generally includes an increase in the dose of the antifungal agents, which would concomitantly increase the drug's therapeutic index, thereby overcoming the resistance [188]. However, a preclinical and a clinical therapeutically effective dose for treating antifungal resistant strains needs to be studied. To overcome the antifungal resistance, research is focused on novel drug delivery systems like nanocarriers, lipid carriers, and nanoparticles which improves the precorneal residence, enhancing the drug permeation and bioavailability at the target site.

Beyond modifying the existing treatment regimens, exploring novel antifungal classes with novel targets within the fungal cell wall has recently emerged. For instance, echinocandins that target cell wall biosynthesis are being studied for their potential in treating resistant fungal strains. In addition, combination therapy with antifungal agents having different mechanisms of action can provide synergistic effects, potentially overcome resistance, and improve clinical outcomes. Reports show synergism of amphotericin B with terbinafine, amphotericin B with itraconazole [51], and natamycin with voriconazole [106, 107]. These combinations could decrease the dosage regimen, thereby decreasing the likelihood of developing resistance. With the clinical paradigm of collagen cross-linking and photodynamic therapy, investigating their use to enhance the antifungal effects and improve patient outcomes in severe or resistant cases is being explored [189].

2.6 Conclusion

Effective management of ocular fungal infections requires a thorough understanding of both the fungal strain and the pharmacological properties of current antifungals. Although topical eye drops are still the primary treatment for anterior segment infections due to their ease and safety, their limitations, particularly in solubility and corneal penetration, require alternative or additional treatment in more severe or refractory cases. Antifungal therapy must therefore be tailored to the species involved, in vitro drug susceptibility, site and degree of infection, and the drug's pharmacokinetic features. In order to improve ocular bioavailability and therapeutic outcomes, future research should focus on developing new delivery systems and optimizing existing ones, as changing resistance patterns and the need for more efficient delivery systems become more apparent.

Acknowledgments The authors would like to thank Indian Council of Medical Research, India—Centre for Advanced Research, India (ICMR-CAR-2024-01-000365) and ICMR (2021-9766) for funding support.

References

1. Thomas PA, Kaliamurthy J. Mycotic keratitis: epidemiology, diagnosis and management. Clin Microbiol Infect. 2013;19(3):210–20.
2. Toumasis P, Tsantes AG, Tsiogka A, Samonis G, Vrioni G. From clinical suspicion to diagnosis: a review of diagnostic approaches and challenges in fungal keratitis. Vol. 13, J Clin Med Multidiscipl Digit Pub Inst (MDPI); 2024.
3. Reginatto P, de Agostinetto GJ, do Fuentefria RN, Marinho DR, Pizzol MD, Fuentefria AM. Eye fungal infections: a mini review. Arch Microbiol. 2023;205(6):236.
4. Lakhani P, Patil A, Majumdar S. Challenges in the polyene- and azole-based pharmacotherapy of ocular fungal infections. J Ocul Pharmacol Ther. 2019;35(1):6–22.
5. Kaur IP, Kakkar S. Topical delivery of antifungal agents. Expert Opin Drug Deliv. 2010;7(11):1303–27.
6. Sathe P, Kailasam V, Nagarjuna V, Sharma H, Velpandian T, Garg P, et al. Nanomicelles empower natamycin in treating fungal keratitis: an in vitro, ex vivo and in vivo study. Int J Pharm. 2024;656:124118.
7. Kailasam V, Sai Veda Koduganti S, Dasgupta O, Garg P, Nirmal J. Ocular delivery of amphotericin B: current challenges and future perspectives. Expert Opin Drug Deliv. 2024;21(12):1793–805.
8. Ansari Z, Miller D, Galor A. Current thoughts in fungal keratitis: diagnosis and treatment. Curr Fungal Infect Rep. 2013;7(3):209–18.
9. Sahay P, Singhal D, Nagpal R, Maharana PK, Farid M, Gelman R, et al. Pharmacologic therapy of mycotic keratitis. Surv Ophthalmol. 2019;64(3):380–400.
10. Reddy PRRPRASN. A comparative evaluation of nystatin, Amphotericin-B and miconazole in Keratomycosis. Indian J Ophthalmol. 1982;30(4):249–50.
11. Bernauer W, Allan BDS, Dart JKG. Successful management of aspergillus scleritis by medical and surgical treatment. Eye. 1998;12(2):311–6.
12. Qiu S, Zhao G-Q, Lin J, Wang X, Hu L-T, Du Z-D, Wang Q, Zhu C-C. Natamycin in the treatment of fungal keratitis: a systematic review and meta-analysis. Int J Ophthalmol. 2015;8(3):597–602.
13. Lalitha P, Vijaykumar R, Prajna NV, Fothergill AW. In vitro natamycin susceptibility of ocular isolates of *Fusarium* and *Aspergillus* species: comparison of commercially formulated natamycin eye drops to pharmaceutical-grade powder. J Clin Microbiol. 2008;46(10):3477–8.
14. Prajna NV, Mascarenhas J, Krishnan T, Reddy PR, Prajna L, Srinivasan M, et al. Comparison of natamycin and voriconazole for the treatment of fungal keratitis. Arch Ophthalmol. 2010;128(6):672–8.
15. Prajna NV, Krishnan T, Mascarenhas J, Rajaraman R, Prajna L, Srinivasan M, et al. The mycotic ulcer treatment trial. JAMA Ophthalmol. 2013;131(4):422.
16. Sharma N, Bagga B, Singhal D, Nagpal R, Kate A, Saluja G, et al. Fungal keratitis: a review of clinical presentations, treatment strategies and outcomes. Ocul Surf. 2022;24:22–30.
17. Obrien T. Therapy of ocular fungal infections. Ophthalmol Clin North Am. 1999;12(1):33–50.

18. Gallis HA, Drew RH, Pickard WW. Amphotericin B: 30 years of clinical experience. Rev Infect Dis. 1990;12(2):308–29.
19. Khoo SH, Bond J, Denning DW. Administering amphotericin B–a practical approach. J Antimicrob Chemother 1994 33(2):203–213.
20. Qu L, Li L, Xie H. Corneal and aqueous humor concentrations of amphotericin B using three different routes of administration in a rabbit model. Ophthalmic Res. 2010;43(3):153–8.
21. Hirose H, Terasaki H, Awaya S, Yasuma T. Treatment of fungal corneal ulcers with amphotericin B ointment. Am J Ophthalmol. 1997;124(6):836–8.
22. O'Day DM, Ray WA, Robinson RD, Head WS, Williams TE. Differences in response in vivo to amphotericin B among Candida albicans strains. Invest Ophthalmol Vis Sci. 1991;32(5):1569–72.
23. Nett JE, Andes DR. Antifungal agents: Spectrum of activity, pharmacology, and clinical indications. In: Infectious disease clinics of North America, vol. 30. W.B. Saunders; 2016. p. 51–83.
24. Garcia-Valenzuela E, Song CD. Intracorneal injection of amphothericin B for recurrent fungal keratitis and endophthalmitis. Arch Ophthalmol. 2005;123(12):1721–3.
25. Yoon KC, Jeong IY, Im SK, Chae HJ, Yang SY. Therapeutic effect of intracameral amphotericin B injection in the treatment of fungal keratitis. Cornea. 2007;26(7):814–8.
26. Kuriakose T, Kothari M, Paul P, Jacob P, Thomas R. Intracameral amphotericin B injection in the management of deep Keratomycosis. Cornea. 2002;21(7):653–6.
27. Yamaguchi H, Abe S, Tokuda Y. Immunomodulating activity of antifungal drugs. Ann N Y Acad Sci. 1993;685:447–57.
28. Joseph J, Sharma S. Antifungal therapy in eye infections: new drugs, new trends. In: Recent trends in antifungal agents and antifungal therapy. New Delhi: Springer; 2016. p. 217–36.
29. Bunya VY, Hammersmith KM, Rapuano CJ, Ayres BD, Cohen EJ. Topical and oral Voriconazole in the treatment of fungal keratitis. Am J Ophthalmol. 2007;143(1):151–3.
30. Parchand S, Gupta A, Ram J, Gupta N, Chakrabarty A. Voriconazole for fungal corneal ulcers. Ophthalmology. 2012;119(5):1083.
31. Diekema DJ, Messer SA, Hollis RJ, Jones RN, Pfaller MA. Activities of Caspofungin, Itraconazole, Posaconazole, Ravuconazole, Voriconazole, and amphotericin B against 448 recent clinical isolates of filamentous fungi. J Clin Microbiol. 2003;41(8):3623–6.
32. Pfaller MA, Messer SA, Boyken L, Rice C, Tendolkar S, Hollis RJ, et al. Global trends in the antifungal susceptibility of Cryptococcus neoformans (1990 to 2004). J Clin Microbiol. 2005;43(5):2163–7.
33. Purkins L, Wood N, Ghahramani P, Greenhalgh K, Allen MJ, Kleinermans D. Pharmacokinetics and safety of voriconazole following intravenous-to oral-dose escalation regimens. Antimicrob Agents Chemother. 2002;46(8):2546–53.
34. Purkins L, Wood N, Greenhalgh K, Allen MJ, Oliver SD. Voriconazole, a novel wide-spectrum triazole: oral pharmacokinetics and safety. Br J Clin Pharmacol. 2003;56(Suppl 1):10–6.
35. Hariprasad SM, Mieler WF, Lin TK, Sponsel WE, Graybill JR. Voriconazole in the treatment of fungal eye infections: a review of current literature. Br J Ophthalmol. 2008;92(7):871–8.
36. Al-Badriyeh D, Neoh CF, Stewart K, Kong DCM. Clinical utility of voriconazole eye drops in ophthalmic fungal keratitis. Clin Ophthalmol. 2010;6(4):391–405.
37. Dupuis A, Tournier N, Le Moal G, Venisse N. Preparation and stability of voriconazole eye drop solution. Antimicrob Agents Chemother. 2009;53(2):798–9.
38. Clode AB, Davis JL, Salmon J, Michau TM, Gilger BC. Evaluation of concentration of voriconazole in aqueous humor after topical and oral administration in horses. Am J Vet Res. 2006;67(2):296–301.
39. Prakash G, Sharma N, Goel M, Titiyal JS, Vajpayee RB. Evaluation of intrastromal injection of Voriconazole as a therapeutic adjunctive for the Management of Deep Recalcitrant Fungal Keratitis. Am J Ophthalmol. 2008;146(1):56–59.e2.

40. Siatiri H, Daneshgar F, Siatiri N, Khodabande A. The effects of intrastromal voriconazole injection and topical voriconazole in the treatment of recalcitrant *Fusarium* keratitis. Cornea. 2011;30(8):872–5.
41. Sharma N, Agarwal P, Sinha R, Titiyal JS, Velpandian T, Vajpayee RB. Evaluation of intrastromal voriconazole injection in recalcitrant deep fungal keratitis: case series. Br J Ophthalmol. 2011;95(12):1735–7.
42. Barasch A, Griffin AV. Miconazole revisited: new evidence of antifungal efficacy from laboratory and clinical trials. Future Microbiol. 2008;3(3):265–9.
43. Thevissen K, Ayscough KR, Aerts AM, Du W, De Brucker K, Meert EMK, et al. Miconazole induces changes in actin cytoskeleton prior to reactive oxygen species induction in yeast. J Biol Chem. 2007;282(30):21592–7.
44. Foster CS, Stefanyszyn M. Intraocular penetration of miconazole in rabbits. Arch Ophthalmol. 1979;97(9):1703–6.
45. O'Day DM, Foulds G, Williams TE, Robinson RD, Allen RH, Head WS. Ocular uptake of fluconazole following oral administration. Arch Ophthalmol. 1990;108(7):1006–8.
46. Thakar M. Oral fluconazole therapy for keratomycosis. Acta Ophthalmol. 1994;72(6):765–7.
47. Avunduk AM, Beuerman RW, Warnel ED, Kaufman HE, Greer D. Comparison of efficacy of topical and oral fluconazole treatment in experimental aspergillus keratitis. Curr Eye Res. 2003;26(2):113–7.
48. Mahdy RA, Nada WM, Wageh MM. Topical amphotericin B and subconjunctival injection of fluconazole (combination therapy) versus topical amphotericin B (monotherapy) in treatment of Keratomycosis. J Ocul Pharmacol Ther. 2010;26(3):281–5.
49. Mahdy RA, Nada WM, Wageh MM, Kader MA, Saleh MM, Alswad MM. Assessment safety and efficacy of a combination therapy of topical amphotericin B and subconjunctival fluconazole for the treatment of fungal keratitis. Cutan Ocul Toxicol. 2010;29(3):193–7.
50. Yilmaz S, Maden A. Severe fungal keratitis treated with subconjunctival fluconazole. Am J Ophthalmol. 2005;140(3):454–8.
51. Li L, Wang Z, Li R, Luo S, Sun X. In vitro evaluation of combination antifungal activity against *Fusarium* species isolated from ocular tissues of Keratomycosis patients. Am J Ophthalmol. 2008;146(5):724–728.e1.
52. Müller GG, Kara-José N, de Castro RS. Antifúngicos em infecções oculares: drogas e vias de administração. Rev Bras Oftalmol. 2013 Apr;72(2):132–41.
53. Thomas PA, Kalavathy CM, Abraham DJ, Rajasekaran J. Oral ketoconazole in Keratomycosis. Indian J Ophthalmol. 1987;35(4):197–203.
54. Gupta AK, Lyons DCA. The rise and fall of Oral ketoconazole. J Cutan Med Surg. 2015;19(4):352–7.
55. Ishibashi Y. Oral ketoconazole therapy for Keratomycosis. Am J Ophthalmol. 1983;95(3):342–5.
56. Daneshmend TK, Warnock DW. Clinical pharmacokinetics of ketoconazole. Clin Pharmacokinet. 1988;14(1):13–34.
57. Hemady RK, Chu W, Foster CS. Intraocular penetration of ketoconazole in rabbits. Cornea. 1992;11(4):329–33.
58. Rajaraman R, Bhat P, Vaidee V, Maskibail S, Raghavan A, Sivasubramaniam S, et al. Topical 5% Natamycin with Oral ketoconazole in filamentous fungal keratitis. Asia-Pacific J Ophthal. 2015;4(3):146–50.
59. Nett JE, Andes DR. Antifungal Agents. Infect Dis Clin N Am. 2016;30(1):51–83.
60. Altun A, Kurna SA, Sengor T, Altun G, Olcaysu OO, Aki SF, et al. Effectiveness of Posaconazole in recalcitrant fungal keratitis resistant to conventional antifungal drugs. Case Rep Ophthalmol Med. 2014;2014:1–4.
61. Cuenca-Estrella M, Gomez-Lopez A, Mellado E, Buitrago MJ, Monzon A, Rodriguez-Tudela JL. Head-to-Head comparison of the activities of currently available antifungal agents against 3,378 Spanish clinical isolates of yeasts and filamentous fungi. Antimicrob Agents Chemother. 2006;50(3):917–21.

62. Tu EY, McCartney DL, Beatty RF, Springer KL, Levy J, Edward D. Successful treatment of resistant ocular Fusariosis with Posaconazole (SCH-56592). Am J Ophthalmol. 2007;143(2):222–227.e1.
63. Sponsel WE, Graybill JR, Nevarez HL, Dang D. Ocular and systemic posaconazole(SCH-56592) treatment of invasive *Fusarium solani* keratitis and endophthalmitis. Br J Ophthalmol. 2002;86(7):829–30.
64. Pilmis B, Jullien V, Sobel J, Lecuit M, Lortholary O, Charlier C. Antifungal drugs during pregnancy: an updated review. J Antimicrob Chemother. 2015;70(1):14–22.
65. Thomas PA, Abraham DJ, Kalavathy CM, Rajasekaran J. Oral Itraconazole therapy for mycotic keratitis/Orale Itraconazol-Therapie bei mykotischer keratitis. Mycoses. 1988;31(5):271–9.
66. Li RK, Ciblak MA, Nordoff N, Pasarell L, Warnock DW, McGinnis MR. In Vitro Activities of Voriconazole, Itraconazole, and Amphotericin B against *Blastomyces dermatitidis*, *Coccidioides immitis*, and *Histoplasma capsulatum*. Antimicrob Agents Chemother. 2000;44(6):1734–6.
67. Agarwal PK, Roy P, Das A, Banerjee A, Maity PK, Banerjee AR. Efficacy of topical and systemic itraconazole as a broad-spectrum antifungal agent in mycotic corneal ulcer. A preliminary study. Indian J Ophthalmol. 2001:173–6.
68. Van Peer A, Woestenborghs R, Heykants J, Gasparini R, Gauwenbergh G. The effects of food and dose on the oral systemic availability of itraconazole in healthy subjects. Eur J Clin Pharmacol. 1989;36(4):423–6.
69. Willems L, van der Geest R, de Beule K. Itraconazole oral solution and intravenous formulations: a review of pharmacokinetics and pharmacodynamics. J Clin Pharm Ther. 2001;26(3):159–69.
70. Patil A, Majumdar S. Echinocandins in ocular therapeutics. J Ocul Pharmacol Ther. 2017;33(5):340–52.
71. Neoh CF, Jacob J, Leung L, Li J, Stathopoulos A, Stewart K, et al. Stability of extemporaneously prepared 0.5-percent Caspofungin eye drops: a potential cost-savings exercise. Antimicrob Agents Chemother. 2012;56(6):3435–7.
72. Neoh CF, Leung L, Vajpayee RB, Stewart K, Kong DC. Treatment of Alternaria keratitis with intrastromal and topical Caspofungin in combination with intrastromal, topical, and Oral Voriconazole. Ann Pharmacother. 2011;45(5):681.
73. Goldblum D, Frueh BE, Sarra GM, Katsoulis K, Zimmerli S. Topical Caspofungin for treatment of keratitis caused by *Candida albicans* in a rabbit model. Antimicrob Agents Chemother. 2005;49(4):1359–63.
74. Ozturk F, Yavas GF, Kusbeci T, Cetinkaya Z, Inan UU, Ermis SS, et al. Efficacy of topical Caspofungin in experimental *Fusarium keratitis*. Cornea. 2007;26(6):726–8.
75. Joseph JM, Jain R, Danziger LH. Micafungin: a new Echinocandin antifungal. Pharmacotherapy: the Journal of human pharmacology and drug. Therapy. 2007;27(1):53–67.
76. Matsumoto Y, Dogru M, Goto E, Fujishima H, Tsubota K. Successful topical application of a new antifungal agent, micafungin, in the treatment of refractory fungal corneal ulcers. Cornea. 2005;24(6):748–53.
77. Matsumoto Y, Murat D, Kojima T, Shimazaki J, Tsubota K. The comparison of solitary topical micafungin or fluconazole application in the treatment of Candida fungal keratitis. Br J Ophthalmol. 2011;95(10):1406–9.
78. Trujillo F, Paris G, Woodward L, Graybill J, Pena M, Najvar L, Trigo Y, Sponsel WE, et al. Comparison of two antifungal agents, Natamycin and micafungin, for fungal keratitis. Invest Ophthalmol Vis Sci. 2004;45(13):113.
79. Vermes A. Flucytosine: a review of its pharmacology, clinical indications, pharmacokinetics, toxicity and drug interactions. J Antimicrob Chemother. 2000;46(2):171–9.
80. Riddell J, Comer GM, Kauffman CA. Treatment of endogenous fungal Endophthalmitis: focus on new antifungal agents. Clin Infect Dis. 2011;52(5):648–53.
81. Pappas PG, Kauffman CA, Andes DR, Clancy CJ, Marr KA, Ostrosky-Zeichner L, et al. Clinical practice guideline for the Management of Candidiasis: 2016 update by the Infectious Diseases Society of America. Clin Infect Dis. 2016;62(4):e1–50.

82. Louie A, Liu W, Miller DA, Sucke AC, Liu QF, Drusano GL, et al. Efficacies of high-dose fluconazole plus amphotericin B and high-dose fluconazole plus 5-Fluorocytosine versus amphotericin B, fluconazole, and 5-Fluorocytosine monotherapies in treatment of experimental endocarditis, Endophthalmitis, and pyelonephritis due to *Candida albicans*. Antimicrob Agents Chemother. 1999;43(12):2831–40.
83. O'day DM, Head WS, Robinson RD, Stern WH, Freeman JM. Intraocular penetration of systemically administered antifungal agents. Curr Eye Res. 1985;4(2):131–4.
84. Saluja G, Sharma N, Agarwal R, Sharma HP, Maharana P, Satpathy G, et al. Determination of surgical outcomes with a novel formulation of intrastromal natamycin in recalcitrant fungal keratitis: a pilot study. Indian J Ophthalmol. 2021;69(10):2670–4.
85. Morand K, Bartoletti AC, Bochot A, Barratt G, Brandely ML, Chast F. Liposomal amphotericin B eye drops to treat fungal keratitis: Physico-chemical and formulation stability. Int J Pharm. 2007;344(1–2):150–3.
86. Carrasco MA, Genesoni G. Treatment of severe fungal keratitis with subconjunctival amphotericin B. Cornea. 2011;30(5):608–11.
87. Haddad R, El-Mollayess G. Combination of intracameral and intrastromal voriconazole in the treatment of recalcitrant *Acremonium* fungal keratitis. Middle East Afr J Ophthalmol. 2012;19(2):265.
88. Foster CS. Miconazole therapy for Keratomycosis. Am J Ophthalmol. 1981;91(5):622–9.
89. Tsai SH, Lin YC, Hsu HC, Chen YM. Subconjunctival injection of fluconazole in the treatment of fungal *Alternaria* keratitis. Ocul Immunol Inflamm. 2016;24(1):103–6.
90. Atighehchian M, Ghassemi H, Latifi G, Ouano D, Abedinifar Z, Zarei-Ghanavati M. Topical Caspofungin 0.5% monotherapy for filamentous fungal keratitis. Cornea. 2025;
91. Danielescu C, Cantemir A, Chiselita D. Successful treatment of fungal endophthalmitis using intravitreal caspofungin. Arq Bras Oftalmol. 2017;80(3):196–8.
92. von Jagow B, Kurzai O, Kakkassery V. Case report: beyond the blood-retina barrier: intravitreal Caspofungin for fungal Endophthalmitis. Optom Vis Sci. 2020;97(7):473–6.
93. Nakhwa C. Endogenous fungal endophthalmitis treated with intravitreal caspofungin in a COVID-19 recovered patient: a case report. Indian J Ophthalmol. 2021;69(12):3759–61.
94. Dwivedi S, Rudramurthy SM. Caspofungin. Indian J Ophthal – Case Reports. 2021;1(1):43.
95. Ramos JT, Romero CA, Belda S, Candel FJ, Carazo Gallego B, Fernández-Polo A, et al. Clinical practice update of antifungal prophylaxis in immunocompromised children. Rev Esp Quimioter. 2019;32(5):410–25.
96. Badiee P, Nejabat M, Choopanizadeh M. Management of Fungal Keratitis in pediatric patients. Arch. Pediatr Infect Dis. 2017; Oct 3; In Press (In Press)
97. Ferreras-Antolín L, Irwin A, Atra A, Chapelle F, Drysdale SB, Emonts M, et al. Pediatric antifungal prescribing patterns identify significant opportunities to rationalize antifungal use in children. Pediatr Infect Dis J. 2022;41(3):E69–74.
98. Groll AH, Castagnola E, Cesaro S, Dalle JH, Engelhard D, Hope W, et al. Fourth European conference on infections in Leukaemia (ECIL-4): guidelines for diagnosis, prevention, and treatment of invasive fungal diseases in paediatric patients with cancer or allogeneic haemopoietic stem-cell transplantation. Lancet Oncol. 2014;15(8):e327–40.
99. Lehrnbecher T. Antifungal prophylaxis in pediatric patients undergoing therapy for cancer. Curr Opin Infect Dis. 2015;28(6):523–31.
100. Mellinghoff SC, Panse J, Alakel N, Behre G, Buchheidt D, Christopeit M, et al. Primary prophylaxis of invasive fungal infections in patients with haematological malignancies: 2017 update of the recommendations of the infectious diseases working party (AGIHO) of the German Society for Haematology and Medical Oncology (DGHO). Ann Hematol. 2018;97(2):197–207.
101. Taplitz RA, Kennedy EB, Bow EJ, Crews J, Gleason C, Hawley DK, et al. Antimicrobial prophylaxis for adult patients with cancer-related immunosuppression: ASCO and IDSA clinical practice guideline update. J Clin Oncol. 2018;36(30):3043–54.
102. Patel MA, Aliporewala VM, Patel DA. Common antifungal drugs in pregnancy: risks and precautions. J Obs Gynecol India. Springer. 2021;71:577–82.

103. Demarinis G, Tatti F, Taloni A, Giugliano AV, Panthagani J, Myerscough J, et al. Treatments for ocular diseases in pregnancy and breastfeeding: a narrative review. Pharmaceuticals (Basel). 2023;16(10)
104. Patel VM, Schwartz RA, Lambert WC. Topical antiviral and antifungal medications in pregnancy: a review of safety profiles. Vol. 31, J European Acad Dermatol Venereol. Blackwell Publishing Ltd; 2017. p. 1440–1446.
105. Johnson MD, Perfect JR. Use of antifungal combination therapy: agents, order, and timing. Curr Fungal Infect Rep. 2010;4(2):87–95.
106. Sradhanjali S, Yein B, Sharma S, Das S. In vitro synergy of natamycin and voriconazole against clinical isolates of *Fusarium*, *Candida*, *Aspergillus* and *Curvularia* spp. Br J Ophthalmol. 2018;102(1):142–5.
107. Al-Hatmi AMS, Meletiadis J, Curfs-Breuker I, Bonifaz A, Meis JF, De Hoog GS. *In vitro* combinations of natamycin with voriconazole, itraconazole and micafungin against clinical *Fusarium* strains causing keratitis: Table 1. J Antimicrob Chemother. 2016;71(4):953–5.
108. El-Mofty HM, Abdelhakim MASE, El-Miligi MF, El-Nabarawi MA, Khalil IAH. A new combination formula for treatment of fungal keratitis: an experimental study. J Ophthalmol. 2014;2014:1–7.
109. Deren YT, Özdek Ş, Kalkanci A, Akyürek N, Hasanreisoğlu B. Comparison of antifungal efficacies of moxifloxacin, liposomal amphotericin B, and combination treatment in experimental Candida albicans endophthalmitis in rabbits. Can J Microbiol. 2010;56(1):1–7.
110. Guo H, Zhou L, He Y, Gao C, Han L, Xu Y. Natamycin and azithromycin are synergistic *in vitro* against ocular pathogenic *Aspergillus flavus* species complex and *Fusarium solani* species complex isolates. Antimicrob Agents Chemother. 2018;62(7)
111. Choudhury H, Mithal K, Pathengay A, Bawdekar A, Jindal A, Vira D, et al. Filamentous fungal endophthalmitis: results of combination therapy with intravitreal amphotericin B and voriconazole. Clin Ophthalmol. 2015;649
112. Fitzsimons R, Peters AL. Miconazole and ketoconazole as a satisfactory first-line treatment for Keratomycosis. Am J Ophthalmol. 1986;101(5):605–8.
113. Wang D, Peng Y, Zhang Q, Pu Y, Gao X, Zeng L, et al. Ocular safety evaluation of toplic and systemic antifungal medications: a multi-source pharmacovigilance and genomic study. Eur J Pharmacol [Internet] 2025 [cited 2025 Sep 9];1005. Available from: https://pubmed.ncbi.nlm.nih.gov/40876614/.
114. Kimakura M, Usui T, Yokoo S, Nakagawa S, Yamagami S, Amano S. Toxicity of topical antifungal agents to stratified human cultivated corneal epithelial sheets. J Ocular Pharmacol Therap [Internet] 2014 [cited 2025 Sep 9];30(10):810. Available from: https://pmc.ncbi.nlm.nih.gov/articles/PMC4259201/.
115. Mounier A, Douma I, Chehab H EL, Vie A, Agard E, Russo A, et al. Ocular toxicity of voriconazole: a case report and review of litterature. Acta Ophthalmol [Internet] 2014 [cited 2025 Sep 9];92(s253):0–0. Available from: https://onlinelibrary.wiley.com/doi/full/10.1111/j.1755-3768.2014.F015.x.
116. Mascarenhas M, Chaudhari P, Lewis SA. Natamycin Ocular Delivery: Challenges and Advancements in Ocular Therapeutics. Adv Ther [Internet]. 2023 [cited 2025 Sep 9];40(8):3332. Available from: https://pmc.ncbi.nlm.nih.gov/articles/PMC10329963/.
117. Delves-Broughton J. Preservatives: permitted preservatives – Natamycin. In: Encyclopedia of Food Microbiology: Second Edition; 2014. p. 87–91.
118. Patil A, Lakhani P, Majumdar S. Current perspectives on natamycin in ocular fungal infections. J Drug Deliv Sci Technol [Internet]. 2017 [cited 2025 Sep 9];41:206–12. Available from: https://www.sciencedirect.com/science/article/pii/S177322471730504X.
119. Noor A, Preuss C V. Amphotericin B. StatPearls [Internet]. 2024 [cited 2025 Sep 9]; Available from: https://www.ncbi.nlm.nih.gov/books/NBK482327/.
120. Heralgi MM, Badami A, Vokuda H, Venkatachalam K. An update on Voriconazole in ophthalmology. Delhi J Ophthal. 2016 Jul;27(1):9–15.
121. Miconazole. Meyler's Side Effects of Drugs [Internet]. 2016 [cited 2025 Sep 9];1015–6. Available from: https://linkinghub.elsevier.com/retrieve/pii/B9780444537171010829.

122. Mehrandish S, Mirzaeei S. A review on ocular novel drug delivery Systems of Antifungal Drugs: functional evaluation and comparison of conventional and novel dosage forms. Adv Pharm Bull [Internet]. 2020; [cited 2025 Sep 9];11(1):28. Available from: https://pmc.ncbi.nlm.nih.gov/articles/PMC7961232/.
123. Uchiyama K, Asano N, Ogata M, Tanahashi T, Torisaki M, Mochizuki K, et al. Topical Fluconazole: high penetration without corneal toxicity. Ocular Toxicol [Internet] 1995 [cited 2025 Sep 9];181–90. Available from: https://link.springer.com/chapter/10.1007/978-1-4615-1887-7_19.
124. Sponsel WE, Graybill JR, Nevarez HL, Dang D. Ocular and systemic posaconazole (SCH-56592) treatment of invasive *Fusarium solani* keratitis and endophthalmitis. Br J Ophthalmol [Internet] 2002 [cited 2025 Sep 9];86(7):829. Available from: https://pmc.ncbi.nlm.nih.gov/articles/PMC1771206/.
125. Phatak KM, Yawalkar AN, Sole SS, Vavia PR. Overcoming corneal barriers: Posaconazole loaded cationic surfactant vesicles for enhanced ocular permeability and anti-fungal efficacy. Asian J Pharm Sci [Internet] 2025 [cited 2025 Sep 9];101087. Available from: https://linkinghub.elsevier.com/retrieve/pii/S1818087625000716.
126. Tucker RM, Haq Y, Denning DW, Stevens DA. Adverse events associated with itraconazole in 189 patients on chronic therapy. J Antimicrob Chemother [Internet]. 1990 [cited 2025 Sep 15];26(4):561–6. Available from: https://pubmed.ncbi.nlm.nih.gov/2174854/.
127. Schulman JA, Peyman GA, Dietlein J, Fiscella R. Ocular toxicity of experimental intravitreal itraconazole. Int Ophthalmol [Internet] 1991 [cited 2025 Sep 15];15(1):21–24. Available from: https://pubmed.ncbi.nlm.nih.gov/1849126/.
128. Espinel-Ingroff A. Antifungal agents. In: Encyclopedia of microbiology. 3rd ed; 2009. p. 205–22.
129. Goldblum D, Frueh BE, Sarra GM, Katsoulis K, Zimmerli S. Topical Caspofungin for Treatment of Keratitis Caused by *Candida albicans* in a Rabbit Model. Antimicrob Agents Chemother [Internet]. 2005 [cited 2025 Sep 9];49(4):1359. Available from: https://pmc.ncbi.nlm.nih.gov/articles/PMC1068631/.
130. Gaudana R, Ananthula HK, Parenky A, Mitra AK. Ocular drug delivery. AAPS J. 2010;12:348–60.
131. Barar J, Reza Javadzadeh A, Omidi Y. Ocular novel drug delivery: impacts of membranes and barriers. Expert Opin Drug Deliv. 2008;5(5):567–81.
132. Muhammad Faris, Adrianto Febri, Annuryanti Clive G., Wilson Ravi, Sheshala Raghu Raj Singh, Thakur (2022) In vitro dissolution testing models of ocular implants for posterior segment drug delivery Abstract Drug Delivery and Translational Research 12(6) 1355–75 https://doi.org/10.1007/s13346-021-01043-z.
133. Chandel A, Kandav G. Insights into ocular therapeutics: a comprehensive review of anatomy, barriers, diseases and nanoscale formulations for targeted drug delivery. J Drug Deliv Sci Technol. 2024;97:105785.
134. Montgomery SA, McAuley R, Montgomery DB, Brunswick DJ, Amsterdam JD, Mendels J, et al. M. Gibaldi and D. Perrier a s, Dekker, New (13) A. Amidsen. Vol. 5, 1268 I Journal of Pharmaceutical Sciences. Duxbury Press; 1981.
135. Prausnitz MR, Noonan JS. Permeability of cornea, sclera, and conjunctiva: a literature analysis for drug delivery to the eye. J Pharm Sci. 1998;87(12):1479–88.
136. Mun EA, Morrison PWJ, Williams AC, Khutoryanskiy VV. On the barrier properties of the cornea: a microscopy study of the penetration of fluorescently labeled nanoparticles, polymers, and sodium fluorescein. Mol Pharm. 2014;11(10):3556–64.
137. Jumelle C, Gholizadeh S, Annabi N, Dana R. Advances and limitations of drug delivery systems formulated as eye drops, vol. 321., J Controlled Release. Elsevier B.V; 2020. p. 1–22.
138. Tavakoli S, Peynshaert K, Lajunen T, Devoldere J, del Amo EM, Ruponen M, et al. Ocular barriers to retinal delivery of intravitreal liposomes: impact of vitreoretinal interface. J Control Release. 2020;328:952–61.
139. Campbell M, Humphries P. The blood-retina barrier tight Junctions and barrier modulation introduction: general anatomy of the human eye.

140. Sánchez-López E, Espina M, Doktorovova S, Souto EB, García ML. Lipid nanoparticles (SLN, NLC): overcoming the anatomical and physiological barriers of the eye—part II - ocular drug-loaded lipid nanoparticles. Eur J Pharm Biopharm. 2017;110:58–69.
141. Tiffany JM. The Normal tear film, vol. 41. Basel, Karger: Dev Ophthalmol; 2008.
142. Dartt DA. Tear lipocalin: structure and function. In: Ocular surface, vol. 9. Elsevier Inc.; 2011. p. 126–38.
143. Mudgil P. Antimicrobial tear lipids in the ocular surface defense, vol. 12., Front Cellular Infection Microbiol. Frontiers Media S.A.; 2022.
144. Shell JW. Therapeutic review pharmacokinetics of topically applied ophthalmic drugs. Vol. 26, Surv Ophthalmol.
145. Lanier OL, Manfre MG, Bailey C, Liu Z, Sparks Z, Kulkarni S, et al. Review of approaches for increasing ophthalmic bioavailability for eye drop formulations. In: AAPS PharmSciTech, vol. 22. Springer Science and Business Media Deutschland GmbH; 2021.
146. Kulkarni NS, Josowitz A, James R, Liu Y, Rayaprolu B, Sagdullaev B, et al. Latest trends & strategies in ocular drug delivery. Methods. 2025;235:100–17.
147. Grassiri B, Zambito Y, Bernkop-Schnürch A. Strategies to prolong the residence time of drug delivery systems on ocular surface. In: Advances in colloid and interface science, vol. 288. Elsevier B.V; 2021.
148. Ramsay E, Ruponen M, Picardat T, Tengvall U, Tuomainen M, Auriola S, et al. Impact of chemical structure on conjunctival drug permeability: adopting porcine conjunctiva and cassette dosing for construction of in silico model. J Pharm Sci. 2017;106(9):2463–71.
149. Hosoya KI, Lee VHL, Kim KJ. Roles of the conjunctiva in ocular drug delivery: a review of conjunctival transport mechanisms and their regulation. Eur J Pharm Biopharm. 2005:227–40.
150. Dave VS. Formulation approaches for ocular drug delivery. In: Nano-biomaterials for ophthalmic drug delivery. Springer; 2016. p. 147–75.
151. Janga KY, Tatke A, Balguri SP, Lamichanne SP, Ibrahim MM, Maria DN, et al. Ion-sensitive *in situ* hydrogels of natamycin bilosomes for enhanced and prolonged ocular pharmacotherapy: *in vitro* permeability, cytotoxicity and *in vivo* evaluation. Artif Cells Nanomed Biotechnol. 2018;46(sup1):1039–50.
152. Diebold Y, Calonge M. Applications of nanoparticles in ophthalmology. Prog Retin Eye Res. 2010;29(6):596–609.
153. Das S, Suresh PK, Desmukh R. Design of Eudragit RL 100 nanoparticles by nanoprecipitation method for ocular drug delivery. Nanomedicine. 2010;6(2):318–23.
154. Chhonker YS, Prasad YD, Chandasana H, Vishvkarma A, Mitra K, Shukla PK, et al. Amphotericin-B entrapped lecithin/chitosan nanoparticles for prolonged ocular application. Int J Biol Macromol. 2015;72:1451–8.
155. Mohsen AM. Cationic polymeric nanoparticles for improved ocular delivery and Antimycotic activity of Terconazole. J Pharm Sci. 2022;111(2):458–68.
156. Mishra GP, Bagui M, Tamboli V, Mitra AK. Recent applications of liposomes in ophthalmic drug delivery. J Drug Deliv. 2011;2011:1–14.
157. Tsukada K, Ueda S, Okada R. Preparation of liposome-encapsulated anti-tumor drugs; relationship between lipophilicity of drugs and in vitro drug release. Chem Pharm Bull (Tokyo). 1984;32(5):1929–35.
158. Mishra A, Bano M, Bisen AC, Verma S, Sanap SN, Kishor R, et al. Topical corneal targeted sustained release amphotericin B liposomal formulation for the treatment of fungal keratitis and its PK-PD evaluation. J Drug Deliv Sci Technol. 2020;60:101944.
159. Habib FS, Fouad EA, Abdel-Rhaman MS, Fathalla D. Liposomes as an ocular delivery system of fluconazole: *in-vitro* studies. Acta Ophthalmol. 2010;88(8):901–4.
160. Liang Z, Zhang Z, Yang J, Lu P, Zhou T, Li J, et al. Assessment to the antifungal effects in vitro and the ocular pharmacokinetics of solid-lipid nanoparticle in rabbits. Int J Nanomedicine. 2021;16:7847–57.
161. Khames A, Khaleel MA, El-Badawy MF, El-Nezhawy AOH. Natamycin solid lipid nanoparticles- sustained ocular delivery system of higher corneal penetration against deep fungal keratitis: preparation and optimization. Int J Nanomedicine. 2019;14:2515–31.

162. Mahal RK, Al-Gawhari F. Design and evaluation of solid lipid nanoparticle eye drops containing VRN for ocular drug delivery. Int J Drug Delivery Technol. 2022;12(04):1702–16.
163. Li Z, Liu M, Ke L, Wang LJ, Wu C, Li C, et al. Flexible polymeric nanosized micelles for ophthalmic drug delivery: research progress in the last three years. Nanoscale Adv. 2021;3(18):5240–54.
164. Durgun ME, Kahraman E, Hacıoğlu M, Güngör S, Özsoy Y. Posaconazole micelles for ocular delivery: in vitro permeation, ocular irritation and antifungal activity studies. Drug Deliv Transl Res. 2022;12(3):662–75.
165. Han Y, Xu C, Shi H, Yu F, Zhong Y, Liu Z, et al. Engineered bio-adhesive polyhedral oligomeric silsesquioxane hybrid nanoformulation of amphotericin B for prolonged therapy of fungal keratitis. Chem Eng J. 2021;421:129734.
166. Fang G, Yang X, Wang Q, Zhang A, Tang B. Hydrogels-based ophthalmic drug delivery systems for treatment of ocular diseases. Mater Sci Eng C. 2021;127:112212.
167. Banshoya K, Fujita C, Hokimoto Y, Ohnishi M, Inoue A, Tanaka T, et al. Amphotericin B nanohydrogel ocular formulation using alkyl glyceryl hyaluronic acid: formulation, characterization, and in vitro evaluation. Int J Pharm. 2021 Dec;610:121061.
168. Díaz-Tomé V, Luaces-Rodríguez A, Silva-Rodríguez J, Blanco-Dorado S, García-Quintanilla L, Llovo-Taboada J, et al. Ophthalmic Econazole hydrogels for the treatment of fungal keratitis. J Pharm Sci. 2018;107(5):1342–51.
169. Almehmady AM, El-Say KM, Mubarak MA, Alghamdi HA, Somali NA, Sirwi A, et al. Enhancing the antifungal activity and ophthalmic transport of fluconazole from PEGylated Polycaprolactone loaded nanoparticles. Polymers (Basel). 2022;15(1):209.
170. Ilochonwu BC, Urtti A, Hennink WE, Vermonden T. Intravitreal hydrogels for sustained release of therapeutic proteins. J Control Release. 2020;326:419–41.
171. Li CC, Chauhan A. Modeling ophthalmic drug delivery by soaked contact lenses. Ind Eng Chem Res. 2006;45(10):3718–34.
172. Xu J, Xue Y, Hu G, Lin T, Gou J, Yin T, et al. A comprehensive review on contact lens for ophthalmic drug delivery. J Control Release. 2018;281:97–118.
173. Phan CM, Subbaraman LN, Jones L. In vitro uptake and release of Natamycin from conventional and silicone hydrogel contact lens materials. Eye Contact Lens: Sci Clin Pract. 2013;39(2):162–8.
174. Peng CC, Kim J, Chauhan A. Extended delivery of hydrophilic drugs from silicone-hydrogel contact lenses containing vitamin E diffusion barriers. Biomaterials. 2010;31(14):4032–47.
175. Ciolino JB, Hudson SP, Mobbs AN, Hoare TR, Iwata NG, Fink GR, et al. A prototype antifungal contact lens. Investigat Opthal Visual Sci. 2011;52(9):6286.
176. Kailasam V, Hiremath MS, Sudharsan P, Nagarjuna V, Garg P, Nirmal J. Stability enhancement of amphotericin B using 3D printed biomimetic polymeric corneal patch to treat fungal infections. Int J Pharm. 2025;670:125149.
177. Glover K, Mishra D, Gade S, Vora LK, Wu Y, Paredes AJ, et al. Microneedles for advanced ocular drug delivery. Adv Drug Deliv Rev. 2023;201:115082.
178. Thakur RRS, Fallows SJ, McMillan HL, Donnelly RF, Jones DS. Microneedle-mediated intrascleral delivery of *in situ* forming thermoresponsive implants for sustained ocular drug delivery. J Pharm Pharmacol. 2014;66(4):584–95.
179. Thakur Singh RR, Tekko I, McAvoy K, McMillan H, Jones D, Donnelly RF. Minimally invasive microneedles for ocular drug delivery. Expert Opin Drug Deliv. 2017;14(4):525–37.
180. Roy G, Galigama RD, Thorat VS, Mallela LS, Roy S, Garg P, et al. Amphotericin B containing microneedle ocular patch for effective treatment of fungal keratitis. Int J Pharm. 2019;572:118808.
181. Albadr AA, Tekko IA, Vora LK, Ali AA, Laverty G, Donnelly RF, et al. Rapidly dissolving microneedle patch of amphotericin B for intracorneal fungal infections. Drug Deliv Transl Res. 2022;12(4):931–43.
182. Hu J, Zhang D, Chen S, Wang X, Zheng Z, Gui S, et al. Minimally invasive treatment of fungal keratitis with voriconazole microneedle corneal patch. Eur J Pharm Biopharm. 2025;211:114717.

183. Kumari A, Sharma P, Garg V, Garg G. Ocular inserts – advancement in therapy of eye diseases. J Adv Pharm Technol Res. 2010;1(3):291.
184. Said M, Elsayed I, Aboelwafa AA, Elshafeey AH, Hassan M. Ocular Mucoadhesive and biodegradable sponge-like inserts for the sustained and controlled delivery of Voriconazole; preparation, D-optimal factorial optimization and in-vivo evaluation. J Pharm Sci. 2024;113(4):961–73.
185. Teba HE, Khalil IA, Gebreel RM, Fahmy LI, El SHM. Development of antifungal fibrous ocular insert using freeze-drying technique. Drug Deliv Transl Res. 2024;14(9):2520–38.
186. Bourges JL, Bloquel C, Thomas A, Froussart F, Bochot A, Azan F, et al. Intraocular implants for extended drug delivery: therapeutic applications. Adv Drug Deliv Rev. 2006;58(11):1182–202.
187. Yang L, Dong X, Wu X, Xie L, Min X. Intravitreally implantable voriconazole delivery system for experimental fungal endophthalmitis. Retina. 2011;31(9):1791–800.
188. Wiederhold NP. Antifungal resistance: current trends and future strategies to combat. Infect Drug Resist. 2017;10:249–59.
189. Chou B, Krishna K, Durkee H, Echeverri Tribin F, Ahmed A, Lai J, et al. Photodynamic antimicrobial therapy with Erythrosin B, Eosin Y, and Rose Bengal for the inhibition of fungal keratitis isolates: an in vitro study. J Photochem Photobiol B. 2025;263:113090.

Emerging Antifungal Resistance in Ocular Infections

3

Haroldo Cesar de Oliveira, Aileen Miwa Tabuse, Ana Luisa Hofling-Lima, and Anderson Messias Rodrigues

3.1 Introduction

Fungal infections of the eye, while less common than those caused by bacteria or viruses, represent a significant and often devastating clinical challenge owing to their diagnostic complexity and potential for severe visual impairment [1]. These infections primarily manifest as fungal keratitis, infection of the cornea, or fungal endophthalmitis, which involves intraocular compartments such as the vitreous and aqueous humor [2, 3].

Fungal keratitis, in particular, is a global ocular emergency that affects an estimated one million individuals annually [4]. The burden of fungal keratitis is disproportionately high in the tropical and subtropical regions of Asia and Africa, where it frequently affects young agricultural workers [5]. Ocular trauma involving plant matter is a common inciting event in which ubiquitous environmental fungi, such as *Fusarium* and *Aspergillus* species, are directly inoculated into the cornea. The profound socioeconomic impact of resulting blindness in working-age individuals has led to compelling arguments for its classification as a neglected tropical disease (NTD) [6, 7].

H. C. de Oliveira
Department of Microbiology, Immunology, and Parasitology, Discipline of Cellular Biology, Federal University of São Paulo (UNIFESP), São Paulo, Brazil

A. M. Tabuse · A. L. Hofling-Lima
Department of Ophthalmology and Visual Sciences, Escola Paulista de Medicina (EPM), Federal University of São Paulo (UNIFESP), Sao Paulo, Brazil

A. M. Rodrigues (✉)
Department of Microbiology, Immunology, and Parasitology, Discipline of Cellular Biology, Federal University of São Paulo (UNIFESP), São Paulo, Brazil

National Institute of Science and Technology in Human Pathogenic Fungi, São Paulo, Brazil
e-mail: amrodrigues@unifesp.br

M. C. Ramírez-Soto (ed.), *Fungal Eye Infections*,
https://doi.org/10.1007/978-3-032-19923-2_3

Fungal endophthalmitis, by contrast, can arise either exogenously following ocular trauma or surgery or endogenously from the hematogenous spread of pathogens such as *Candida* species from a systemic infection [8, 9]. The diverse range of fungi implicated in both keratitis and endophthalmitis underscores the critical need for timely recognition and tailored management to prevent vision loss.

The clinical management of fungal keratitis is complex, as the infection often presents with an insidious onset and nonspecific symptoms, such as pain, redness, and blurred vision, that closely mimic the more common bacterial keratitis [10]. These clinically nonspecific signs and symptoms frequently lead to initial misdiagnosis and the inappropriate administration of topical antibiotics and, more detrimentally, corticosteroids, which can suppress the host immune response and accelerate fungal proliferation [11].

When a fungal etiology is suspected, the infection is often deep-seated and significantly more challenging to eradicate. This diagnostic delay is exacerbated by a therapeutic arsenal that is both antiquated and limited [12]. The only topical agent approved by the U.S. Food and Drug Administration (FDA) for fungal keratitis is natamycin, a polyene antifungal that has been the standard of care since the 1960s [13]. Other agents, such as amphotericin B and voriconazole, are commonly used off-label in ophthalmology [14]. Because no commercial ophthalmic formulations are widely approved, they typically require preparation by compounding pharmacies or hospital pharmacies, which can delay the initiation of topical therapy, especially outside tertiary centers with onsite compounding capabilities.

Adding to the above longstanding challenges is the emergent and escalating threat of antifungal resistance [15]. Fungal keratitis treatment often requires prolonged, intensive application of topical agents, creating an environment favorable for the selection of resistant organisms [16]. Furthermore, the poor ocular penetration of most antifungal molecules means that achieving fungicidal concentrations at the site of a deep stromal infection is a significant barrier, often resulting in subinhibitory drug levels that promote resistance development [3].

A silent pandemic of antifungal resistance is on the move, and it is not confined to the clinic but is fundamentally a "One Health" issue, wherein the health of humans, animals, and the environment are closely linked [17]. The most compelling evidence for this paradigm is the environmental selection of azole-resistant fungi driven by agricultural practices [18].

Azole fungicides used extensively in crop protection are structurally and mechanistically almost identical to the frontline azole drugs used in human medicine [15]. This creates powerful, nontarget selective pressure on ubiquitous environmental molds such as *Aspergillus fumigatus*. Consequently, specific resistance mechanisms, such as the TR34/L98H mutation in the *cyp51A* gene, evolve in agricultural settings and are subsequently acquired by azole-*naïve* patients, leading to clinical treatment failure [19]. The environmental origin of these clinical isolates is further substantiated by the presence of genetic markers conferring resistance to fungicides used exclusively in agriculture, providing evidence of a pathway from the farm field to the hospital ward [20, 21].

Compounding this environmental pressure is a multifaceted global crisis characterized by social and political inertia [22]. Antifungal resistance disproportionately harms the world's most vulnerable populations, particularly in low- and middle-income countries, where a profound "diagnostic void" prevents accurate identification of pathogens and targeted therapy [22–24].

This crisis converges with a near-total market failure in the research and development of new antifungal agents; with only a handful of candidates in late-stage clinical trials, very few new drugs are expected to reach patients in the next decade [25, 26]. This therapeutic stagnation is made more dangerous by the emergence of novel pathogens such as *Candidozyma auris* (formerly *Candida auris*), a multidrug-resistant yeast that has emerged nearly simultaneously on multiple continents [27]. The unprecedented global spread and high mortality associated with *C. auris* signal a new and more dangerous paradigm in fungal threats, underscoring the urgent need for a globally coordinated response [27, 28].

Recent analyses of fungal ocular isolates from large clinical trials have provided stark evidence of this trend, demonstrating a significant increase in the in vitro resistance of fungal pathogens to both natamycin and voriconazole over recent decades [29–32]. This rising resistance is particularly alarming for pathogens such as *Fusarium* and allied fusarioid genera, which already exhibit high intrinsic resistance to azoles, complicating treatment decisions and contributing to high rates of medical therapy failure [16].

The convergence of a high global disease burden, limited therapeutic tools, and increasing microbial resistance creates a risk for patients and a complex challenge for the entire healthcare ecosystem [33, 34]. In this chapter, we systematically address the issue of antifungal resistance in ocular infections by reviewing the epidemiological landscape and the pharmacological obstacles that define current treatments. We explored the clinical evidence and molecular mechanisms of resistance in key pathogens, such as *Aspergillus*, *Candida*, and *Fusarium*. Finally, the chapter explores essential strategies such as antifungal stewardship and novel therapies designed to manage resistance and preserve vision.

3.2 Antifungal Classes, Mechanisms, and Challenges in Treating Fungal Infections

Approximately 3.8 million people die each year as a result of fungal infections, making these diseases increasingly serious threats to global public health [35]. In addition, fungal diseases remain largely neglected by both the scientific community and healthcare systems and are characterized by structural failures, such as limited knowledge of many pathogenic fungal species and chronically low investment in related research. Market barriers further exacerbate this issue, including the high cost of antifungal medications, logistical challenges in distribution, and insufficient government action to implement public health policies that ensure early diagnosis and adequate treatment, particularly in low- and middle-income countries [36–38].

The emergence of fungal crisis is further compounded by the limited diversity of available antifungal agents, which restricts therapeutic options and increases the vulnerability of patients, particularly those who are immunocompromised or affected by specific conditions such as fungal eye infections [17, 26].

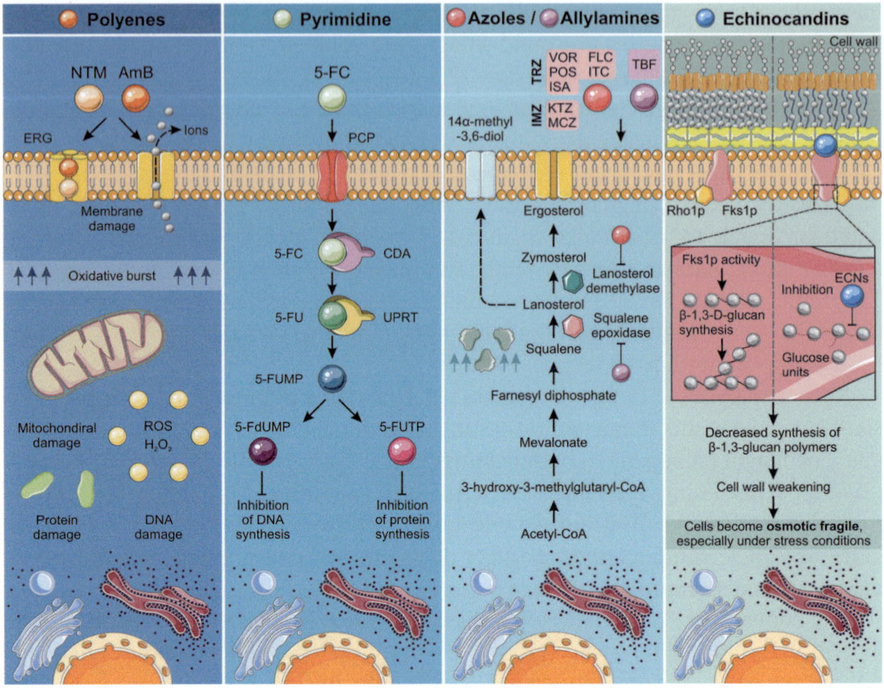

Fig. 3.1 Mechanisms of action of antifungal agents. Polyenes target ergosterol, a key component of the fungal cell membrane, creating pores that cause lethal leakage of cellular contents. Pyrimidine analogs act within the cell to interfere with the synthesis of fungal DNA and RNA. Both azoles and allylamines disrupt the production of ergosterol by inhibiting critical enzymes in its synthesis pathway, lanosterol 14-α-demethylase and squalene epoxidase, respectively, thereby compromising the integrity of the cell membrane. In contrast, echinocandins target the fungal cell wall by inhibiting β-(1,3)-D-glucan synthase, which disrupts cell wall synthesis and leads to osmotic instability. Abbreviations: 5-FC, 5-fluorocytosine; 5-FdUMP, 5-fluoro-deoxyuridine monophosphate; 5-FU, 5-fluorouracil; 5-FUMP, 5-fluorouridine monophosphate; 5-FUTP, 5-fluorouridine triphosphate; AmB, amphotericin B; CDA, cytosine deaminase; ECNs, echinocandins; ERG, ergosterol; FLC, fluconazole; Fks1p, Fks1 protein; IMZ, imidazoles; ISA, isavuconazole; ITC, itraconazole; KTZ, ketoconazole; MCZ, miconazole; NTM, natamycin; PCP, cytosine permease; POS, posaconazole; Rho1p, Rho1 protein; ROS, reactive oxygen species; TBF, terbinafine; TRZ, triazoles; UPRT, uracil phosphoribosyltransferase; VOR, voriconazole. The illustration was partially based on Servier Medical Art elements and licensed under a Creative Commons Attribution 4.0 Unported License

Most current antifungal medications fall into only a few classes, each with distinct limitations in terms of toxicity, spectrum of activity, drug interactions, and delivery methods. The narrow pipeline of new antifungal compounds has not kept pace with the increasing burden of fungal diseases or with the emergence of resistant isolates or intrinsically resistant pathogens [39–41]. These factors collectively intensify the global challenge of antifungal resistance, leading to higher rates of treatment failure, complications, and mortality. In this context, antifungal agents play a vital and increasingly complex role in clinical practice, highlighting the urgent need for innovation, surveillance, and equitable access to effective therapies.

Currently, there are five main classes of clinically available antifungal agents: polyenes, azoles, allylamines, echinocandins, and pyrimidine analogs (Fig. 3.1) [17, 38, 42]. However, despite this apparent variety, the use of these drugs faces several challenges, including high treatment costs, the need for hospitalization due to intravenous administration, limited availability in many countries, significant toxicity, and the emergence of antifungal resistance, which collectively hinder effective management of fungal infections.

3.2.1 Polyenes

The first clinically relevant class of antifungals to be discovered and used was polyenes (1950s), which are composed primarily of amphotericin B, nystatin, and natamycin [43–45]. Amphotericin B, which was isolated in 1955 from *Streptomyces nodosus*, was introduced into clinical practice in 1958 and rapidly became the gold standard for the treatment of life-threatening systemic mycoses. Its broad antifungal spectrum and fungicidal activity have made it indispensable in the management of invasive fungal infections, despite its well-documented nephrotoxicity and infusion-related adverse effects [46]. Over the past few decades, the safety profile of lipid-based formulations has improved, although their high cost limits access in many regions [46].

Natamycin (originally named pimaricin) was also isolated in 1955 from *Streptomyces natalensis* and was introduced into clinical use in the early 1960s, primarily as a topical ophthalmic agent for the treatment of fungal keratitis and other superficial fungal infections [45, 47, 48]. To date, natamycin eye drops remain the first-line treatment for filamentous fungal keratitis, particularly that caused by *Fusarium* spp., and are recommended by the World Health Organization for this purpose [49–51].

Polyenes exert their antifungal effects by targeting the fungal cell membrane, specifically by binding to ergosterol, a key structural component unique to fungal membranes. This binding leads to the formation of membrane-spanning pores, which disrupt membrane integrity, cause the loss of essential ions, and lead to cytoplasmic damage, ultimately resulting in fungal cell death [52, 53]. In addition to membrane disruption, polyenes also induce oxidative stress within fungal cells by promoting the generation of reactive oxygen species [54], further contributing to cellular injury. Natamycin, however, appears to act through a distinct mechanism, binding to ergosterol without forming large membrane pores, thereby impairing membrane transport functions rather than causing extensive leakage [55] (Fig. 3.1).

These combined mechanisms make polyenes highly effective antifungal agents. However, owing to the structural similarity between ergosterol and cholesterol found in mammalian cell membranes, polyenes, especially amphotericin B, are associated with significant toxicity, most notably nephrotoxicity [53]. Although the development of liposomal and lipid-based formulations has helped reduce toxicity, their prohibitive cost and limited availability in low- and middle-income countries continue to pose major barriers to treatment [38, 56]. As a result, the use of polyenes remains a critical challenge in the fight against severe fungal infections.

3.2.2 Pyrimidine Derivatives

In the 1960s, a new class of antifungal agents, pyrimidine derivatives, with 5-fluorocytosine (5-FC) as their primary representative, emerged [57, 58]. This compound introduced a novel mechanism of action by inhibiting fungal DNA and protein synthesis, offering a promising alternative to existing therapies at the time [59]. 5-FC is a prodrug, meaning that it requires activation inside fungal cells to exert its antifungal effects. This activation depends on two enzymes that are absent in mammalian cells, which contributes to its selective toxicity and favorable safety profile [42].

First, cytosine permease (PCP) facilitates the entry of 5-FC into fungal cells. Then, cytosine deaminase (CDA) converts 5-FC into 5-fluorouracil (5-FU), the active metabolite. Once inside the cell, 5-FU undergoes further metabolic processing: it is converted into 5-fluorouridine triphosphate (5-FUTP), which becomes incorporated into fungal RNA in place of uridylic acid, thereby disrupting protein synthesis. Additionally, 5-FU can be metabolized into 5-fluoro-deoxyuridine monophosphate (5-FdUMP), which inhibits thymidylate synthase, a crucial enzyme in DNA synthesis, further impairing fungal cell replication [60–62]. These dual mechanisms make 5-FC an effective antifungal agent with relatively low toxicity to the host (Fig. 3.1).

However, despite its promising pharmacological profile, 5-FC has a narrow spectrum of activity [63] and is rarely used as monotherapy due to the rapid emergence of resistance when it is used alone [58, 63]. Its clinical utility is often limited to combination therapy, particularly with amphotericin B, for treating severe infections such as cryptococcal meningitis [58, 63, 64]. Furthermore, limited availability, especially in low- and middle-income countries, severely restricts access to 5-FC in regions with a high burden of fungal diseases, posing a major obstacle to the effective treatment of medically important mycoses [38, 63].

3.2.3 Azoles

Azoles emerged in the 1970s as a new class of antifungal agents that target ergosterol, a key component of the fungal cell membrane [65–67]. Unlike polyenes, which bind directly to ergosterol, azoles exert their antifungal activity by inhibiting their biosynthesis [68, 69]. Specifically, they block the enzyme 14-α-demethylase (a cytochrome P450-dependent enzyme), which is essential for converting lanosterol into ergosterol. Inhibition of this enzyme results not only in the depletion of ergosterol but also in the accumulation of a toxic sterol intermediate, 14α-methyl-3,6-diol, which disrupts membrane integrity and fluidity [38, 70, 71]. The replacement of ergosterol with this faulty sterol impairs membrane organization and permeability, ultimately inhibiting fungal cell growth and viability (Fig. 3.1).

Azoles are subdivided into imidazoles (IMZs) and triazoles (TRZs), which are distinguished by the presence of an imidazole or triazole ring in their chemical structure [72]. They represent significant success in rational drug design, with successive structural modifications resulting in improved agents that exhibit greater antifungal potency, better aqueous solubility, lower serum protein binding, enhanced pharmacokinetics, increased tissue and central nervous system penetration, greater selectivity, and broader spectra of activity [67, 73, 74].

Among the triazoles, fluconazole has become a cornerstone antifungal agent for many infections because of its favorable properties, including high oral bioavailability, good central nervous system penetration, and low toxicity [75–77]. However, its limited spectrum of activity, especially against filamentous fungi such as *Aspergillus* spp. and *Fusarium* spp., has significantly restricted its use in treating invasive mold infections [78–80]. The limited efficacy of fluconazole prompted the development of newer-generation azoles, such as itraconazole, voriconazole, posaconazole, and, more recently, isavuconazole, with improved activity against a broader range of pathogenic molds.

Despite these advancements, emerging resistance remains a significant concern across all azole compounds, increasingly compromising their clinical efficacy. This increasing resistance is compounded by the widespread use of azole-based fungicides in agriculture, which exposes environmental fungal populations to subtherapeutic levels of azoles, fostering cross-resistance to clinically important drugs [81–83]. This phenomenon exemplifies the One Health challenge, highlighting the interconnectedness between human health, agriculture, and the environment, and underscores the urgent need for coordinated surveillance and stewardship of antifungal use in both medical and agricultural contexts.

3.2.4 Allylamines

In addition to targeting ergosterol biosynthesis, allylamines emerged in the 1980s as an important alternative for the treatment of superficial mycoses. Unlike azoles, which inhibit ergosterol synthesis at a later step, allylamines act earlier in the pathway by inhibiting the enzyme squalene epoxidase [84–86]. This enzyme is responsible for converting squalene into lanosterol, a precursor that is subsequently transformed into ergosterol by 14-α-demethylase. Inhibiting squalene epoxidase leads to two antifungal effects: depletion of ergosterol in the fungal membrane, which compromises its integrity and organization, and accumulation of intracellular squalene, which becomes toxic to fungal cells [84, 87] (Fig. 3.1).

The main representatives of this class are terbinafine, naftifine, and butenafine. Among them, terbinafine is the most widely used allylamine in clinical practice, particularly for the treatment of dermatophyte infections such as tinea pedis, tinea corporis, and onychomycosis. Although allylamines exhibit a moderately broad antifungal spectrum, their use is primarily indicated for cutaneous and superficial fungal infections. This is due to their pharmacokinetic profile, which favors accumulation in skin, nails, and adipose tissue but does not achieve adequate therapeutic levels in deep organs or the central nervous system [84]. As a result, they are not recommended for invasive fungal infections or for use in immunocompromised patients. Additionally, terbinafine use has been associated with hepatotoxicity, requiring liver function monitoring in long-term treatments [88]. Studies have also reported the emergence of resistance, especially in dermatophytes, raising concerns about their future efficacy [89–91].

3.2.5 Echinocandins

Echinocandins represent the most recent class of antifungal agents to be introduced into clinical use and became available in the early 2000s [92]. They marked a significant advancement in antifungal therapy by targeting the fungal cell wall, a structure that is unique to fungi and absent in mammalian cells, offering high specificity and low toxicity for the host.

The fungal cell wall is a complex and essential structure that provides shape, rigidity, and protection against osmotic stress. One of its critical components is β-(1,3)-D-glucan, a polysaccharide composed of glucose molecules linked by β-(1 → 3) glycosidic bonds, forming long linear or branched chains that are essential for maintaining the integrity and strength of the cell wall [93–95]. This is precisely where echinocandins exert their action, as they inhibit the enzyme β-(1,3)-D-glucan synthase (encoded by the *FKS1* gene), thereby disrupting the synthesis of β-(1,3)-D-glucan. As a result, the fungal cell wall becomes weakened, compromising structural stability and ultimately leading to cell lysis and death, especially in actively growing cells [96–99] (Fig. 3.1).

The main drugs in this class are caspofungin, micafungin, anidulafungin, and, recently, rezafungin. Echinocandins exhibit fungicidal activity against most *Candida* species and fungistatic activity against *Aspergillus* spp. [94, 100–103], making them particularly useful for treating invasive candidiasis and aspergillosis, especially in immunocompromised patients. They are generally well tolerated, with minimal drug interactions and a low risk of systemic toxicity.

However, despite their advantages, echinocandins have limitations, including a lack of oral formulations, restricted activity against certain fungi (e.g., *Cryptococcus* spp. and *Fusarium* spp.), and the emergence of resistance, mainly due to mutations in *FKS* genes [104–106]. Nevertheless, their unique mechanism of action, safety profile, and clinical efficacy make echinocandins indispensable tools in the current antifungal arsenal.

3.3 Treatment of Fungal Ocular Infections

3.3.1 Topical Treatment

Fungal keratitis treatment varies according to the species detected. Natamycin and voriconazole are the two most commonly prescribed drugs. Other antifungal agents include amphotericin B, ketoconazole, itraconazole, and fluconazole [107, 108].

Natamycin has a broad spectrum of antifungal activity and works well against various fungal species, such as *Fusarium*, *Aspergillus*, *Candida*, *Cephalosporium*,

Colletotrichum, *Curvularia*, *Lasiodiplodia*, *Scedosporium*, *Trichophyton*, and *Penicillium*. According to the Mycotic Ulcer Treatment Trial I (MUTT I), published in 2016, natamycin was more effective for treating *Fusarium* spp. than voriconazole was [108, 109]. In a secondary analysis of MUTT I, a nearly twofold annual increase in azole resistance was observed, whereas no increase in natamycin resistance was detected [109]. One of the advantages of natamycin has been the apparent lack of resistance development among fungal pathogens [110]. However, studies have shown that fungal strains can develop resistance to natamycin with prolonged in vitro exposure (i.e., through adaptive training) [111].

Voriconazole is the second-best topical drug available for the treatment of fungal keratitis. It is available in both oral and parenteral formulations and is approved by the US FDA for the treatment of invasive aspergillosis and refractory infections with *Fusarium* species and *S. apiospermum*. Like natamycin, voriconazole displays a broad spectrum of activity against various species of *Aspergillus*, *Candida*, *Cryptococcus*, *Fusarium*, and *Scedosporium* [107].

Amphotericin B is also used as an alternative; however, there is limited evidence concerning its efficacy [112–114]. In its standard form, amphotericin B cannot penetrate the intact cornea. Amphotericin B has been shown to be more effective against yeasts than against *Fusarium* species [115]. There have been no head-to-head trials published to date comparing topical amphotericin B to other topical agents [49]. However, liposomal amphotericin B has better antifungal action than the conventional form of amphotericin B. The conventional technique results in poor ocular penetration and is epitheliotoxic. Liposomes can increase the affinity between amphotericin B and sterols in fungal cells and reduce the affinity of the mammalian cell membrane for cholesterol. Therefore, they not only increase antifungal activity but also reduce damage to host tissues in experimental rabbit models [14, 116, 117].

3.3.2 Oral Treatment

Adjunctive oral antifungal therapy for fungal keratitis, including itraconazole, ketoconazole, and voriconazole, has been investigated, although its added benefit remains uncertain [107]. Although several case reports support voriconazole use as an adjunct to topical therapy [118, 119] and pharmacokinetic considerations suggest that it may help maintain therapeutic drug levels between topical doses [120], the MUTT 2 trial demonstrated no significant difference in the primary outcome (corneal perforation or need for therapeutic keratoplasty) at 3 months, comparing voriconazole and placebo, whereas adverse effects were more common in the voriconazole group, leading to the conclusion that oral voriconazole provided no additional benefit. A subgroup analysis suggested a possible, although not statistically significant, benefit in terms of *Fusarium* infections [108]. Conversely, some supportive evidence exists. The TST (topical, systemic, and targeted) protocol by Sharma et al. included oral ketoconazole or voriconazole alongside topical natamycin in patients with large ulcers (>5 mm), deep stromal involvement (>50%), or impending perforation. In this five-year study of 223 patients, a treatment success rate of 79.8% was reported, comparable to other published outcomes [121].

An earlier randomized control trial involving 54 fungal keratitis patients revealed no difference in healing at 6 weeks between those receiving oral itraconazole and those who did not [122]. A more recent study of 50 patients on topical natamycin compared oral voriconazole and oral ketoconazole, showing a modest visual benefit with voriconazole, although the perforation rates were similar [123].

Oral antifungals can cause serious adverse effects, particularly hepatotoxicity. Liver function tests are essential at baseline and weekly during the first month and then monthly if stable. Visual disturbances, including changes in color vision, photophobia, and transient hallucinations, occur in up to one-third of patients, typically within 30 minutes of dosing [124].

3.3.3 Injected Drug Delivery

Intrastromal and intracameral antifungal injections have been explored as adjunctive treatments for severe fungal keratitis, particularly in patients who are unresponsive to topical therapy [125]. The agents used include amphotericin B and voriconazole via both routes. Natamycin has generally been avoided for targeted injection due to formulation limitations, although recent studies using a soluble form (0.01% Natasol) suggest potential utility, pending further evaluation [126, 127].

Intrastromal injections involve depositing antifungal agents such as voriconazole (50 μg/0.1 mL) circumferentially around the ulcer in the mid-stroma via a 30-gauge needle. Although these can be repeated every 72 hours, complications may include infection spread, intraocular inflammation, cataracts, perforation, elevated IOP, hyphema, and endothelial damage [107].

Two randomized controlled trials have assessed the use of intrastromal voriconazole. The first compared topical to intrastromal in patients unresponsive to natamycin, with better BSCVA and higher healing rates in the topical group [128]. The second study compared natamycin monotherapy to natamycin plus intrastromal voriconazole, finding no difference in outcomes and suggesting a limited benefit of intrastromal voriconazole in fungal keratitis [129]. Although some case series have reported success with intrastromal voriconazole in deep or refractory cases [128, 130], clinical trial evidence remains insufficient to support its routine use.

The intracameral voriconazole is even less studied. A case series reported resolution of anterior chamber fungal infection with a single 50 μg/0.1 mL dose followed by topical therapy [130], whereas another series used up to eight 100 μg/0.1 mL doses in patients with fungal endophthalmitis, achieving infection control, although several required therapeutic keratoplasty [131]. These findings suggest a potential, but limited, role for intracameral voriconazole in deep fungal keratitis with anterior chamber involvement.

There is growing interest in the use of intracameral amphotericin B (ICAB) for recalcitrant filamentous fungal keratitis. Two prospective interventional studies reported improved BSCVA, faster hypopyon clearance, fewer complications, and significantly lower perforation rates when ICAB was used earlier [132]. Several case series also reported favorable outcomes with ICAB [133–135], suggesting that ICAB may be a viable option in deep fungal keratitis patients with hypopyon or anterior chamber involvement. Another three-arm trial, however, reported no significant difference between ICAB arms and medical therapy alone, although the small sample size may have limited conclusions [136].

The use of intrastromal amphotericin B has limited standalone evidence. Most studies use it in combination with other agents. One audit reported faster healing with amphotericin B and fluconazole than with amphotericin B alone [137]. Another case series of 32 patients with progressive fungal keratitis despite combined topical therapy reported an 87.5% resolution rate following 1–18 intrastromal injections (mean 9.3 ± 6.4) [138].

A recent study compared intrastromal amphotericin B, voriconazole, and natamycin in patients unresponsive to natamycin after 2 weeks. Although the healing duration was significantly shorter in the intrastromal natamycin group, no differences in overall healing rates were found. Deep corneal vascularization was more common with amphotericin B [139].

Intrastromal and intracameral antifungal injections may benefit select, deep, or recalcitrant fungal keratitis cases; however, current evidence does not support their routine use. However, further robust clinical trials are needed to clarify their roles.

3.4 Factors Driving the Emergence of Antifungal Resistance

Following the development and widespread use of antifungal agents across clinical and agricultural settings, the emergence of antifungal resistance has become a growing public health concern [140]. The emergence and spread of antifungal resistance are particularly alarming in the context of ocular fungal infections, where early and effective treatment is critical for preventing irreversible damage and vision loss [41, 141–143]. Unlike systemic infections, ocular mycoses present unique therapeutic challenges due to limited drug penetration into ocular tissues, the need for localized treatment, and the fragility of the eye's anatomical structures [3, 107]. The increasing incidence of multidrug-resistant fungal species involved in ocular infections has led to further complicated clinical management, often leading to prolonged therapy, increased morbidity, and the need for surgical interventions.

Among these pathogens, *Fusarium* and related fusarioid genera are especially problematic, as they are among the most common causes of fungal keratitis globally [5, 144, 145] and are intrinsically resistant to many antifungals, including azoles, echinocandins, and, in some cases, polyenes [79, 146–148]. This intrinsic multiresistance is not the result of recent selective pressure but is an evolutionarily ingrained trait that presents the principal challenge to effective clinical management [149]. This baseline resistance is observed even in isolates from patients with no prior antifungal exposure and complicates the selection of empirical therapy, necessitating rapid species identification and susceptibility testing whenever possible. Infections caused by *Fusarium* are often associated with trauma, agricultural exposure, or contact lens use and are notorious for their aggressive course and poor therapeutic response [150–152]. Similarly, *Aspergillus* spp., particularly *A. flavus*, are frequent causes of ocular infections in tropical regions and exhibit variable susceptibility to azoles and polyenes, often necessitating combination therapy or surgical removal of infected tissue [153–155].

Mucorales fungi, although less commonly associated with keratitis, can cause rapidly progressive and destructive infections of the orbit and eye in immunocompromised patients, especially following trauma or surgery [156, 157]. These organisms are typically resistant to azoles and echinocandins, leaving liposomal amphotericin B as the main treatment option, although its use is limited by its toxicity and availability in resource-poor settings [158]. On the other hand, *Candida* spp., while better studied in systemic infections, are important agents of endophthalmitis, particularly in hospitalized or immunosuppressed individuals [9, 159]. Resistance to fluconazole and echinocandins has emerged in several non*albicans Candida* species, complicating the management of these deep ocular infections [160, 161]. *Cryptococcus neoformans*, although rare as a direct cause of keratitis, may reach ocular structures during disseminated infections and is intrinsically resistant to echinocandins, requiring prolonged therapy with amphotericin B and 5-FC [162].

Ultimately, the increasing prevalence of antifungal-resistant pathogens in ocular infections [144, 163, 164] highlights the urgent need for new therapeutic strategies, including the development of novel antifungal agents, drug delivery systems with better ocular penetration, and improved diagnostic tools for rapid identification and susceptibility testing. We also reinforce the importance of a One Health approach that addresses antifungal resistance not only in clinical settings but also in environmental and agricultural contexts, where selective pressure from widespread azole use may contribute to the rise of resistant strains that impact human health.

Understanding the clinical and environmental factors contributing to antifungal resistance, particularly in challenging infections such as *Fusarium*-related keratitis, is only part of the picture. To effectively combat this growing threat, it is essential to explore the molecular underpinnings of resistance and tolerance that allow fungal pathogens to evade antifungal action more deeply. In the next section, we explore the cellular and genetic mechanisms that drive these phenotypes, including mutations in drug targets, efflux pump activation, biofilm formation, and stress response pathways (Fig. 3.2).

3.4.1 Molecular Mechanisms of Drug Resistance and Tolerance

3.4.1.1 Polyene Resistance

Resistance to polyene antifungals, such as amphotericin B, is remarkably rare in both clinical and laboratory settings. This phenomenon is attributed primarily to the substantial biological costs associated with the genetic mutations required for resistance. To evade the mechanism of action of polyene, fungi must reduce or replace ergosterol with alternative sterols, compromising membrane integrity, fluidity, and overall function [70, 165]. Experimental studies have shown that such modifications severely impair fungal fitness by reducing the growth rate, stress tolerance, and

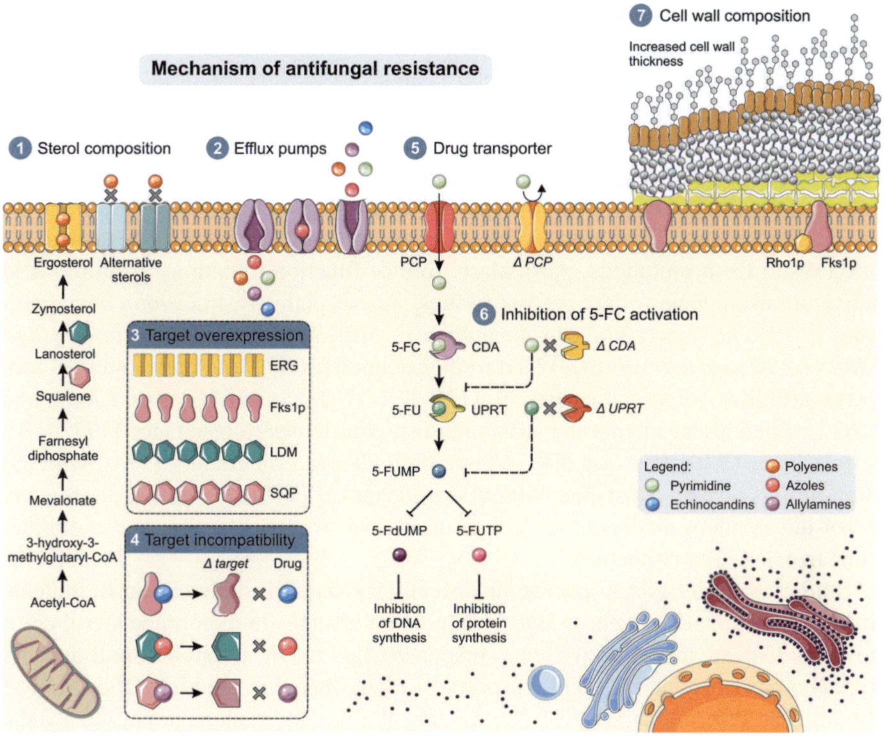

Fig. 3.2 An overview of the primary molecular mechanisms that confer antifungal resistance in fungal pathogens. These strategies include [1] alterations in the ergosterol biosynthesis pathway that modify the sterol composition of the cell membrane; [2] overexpression of efflux pumps that actively expel antifungal agents; [3] increased production of the drug's molecular target protein; [4] mutations that change the target's structure, leading to drug incompatibility and reduced binding; [5] loss of function in membrane transporters, which reduces drug uptake; [6] inhibition of the metabolic pathway required to activate prodrugs such as 5-fluorocytosine (5-FC); and [7] structural modifications of the cell wall, such as increased thickness, which limits drug penetration. Abbreviations: 5-FC, 5-fluorocytosine; 5-FdUMP, 5-fluoro-deoxyuridine monophosphate; 5-FU, 5-fluorouracil; 5-FUMP, 5-fluorouridine monophosphate; 5-FUTP, 5-fluorouridine triphosphate; CDA, cytosine deaminase; ERG, ergosterol; Fks1p, Fks1 protein; LDM, lanosterol 14-α-demethylase; PCP, cytosine permease; Rho1p, Rho1 protein; SQP, squalene epoxidase; UPRT, uracil phosphoribosyltransferase; Δ, mutation or loss of function. The illustration was partially based on Servier Medical Art elements and licensed under a Creative Commons Attribution 4.0 Unported License

virulence of fungi [166, 167]. Consequently, resistant strains are less competitive and are typically outcompeted by sensitive strains under natural or infectious conditions. This negative relationship between resistance and fitness, known as a fitness trade-off, effectively constrains the emergence and persistence of resistance to polyenes, even after decades of clinical use [165, 167].

Although rare, reports of isolates with elevated minimum inhibitory concentrations of amphotericin B have increased in recent years. These isolates have been associated with therapeutic failure, suggesting a clinically significant impact even in the absence of fully established resistance [25, 168]. Owing to the complex interaction between amphotericin B and the plasma membrane, the development of resistance may require multiple cellular changes to prevent the drug's membrane-disrupting action [169], and understanding the molecular mechanisms underlying this resistance phenotype is therefore critically important in light of future challenges in the treatment of fungal infections.

Alterations in the composition of plasma membrane sterols are key mechanisms of fungal resistance to polyenes such as amphotericin B (Fig. 3.2). These changes often result from mutations, particularly loss-of-function mutations or amino acid substitutions, in genes of the ergosterol biosynthesis pathway. In *C. albicans*, mutations in *ERG11* (*lanosterol 14α-demethylase*), *ERG3* (*C-5 sterol desaturase*), and *ERG5* (*C-22 sterol desaturase*) lead to the accumulation of alternative sterols with lower affinities for amphotericin B [167, 170, 171]. Inactivation of *ERG6* and *ERG2*, which affect membrane structure, also contributes to resistance [172, 173]. Similarly, in *C. neoformans*, *ERG2* disruption alters sterol content [174], whereas some strains display resistance without sterol changes [175], suggesting alternative, sterol-independent mechanisms such as oxidative stress adaptation and modifications in cell wall architecture.

Studies on *A. terreus*, a species intrinsically resistant to amphotericin B, indicate that resistance is not primarily due to significant changes in membrane sterol composition. Instead, the oxidative stress response triggered by amphotericin B appears to play a more critical role. This response is likely linked to the high production of catalase, an enzyme capable of neutralizing the oxidative damage caused by the drug by breaking down reactive oxygen species (ROS) [176]. The importance of oxidative stress resistance in polyene resistance is further supported by observations in rare *A. terreus* isolates that are susceptible to amphotericin B. When exposed to the drug, these isolates show a significant increase in mitochondrial ROS production [176–178], suggesting that their inability to manage oxidative stress effectively may underlie their susceptibility.

The thickening of the fungal cell wall due to the abnormal accumulation of glucans has also been associated with resistance to polyenes. In *A. flavus*, isolates exhibiting increased resistance to amphotericin B presented an increased proportion of 1,3-α-glucan in the cell wall [179]. Similarly, in amphotericin B-resistant *C. tropicalis* isolates, cell wall thickening is observed with an increased fraction of 1,3-β-glucan [180]. This thickening may physically hinder the drug's interaction with membrane sterols, thereby protecting fungal cells by limiting drug penetration through the cell wall.

In summary, while resistance to polyenes remains uncommon, accumulating evidence highlights a multifactorial basis for the reduced susceptibility observed in certain fungal isolates. These mechanisms include alterations in sterol biosynthesis, enhanced oxidative stress responses, and structural remodeling of the cell wall, all of which may act synergistically to diminish drug efficacy. Understanding these diverse and sometimes overlapping strategies is essential for improving diagnostics, optimizing antifungal therapy, and guiding the development of next-generation polyene formulations better equipped to overcome emerging resistance.

3.4.1.2 Pyrimidine Derivative Resistance

Resistance to 5-fluorocytosine (5-FC) in pathogenic fungi is an emerging concern in clinical medicine. Although primary resistance remains relatively uncommon (as detected in a few *Candida* spp. isolates [181]), acquired resistance during treatment has become increasingly common across various fungal species [58, 63].

Resistance to 5-FC arises from a few molecular mechanisms that impair the intracellular activation of the drug. These resistance mechanisms typically involve mutations in genes encoding key proteins responsible for drug transport and metabolism, impairing their mechanism of action (Fig. 3.2) [63, 182].

One primary resistance mechanism involves mutations in the *FCY2* gene, which encodes cytosine permease, a membrane protein responsible for importing 5-FC into fungal cells. Loss-of-function mutations in this transporter prevent adequate intracellular concentrations of the drug, leading to therapeutic failure [183–190].

A second mechanism involves the *FCY1* gene, which encodes cytosine deaminase, the enzyme responsible for converting 5-FC into 5-fluorouracil (5-FU), the first toxic metabolite. Point mutations in the *FCY1* gene can result in alterations to the cytosine deaminase enzyme, limiting or abolishing its catalytic activity and thereby impairing the conversion of 5-FC to 5-FU (Fig. 3.2) [186, 191, 192].

Another well-documented mechanism of resistance involves a deficiency in uracil phosphoribosyltransferase, the enzyme encoded by the *FUR1* gene, which catalyzes the conversion of 5-FU to 5-fluorouridine monophosphate (5-FUMP). Mutations in *FUR1*, including missense mutations, disrupt this step and block the formation of the active nucleotide analog, thus preventing disruption of nucleic acid synthesis [185, 193–201].

In addition to mutations in the *FCY2*, *FCY1*, and *FUR1* genes, another proposed mechanism involves the upregulation of endogenous pyrimidine synthesis, which competes with fluorinated metabolites such as 5-FUMP and reduces their incorporation into RNA, thereby diminishing the drug's cytotoxic effect [58, 60, 202].

These mechanisms may occur individually or in combination, resulting in varying degrees of resistance. Understanding the molecular basis of 5-FC resistance is critical for guiding antifungal therapy, especially in systemic mycoses such as cryptococcal meningitis, where 5-FC is commonly used in combination regimens.

3.4.1.3 Azole Resistance

Azole resistance is generally associated with alterations in genes encoding the 14-α-demethylase enzyme (Fig. 3.2). In *C. albicans*, distinct mutations in the Erg11 protein, which mostly cluster in three high-frequency mutation regions, have been linked to resistance in clinical isolates [203, 204]. Mutations in *ERG11* have also been implicated in reduced azole susceptibility in *C. auris* [205, 206]. In *A. fumigatus*, mutations in the cyp51A gene, which encodes the 14-α-demethylase enzyme in filamentous fungi, are widely recognized as the primary mechanism of azole resistance. Furthermore, duplications in the promoter regions of cyp51A are associated with high levels of resistance, and studies indicate that azole use in agriculture is linked to the emergence of resistance both in environmental isolates and in clinical isolates from patients without prior azole exposure [207–211].

Unlike *Aspergillus*, *Fusarium* possesses a unique three-paralog system: *CYP51A*, *CYP51B*, and *CYP51C* [79]. This genetic redundancy provides a high level of intrinsic resistance. Transcriptomic studies have revealed that these paralogs play distinct roles in which *CYP51B* appears to be the primary housekeeping gene, whereas *CYP51A* functions as a highly inducible gene that is strongly upregulated in response to azole exposure, suggesting a key role in adaptive resistance [212]. This contrasts sharply with the paradigm in *A. fumigatus*, where acquired resistance is often driven by point mutations and promoter tandem repeats in a single *CYP51A* gene. In fact, in *F. graminearum*, deletion of *CYP51A* paradoxically increases susceptibility to azoles, further highlighting the unique biology of *Fusarium* [79]. Although point mutations and amino acid alterations have been identified in the *Fusarium CYP51* genes, their direct contribution to clinical resistance profiles is less characterized than that in *Aspergillus* and remains an area of active investigation [212].

The overexpression of the azole target enzyme is also a significant mechanism of resistance to these drugs (Fig. 3.2). This overexpression is often associated with mutations in key transcriptional regulators of genes involved in the ergosterol biosynthesis pathway, leading to increased expression of critical genes such as *ERG11* [68, 165, 213]. The transcription factor Upc2, a zinc cluster protein, plays a central role in regulating the expression of *ERG11* and other sterol metabolism-related genes [214, 215]. Under normal physiological conditions, Upc2 is activated in response to decreased ergosterol levels [215]. However, gain-of-function mutations in the *UPC2* gene can cause constitutive activation of the protein, leading to sustained *ERG11* overexpression even in the absence of azole exposure [216, 217]. These mutations typically affect the ligand-binding domain (LBD) of Upc2, which is responsible for sensing intracellular ergosterol. Alterations in this domain disrupt normal feedback inhibition, allowing Upc2 to remain active regardless of sterol concentration. As a result, elevated expression levels of *ERG11* increase the production of the target enzyme, reducing the effectiveness of azole drugs, which can no longer efficiently inhibit the enzyme. Studies have identified specific gain-of-function mutations in *UPC2* in azole-resistant clinical isolates of *C. albicans*, clearly linking these mutations to *ERG11* upregulation and fluconazole resistance [214, 216–218]. Moreover, deletion of *UPC2* has been shown to increase azole susceptibility, further confirming its crucial role in mediating azole resistance [214].

Another key factor in regulating sterol biosynthesis is sterol regulatory element-binding proteins (SREBPs) in pathogenic fungi, whose activation is closely linked to resistance to azole antifungals [219–221]. In *A. fumigatus*, the SREBP homolog SrbA is essential for the expression of ergosterol biosynthesis genes, including cyp51A [220–222]. Deletion of SrbA leads to increased azole sensitivity, accumulation of toxic sterol intermediates, and reduced virulence [219–221]. SrbA also interacts with the CCAAT-binding complex (CBC), and the balance between these regulatory systems influences azole tolerance [222]. In *C. neoformans*, the SREBP protein Sre1 becomes activated in response to low oxygen levels. When sre1 or its associated activator genes, such as scp1 and stp1, are deleted, the fungus shows decreased ergosterol production, increased susceptibility to azoles, and reduced virulence [223].

Azole resistance arises through a combination of genetic mutations, the overexpression of key biosynthetic enzymes, and the activation of regulatory pathways that increase survival under antifungal pressure (Fig. 3.2). These mechanisms frequently coexist, making resistance more robust and harder to manage clinically. Importantly, the emergence of resistance is not confined to clinical settings. The extensive use of azole-based fungicides in agriculture creates environmental reservoirs of resistant strains, which can infect humans later [15]. This highlights the need for integrated surveillance and more thoughtful use of azoles across human, animal, and environmental contexts to limit the spread of resistance and preserve the efficacy of these essential drugs.

3.4.1.4 Allylamine Resistance

Although resistance to allylamines remains relatively uncommon, especially compared with other antifungal classes, such as azoles, which also target ergosterol synthesis, there is growing evidence that fungi can develop resistance through several distinct mechanisms. Given the increasing global use of terbinafine and related agents, understanding these mechanisms is crucial for monitoring and managing potential resistance in clinical and veterinary contexts.

One well-documented mechanism of resistance involves the overexpression of efflux pumps (Fig. 3.2), where the overexpression of genes encoding efflux pumps has been observed in resistant strains of *Trichophyton* species [224–226]. These membrane proteins actively transport antifungal compounds out of fungal cells, reducing intracellular drug concentrations and thereby diminishing their efficacy.

Another key resistance mechanism is the presence of point mutations in the squalene epoxidase (*SQLE*) gene [227–232]. These mutations can lead to structural changes in the enzyme, impairing its binding affinity for allylamines. Specific amino acid substitutions in the active site of the enzyme reduce the inhibitory effects of terbinafine without significantly affecting its catalytic function, allowing the fungus to maintain ergosterol synthesis in the presence of the drug. Such mutations have been frequently reported in terbinafine-resistant dermatophyte isolates, particularly *T. rubrum* and *T. interdigitale* [227–230, 232].

More recently, a less conventional mechanism has been identified, which is based on the overexpression of salicylate 1-monooxygenase [233, 234]. The specific role of this enzyme in antifungal resistance is not fully understood, and its overexpression has been associated with decreased susceptibility to terbinafine in *T. rubrum* [234], highlighting the complexity and adaptability of fungal resistance mechanisms.

3.4.1.5 Echinocandin Resistance

Echinocandin resistance in pathogenic fungi is primarily associated with mutations in genes encoding the β-1,3-D-glucan synthase enzyme complex, which is essential for fungal cell wall biosynthesis (Fig. 3.2).

In *C. albicans* and *Nakaseomyces glabratus* (formerly *C. glabrata*), resistance has been most strongly linked to mutations in the *FKS1* and *FKS2* genes, which encode catalytic subunits of the glucan synthase complex [98]. These mutations cluster within two highly conserved regions of the Fks proteins, designated hot spot 1 (HS1) and hot spot 2 (HS2), resulting in reduced binding affinity of the drug to its target. In *C. albicans*, common substitutions such as S645P, R1361H, and F641S in *FKS1* are frequently observed in resistant clinical isolates [98, 106, 235]. In *N. glabratus*, resistance is most often associated with mutations in *FKS2*, and isolates harboring these mutations are strongly linked to clinical failure of echinocandin therapy [236, 237].

Intrinsic resistance mechanisms also exist. Species such as *C. parapsilosis* and *Meyerozyma guilliermondii* (formerly *C. guilliermondii*) naturally exhibit relatively high minimum inhibitory concentrations (MICs) of echinocandins due to polymorphisms in *FKS1*, such as P660A or T634A, although these species remain clinically susceptible in many contexts [238, 239]. The intrinsic resistance of *Cryptococcus* spp. to echinocandins is a well-established phenomenon and presents a significant therapeutic limitation in the treatment of cryptococcal infections. *Cryptococcus* strains exhibit naturally high MICs for echinocandins and are considered intrinsically resistant in vitro, even without prior exposure to these drugs. This resistance is attributed primarily to the low expression of the *FKS1* gene, as well as to the unique composition of the cryptococcal cell wall, which contains relatively low levels of β-1,3-glucan and a relatively high proportion of other components, such as chitin and mannans [238, 240–242]. Additionally, the calcineurin signaling pathway, which is crucial for cell wall stress adaptation, is highly active in *Cryptococcus* and further contributes to its tolerance to multiple antifungal agents, including echinocandins [243]. As a result, echinocandins are not recommended for the treatment of cryptococcal infections, underscoring the need for alternative antifungal therapies that are more effective against this genus.

In fusarioid species, naturally occurring polymorphisms, or mutations, within conserved "hot spot" regions of the *FKS1* gene are believed to alter the conformation of the drug-binding site. Specific substitutions, such as P647A and F639Y, identified in *N. solani* prevent the echinocandin molecule from effectively binding to and inhibiting the enzyme, rendering the entire drug class ineffective [79].

In addition to mutations in *FKS* genes, adaptive responses to cell wall stress also contribute to echinocandin tolerance. Echinocandin-induced inhibition of β-glucan synthesis triggers the activation of stress-response pathways, including protein kinase C (PKC), calcineurin, and HOG MAPK signaling, which in turn upregulate chitin biosynthesis as a compensatory mechanism [223, 238]. This increase in chitin content strengthens the cell wall and enables fungal survival even in the presence of echinocandins, a phenomenon known as the "paradoxical effect" [244, 245]. The molecular chaperone Hsp90 plays a critical role in stabilizing components of these stress-response pathways. Hsp90 maintains the functional integrity of calcineurin and PKC signaling, and its inhibition has been shown to reverse resistance or tolerance to echinocandins in *Candida* spp. and *A. fumigatus* [246, 247].

3.4.2 Efflux Pump Overexpression

Efflux pumps play pivotal roles in mediating antifungal resistance among various pathogenic fungi (Fig. 3.2). These membrane-associated proteins actively transport a wide range of substrates, including antifungal agents, out of the cell, thereby reducing intracellular drug concentrations and compromising therapeutic efficacy. Two major families of efflux pumps, ATP-binding cassette (ABC) transporters and major facilitator superfamily (MFS) transporters, have been implicated in antifungal resistance [248].

In *Candida* species, particularly *C. albicans*, the overexpression of ABC transporters such as Cdr1p and Cdr2p and MFS transporters such as Mdr1p has been extensively documented as a key mechanism of resistance to azole antifungals [249–252]. These pumps are capable of extruding fluconazole and other azoles from fungal cells, significantly diminishing drug accumulation and facilitating survival under antifungal pressure. Notably, efflux-mediated resistance is often associated with mutations in or transcriptional upregulation of regulatory genes such as *TAC1*, *MRR1*, and *UPC2* [253]. In *A. fumigatus* and *A. flavus,* the ABC transporter Cdr1B has been directly implicated in azole resistance [254, 255], whereas members of the MSF transporters have received less attention, with mdrA being the only transporter linked to increased susceptibility to itraconazole and voriconazole in *A. fumigatus* [256].

In the *Fusarium* and allied fusarioid genera, this mechanism is considered an important contributor to intrinsic multidrug resistance [79]. These pumps can recognize and extrude a broad range of xenobiotics, including azole antifungals, thereby lowering the intracellular drug concentration to sublethal levels [212]. Studies on *N. solani* and related species have provided indirect evidence of efflux pump activity, showing that pump inhibitors can increase susceptibility to antifungals [257]. Furthermore, proteomic analyses of *F. oxysporum* exposed to amphotericin B have demonstrated high expression levels of efflux proteins, confirming their role as part of the fungus's adaptive response to drug-induced stress [258].

The clinical importance of efflux pump-mediated resistance highlights the urgent need for novel therapeutic strategies. These may include the development of efflux pump inhibitors (EPIs) as adjuvants to existing antifungal drugs or the use of compounds that bypass efflux mechanisms altogether. Understanding the regulatory networks and environmental triggers that induce efflux pump expression is also essential for designing targeted interventions aimed at curbing antifungal resistance.

3.4.3 Biofilm Formation: A Multifaceted Resistance Strategy

Biofilm formation is a critical virulence factor and a powerful resistance strategy for many microbial pathogens, including *Fusarium.* Biofilms are structured, surface-adherent communities of fungal cells encased within a self-produced extracellular polymeric matrix [259]. This matrix, which is composed of polysaccharides, proteins, lipids, and extracellular DNA, acts as a physical barrier, impeding the penetration of antifungal agents and shielding the embedded fungal cells from host immune defenses [260].

The clinical consequence of this phenotype is a dramatic increase in drug tolerance. Studies have shown that sessile, biofilm-forming fusarioid strains, particularly within *N. solani*, present significantly higher MICs for amphotericin B, voriconazole, and posaconazole than their free-floating (planktonic) counterparts do [261]. This phenomenon helps explain the recalcitrant nature of biofilm-associated infections such as keratitis (especially on contact lenses) and onychomycosis, where therapies that are active against planktonic cells often fail. Recent research has indicated that the composition of the fusarioid biofilm matrix is dynamic, shifting from lipid-dominant in early stages to polysaccharide-dominant in mature biofilms, an adaptability that may further contribute to its resistance [259].

3.5 Assessment of Antifungal Resistance and Surveillance

The development of standardized antifungal susceptibility testing (AFST) has been pivotal for advancing clinical mycology, enabling evidence-based therapeutic decisions and supporting antifungal drug development and surveillance efforts. For much of the twentieth century, AFSTs were rarely performed in routine settings, as treatment options were limited and dominated by amphotericin B. Early laboratory techniques, such as Alexander Fleming's ditch plate method, were qualitative and lacked the rigor required for clinical application. With the advent of new antifungal classes such as flucytosine and azoles, the clinical relevance of susceptibility testing has become increasingly apparent. However, the field was soon challenged by a lack of standardization, and laboratories employed disparate in-house methods with variable media, inoculum sizes, incubation conditions, and result interpretation criteria, leading to poor reproducibility and unreliable data across institutions.

This fragmented landscape prompted a critical turning point in 1985, when a report by the National Committee for Clinical Laboratory Standards (NCCLS, now CLSI) declared the state of AFST reproducibility "unacceptable." This led to the creation of standardized, consensus-driven reference methods, which would later be adopted and refined by leading organizations such as CLSI and the European Committee on Antimicrobial Susceptibility Testing (EUCAST). Although each group developed distinct methodological approaches, both contributed significantly to the establishment of reliable, clinically meaningful AFST protocols. Their parallel evolution reflects ongoing efforts to address the complexity of invasive fungal infections and the limitations of current antifungal therapies while also underscoring the global need for methodological harmonization.

3.5.1 Clinical and Laboratory Standards Institute (CLSI)

The CLSI was established in 1968, originally the NCCLS, with a broad mission to develop voluntary consensus standards for the entire clinical laboratory community in response to the rapid technological advancements of the era. Its foundational philosophy is a unique consensus process that brings together experts from three key sectors: government (including the U.S. Food and Drug Administration and Centers for Disease Control and Prevention), private industry (including diagnostic and pharmaceutical companies), and healthcare professions (academia and clinical laboratories) [262, 263]. This tripartite structure ensures that the resulting standards are not only scientifically sound but also practical for routine use, commercially viable, and aligned with regulatory requirements.

Although CLSI's initial focus was broader laboratory standards, with its first antimicrobial susceptibility testing (AST) document for bacteria published in 1975 [262], the growing crisis in mycology urged dedicated action. In direct response to the 1985 report on testing inconsistency, the Subcommittee on Antifungal Susceptibility Tests (AFUNG) was formed that same year [264]. This group was tasked with developing a reference method for the AFST. Their work culminated in a series of landmark documents that would become the standard in North America and many other parts of the world.

The first major output was the M27 document, "Reference Method for Broth Dilution Antifungal Susceptibility Testing of Yeast" [265], which was first published as a proposed standard in 1992, progressed to a tentative standard in 1995, and was finalized as an approved standard (M27-A) in 1997 [266]. This document, and its subsequent major revisions, M27-A2 in 2002 [265], M27-A3 in 2008 [267], and the fourth edition in 2017 [268], provided a meticulously detailed protocol for testing yeasts such as *Candida* spp. and *C. neoformans*.

A parallel effort for filamentous fungi (molds) led to the publication of document M38-A in 2002, which was similarly updated with M38-A2 in 2008 and a third edition in 2017 [266]. These studies established the broth microdilution (BMD) method as the reference standard. Although it originated in the United States, the CLSI's influence quickly became global; it was designated a World Health Organization Collaborating Center as early as 1985, and its standards are now adopted in more than 155 countries [262, 263].

3.5.2 European Committee on Antimicrobial Susceptibility Testing (EUCAST)

The development of standardized AFSTs in Europe followed a different trajectory. Rather than creating a standard where none existed, the challenge was to unify a continent where multiple, often sophisticated, national standards were already in use. EUCAST was formed in 1997 as a joint committee of the European Society of Clinical Microbiology and Infectious Diseases (ESCMID), the European Centre for Disease Prevention and Control (ECDC), and various European National Breakpoint Committees [264]. Its primary objective was to harmonize these disparate national guidelines into a single, cohesive European standard [264].

The EUCAST Subcommittee on Antifungal Susceptibility Testing (AFST-EUCAST) was also established in 1997, and its first standards for both yeasts and molds were published in 2008 [264]. EUCAST disseminates its methodologies through a series of "Definitive Documents" (E.Def). The methods for yeasts are detailed in the E.Def 7 series, and those for molds are in the E.Def 9 series. These documents are living standards and are subject to frequent review and updates to incorporate new data and refine techniques. For example, the yeast method was updated to version 7.4 in 2023, and the mold method was updated to version 9.4 in 2022 [269].

EUCAST distinguishes itself from CLSI in several key feature aspects. All EUCAST documents, including detailed rationale documents explaining the basis for every breakpoint decision, are freely and publicly available on its website. Furthermore, its decision-making committees do not include formal voting representations from industry, a structure intended to ensure that scientific and clinical considerations are the primary drivers of its recommendations [270].

3.5.3 Comparative Analysis of the CLSI and EUCAST Methodologies

At the heart of standardized antifungal susceptibility testing lies the reference broth microdilution (BMD) methods developed by CLSI and EUCAST. Although both methods aim to determine the MIC, they employ different procedures to achieve this goal. These differences, although subtle in some cases, can significantly affect the final MIC value and its interpretation. Box 3.1 provides a side-by-side comparison of the CLSI and EUCAST reference methodologies for both yeasts and molds.

Box 3.1

A comparative analysis of reference broth microdilution (BMD) methodologies for antifungal susceptibility testing was developed by the Clinical and Laboratory Standards Institute (CLSI) and the European Committee on Antimicrobial Susceptibility Testing (EUCAST).

Parameter	CLSI (Mold - M38)	EUCAST (Mold - E.Def 9.4)	CLSI (Yeast - M27)	EUCAST (Yeast - E.Def 7.4)
Culture medium	RPMI 1640 + **0.2% glucose**, buffered with MOPS	RPMI 1640 + **2.0% glucose**, buffered with MOPS	RPMI 1640 + **0.2% glucose**, buffered with MOPS	RPMI 1640 + **2.0% glucose**, buffered with MOPS
Inoculum preparation	Spectrophotometric adjustment of conidial suspension	Conidia adjustment via hemacytometer or spectrophotometry	Spectrophotometric adjustment of yeast suspension	Yeast adjustment via hemacytometer or spectrophotometry
Final inoculum size	**0.4–5×10^4 CFU/mL**	**1–2.5×10^5 CFU/mL**	**0.5–2.5×10^3 CFU/mL**	**1–5×10^5 CFU/mL**
Plate type	**Round-bottom** microdilution plates	**Flat-bottom** microdilution plates	**Round-bottom** microdilution plates	**Flat-bottom** microdilution plates
Incubation time	24–72 hours (species dependent)	48 hours (most molds); 24h for Mucorales	24–48 hours (species dependent)	24 hours (most yeasts)
Incubation temp.	**35±2°C**	**35±1°C**	**35±2°C**	**35±1°C**
Endpoint reading	**Visual** (100% inhibition for most; MEC for echinos)	**Visual** (100% AMB/ azoles); MEC: echino.; OD val. *A. fumigatus*	**Visual** (inhibition, ≈50% for azoles/echinos; 100% for AMB)	**Spectrophotometric** (50% inhibition of growth vs control)
Interpretation	CBPs (limited) & ECVs	CBPs (limited) & ECOFFs	CBPs & ECVs	CBPs & ECOFFs
Reproducibility	High intra/inter-lab reproducibility with standardized QC	High intra/inter-lab reproducibility.	High intra/inter-lab reproducibility with standardized QC	High intra/inter-lab reproducibility
Limitations	Difficult endpoint for some molds; long incubation	Vis. reading of molds is challenging; MEC reading is subjective	Visual reading is subjective; trailing growth with azoles	Spectrophotometry requires costly equipment; high inoculum may mask subtle effects

3.5.3.1 Culture Media and Growth Conditions

The choice of culture medium is fundamental to any microbiology assay, as it must support the reliable growth of the target organism. Both CLSI and EUCAST have standardized Roswell Park Memorial Institute (RPMI) 1640 media buffered to a physiological pH of 7.0 with 3-(N-morpholino)propanesulfonic acid (MOPS) [262, 264]. The critical point of divergence, however, is the concentration of glucose supplementation. The CLSI M27 and M38 documents specify a final glucose concentration of 0.2%, whereas the EUCAST E.Def documents mandate a ten-fold higher concentration of 2.0% (Box 3.1) [264, 271].

This difference is a deliberate choice with significant consequences. The 2.0% glucose concentration in the EUCAST method promoted more robust, rapid, and luxuriant fungal growth. This was a strategic decision by the EUCAST committee to ensure that a wide variety of fungal species, including more fastidious ones, would grow reliably and consistently in laboratories across Europe, thereby improving interlaboratory agreement [271]. However, this richer medium can alter the outcome of the susceptibility test. For certain organism-drug combinations, more vigorous growth can lead to higher MIC values. A notable example is in the testing of *Mucorales*, where the more luxuriant growth observed with the EUCAST method is thought to contribute to the higher amphotericin B MICs generated compared with those of the CLSI method [272].

A more subtle, yet important, difference lies in the specific incubation temperature. CLSI documents recommend a temperature of 35 ± 2 °C, allowing for a range of acceptable temperatures of 4 degrees. In contrast, EUCAST specifies a much tighter tolerance of 35 ± 1 °C (Box 3.1) [270]. Although seemingly minor, this reflects EUCAST's more stringent approach to standardizing every possible variable to minimize environmental factors that could contribute to testing variability and enhance reproducibility.

3.5.3.2 Inoculum Preparation and Density

Perhaps the most impactful methodological difference between the two standards is the size of the initial fungal inoculum. For testing yeasts, the CLSI M27 method specifies a final inoculum concentration in the microdilution well of 0.5×10^3 to 2.5×10^3 colony-forming units per milliliter (CFU/mL). The EUCAST E.Def 7.4 method, however, requires a final concentration of 1×10^5 to 5×10^5 CFU/mL, a difference of approximately 100-fold (Box 3.1) [264, 271, 273]. Similarly, although less pronounced, disparity exists for molds, with EUCAST again requiring a higher inoculum density than CLSI does [264, 273].

This vast difference in the starting number of fungal cells has profound implications. The greater inoculum used in the EUCAST method presents a much greater biological challenge to the antifungal agent being tested. This may better simulate the high fungal burden often present in patients with severe, invasive fungal infections, potentially offering a more clinically relevant assessment of antifungal potency. However, this higher density can also lead to a more pronounced "inoculum effect," where the efficacy of certain drugs decreases as the number of fungal cells increases. This can result in higher MICs and may mask the activity of some compounds, particularly those that are fungistatic rather than fungicidal.

Conversely, the lower inoculum specified by the CLSI may be more sensitive for detecting subtle antifungal activity and may yield lower MICs. The criticism of this approach is that it may not accurately reflect the in vivo conditions of a deep-seated infection and could overestimate the effectiveness of an antifungal agent. This fundamental disagreement on the optimal starting population of fungal cells is a major source of the observed differences in MIC values between the two systems and represents a significant hurdle to harmonization.

3.5.3.3 Endpoint: Visual Versus Spectrophotometric Reading

After incubation, the final and most critical step is determining the MIC by assessing the extent of fungal growth in each well. Here, again, CLSI and EUCAST have historically taken different paths. The CLSI standards for both yeasts and molds have traditionally relied on visual endpoint determination [274]. For most fungistatic drugs, such as azoles and echinocandins, the MIC is defined as the lowest drug concentration that causes a significant decrease in turbidity (approximately 50% inhibition) compared with the drug-free growth control well. For fungicidal drugs such as amphotericin B, a more stringent endpoint of 100% inhibition (no visible growth) is used [274].

The primary limitation of this approach is its subjectivity. The visual estimation of "50% inhibition" can vary considerably between technicians and laboratories, introducing a significant source of variability. This is particularly problematic when azoles are tested against *Candida* species, which often exhibit a phenomenon known as "trailing," the persistence of some reduced, hazy growth even at high drug concentrations, making a clear endpoint difficult to determine [275].

To overcome this subjectivity, EUCAST mandates spectrophotometric reading for yeast susceptibility testing [276]. An automated plate reader was used to measure the optical density (OD) of each well, and the MIC was defined as the lowest drug concentration that reduced the OD by 50% compared with the OD of the growth control. This provides an objective, quantitative, and highly reproducible measure of growth inhibition [277]. EUCAST has also validated spectrophotometric readings for testing azoles against *A. fumigatus*, further promoting objectivity in mold testing [277]. This commitment to objectivity, even at the cost of requiring more specialized equipment, is a hallmark of the EUCAST approach.

A special case exists for the testing of echinocandins against molds. Owing to a paradoxical effect where growth can sometimes resume at high drug concentrations, a traditional MIC is often unreadable. Both CLSI and EUCAST have therefore adopted the concept of the minimum effective concentration (MEC). The MEC is defined as the lowest drug concentration that produces a visible morphological change, specifically, the growth of small, aberrant, compact hyphal forms instead of the normal long, filamentous hyphae seen in the control well [278, 279]. Although this provides a workable alternative to the MIC, MEC determination is itself a subjective microscopic or macroscopic assessment and can be challenging to perform consistently, particularly with the high inoculum density used in the EUCAST method, which can obscure the morphology of individual hyphae (Box 3.1) [280].

3.5.3.4 The Ripple Effect of Methodological Choices on MIC Concordance

Importantly, the individual methodological differences in terms of the medium, inoculum, plate type, and reading method do not affect isolation. They interact to create a complex system where the final MIC value is a net result of multiple, sometimes competing, influences. This explains why the difference between the CLSI and EUCAST MICs is not a simple, unidirectional shift but rather a complex, drug- and species-dependent pattern. Although overall essential agreement (defined as MICs within ±2 $\log_2$ dilutions) between the two methods is often high, frequently exceeding 90% for common pathogens, specific "problem areas" emerge where these methodological choices have the greatest impact [281].

One might hypothesize that the combination of higher glucose and a 100-fold higher inoculum in the EUCAST method would invariably lead to higher MICs. Indeed, for some combinations, this holds true. For example, when amphotericin B is tested against *Mucorales*, the growth-promoting conditions of the EUCAST method appear to dominate, resulting in significantly higher and potentially more clinically relevant MICs than those of CLSI [272].

However, for many other combinations, the CLSI MICs tend to be one or more dilutions higher than the EUCAST MICs [274]. This seemingly contradictory outcome can be explained by other countervailing factors. The objective, mathematically defined 50% inhibition cutoff determined by spectrophotometry via the EUCAST yeast method, may yield a more consistent and sometimes lower MIC value than the subjective visual estimation of ~50% inhibition required by CLSI, especially in cases of trailing growth with azoles. Furthermore, the standard 24-hour reading time for EUCAST yeast testing is shorter than the 48-hour incubation allowed for some slower-growing yeasts by CLSI, allowing the drug less time to be overcome by fungal growth.

For caspofungin, the pattern is often reversed, with EUCAST yielding higher MICs than CLSI does [274]. The reasons for this are not fully understood but may be related to differential drug binding to plastic flat-bottom (EUCAST) versus round-bottom (CLSI) plates or specific interactions between the drug and the high-glucose medium that are not observed with other echinocandins [273].

This complex interplay of factors demonstrates why harmonization is such a formidable challenge. Adjusting a single parameter, such as inoculum size, to align the methods for one drug class could have unpredictable and deleterious effects on the results for another. The current state is one of high overall concordance punctuated by specific, well-documented areas of disagreement. This reality necessitates that laboratories, researchers, and surveillance programs are acutely aware of which method is used to generate a given MIC value, as the results from the two systems are not always interchangeable.

3.5.4 Translating MICs into Clinical Action: The Role of Breakpoints and Cutoff Values in the AFST

Standardized AFSTs play a critical role in bridging laboratory data with clinical decision-making, public health surveillance, and antifungal drug development. Its main clinical utility lies in translating raw MIC values into actionable outcomes, primarily through two interpretive tools, including clinical breakpoints (CBPs) and epidemiological cutoff values (ECVs).

CBPs are specific MIC thresholds that categorize a fungal isolate as "susceptible" (S), "intermediate" or "susceptible-increased exposure" (I), or "resistant" (R). These categories are designed to predict the likelihood of a successful clinical outcome with a standard dosing regimen of the antifungal agent [282]. The process of setting a CBP is complex and rigorous, integrating data from three domains: [1] the MIC distributions of the fungal species against the drug; [2] pharmacokinetic/pharmacodynamic (PK/PD) data, which model the drug's concentration in the body over time and its killing activity; and [3] clinical outcome data from patients with documented infections, correlating their treatment success or failure with the MIC of their infecting isolate [266].

A significant evolution in the use of CBPs was EUCAST's 2019 redefinition of the "I" category. Previously defined as "Intermediate," a zone of uncertain therapeutic effect, it was redefined as "Susceptible, Increased Exposure." This paradigm shift explicitly states that an infection with an isolate in the "I" category can be treated successfully if exposure to the antifungal agent is increased, either by administering a higher dose or because the drug naturally concentrates at the site of infection (e.g., fluconazole in the urinary tract) [283]. This change transformed "I" from a category of uncertainty into a conditional "susceptible" category, providing clearer guidance to clinicians and preserving the utility of valuable antifungal agents that might otherwise have been discarded.

Epidemiological cutoff values (ECVs or ECOFFs) are utilized when there are insufficient clinical or PK/PD data to establish a formal CBP. An ECV is a statistically determined MIC value that separates the "wild-type" (WT) population of a fungal species, those without detectable acquired resistance mechanisms, from the "nonwild-type" (non-WT) population, which may harbor such mechanisms [265]. ECV is fundamentally a microbiological tool for resistance surveillance, as it is not designed to predict the outcome for an individual patient. However, it provides valuable information to clinicians. Identifying an isolate as non-WT raises the red flag that it possesses reduced susceptibility, making it a less reliable candidate for therapy and prompting the consideration of alternative agents [284].

Beyond individual patient care, AFST underpins antifungal stewardship, informs local empirical therapy through cumulative susceptibility reports ("antifungigrams"), and supports national and international resistance surveillance programs. In the pharmaceutical context, standardized testing methods are integral at all stages of antifungal development, from early discovery and MIC profiling to regulatory submission and breakpoint setting. However, the coexistence of two major, nonharmonized standards poses logistical and financial challenges. Drug and diagnostic developers must produce and validate dual datasets for global approval, potentially delaying the release of novel antifungal agents and susceptibility testing systems. Despite these barriers, CBPs and ECVs remain indispensable pillars in the global response to invasive fungal infections and antifungal resistance.

3.5.5 Challenges in Antifungal Susceptibility Testing of Fusarium spp.: Methodological and Interpretive Limitations

Although the standardization efforts of the CLSI and EUCAST have brought remarkable clarity and reproducibility to the testing of common yeasts and *Aspergillus* species, some fungal pathogens remain exceptionally challenging. Among the most difficult species are *Fusarium* and related fusarioid genera. For fusarioids, the application of standard AFST protocols is fraught with methodological difficulties, and the interpretation of the results is hampered by a critical lack of validated clinical data, creating a true diagnostic and therapeutic conundrum.

3.5.5.1 The Clinical Imperative: Why Does Fusarioid Testing Matter?

The need for accurate susceptibility testing for fusarioids is driven by the genus's intrinsic and highly species-specific resistance profiles. Unlike *C. albicans*, where susceptibility to common agents can often be presumed, the susceptibility of a fusarioid isolate cannot be predicted from the genus name alone. For example, members of *Neocosmospora* are frequently less susceptible to amphotericin B and have higher voriconazole MICs than are members of the *F. oxysporum* species complex (FOSC) [285]. Given that both entities can cause life-threatening disease, knowledge of the species identity and its associated in vitro susceptibility profile is paramount for selecting an appropriate antifungal agent and avoiding the use of an ineffective agent [285].

3.5.5.2 Methodological Challenges with the CLSI and EUCAST Protocols

Both CLSI and EUCAST include fusarioid species within the scope of their reference methods for mold testing [278, 279]. However, applying these protocols to fusarioids presents significant practical challenges.

The CLSI M38-A2 document outlines specific parameters, but achieving consistent and timely sporulation to prepare the standardized conidial inoculum can be difficult and may require extended or dual-temperature incubation schemes [278, 279]. The incubation times for the test itself are long, typically requiring 46 to 50 hours or more to achieve sufficient growth for reading.

Furthermore, the filamentous, often cottony growth of fusarioids in microdilution wells can make visual determination of the MIC endpoint exceptionally difficult and subjective. Owing to its relatively high inoculum and glucose concentrations, the EUCAST method faces similar issues with inoculum preparation and endpoint reading, and more luxuriant growth may further obscure the endpoint. The slow, variable, and morphologically challenging growth of fusarioids makes both reference methods more laborious and less reproducible than yeasts or even *Aspergillus* species [285].

3.5.5.3 The Absence of Clinical Breakpoints: Implications for Antifungal Susceptibility Interpretation

The most significant challenge in fusarioid AFSTs is not methodological but rather interpretive. Despite the existence of reference testing methods, there are no established clinical breakpoints for any antifungal agent against any fusarioid species from either the CLSI or EUCAST [279, 285]. This creates a profound "interpretive vacuum" for clinicians. A laboratory can perform a test and generate an MIC value, but there is no validated threshold against which to interpret that value as "susceptible" or "resistant."

The reason for this absence is the relative rarity of invasive fusariosis compared with candidiasis or aspergillosis. Establishing a robust clinical breakpoint requires large-scale clinical studies that correlate patient outcomes (e.g., survival, clearance of infection) with the MICs of the infecting isolates. The low incidence of fusariosis makes accruing a sufficient number of cases for such a study statistically prohibitive [286]. Without these essential in vitro–in vivo correlation data, neither the CLSI nor EUCAST can confidently define an MIC value that can predict therapeutic success or failure. Consequently, treatment decisions for fusariosis must be based on the available in vitro data, published case series, and expert opinions, without the guidance and confidence provided by a formal CBP.

3.5.5.4 Role of Epidemiological Cutoff Values (ECVs)

In the absence of CBPs, the mycological community has focused on establishing ECVs to achieve some level of standardized interpretation of fusarioid MICs. An ECV, as previously described, is a microbiological threshold that distinguishes wild-type isolates from those that may harbor acquired or intrinsic resistance mechanisms. A major international collaborative study successfully defined CLSI-based ECVs for several important *Fusarium* and related fusarioid genera against a range of antifungal agents [286].

These ECVs are valuable tools, as they formally quantify the innate differences in susceptibility between species complexes. For example, the higher voriconazole ECV for the *Neocosmospora* species than for the *F. oxysporum* species complex provides a standardized measure of their differing intrinsic susceptibility. For surveillance, ECVs allow laboratories to identify and track the emergence of nonwild-type isolates that exhibit unusually high MICs for their species [286].

However, it is critical to remember the limitations of ECVs. An ECV is not a clinical breakpoint. An isolate with an MIC above the ECV is classified as nonwild type, suggesting that it may be less likely to respond to therapy, but this does not guarantee clinical failure. Conversely, an isolate with an MIC at or below the ECV is considered the wild type, but treatment may still fail owing to host factors, the severity of the infection, or inadequate drug delivery to the site of infection. Until the arduous challenge of collecting sufficient clinical outcome data is overcome, ECVs remain the best, albeit imperfect, tool for interpreting the susceptibility of this difficult-to-treat pathogen.

3.6 Therapeutic Approaches for Overcoming Antifungal Resistance

Emerging strategies to combat antifungal resistance in keratitis are increasingly diverse and include photodynamic interventions, novel antifungal classes, drug repurposing, advanced delivery systems, host-directed therapies, and gene-editing technologies.

Photodynamic therapies such as photoactivated chromophores for keratitis-corneal collagen cross-linking (PACK-CXL) and Rose Bengal photodynamic antimicrobial therapy (RB-PDAT) have attracted significant interest. PACK-CXL involves riboflavin application followed by ultraviolet A (UV-A) light exposure, which results in the production of reactive oxygen species (ROS) that create covalent cross-links between stromal collagen fibrils [287]. This process strengthens the cornea and increases resistance to enzymatic degradation by collagenases [288]. In contrast, RB-PDAT uses Rose Bengal activated by green light (500–550 nm) to generate ROS, particularly singlet oxygen, with potent antimicrobial effects [289]. Two principal ROS-mediated mechanisms underpin both therapies: Type I reactions, in which electron transfer generates free radicals, and Type II reactions, in which energy transfer to oxygen produces singlet oxygen [290]. Owing to their ROS-dependent mode of action, these therapies are unlikely to be affected by conventional antifungal resistance mechanisms and may be valuable for recalcitrant infections [291, 292].

Novel antifungal agents, including those that target pathways distinct from those affected by current drugs, are expanding treatment possibilities. These include the triterpenoid ibrexafungerp (which is active against echinocandin-resistant strains) [293, 294]; the GPI-anchor synthesis inhibitor fosmanogepix (which is potent against *Aspergillus*, *Fusarium*, and *C. auris*) [295, 296]; and the orotomide olorofim (which is effective against azole-resistant *Aspergillus*, *Sporothrix*, and *Scedosporium* spp.) [293, 297, 298]. Additional innovations include once-weekly intravenous rezafungin, orally bioavailable inhaled amphotericin B (MAT2203), and structurally improved polyene analogs designed to minimize toxicity [293, 299, 300]. These agents hold promise for both topical ophthalmic compounding and systemic therapy in deep or refractory keratitis.

Combination therapy and drug repurposing represent pragmatic means of enhancing efficacy and overcoming resistance [301]. Synergistic combinations, such as natamycin with voriconazole or azoles with efflux pump inhibitors such as minocycline, can improve fungicidal activity and overcome specific resistance mechanisms [302, 303]. Repurposed agents, including tacrolimus and amantadine, may inhibit biofilm formation or interfere with resistance pathways [304]. Artificial intelligence and machine learning-based drug screening platforms are accelerating the discovery of such combinations by integrating molecular structure, target profiles, and pathway analyses [305].

Advanced drug delivery systems developed through nanotechnology offer targeted, sustained release to the cornea, improving drug penetration and residence time while reducing dosing frequency. Examples include chitosan-coated polymeric nanoparticles [306], penetratin-decorated liposomes [307, 308], and thermosensitive hydrogels [309]. Host-directed therapies aim to augment innate and adaptive antifungal immunity. These include antifungal peptides (e.g., synthetic branched peptides) [310, 311], monoclonal antibodies (e.g., VX-01, anti-PNAG mAb, and anti-Pmt4p mAb), and immune checkpoint inhibitors (e.g., anti-PD-1 and anti-CTLA-4) that enhance pathogen clearance [312, 313].

Finally, gene-editing platforms such as CRISPR-Cas present a highly specific, precision-based antifungal strategy [314]. By designing guide RNAs (gRNAs) with no homology to human or commensal microbial genomes, CRISPR-based systems can target a single fungal species or even a strain, minimizing off-target effects [314, 315]. Major translational challenges remain, particularly the development of safe and efficient delivery systems to transport the CRISPR-Cas machinery into fungal cells in vivo [316]. Collectively, these approaches mark a paradigm shift toward integrated, targeted, and resistance-resilient strategies for the management of fungal keratitis.

3.7 Clinical Case

To illustrate antifungal resistance, we present the clinical case of a 38-year-old female patient with keratoconus who underwent deep anterior lamellar keratoplasty (Fig. 3.3a). Four months post-surgery, she developed keratitis caused by resistant *Neocosmospora solani* (Fig. 3.3b). The patient had a medical history of psoriasis treated with adalimumab and subsequently developed onychomycosis (Fig. 3.3c) and corneal keratitis due to resistant *N. solani*. She received both topical and systemic voriconazole, as well as systemic amphotericin B. However, the isolate demonstrated resistance to the administered antifungal agents, with an MIC of 32 μg/mL for voriconazole. Given the rapid progression of the infection (Fig. 3.3d), the patient underwent rose bengal photodynamic antimicrobial therapy (RB-PDAT); an in vitro study demonstrated growth inhibition after RB-PDAT (Fig. 3.3e). However, owing to the severity of the infection, therapeutic penetrating keratoplasty (TPK) was performed after 20 days of clinical treatment, successfully controlling the infection (Fig. 3.3f). No signs of reinfection were observed.

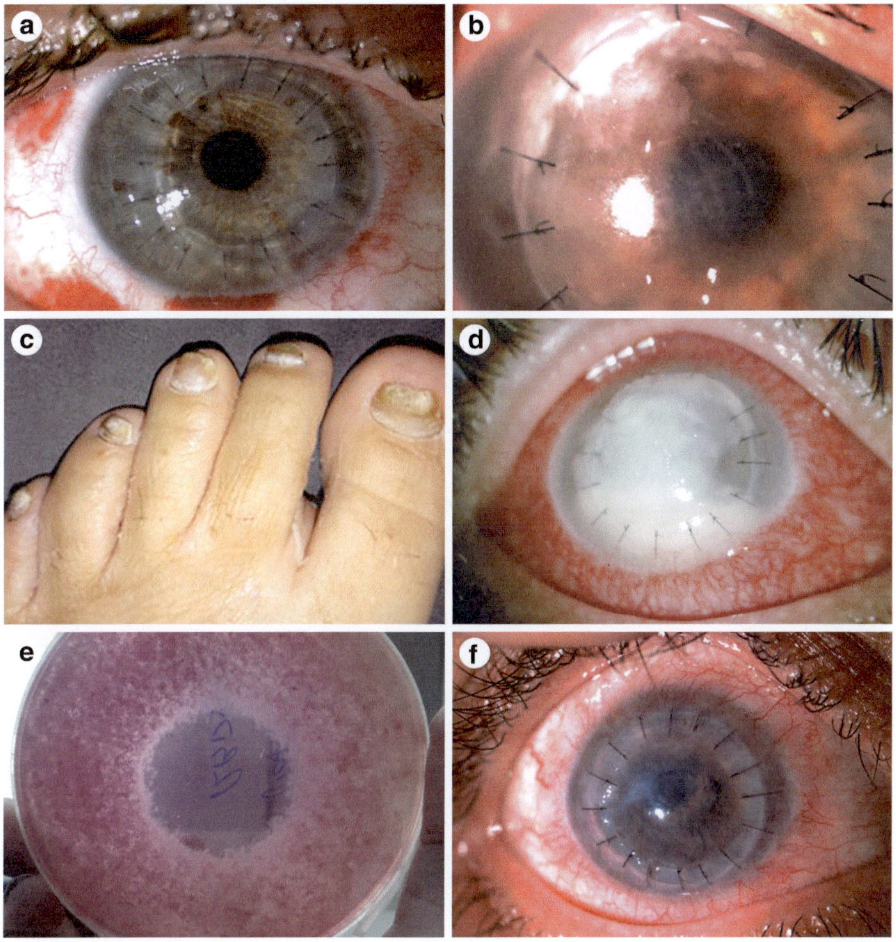

Fig. 3.3 Clinical case of antifungal-resistant *Neocosmospora solani* keratitis in a 38-year-old female with keratoconus. (**a**) Postdeep anterior lamellar keratoplasty performed for keratoconus. (**b**) Temporal-superior corneal infiltrate observed 4 months after surgery. (**c**) Onychomycosis in the same patient, with a history of psoriasis treated with adalimumab. (**d**) Rapid progression to diffuse corneal infiltration with hypopyon after 14 days of antifungal treatment. (**e**) In vitro inhibition of *N. solani* growth following Rose Bengal photodynamic antimicrobial therapy (RB-PDAT). (**f**) Clear graft with no signs of reinfection following therapeutic penetrating keratoplasty performed after 20 days of clinical management

3.8 Conclusions

In conclusion, the increasing challenge of antifungal resistance demands a coordinated and targeted response within ophthalmology. Efforts must focus on the development of rapid, point-of-care diagnostic tools that can facilitate timely and accurate identification of pathogens, alongside refinement of susceptibility testing methods to ensure that results are clinically relevant. Advancements in antifungal management strategies, combined with increased clinician awareness of evolving resistance patterns, are essential for guiding effective treatment choices. Equally important is support for pragmatic clinical trials that address the realities of managing resistant ocular mycoses in diverse healthcare settings. Together, these measures hold the potential to significantly improve outcomes in fungal keratitis, particularly in regions where the disease burden is high and access to specialized resources remains limited.

References

1. Klotz SA, Penn CC, Negvesky GJ, Butrus SI. Fungal and parasitic infections of the eye. Clin Microbiol Rev. 2000;13(4):662–85.
2. Słowik M, Biernat MM, Urbaniak-Kujda D, Kapelko-Słowik K, Misiuk-Hojło M. Mycotic infections of the eye. Adv Clin Exp Med. 2015;24(6):1113–7.
3. Reginatto P, Agostinetto GJ, Fuentefria RDN, Marinho DR, Pizzol MD, Fuentefria AM. Eye fungal infections: a mini review. Arch Microbiol. 2023;205(6):236.
4. Brown L, Leck AK, Gichangi M, Burton MJ, Denning DW. The global incidence and diagnosis of fungal keratitis. Lancet Infect Dis. 2021;21(3):e49–57.
5. Ahmadikia K, Aghaei Gharehbolagh S, Fallah B, Naeimi Eshkaleti M, Malekifar P, Rahsepar S, et al. Distribution, prevalence, and causative agents of fungal keratitis: a systematic review and meta-analysis (1990 to 2020). Front Cell Infect Microbiol. 2021;11:698780.
6. Bourcier T, Sauer A, Dory A, Denis J, Sabou M. Fungal keratitis. J Fr Ophtalmol. 2017;40(9):e307–e13.
7. Bisen AC, Sanap SN, Agrawal S, Biswas A, Mishra A, Verma SK, et al. Etiopathology, epidemiology, diagnosis, and treatment of fungal keratitis. ACS Infect Dis. 2024;10(7):2356–80.
8. Chhablani J. Fungal endophthalmitis. Expert Rev Anti-Infect Ther. 2011;9(12):1191–201.
9. Haseeb AA, Elhusseiny AM, Siddiqui MZ, Ahmad KT, Sallam AB. Fungal endophthalmitis: a comprehensive review. J Fungi. 2021;7(11).
10. Bourcier T, Thomas F, Borderie V, Chaumeil C, Laroche L. Bacterial keratitis: predisposing factors, clinical and microbiological review of 300 cases. Br J Ophthalmol. 2003;87(7):834.
11. Dinesh S, Prajna L, Venkatesh PN, Dharmalingam K, Devarajan B. Fusarium spp. and aspergillus flavus infection induces pathogen-specific and pathogen-independent host immune response in patients with fungal keratitis. Front Cell Infect Microbiol. 2025;15:1560628.
12. van Rhijn N, Arikan-Akdagli S, Beardsley J, Bongomin F, Chakrabarti A, Chen SC, et al. Beyond bacteria: the growing threat of antifungal resistance. Lancet. 2024;404(10457):1017–8.
13. Qiu S, Zhao GQ, Lin J, Wang X, Hu LT, Du ZD, et al. Natamycin in the treatment of fungal keratitis: a systematic review and meta-analysis. Int J Ophthalmol. 2015;8(3):597–602.
14. Morand K, Bartoletti AC, Bochot A, Barratt G, Brandely ML, Chast F. Liposomal amphotericin B eye drops to treat fungal keratitis: Physico-chemical and formulation stability. Int J Pharm. 2007;344(1):150–3.
15. Fisher MC, Hawkins NJ, Sanglard D, Gurr SJ. Worldwide emergence of resistance to antifungal drugs challenges human health and food security. Science. 2018;360(6390):739–42.
16. Al-Hatmi AMS, Bonifaz A, Ranque S, Sybren de Hoog G, Verweij PE, Meis JF. Current antifungal treatment of fusariosis. Int J Antimicrob Agents. 2018;51(3):326–32.
17. Fisher MC, Alastruey-Izquierdo A, Berman J, Bicanic T, Bignell EM, Bowyer P, et al. Tackling the emerging threat of antifungal resistance to human health. Nat Rev Microbiol. 2022;20(9):557–71.

18. Bédard C, Pageau A, Fijarczyk A, Mendoza-Salido D, Alcañiz AJ, Després PC, et al. FungAMR: a comprehensive database for investigating fungal mutations associated with antimicrobial resistance. Nat Microbiol. 2025;10(9):2338–52.
19. Chowdhary A, Kathuria S, Xu J, Sharma C, Sundar G, Singh PK, et al. Clonal expansion and emergence of environmental multiple-triazole-resistant aspergillus fumigatus strains carrying the TR34/L98H mutations in the cyp51A gene in India. PLoS One. 2012;7(12):e52871.
20. Kang SE, Sumabat LG, Melie T, Mangum B, Momany M, Brewer MT. Evidence for the agricultural origin of resistance to multiple antimicrobials in aspergillus fumigatus, a fungal pathogen of humans. G3. 2022;12(2).
21. Barber AE, Riedel J, Sae-Ong T, Kang K, Brabetz W, Panagiotou G, et al. Effects of agricultural fungicide use on aspergillus fumigatus abundance, antifungal susceptibility, and population structure. MBio. 2020;11(6) https://doi.org/10.1128/mbio.02213-20.
22. Bongomin F, Denning DW. Addressing the fungal diagnostic gap in LMICs. Nat Rev Microbiol. 2025;23(9):543–4.
23. World Health Organization. Landscape analysis of commercially available and pipeline in vitro diagnostics for fungal priority pathogens. Geneva: World Health Organization; 2025.
24. Lass-Flörl C. Beyond guidelines: what do I need to know when dealing with fungal diagnostics? Clin Microbiol Infect. 2025;31:1980.
25. Denning DW. Antifungal drug resistance: An update. Eur J Hosp Pharm. 2022;29(2):109.
26. Kneale M, Bartholomew JS, Davies E, Denning DW. Global access to antifungal therapy and its variable cost. J Antimicrob Chemother. 2016;71(12):3599–606.
27. Garcia-Bustos V, Cabañero-Navalon MD, Ruiz-Gaitán A, Salavert M, Tormo-Mas M, Pemán J. Climate change, animals, and Candida auris: insights into the ecological niche of a new species from a one health approach. Clin Microbiol Infect. 2023;29(7):858–62.
28. Liu D, Zhou R, Gao X. Recent innovations and challenges in the treatment of fungal infections. Front Cell Infect Microbiol. 2025;15:1676009.
29. Tandra P, Mitra S, Madduri B, Tarini S. Macrophomina phaseolina keratitis: treatment approach for poor response to topical natamycin. BMJ Case Rep. 2025;18(5).
30. Blaize M, Normand A-C, Imbert S, Al-Hatmi Abdullah MS, Chryssanthou E, Cassaing S, et al. Antifungal susceptibility of 182 Fusarium species isolates from 20 European centers: comparison between EUCAST and gradient concentration strip methods. Antimicrob Agents Chemother. 2021;65(12):10.1128/aac.01495-21.
31. Alastruey-Izquierdo A, Cuenca-Estrella M, Monzón A, Mellado E, Rodríguez-Tudela JL. Antifungal susceptibility profile of clinical Fusarium spp. isolates identified by molecular methods. J Antimicrob Chemother. 2008;61(4):805–9.
32. Espinel-Ingroff A, Colombo AL, Cordoba S, Dufresne PJ, Fuller J, Ghannoum M, et al. International evaluation of MIC distributions and epidemiological cutoff value (ECV) definitions for Fusarium species identified by molecular methods for the CLSI broth microdilution method. Antimicrob Agents Chemother. 2016;60(2):1079–84.
33. Awad R, Ghaith AA, Awad K, Mamdouh Saad M, Elmassry AA. Fungal keratitis: diagnosis, management, and recent advances. Clin Ophthalmol. 2024;18:85–106.
34. Atta S, Perera C, Kowalski RP, Jhanji V. Fungal keratitis: clinical features, risk factors, treatment, and outcomes. J Fungi. 2022;8(9).
35. Denning DW. Global incidence and mortality of severe fungal disease. Lancet Infect Dis. 2024;24(7):e428–e38.
36. Rodrigues ML. Funding and innovation in diseases of neglected populations: the paradox of cryptococcal meningitis. PLoS Negl Trop Dis. 2016;10(3):e0004429.
37. Rodrigues ML, Nosanchuk JD. Fungal diseases as neglected pathogens: a wake-up call to public health officials. PLoS Negl Trop Dis. 2020;14(2):e0007964.
38. de Oliveira HC, Bezerra BT, Rodrigues ML. Antifungal development and the urgency of minimizing the impact of fungal diseases on public health. ACS Bio Med Chem Au. 2023;3(2):137–46.

39. Hoenigl M, Seidel D, Carvalho A, Rudramurthy SM, Arastehfar A, Gangneux J-P, et al. The emergence of COVID-19 associated mucormycosis: a review of cases from 18 countries. Lancet Microbe. 2022;3(7):e543–e52.
40. Forsberg K, Woodworth K, Walters M, Berkow EL, Jackson B, Chiller T, et al. Candida auris: the recent emergence of a multidrug-resistant fungal pathogen. Med Mycol. 2019;57(1):1–12.
41. Lockhart SR, Chowdhary A, Gold JAW. The rapid emergence of antifungal-resistant human-pathogenic fungi. Nat Rev Microbiol. 2023;21(12):818–32.
42. Souza CMD, Bezerra BT, Mellon DA, de Oliveira HC. The evolution of antifungal therapy: traditional agents, current challenges and future perspectives. Curr Res Microb Sci. 2025;8:100341.
43. Carmo A, Rocha M, Pereirinha P, Tomé R, Costa E. Antifungals: from pharmacokinetics to clinical practice. Antibiotics. 2023;12(5).
44. Smith EB. History of antifungals. J Am Acad Dermatol. 1990;23(4, Part 2):776–8.
45. Meena M, Prajapati P, Ravichandran C, Sehrawat R. Natamycin: a natural preservative for food applications-a review. Food Sci Biotechnol. 2021;30(12):1481–96.
46. Hamill RJ. Amphotericin B formulations: a comparative review of efficacy and toxicity. Drugs. 2013;73(9):919–34.
47. Vardanyan RS, Hruby VJ. Antifungal drugs. In: Vardanyan RS, Hruby VJ, editors. Synthesis of essential drugs. Amsterdam: Elsevier; 2006. p. 535–47.
48. Stanley RG. Ocular clinical pharmacology. In: Maddison JE, Page SW, Church DB, editors. Small animal clinical pharmacology. 2nd ed. Edinburgh: Elsevier; 2008. p. 557–73.
49. Hoffman JJ, Arunga S, Mohamed Ahmed AHA, Hu VH, Burton MJ. Management of filamentous fungal keratitis: a pragmatic approach. J Fungi. 2022;8(10).
50. World Health Organization. WHO Model List of Essential Medicines - 22nd list, 2021. WHO Technical document, Report No.: WHO/MHP/HPS/EML/2021.02. Geneva: World Health Organization; 2021.
51. Prajna NV, Krishnan T, Mascarenhas J, Rajaraman R, Prajna L, Srinivasan M, et al. The mycotic ulcer treatment trial: a randomized trial comparing natamycin vs voriconazole. JAMA Ophthalmol. 2013;131(4):422–9.
52. Carolus H, Pierson S, Lagrou K, Van Dijck P. Amphotericin B and other polyenes-discovery, clinical use, mode of action and drug resistance. J Fungi. 2020;6(4).
53. Cavassin FB, Baú-Carneiro JL, Vilas-Boas RR, Queiroz-Telles F. Sixty years of amphotericin B: an overview of the main antifungal agent used to treat invasive fungal infections. Infect Dis Ther. 2021;10(1):115–47.
54. Sangalli-Leite F, Scorzoni L, Mesa-Arango AC, Casas C, Herrero E, Soares Mendes Gianinni MJ, et al. Amphotericin B mediates killing in Cryptococcus neoformans through the induction of a strong oxidative burst. Microbes Infect. 2011;13(5):457–67.
55. te Welscher YM, ten Napel HH, Balagué MM, Souza CM, Riezman H, de Kruijff B, et al. Natamycin blocks fungal growth by binding specifically to ergosterol without permeabilizing the membrane. J Biol Chem. 2008;283(10):6393–401.
56. Borba HHL, Steimbach LM, Riveros BS, Tonin FS, Ferreira VL, Bagatim BAQ, et al. Cost-effectiveness of amphotericin B formulations in the treatment of systemic fungal infections. Mycoses. 2018;61(10):754–63.
57. AsheJr WD, Van Reken DE. 5-Fluorocytosine: a brief review. Clin Pediatr. 1977;16(4):364–6.
58. Delma FZ, Al-Hatmi AMS, Brüggemann RJM, Melchers WJG, de Hoog S, Verweij PE, et al. Molecular mechanisms of 5-fluorocytosine resistance in yeasts and filamentous fungi. J Fungi. 2021;7(11).
59. Bennett JE, Dismukes WE, Duma RJ, Medoff G, Sande MA, Gallis H, et al. A comparison of amphotericin B alone and combined with flucytosine in the treatment of cryptoccal meningitis. N Engl J Med. 1979;301(3):126–31.
60. Vermes A, Guchelaar HJ, Dankert J. Flucytosine: a review of its pharmacology, clinical indications, pharmacokinetics, toxicity and drug interactions. J Antimicrob Chemother. 2000;46(2):171–9.

61. Polak A, Scholer HJ. Mode of action of 5-fluorocytosine and mechanisms of resistance. Chemotherapy. 2009;21(3–4):113–30.
62. Waldorf AR, Polak A. Mechanisms of action of 5-fluorocytosine. Antimicrob Agents Chemother. 1983;23(1):79–85.
63. Sigera LSM, Denning DW. Flucytosine and its clinical usage. Ther Adv Infect Dis. 2023;10:20499361231161387.
64. Zobi C, Algul O. The significance of mono- and dual-effective agents in the development of new antifungal strategies. Chem Biol Drug Des. 2025;105(1):e70045.
65. Sheehan DJ, Hitchcock CA, Sibley CM. Current and emerging azole antifungal agents. Clin Microbiol Rev. 1999;12(1):40–79.
66. Zavrel M, Esquivel BD, White TC. The ins and outs of azole antifungal drug resistance: molecular mechanisms of transport. In: Berghuis A, Matlashewski G, Wainberg MA, Sheppard D, Gotte M, editors. Handbook of antimicrobial resistance. New York: Springer; 2017. p. 423–52.
67. Shafiei M, Peyton L, Hashemzadeh M, Foroumadi A. History of the development of antifungal azoles: a review on structures, SAR, and mechanism of action. Bioorg Chem. 2020;104:104240.
68. Song L, Wang S, Zou H, Yi X, Jia S, Li R, et al. Regulation of ergosterol biosynthesis in pathogenic Ffungi: opportunities for therapeutic development. Microorganisms. 2025;13(4).
69. Francois IEJA, Cammue BPA, Borgers M, Ausma J, Dispersyn GD, Thevissen K. Azoles: mode of antifungal action and resistance development. Effect of miconazole on endogenous reactive oxygen species production in Candida albicans. Anti-Infect Agents Med Chem. 2006;5(1):3–13.
70. Kanafani ZA, Perfect JR. Resistance to antifungal agents: mechanisms and clinical impact. Clin Infect Dis. 2008;46(1):120–8.
71. Xiao L, Madison V, Chau Andrew S, Loebenberg D, Palermo Robert E, McNicholas Paul M. Three-dimensional models of wild-type and mutated forms of cytochrome P450 14α-sterol demethylases from aspergillus fumigatus and Candida albicans provide insights into posaconazole binding. Antimicrob Agents Chemother. 2004;48(2):568–74.
72. Mast N, Zheng W, Stout CD, Pikuleva IA. Antifungal azoles: structural insights into undesired tight binding to cholesterol-metabolizing CYP46A1. Mol Pharmacol. 2013;84(1):86–94.
73. Wirth F, Ishida K. Antifungal drugs: an updated review of central nervous system pharmacokinetics. Mycoses. 2020;63(10):1047–59.
74. Che X, Sheng C, Wang W, Cao Y, Xu Y, Ji H, et al. New azoles with potent antifungal activity: design, synthesis and molecular docking. Eur J Med Chem. 2009;44(10):4218–26.
75. Tucker RM, Williams PL, Arathoon EG, Levine BE, Hartstein AI, Hanson LH, et al. Pharmacokinetics of fluconazole in cerebrospinal fluid and serum in human coccidioidal meningitis. Antimicrob Agents Chemother. 1988;32(3):369–73.
76. Lewis RE. Current concepts in antifungal pharmacology. Mayo Clin Proc. 2011;86(8):805–17.
77. Brammer KW, Farrow PR, Faulkner JK. Pharmacokinetics and tissue penetration of fluconazole in humans. Rev Infect Dis. 1990;12(Suppl_3):S318–S26.
78. Cuenca-Estrella M, Gomez-Lopez A, Mellado E, Buitrago Maria J, Monzon A, Rodriguez-Tudela JL. Head-to-head comparison of the activities of currently available antifungal agents against 3,378 spanish clinical isolates of yeasts and filamentous fungi. Antimicrob Agents Chemother. 2006;50(3):917–21.
79. AMS A-H, Meis JF, de Hoog GS. Fusarium: molecular diversity and intrinsic drug resistance. PLoS Pathog. 2016;12(4):e1005464.
80. Pfaller MA, Diekema DJ. Epidemiology of invasive mycoses in North America. Crit Rev Microbiol. 2010;36(1):1–53.
81. European Food Safety A, European Centre for Disease P, Control, European Chemicals A, European Environment A, European Medicines A, et al. Impact of the use of azole fungicides, other than as human medicines, on the development of azole-resistant Aspergillus spp. EFSA J. 2025;23(1):e9200.

82. Molinero RL, Hermida Alava KS, Brito Devoto T, Sautua F, Carmona M, Cuestas ML, et al. Prevalence of azole-resistant aspergillus fumigatus and other aspergilli in the environment from Argentina. Med Mycol. 2024;62(10):myae098.
83. Fisher MC, Burnett F, Chandler C, NAR G, Gurr S, Hart A, et al. A one health roadmap towards understanding and mitigating emerging fungal antimicrobial resistance: fAMR. NPJ Antimicrob Resist. 2024;2(1):36.
84. Hammoudi Halat D, Younes S, Mourad N, Rahal M. Allylamines, benzylamines, and fungal cell permeability: a review of mechanistic effects and usefulness against fungal pathogens. Membranes. 2022;12(12).
85. Petranyi G, Ryder NS, Stütz A. Allylamine derivatives: new class of synthetic antifungal agents inhibiting fungal squalene epoxidase. Science. 1984;224(4654):1239–41.
86. Birnbaum JE. Pharmacology of the allylamines. J Am Acad Dermatol. 1990;23(4, Part 2):782–5.
87. Leyden J. Pharmacokinetics and pharmacology of terbinafine and itraconazole. J Am Acad Dermatol. 1998;38(5, Suppl 2):S42–S7.
88. Perveze Z, Johnson MW, Rubin RA, Sellers M, Zayas C, Jones JL, et al. Terbinafine-induced hepatic failure requiring liver transplantation. Liver Transpl. 2007;13(1):162–4.
89. Gupta AK, Wang T, Mann A, Piguet V, Chowdhary A, Bakotic WL. Mechanisms of resistance against allylamine and azole antifungals in Trichophyton: a renewed call for innovative molecular diagnostics in susceptibility testing. PLoS Pathog. 2025;21(2):e1012913.
90. Gaurav V, Bhattacharya SN, Sharma N, Datt S, Kumar P, Rai G, et al. Terbinafine resistance in dermatophytes: time to revisit alternate antifungal therapy. J Med Mycol. 2021;31(1):101087.
91. Cañete-Gibas CF, Mele J, Patterson Hoja P, Sanders CJ, Ferrer D, Garcia V, et al. Terbinafine-resistant dermatophytes and the presence of Trichophyton indotineae in North America. J Clin Microbiol. 2023;61(8):e00562-23.
92. Sucher AJ, Chahine EB, Balcer HE. Echinocandins: the newest class of antifungals. Ann Pharmacother. 2009;43(10):1647–57.
93. Du B, Meenu M, Liu H, Xu B. A concise review on the molecular structure and function relationship of β-Glucan. Int J Mol Sci. 2019;20(16):4032.
94. Douglas CM. Fungal β(1,3)-d-glucan synthesis. Med Mycol. 2001;39(1):55–66.
95. Ruiz-Herrera J, Ortiz-Castellanos L. Cell wall glucans of fungi. A review. Cell Surf. 2019;5:100022.
96. Hori Y, Shibuya K. Role of FKS gene in the susceptibility of pathogenic fungi to echinocandins. Med Mycol J. 2018;59(2):E31–40.
97. Patil A, Majumdar S. Echinocandins in antifungal pharmacotherapy. J Pharm Pharmacol. 2017;69(12):1635–60.
98. Perlin DS. Echinocandin resistance in Candida. Clin Infect Dis. 2015;61(Suppl_6):S612–S7.
99. Li J, Liu H, Li J, Liu J, Dai X, Zhu A, et al. Cryo-EM structure of the β-1,3-glucan synthase FKS1-Rho1 complex. Nat Commun. 2025;16(1):2054.
100. Perlin DS. Current perspectives on echinocandin class drugs. Future Microbiol. 2011;6(4):441–57.
101. Kurtz MB, Rex JH. Glucan synthase inhibitors as antifungal agents. Adv Protein Chem. 2001;56:423–75.
102. Kurtz MB, Heath IB, Marrinan J, Dreikorn S, Onishi J, Douglas C. Morphological effects of lipopeptides against Aspergillus fumigatus correlate with activities against (1,3)-beta-D-glucan synthase. Antimicrob Agents Chemother. 1994;38(7):1480–9.
103. Douglas CM. Understanding the microbiology of the aspergillus cell wall and the efficacy of caspofungin. Med Mycol. 2006;44(Suppl_1):S95–9.
104. Perlin DS. Mechanisms of echinocandin antifungal drug resistance. Ann N Y Acad Sci. 2015;
105. Mroczyńska M, Brillowska-Dąbrowska A. Review on current status of echinocandins use. Antibiotics. 2020;9(5).
106. Park S, Kelly R, Kahn JN, Robles J, Hsu MJ, Register E, et al. Specific substitutions in the echinocandin target Fks1p account for reduced susceptibility of rare laboratory and clinical Candida sp. isolates. Antimicrob Agents Chemother. 2005;49(8):3264–73.

107. Sharma N, Bagga B, Singhal D, Nagpal R, Kate A, Saluja G, et al. Fungal keratitis: a review of clinical presentations, treatment strategies and outcomes. Ocul Surf. 2022;24:22–30.
108. Prajna NV, Krishnan T, Rajaraman R, Patel S, Srinivasan M, Das M, et al. Effect of oral voriconazole on fungal keratitis in the mycotic ulcer treatment trial II (MUTT II): a randomized clinical trial. JAMA Ophthalmol. 2016;134(12):1365–72.
109. Prajna NV, Lalitha P, Rajaraman R, Krishnan T, Raghavan A, Srinivasan M, et al. Changing azole resistance: a secondary analysis of the MUTT I randomized clinical trial. JAMA Ophthalmol. 2016;134(6):693–6.
110. Welscher YM, Napel HH, Balagué MM, Souza CM, Riezman H, de Kruijff B, et al. Natamycin blocks fungal growth by binding specifically to ergosterol without prmeabilizing the membrane. J Biol Chem. 2008;283(10):6393–401.
111. Streekstra H, Verkennis AEE, Jacobs R, Dekker A, Stark J, Dijksterhuis J. Fungal strains and the development of tolerance against natamycin. Int J Food Microbiol. 2016;238:15–22.
112. Diekema DJ, Messer SA, Hollis RJ, Jones RN, Pfaller MA. Activities of caspofungin, itraconazole, posaconazole, ravuconazole, voriconazole, and amphotericin B against 448 recent clinical isolates of filamentous fungi. J Clin Microbiol. 2003;41(8):3623–6.
113. Lotery AJ, Kerr JR, Page BA. Fungal keratitis caused by Scopulariopsis brevicaulis: successful treatment with topical amphotericin B and chloramphenicol without the need for surgical debridement. Br J Ophthalmol. 1994;78(9):730.
114. Mahdy RA, Nada WM, Wageh MM. Topical Amphotericin B and subconjunctival injection of fluconazole (combination therapy) versus topical amphotericin B (monotherapy) in treatment of keratomycosis. J Ocul Pharmacol Ther. 2010;26(3):281–5.
115. Sun RL, Jones DB, Wilhelmus KR. Clinical characteristics and outcome of Candida keratitis. Am J Ophthalmol. 2007;143(6):1043–5.e1.
116. Zhao-Qin H, Jin-Xin S, Shi-Yin P, Lin Z, Yan C, Xian-Ning L, et al. Corneal collagen cross-linking and liposomal amphotericin B combination therapy for fungal keratitis in rabbits. Int J Ophthalmol. 2016;9(11):1549–54.
117. Ghosh AK, Rudramurthy SM, Gupta A, Choudhary H, Singh S, Thakur A, et al. Evaluation of liposomal and conventional amphotericin B in experimental fungal keratitis rabbit model. Transl Vis Sci Technol. 2019;8(3):35.
118. Freda R. Use of oral voriconazole as adjunctive treatment of severe cornea fungal infection: Case report. Arq Bras Oftalmol. 2006;69:431.
119. Jones A, Muhtaseb M. Use of voriconazole in fungal keratitis. J Cataract Refract Surg. 2008;34(2):183–4.
120. Thiel MA, Zinkernagel AS, Burhenne J, Kaufmann C, Haefeli WE. Voriconazole concentration in human aqueous humor and plasma during topical or combined topical and systemic administration for fungal keratitis. Antimicrob Agents Chemother. 2007;51(1):239–44.
121. Sharma N, Sahay P, Maharana PK, Singhal D, Saluja G, Bandivadekar P, et al. Management algorithm for fungal keratitis: the TST (topical, systemic, and targeted therapy) protocol. Cornea. 2019;38(2):141–5.
122. Agarwal PK, Roy P, Das A, Banerjee A, Maity PK, Banerjee AR. Efficacy of topical and systemic itraconazole as a broad-spectrum antifungal agent in mycotic corneal ulcer. A preliminary study. Indian J Ophthalmol. 2001;49(3):173.
123. Sharma N, Singhal D, Maharana PK, Sinha R, Agarwal T, Upadhyay AD, et al. Comparison of oral voriconazole versus oral ketoconazole as an adjunct to topical natamycin in severe fungal keratitis: a randomized controlled trial. Cornea. 2017;36(12):1521–7.
124. Sahay P, Singhal D, Nagpal R, Maharana PK, Farid M, Gelman R, et al. Pharmacologic therapy of mycotic keratitis. Surv Ophthalmol. 2019;64(3):380–400.
125. Prakash G, Sharma N, Goel M, Titiyal JS, Vajpayee RB. Evaluation of intrastromal injection of voriconazole as a therapeutic adjunctive for the management of deep recalcitrant fungal keratitis. Am J Ophthalmol. 2008;146(1):56–9.e2.
126. Saluja G, Sharma N, Agarwal R, Sharma HP, Maharana P, Satpathy G, et al. Determination of surgical outcomes with a novel formulation of intrastromal natamycin in recalcitrant fungal keratitis: a pilot study. Indian J Ophthalmol. 2021;69(10):2670–4.

127. Mimouni M, Tam G, Paitan Y, Kidron D, Segev F. Safety and efficacy of intrastromal injection of 5% natamycin in experimental Fusarium keratitis. J Ocul Pharmacol Ther. 2014;30(7):543–7.
128. Sharma N, Chacko J, Velpandian T, Titiyal JS, Sinha R, Satpathy G, et al. Comparative evaluation of topical versus intrastromal voriconazole as an adjunct to natamycin in recalcitrant fungal keratitis. Ophthalmology. 2013;120(4):677–81.
129. Narayana S, Krishnan T, Ramakrishnan S, Samantaray PP, Austin A, Pickel J, et al. Mycotic antimicrobial localized injection: a randomized clinical trial evaluating intrastromal injection of voriconazole. Ophthalmology. 2019;126(8):1084–9.
130. Konar P, Joshi S, Mandhare SJ, Thakur R, Deshpande M, Dayal A. Intrastromal voriconazole: an adjuvant approach for recalcitrant mycotic keratitis. Indian J Ophthalmol. 2020;68(1):35.
131. Shen Y-C, Wang C-Y, Tsai H-Y, Lee H-N. Intracameral voriconazole injection in the treatment of fungal endophthalmitis resulting from keratitis. Am J Ophthalmol. 2010;149(6):916–21.
132. Sharma B, Kataria P, Anand R, Gupta R, Kumar K, Kumar S, et al. Efficacy profile of intracameral amphotericin B. The often forgotten step. Asia-Pac J Ophthalmol. 2015;4(6):360–6.
133. Yoon K-C, Jeong I-Y, Im S-K, Chae H-J, Yang S-Y. Therapeutic effect of intracameral amphotericin B injection in the treatment of fungal keratitis. Cornea. 2007;26(7):814–8.
134. Yi S, Yao Y, Chong-Gang P, Ye-Hui T, Qiong Z, Jing-Lin Y, et al. Therapeutic efficacy of intracameral amphotericin B injection for 60 patients with keratomycosis. Int J Ophthalmol. 2010;3(3):257–60.
135. Hu J, Zhang J, Li Y, Han X, Zheng W, Yang J, et al. A combination of intrastromal and intracameral injections of amphotericin B in the treatment of severe fungal keratitis. J Ophthalmol. 2016;2016(1):3436415.
136. Sharma N, Sankaran P, Agarwal T, Arora T, Chawla B, Titiyal JS, et al. Evaluation of intracameral amphotericin B in the management of fungal keratitis: randomized controlled trial. Ocul Immunol Inflamm. 2016;24(5):493–7.
137. Nada WM, Al Aswad MA, El-Haig WM. Combined intrastromal injection of amphotericin B and topical fluconazole in the treatment of resistant cases of keratomycosis: a retrospective study. Clin Ophthalmol. 2017;11:871–4.
138. Aydin B, Cubuk MO, Ucgul A, Ertop M, Ozmen MC, Atalay T, et al. Combined intrastromal voriconazole and amphotericin B treatment for persistent fungal keratitis. Eye Contact Lens. 2020;46(5):269–73.
139. Saluja G, Sharma N, Agarwal R, Sharma HP, Singhal D, Kumar Maharana P, et al. Comparison of safety and efficacy of intrastromal injections of voriconazole, amphotericin B and natamycin in cases of recalcitrant fungal keratitis: a randomized controlled trial. Clin Ophthalmol. 2021;15:2437–46.
140. Case NT, Gurr SJ, Fisher MC, Blehert DS, Boone C, Casadevall A, et al. Fungal impacts on Earth's ecosystems. Nature. 2025;638(8049):49–57.
141. Donovan C, Arenas E, Ayyala RS, Margo CE, Espana EM. Fungal keratitis: mechanisms of infection and management strategies. Surv Ophthalmol. 2022;67(3):758–69.
142. Raj N, Vanathi M, Ahmed NH, Gupta N, Lomi N, Tandon R. Recent perspectives in the management of fungal keratitis. J Fungi. 2021;7(11).
143. Prajna NV, Lalitha P, Krishnan T, Rajaraman R, Radnakrishnan N, Srinivasan M, et al. Patterns of antifungal resistance in adult patients with fungal keratitis in South India: a post hoc analysis of 3 randomized clinical trials. JAMA Ophthalmol. 2022;140(2):179–84.
144. Manikandan P, Abdel-hadi A, Randhir Babu Singh Y, Revathi R, Anita R, Banawas S, et al. Fungal keratitis: epidemiology, rapid detection, and antifungal susceptibilities of Fusarium and aspergillus isolates from corneal scrapings. Biomed Res Int. 2019;2019(1):6395840.
145. Cintra MEC, da Silva DM, Al-Hatmi AMS, Bastos RW, Rossato L. Fusarium keratitis: a systematic review (1969 to 2023). Mycopathologia. 2024;189(5):74.

146. Al-Hatmi AMS, de Hoog GS, Meis JF. Multiresistant Fusarium pathogens on plants and humans: solutions in (from) the antifungal pipeline? Infect Drug Resist. 2019;12(null):3727–37.
147. Chang R, Zhang X, Si H, Zhao G, Yuan X, Liu T, et al. Ophiostomatoid species associated with pine trees (Pinus spp.) infested by Cryphaluspiceae from eastern China, including five new species. MycoKeys. 2021;83:181–208.
148. Lalitha P, Shapiro BL, Srinivasan M, Prajna NV, Acharya NR, Fothergill AW, et al. Antimicrobial susceptibility of Fusarium, aspergillus, and other filamentous fungi isolated from keratitis. Arch Ophthalmol. 2007;125(6):789–93.
149. Al Yazidi LS, Al-Hatmi AMS. Fusariosis: an update on therapeutic options for management. Expert Opin Orphan Drugs. 2021;9(3):95–103.
150. Batista BG, Chaves MA, Reginatto P, Saraiva OJ, Fuentefria AM. Human fusariosis: an emerging infection that is difficult to treat. Rev Soc Bras Med Trop. 2020;53:e20200013.
151. Alfonso EC, Cantu-Dibildox J, Munir WM, Miller D, O'Brien TP, Karp CL, et al. Insurgence of Fusarium keratitis associated with contact lens wear. Arch Ophthalmol. 2006;124(7):941–7.
152. Sáenz V, Alvarez-Moreno C, Pape PL, Restrepo S, Guarro J, Ramírez AMC. A one health perspective to recognize Fusarium as important in clinical practice. J Fungi. 2020;6(4).
153. Costa JLP, Barra D, Ando E, Pogue R. Keratitis by aspergillus flavus infection after cataract surgery. Rev Bras Oftalmol. 2016;75:75.
154. Chakrabarti A, Chatterjee SS, Das A, Shivaprakash MR. Invasive aspergillosis in developing countries. Med Mycol. 2011;49(Suppl_1):S35–47.
155. Rudramurthy SM, Paul RA, Chakrabarti A, Mouton JW, Meis JF. Invasive aspergillosis by aspergillus flavus: epidemiology, diagnosis, antifungal resistance, and management. J Fungi. 2019;5(3).
156. Thomas PA. Current perspectives on ophthalmic mycoses. Clin Microbiol Rev. 2003;16(4):730–97.
157. Trief D, Gray ST, Jakobiec FA, Durand ML, Fay A, Freitag SK, et al. Invasive fungal disease of the sinus and orbit: a comparison between mucormycosis and aspergillus. Br J Ophthalmol. 2016;100(2):184.
158. Dannaoui E. Antifungal resistance in mucorales. Int J Antimicrob Agents. 2017;50(5):617–21.
159. Durand ML. Endophthalmitis. Clin Microbiol Infect. 2013;19(3):227–34.
160. Wiederhold NP. Echinocandin resistance in Candida species: a review of recent developments. Curr Infect Dis Rep. 2016;18(12):42.
161. Pristov KE, Ghannoum MA. Resistance of Candida to azoles and echinocandins worldwide. Clin Microbiol Infect. 2019;25(7):792–8.
162. Tian J, Li D, Dai S, Chen B, Luo J, Liu S, et al. In vivo confocal microscopy findings of a rare Cryptococcus neoformans keratitis. Ocul Immunol Inflamm. 2024;32(10):2575–8.
163. Ansari Z, Miller D, Galor A. Current thoughts in fungal keratitis: diagnosis and treatment. Curr Fungal Infect Rep. 2013;7(3):209–18.
164. Thomas PA, Kaliamurthy J. Mycotic keratitis: epidemiology, diagnosis and management. Clin Microbiol Infect. 2013;19(3):210–20.
165. Lee Y, Robbins N, Cowen LE. Molecular mechanisms governing antifungal drug resistance. NPJ Antimicrob Resist. 2023;1(1):5.
166. Cowen LE, Sanglard D, Howard SJ, Rogers PD, Perlin DS. Mechanisms of antifungal drug resistance. Cold Spring Harb Perspect Med. 2015;5(7):a019752.
167. Vincent BM, Lancaster AK, Scherz-Shouval R, Whitesell L, Lindquist S. Fitness trade-offs restrict the evolution of resistance to amphotericin B. PLoS Biol. 2013;11(10):e1001692.
168. Tanwar J, Das S, Fatima Z, Hameed S. Multidrug resistance: an emerging crisis. Interdiscip Perspect Infect Dis. 2014;2014(1):541340.
169. McCarthy M, O'Shaughnessy EM, Walsh TJ. Amphotericin B: polyene resistance mechanisms. In: Mayers DL, Sobel JD, Ouellette M, Kaye KS, Marchaim D, editors. Antimicrobial drug resistance: mechanisms of drug resistance, Volume 1. Cham: Springer; 2017. p. 387–95.

170. Sanglard D, Ischer F, Parkinson T, Falconer D, Bille J. Candida albicans mutations in the ergosterol biosynthetic pathway and resistance to several antifungal agents. Antimicrob Agents Chemother. 2003;47(8):2404–12.
171. Martel Claire M, Parker Josie E, Bader O, Weig M, Gross U, Warrilow Andrew GS, et al. A clinical isolate of Candida albicans with mutations in ERG11 (encoding sterol 14α-demethylase) and ERG5 (encoding C22 desaturase) is cross resistant to azoles and amphotericin B. Antimicrob Agents Chemother. 2010;54(9):3578–83.
172. Young LY, Hull CM, Heitman J. Disruption of ergosterol biosynthesis confers resistance to amphotericin B in Candida lusitaniae. Antimicrob Agents Chemother. 2003;47(9):2717–24.
173. Ahmad S, Joseph L, Parker Josie E, Asadzadeh M, Kelly SL, Meis JF, et al. ERG6 and ERG2 are major targets conferring reduced susceptibility to amphotericin B in clinical Candida glabrata isolates in Kuwait. Antimicrob Agents Chemother. 2019;63(2):10.1128/aac.01900-18.
174. Kelly SL, Lamb DC, Taylor M, Corran AJ, Baldwin BC, Powderly WG. Resistance to amphotericin B associated with defective sterol Δ8→7 isomerase in a Cryptococcus neoformans strain from an AIDS patient. FEMS Microbiol Lett. 1994;122(1–2):39–42.
175. Joseph-Horne T, Loeffler RST, Hollomon DW, Kelly SL. Amphotericin B resistant isolates of Cryptococcus neoformans without alteration in sterol biosynthesis. J Med Vet Mycol. 1996;34(3):223–5.
176. Posch W, Blatzer M, Wilflingseder D, Lass-Flörl C. Aspergillus terreus: novel lessons learned on amphotericin B resistance. Med Mycol. 2018;56(Suppl_1):S73–82.
177. Andrews FA, Sarosi GA, Beggs WH. Enhancement of amphotericin B activity by a series of compounds related to phenolic antioxidants. J Antimicrob Chemother. 1979;5(2):173–7.
178. Blatzer M, Jukic E, Posch W, Schöpf B, Binder U, Steger M, et al. Amphotericin B resistance in aspergillus terreus is overpowered by coapplication of pro-oxidants. Antioxid Redox Signal. 2015;23(18):1424–38.
179. Seo K, Akiyoshi H, Ohnishi Y. Alteration of cell wall composition leads to amphotericin B resistance in aspergillus flavus. Microbiol Immunol. 1999;43(11):1017–25.
180. Mesa-Arango AC, Rueda C, Román E, Quintin J, Terrón MC, Luque D, et al. Cell wall changes in amphotericin B-resistant strains from Candida tropicalis and relationship with the immune responses elicited by the host. Antimicrob Agents Chemother. 2016;60(4):2326–35.
181. Barchiesi F, Arzeni D, Caselli F, Scalise G. Primary resistance to flucytosine among clinical isolates of Candida spp. J Antimicrob Chemother. 2000;45(3):408–9.
182. Yang D-H, Khanal Lamichhane A, Kwon-Chung Kyung J, Chang YC. Factors influencing the nitrogen-source dependent flucytosine resistance in Cryptococcus species. MBio. 2023;14(1):e03451–22.
183. Billmyre RB, Applen Clancey S, Li LX, Doering TL, Heitman J. 5-fluorocytosine resistance is associated with hypermutation and alterations in capsule biosynthesis in Cryptococcus. Nat Commun. 2020;11(1):127.
184. Chapeland-Leclerc F, Bouchoux J, Goumar A, Chastin C, Villard J, Noël T. Inactivation of the FCY2 gene encoding purine-cytosine permease promotes cross-resistance to flucytosine and fluconazole in Candida lusitaniae. Antimicrob Agents Chemother. 2005;49(8):3101–8.
185. Papon N, Noël T, Florent M, Gibot-Leclerc S, Jean D, Chastin C, et al. Molecular mechanism of flucytosine resistance in Candida lusitaniae: contribution of the FCY2, FCY1, and FUR1 genes to 5-fluorouracil and fluconazole cross-resistance. Antimicrob Agents Chemother. 2007;51(1):369–71.
186. Vu K, Thompson GR III, Roe CC, Sykes JE, Dreibe EM, Lockhart SR, et al. Flucytosine resistance in Cryptococcus gattii is indirectly mediated by the FCY2-FCY1-FUR1 pathway. Med Mycol. 2018;56(7):857–67.
187. Chevallier MR, Jund R, Lacroute F. Characterization of cytosine permeation in Saccharomyces cerevisiae. J Bacteriol. 1975;122(2):629–41.

188. Steier Z, Vermitsky J-P, Toner G, Gygax Scott E, Edlind T, Katiyar S. Flucytosine antagonism of azole activity versus Candida glabrata: role of transcription factor Pdr1 and multidrug transporter Cdr1. Antimicrob Agents Chemother. 2013;57(11):5543–7.
189. Khanal Lamichhane A, Garraffo HM, Cai H, Walter Peter J, Kwon-Chung KJ, Chang YC. A novel role of fungal type I myosin in regulating membrane properties and its association with d-amino acid utilization in Cryptococcus gattii. MBio. 2019;10(4) https://doi.org/10.1128/mbio.01867-19.
190. Chang YC, Lamichhane AK, Cai H, Walter PJ, Bennett JE, Kwon-Chung KJ. Moderate levels of 5-fluorocytosine cause the emergence of high frequency resistance in cryptococci. Nat Commun. 2021;12(1):3418.
191. Kontoyiannis DP, Lewis RE. Antifungal drug resistance of pathogenic fungi. Lancet. 2002;359(9312):1135–44.
192. Nett JE, Andes DR. Antifungal agents: Spectrum of activity, pharmacology, and clinical indications. Infect Dis Clin N Am. 2016;30(1):51–83.
193. Hope William W, Tabernero L, Denning David W, Anderson Michael J. Molecular mechanisms of primary resistance to flucytosine in Candida albicans. Antimicrob Agents Chemother. 2004;48(11):4377–86.
194. Kern L, de Montigny J, Lacroute F, Jund R. Regulation of the pyrimidine salvage pathway by the FUR1 gene product of Saccharomyces cerevisiae. Curr Genet. 1991;19(5):333–7.
195. Whelan WL. The genetic basis of resistance to 5-fluorocytosine in Candida species and Cryptococcus neoformans. Crit Rev Microbiol. 1987;15(1):45–56.
196. Gsaller F, Furukawa T, Carr Paul D, Rash B, Jöchl C, Bertuzzi M, et al. Mechanistic basis of pH-dependent 5-flucytosine resistance in aspergillus fumigatus. Antimicrob Agents Chemother. 2018;62(6) https://doi.org/10.1128/aac.02593-17.
197. Dodgson AR, Dodgson KJ, Pujol C, Pfaller MA, Soll DR. Clade-specific flucytosine resistance is due to a single nucleotide change in the FUR1 gene of Candida albicans. Antimicrob Agents Chemother. 2004;48(6):2223–7.
198. Edlind TD, Katiyar SK. Mutational analysis of flucytosine resistance in Candida glabrata. Antimicrob Agents Chemother. 2010;54(11):4733–8.
199. Chapeland-Leclerc F, Hennequin C, Papon N, Noël T, Girard A, Socié G, et al. Acquisition of flucytosine, azole, and caspofungin resistance in Candida glabrata bloodstream isolates serially obtained from a hematopoietic stem cell transplant recipient. Antimicrob Agents Chemother. 2010;54(3):1360–2.
200. Vandeputte P, Pineau L, Larcher G, Noel T, Brèthes D, Chabasse D, et al. Molecular mechanisms of resistance to 5-fluorocytosine in laboratory mutants of Candida glabrata. Mycopathologia. 2011;171(1):11–21.
201. Rhodes J, Abdolrasouli A, Farrer RA, Cuomo CA, Aanensen DM, Armstrong-James D, et al. Genomic epidemiology of the UK outbreak of the emerging human fungal pathogen Candida auris. Emerg Microbes Infect. 2018;7(1):43.
202. Perfect JR, Dismukes WE, Dromer F, Goldman DL, Graybill JR, Hamill RJ, et al. Clinical practice guidelines for the management of cryptococcal disease: 2010 update by the infectious diseases society of America. Clin Infect Dis. 2010;50(3):291–322.
203. Morio F, Loge C, Besse B, Hennequin C, Le Pape P. Screening for amino acid substitutions in the Candida albicans Erg11 protein of azole-susceptible and azole-resistant clinical isolates: new substitutions and a review of the literature. Diagn Microbiol Infect Dis. 2010;66(4):373–84.
204. Marichal P, Koymans L, Willemsens S, Bellens D, Verhasselt P, Luyten W, et al. Contribution of mutations in the cytochrome P450 14α-demethylase (Erg11p, Cyp51p) to azole resistance in Candida albicans. Microbiology. 1999;145(10):2701–13.
205. Chowdhary A, Prakash A, Sharma C, Kordalewska M, Kumar A, Sarma S, et al. A multicentre study of antifungal susceptibility patterns among 350 Candida auris isolates (2009–17) in India: role of the ERG11 and FKS1 genes in azole and echinocandin resistance. J Antimicrob Chemother. 2018;73(4):891–9.

206. Rybak JM, Sharma C, Doorley LA, Barker KS, Palmer GE, Rogers PD. Delineation of the direct contribution of Candida auris ERG11 mutations to clinical triazole resistance. Microbiol Spectr. 2021;9(3):e01585–21.
207. Sewell TR, Zhu J, Rhodes J, Hagen F, Meis JF, Fisher MC, et al. Nonrandom distribution of azole resistance across the global population of aspergillus fumigatus. MBio. 2019;10(3).
208. Schoustra S, Debets AJM, Rijs AJMM, Zhang J, Snelders E, Leendertse P, et al. Environmental hotspots for azole resistance selection of aspergillus fumigatus, The Netherlands. Emerg Infect Dis. 2019;25(7):1347.
209. Hurst SF, Berkow EL, Stevenson KL, Litvintseva AP, Lockhart SR. Isolation of azole-resistant aspergillus fumigatus from the environment in the South-Eastern USA. J Antimicrob Chemother. 2017;72(9):2443–6.
210. Alvarez-Moreno C, Lavergne R-A, Hagen F, Morio F, Meis JF, Le Pape P. Azole-resistant aspergillus fumigatus harboring TR34/L98H, TR46/Y121F/T289A and TR53 mutations related to flower fields in Colombia. Sci Rep. 2017;7(1):45631.
211. Etienne Kizee A, Berkow EL, Gade L, Nunnally N, Lockhart SR, Beer K, et al. Genomic diversity of azole-resistant aspergillus fumigatus in the United States. MBio. 2021;12(4) https://doi.org/10.1128/mbio.01803-21.
212. Li D, Amburgey-Crovetti K, Applebach E, Steen TY, Calderone R. The dual pathogen Fusarium: diseases, incidence, azole resistance, and biofilms. J Fungi. 2025;11(4):294.
213. Czajka KM, Venkataraman K, Brabant-Kirwan D, Santi SA, Verschoor C, Appanna VD, et al. Molecular mechanisms associated with antifungal resistance in pathogenic Candida species. Cells. 2023;12(22).
214. Vasicek Erin M, Berkow Elizabeth L, Flowers Stephanie A, Barker Katherine S, Rogers PD. UPC2 is universally essential for azole antifungal resistance in Candida albicans. Eukaryot Cell. 2014;13(7):933–46.
215. Yang H, Tong J, Lee CW, Ha S, Eom SH, Im YJ. Structural mechanism of ergosterol regulation by fungal sterol transcription factor Upc2. Nat Commun. 2015;6(1):6129.
216. Flowers SA, Barker KS, Berkow EL, Toner G, Chadwick SG, Gygax SE, et al. Gain-of-function mutations in UPC2 are a frequent cause of ERG11 upregulation in azole-resistant clinical isolates of Candida albicans. Eukaryot Cell. 2012;11(10):1289–99.
217. Heilmann Clemens J, Schneider S, Barker Katherine S, Rogers PD, Morschhäuser J. An A643T mutation in the transcription factor Upc2p causes constitutive ERG11 upregulation and increased fluconazole resistance in Candida albicans. Antimicrob Agents Chemother. 2010;54(1):353–9.
218. Dunkel N, Liu TT, Barker KS, Homayouni R, Morschhäuser J, Rogers PD. A gain-of-function mutation in the transcription factor Upc2p causes upregulation of ergosterol biosynthesis genes and increased fluconazole resistance in a clinical Candida albicans isolate. Eukaryot Cell. 2008;7(7):1180–90.
219. Willger SD, Puttikamonkul S, Kim KH, Burritt JB, Grahl N, Metzler LJ, et al. A sterol-regulatory element binding protein is required for cell polarity, hypoxia adaptation, azole drug resistance, and virulence in aspergillus fumigatus. PLoS Pathog. 2008;4(11):e1000200.
220. Blatzer M, Barker BM, Willger SD, Beckmann N, Blosser SJ, Cornish EJ, et al. SREBP coordinates iron and ergosterol homeostasis to mediate triazole drug and hypoxia responses in the human fungal pathogen aspergillus fumigatus. PLoS Genet. 2011;7(12):e1002374.
221. Blosser SJ, Cramer RA. SREBP-dependent triazole susceptibility in aspergillus fumigatus is mediated through direct transcriptional regulation of erg11a (cyp51A). Antimicrob Agents Chemother. 2012;56(1):248–57.
222. Gsaller F, Hortschansky P, Furukawa T, Carr PD, Rash B, Capilla J, et al. Sterol biosynthesis and azole tolerance is governed by the opposing actions of srba and the CCAAT binding complex. PLoS Pathog. 2016;12(7):e1005775.
223. Chang Yun C, Ingavale Susham S, Bien C, Espenshade P, Kwon-Chung Kyung J. Conservation of the sterol regulatory element-binding protein pathway and

its pathobiological importance in Cryptococcus neoformans. Eukaryot Cell. 2009;8(11):1770–9.
224. Zhang W, Yu L, Yang J, Wang L, Peng J, Jin Q. Transcriptional profiles of response to terbinafine in Trichophyton rubrum. Appl Microbiol Biotechnol. 2009;82(6):1123–30.
225. Kano R. ATP-binding cassette (ABC) transporter proteins in highly terbinafine-resistant strains of Trichophyton indotineae (former species name: Trichophyton interdigitale). Med Mycol. 2021;62(1):21–5.
226. Martins MP, Franceschini ACC, Jacob TR, Rossi A, Martinez-Rossi NM. Compensatory expression of multidrug-resistance genes encoding ABC transporters in dermatophytes. J Med Microbiol. 2016;65(7):605–10.
227. Caplan AS, Todd GC, Zhu Y, Sikora M, Akoh CC, Jakus J, et al. Clinical course, antifungal susceptibility, and genomic sequencing of Trichophyton indotineae. JAMA Dermatol. 2024;160(7):701–9.
228. Haghani I, Babaie M, Hoseinnejad A, Rezaei-Matehkolaei A, Mofarrah R, Yahyazadeh Z, et al. High prevalence of terbinafine resistance among Trichophyton mentagrophytes/T. Interdigitale species complex, a cross-sectional study from 2021 to 2022 in northern parts of Iran. Mycopathologia. 2024;189(4):52.
229. Saunte DML, Hare RK, Jørgensen KM, Jørgensen R, Deleuran M, Zachariae CO, et al. Emerging terbinafine resistance in Trichophyton: clinical characteristics, squalene epoxidase gene mutations, and a reliable EUCAST method for detection. Antimicrob Agents Chemother. 2019;63(10) https://doi.org/10.1128/aac.01126-19.
230. Abastabar M, Babaei M, Mohammadi R, Valadan R, Javidnia J, Zaedi A, et al. Iranian national survey on tinea capitis: antifungal susceptibility profile, epidemiological characteristics, and report of two strains with a novel mutation in SQLE gene with homology modeling. Mycopathologia. 2023;188(5):449–60.
231. Kano R, Nojo H, Noguchi H. Genomic analysis of antifungal drug resistance induced in Trichophyton rubrum after prolonged culture with terbinafine. Mycopathologia. 2023;188(6):1079–83.
232. Rudramurthy Shivaprakash M, Shankarnarayan Shamanth A, Dogra S, Shaw D, Mushtaq K, Paul Raees A, et al. Mutation in the squalene epoxidase gene of Trichophyton interdigitale and Trichophyton rubrum associated with allylamine resistance. Antimicrob Agents Chemother. 2018;62(5) https://doi.org/10.1128/aac.02522-17.
233. Graminha MAS, Rocha EMF, Prade RA, Martinez-Rossi NM. Terbinafine resistance mediated by salicylate 1-monooxygenase in aspergillus nidulans. Antimicrob Agents Chemother. 2004;48(9):3530–5.
234. Santos HL, Lang EAS, Segato F, Rossi A, Martinez-Rossi NM. Terbinafine resistance conferred by multiple copies of the salicylate 1-monooxygenase gene in Trichophyton rubrum. Med Mycol. 2018;56(3):378–81.
235. Dudiuk C, Gamarra S, Jimenez-Ortigosa C, Leonardelli F, Macedo D, Perlin David S, et al. Quick detection of FKS1 mutations responsible for clinical echinocandin resistance in Candida albicans. J Clin Microbiol. 2015;53(7):2037–41.
236. Pham Cau D, Iqbal N, Bolden CB, Kuykendall RJ, Harrison LH, Farley MM, et al. Role of FKS mutations in Candida glabrata: MIC values, echinocandin resistance, and multidrug resistance. Antimicrob Agents Chemother. 2014;58(8):4690–6.
237. Garcia-Effron G, Lee S, Park S, Cleary JD, Perlin DS. Effect of Candida glabrata FKS1 and FKS2 mutations on echinocandin sensitivity and kinetics of 1,3-β-d-glucan synthase: implication for the existing susceptibility breakpoint. Antimicrob Agents Chemother. 2009;53(9):3690–9.
238. Perlin DS. Resistance to echinocandin-class antifungal drugs. Drug Resist Updat. 2007;10(3):121–30.
239. Garcia-Effron G. Rezafungin-mechanisms of action, susceptibility and resistance: similarities and differences with the other echinocandins. J Fungi. 2020;6(4):E262.
240. Papon N, Goldman GH. Unraveling caspofungin resistance in Cryptococcus neoformans. MBio. 2021;12(2) https://doi.org/10.1128/mbio.00156-21.

241. Mukaremera L. The Cryptococcus wall: a different wall for a unique lifestyle. PLoS Pathog. 2023;19(2):e1011141.
242. Iyer KR, Revie NM, Fu C, Robbins N, Cowen LE. Treatment strategies for cryptococcal infection: challenges, advances and future outlook. Nat Rev Microbiol. 2021;19(7):454–66.
243. Pianalto KM, Billmyre RB, Telzrow CL, Alspaugh JA. Roles for stress response and cell wall biosynthesis pathways in caspofungin tolerance in Cryptococcus neoformans. Genetics. 2019;213(1):213–27.
244. Stevens DA, Ichinomiya M, Koshi Y, Horiuchi H. Escape of Candida from caspofungin inhibition at concentrations above the MIC (paradoxical effect) accomplished by increased cell wall chitin; evidence for β-1,6-glucan synthesis inhibition by caspofungin. Antimicrob Agents Chemother. 2006;50(9):3160–1.
245. Rueda C, Cuenca-Estrella M, Zaragoza O. Paradoxical growth of Candida albicans in the presence of caspofungin is associated with multiple cell wall rearrangements and decreased virulence. Antimicrob Agents Chemother. 2014;58(2):1071–83.
246. Singh SD, Robbins N, Zaas AK, Schell WA, Perfect JR, Cowen LE. Hsp90 governs echinocandin resistance in the pathogenic yeast Candida albicans via calcineurin. PLoS Pathog. 2009;5(7):e1000532.
247. Cowen LE. Hsp90 orchestrates stress response signaling governing fungal drug resistance. PLoS Pathog. 2009;5(8):e1000471.
248. Prasad R, Rawal MK. Efflux pump proteins in antifungal resistance. Front Pharmacol. 2014;5:202.
249. Morschhäuser J. Regulation of multidrug resistance in pathogenic fungi. Fungal Genet Biol. 2010;47(2):94–106.
250. Gauthier C, Weber S, Alarco A-M, Alqawi O, Daoud R, Georges E, et al. Functional similarities and differences between Candida albicans Cdr1p and Cdr2p transporters. Antimicrob Agents Chemother. 2003;47(5):1543–54.
251. Smriti KS, Dixit BL, Gupta CM, Milewski S, Prasad R. ABC transporters Cdr1p, Cdr2p and Cdr3p of a human pathogen Candida albicans are general phospholipid translocators. Yeast. 2002;19(4):303–18.
252. Tsao S, Rahkhoodaee F, Raymond M. Relative contributions of the Candida albicans ABC transporters Cdr1p and Cdr2p to clinical azole resistance. Antimicrob Agents Chemother. 2009;53(4):1344–52.
253. Lohberger A, Coste Alix T, Sanglard D. Distinct roles of Candida albicans drug resistance transcription factors TAC1, MRR1, and UPC2 in virulence. Eukaryot Cell. 2014;13(1):127–42.
254. Paul S, Diekema D, Moye-Rowley WS. Contributions of both ATP-binding cassette transporter and Cyp51A proteins are essential for azole resistance in aspergillus fumigatus. Antimicrob Agents Chemother. 2017;61(5) https://doi.org/10.1128/aac.02748-16.
255. Fraczek MG, Bromley M, Buied A, Moore CB, Rajendran R, Rautemaa R, et al. The cdr1B efflux transporter is associated with non-cyp51a-mediated itraconazole resistance in aspergillus fumigatus. J Antimicrob Chemother. 2013;68(7):1486–96.
256. Meneau I, Coste AT, Sanglard D. Identification of aspergillus fumigatus multidrug transporter genes and their potential involvement in antifungal resistance. Med Mycol. 2016;54(6):616–27.
257. Cordeiro Rd A, Portela FVM, Pereira LMG, de Andrade ARC, de Sousa JK, Aguiar ALR, et al. Efflux pump inhibition controls growth and enhances antifungal susceptibility of Fusarium solani species complex. Future Microbiol. 2020;15(1):9–20.
258. Amatto IVS, Simões FAO, Garzon NGR, Marciano CL, Silva RR, Cabral H. Response of Fusarium oxysporum soil isolate to amphotericin B and fluconazole at the proteomic level. Braz. J Microbiol. 2024;55(3):2557–68.
259. Zhang R, Wiederhold N, Calderone R, Li D. Biofilm formation in clinical isolates of Fusarium. J Fungi. 2024;10(11).

260. Nett Jeniel E, David RA. Fungal biofilms: in vivo models for discovery of anti-biofilm drugs. Microbiol Spectr. 2015;3(4):10.1128/microbiolspec.mb-0008-2014.
261. Sav H, Rafati H, Öz Y, Dalyan-Cilo B, Ener B, Mohammadi F, et al. Biofilm formation and resistance to fungicides in clinically relevant members of the fungal genus Fusarium. J Fungi. 2018;4(1).
262. Weinstein MP, Lewis JS. The clinical and laboratory standards institute subcommittee on antimicrobial susceptibility testing: background, organization, functions, and processes. J Clin Microbiol. 2020;58(3) https://doi.org/10.1128/jcm.01864-19.
263. CLSI. History & impact: More than 50 years of laboratory leadership: The Clinical and Laboratory Standards Institute; 2025 [Available from: https://clsi.org/about/history-impact/
264. Berkow EL, Lockhart SR, Ostrosky-Zeichner L. Antifungal susceptibility testing: current approaches. Clin Microbiol Rev. 2020;33(3):10.1128/cmr.00069-19.
265. NCCLS. Reference Method for Broth Dilution Antifungal Susceptibility Testing of Yeasts; Approved Standard-Second edition. 940 West Valley Road, Suite 1400, Wayne, Pennsylvania 19087–1898 USA: NCCLS; 2002.
266. Alastruey-Izquierdo A, Melhem MSC, Bonfietti LX, Rodriguez-Tudela JL. Susceptibility test for fungi: clinical and laboratorial correlations in medical mycology. Rev Inst Med Trop Sao Paulo. 2015;57(Suppl 19):57–64.
267. CLSI. Reference method for broth dilution antifungal susceptibility testing of yeasts; Approved Standard. 3rd ed. Wayne: Clinical and Laboratory Standards Institute; 2008.
268. CLSI. Reference method for broth dilution antifungal susceptibility testing of yeasts. 4th ed. Wayne: Clinical and Laboratory Standards Institute; 2017.
269. Meletiadis J, Guinea J, Arikan-Akdagli S, Meijer EFJ, Meis JF, Arendrup MC. A multicentre study for determination of epidemiological cut-off values for Candida auris with EUCAST broth microdilution reference methodology. J Antimicrob Chemother. 2025;80:dkaf241.
270. Cusack TP, Ashley EA, Ling CL, Roberts T, Turner P, Wangrangsimakul T, et al. Time to switch from CLSI to EUCAST? A southeast Asian perspective. Clin Microbiol Infect. 2019;25(7):782–5.
271. Chryssanthou E, Cuenca-Estrella M. Comparison of the EUCAST-AFST broth dilution method with the CLSI reference broth dilution method (M38-A) for susceptibility testing of posaconazole and voriconazole against Aspergillus spp. Clin Microbiol Infect. 2006;12(9):901–4.
272. Chowdhary A, Singh PK, Kathuria S, Hagen F, Meis JF. Comparison of the EUCAST and CLSI broth microdilution methods for testing isavuconazole, posaconazole, and amphotericin B against molecularly identified Mucorales species. Antimicrob Agents Chemother. 2015;59(12):7882–7.
273. Pfaller M, Boyken L, Hollis R, Kroeger J, Messer S, Tendolkar S, et al. Comparison of the broth microdilution methods of the European committee on antimicrobial susceptibility testing and the clinical and laboratory standards institute for testing itraconazole, posaconazole, and voriconazole against aspergillus isolates. J Clin Microbiol. 2011;49(3):1110–2.
274. Pfaller MA, Castanheira M, Messer SA, Rhomberg PR, Jones RN. Comparison of EUCAST and CLSI broth microdilution methods for the susceptibility testing of 10 systemically active antifungal agents when tested against Candida spp. Diagn Microbiol Infect Dis. 2014;79(2):198–204.
275. Claudino ALR, Peixoto RF, Melhem MSC, Szeszs MW, Lyon JP, Chavasco JK, et al. Correlation between CLSI, EUCAST and Etest methodologies for amphotericin B and fluconazole antifungal susceptibility testing of Candida spp. clinical isolates. Pharmazie. 2008;63(4):286–9.
276. Astvad KM, Arikan-Akdagli S, Arendrup MC. A pragmatic approach to susceptibility classification of yeasts without EUCAST clinical breakpoints. J Fungi. 2022;8(2).
277. Arendrup MC, Guinea J, Meletiadis J. Twenty years in EUCAST anti-fungal susceptibility testing: progress & remaining challenges. Mycopathologia. 2024;189(4):64.

278. CLSI. Reference method for broth dilution antifungal susceptibility testing of filamentous fungi; approved standard. 2nd ed. Wayne: Clinical and Laboratory Standards Institute; 2008. p. 52.
279. EUCAST. EUCAST technical note on the method for the determination of broth dilution minimum inhibitory concentrations of antifungal agents for conidia–forming moulds. Clin Microbiol Infect. 2008;14(10):982–4.
280. Siopi M, Georgiou P-C, Pournaras S, Meletiadis J. Optimization of the EUCAST reference broth microdilution method for echinocandin susceptibility testing of aspergillus fumigatus. J Antimicrob Chemother. 2023;78(12):2830–9.
281. Ceballos-Garzon A, Holzapfel M, Welsch J, Mercer D. Identification and antifungal susceptibility patterns of reference yeast strains to novel and conventional agents: a comparative study using CLSI, EUCAST and Sensititre YeastOne methods. JAC Antimicrob Resist. 2025;7(2):dlaf040.
282. Durand C, Maubon D, Cornet M, Wang Y, Aldebert D, Garnaud C. Can we improve antifungal susceptibility testing? Front Cell Infect Microbiol. 2021;11.
283. EUCAST. Definitions of S, I and R: The European Committee on Antimicrobial Susceptibility Testing; 2019 [Available from: https://www.eucast.org/newsiandr.
284. Sanguinetti M, Posteraro B. Susceptibility testing of fungi to antifungal drugs. J Fungi. 2018;4(3)
285. Al-Hatmi AMS, Curfs-Breuker I, De Hoog GS, Meis JF, Verweij PE. Antifungal susceptibility testing of Fusarium: a practical approach. J Fungi. 2017;3(2)
286. Marinelli T, Kim HY, Halliday CL, Garnham K, Bupha-Intr O, Dao A, et al. Fusarium species, Scedosporium species, and Lomentospora prolificans: a systematic review to inform the World Health Organization priority list of fungal pathogens. Med Mycol. 2024;62(6):myad128.
287. Tsugita A, Okada Y, Uehara K. Photosensitized inactivation of ribonucleic acids in the presence of riboflavin. Biochim Biophys Acta Nucleic Acids Protein Synth. 1965;103(2):360–3.
288. Altamirano D, Martinez J, Leviste KD, Parel JM, Amescua G. Photodynamic therapy for infectious keratitis. Curr Ophthalmol Rep. 2020;8(4):245–51.
289. Kharkwal GB, Sharma SK, Huang Y-Y, Dai T, Hamblin MR. Photodynamic therapy for infections: clinical applications. Lasers Surg Med. 2011;43(7):755–67.
290. Torres-Hurtado SA, Ramírez-Ramírez J, Larios-Morales AC, Ramírez-San-Juan JC, Ramos-García R, Espinosa-Texis AP, et al. Efficient in vitro photodynamic inactivation using repetitive light energy density on Candida albicans and Trichophyton mentagrophytes. Photodiagn Photodyn Ther. 2019;26:203–9.
291. Arboleda A, Miller D, Cabot F, Taneja M, Aguilar MC, Alawa K, et al. Assessment of rose bengal versus riboflavin photodynamic therapy for inhibition of fungal keratitis isolates. Am J Ophthalmol. 2014;158(1):64–70.e2.
292. Halili F, Arboleda A, Durkee H, Taneja M, Miller D, Alawa KA, et al. Rose bengal– and riboflavin-mediated photodynamic therapy to inhibit methicillin-resistant Staphylococcus aureus keratitis isolates. Am J Ophthalmol. 2016;166:194–202.
293. Kriegl L, Egger M, Boyer J, Hoenigl M, Krause R. New treatment options for critically important WHO fungal priority pathogens. Clin Microbiol Infect. 2025;31(6):922–30.
294. Ceballos-Garzon A, Lebrat J, Holzapfel M, Josa DF, Welsch J, Mercer D. Antibiofilm activity of manogepix, ibrexafungerp, amphotericin B, rezafungin, and caspofungin against Candida spp. biofilms of reference and clinical strains. Antimicrob Agents Chemother. 2025;69(6):e0013725.
295. Hodges MR, Tawadrous M, Cornely OA, Thompson GR 3rd, Slavin MA, Maertens JA, et al. Fosmanogepix for the treatment of invasive mold diseases caused by Aspergillus species and rare molds: a phase 2, open-label study (AEGIS). Clin Infect Dis. 2025;
296. Vazquez JA, Pappas PG, Boffard K, Paruk F, Bien PA, Tawadrous M, et al. Clinical efficacy and safety of a novel antifungal, fosmanogepix, in patients with candidemia caused by Candida auris: results from a phase 2 trial. Antimicrob Agents Chemother. 2023;67(5):e0141922.
297. Guinea J. New trends in antifungal treatment: what is coming up? Rev Esp Quimioter. 2023;36 Suppl 1(Suppl 1):59–63.

298. Borba-Santos LP, Rollin-Pinheiro R, da Silva Fontes Y, Dos Santos GMP, de Sousa Araújo GR, Rodrigues AM, et al. Screening of pandemic response box library reveals the high activity of olorofim against pathogenic Sporothrix species. J Fungi. 2022;8(10):1004.
299. Jacobs SE, Zagaliotis P, Walsh TJ. Novel antifungal agents in clinical trials. F1000Res. 2021;10:507.
300. Hoenigl M, Arastehfar A, Arendrup MC, Brüggemann R, Carvalho A, Chiller T, et al. Novel antifungals and treatment approaches to tackle resistance and improve outcomes of invasive fungal disease. Clin Microbiol Rev. 2024;37(2):e00074–23.
301. Jacobs SE, Chaturvedi V. CAF to the rescue! Potential and challenges of combination antifungal therapy for reducing morbidity and mortality in hospitalized patients with serious fungal infections. Open Forum Infect Dis. 2024;11(11):ofae646.
302. Cui J, Ren B, Tong Y, Dai H, Zhang L. Synergistic combinations of antifungals and antivirulence agents to fight against Candida albicans. Virulence. 2015;6(4):362–71.
303. Combination treatment of 5% natamycin and 1% voriconazole in fungal keratitis: A prospective randomized double masked clinical trial [Internet]. 2017. Available from: https://clinicaltrials.gov/study/NCT03230058.
304. Borba-Santos LP, Reis de Sa LF, Ramos JA, Rodrigues AM, de Camargo ZP, Rozental S, et al. Tacrolimus increases the effectiveness of itraconazole and fluconazole against Sporothrix spp. Front Microbiol. 2017;8:1759.
305. Roudbary M, Branquinha MH, Santos ALS. Editorial: drug repurposing to fight resistant fungal species: recent developments as novel therapeutic strategies. Front Cell Infect Microbiol. 2025;15:1633037.
306. Zhu X, Chen Y, Yu D, Fang W, Liao W, Pan W. Progress in the application of nanoparticles for the treatment of fungal infections: a review. Mycology. 2024;15(1):1–16.
307. LaMastro V, Walker D, Liu J, Meng-Saccoccio T, Shukla A. Peptide-decorated liposomes enhance fungal targeting and antifungal drug delivery. Adv Funct Mater. 2025;n/a(n/a):2508570.
308. Wu Q, Cen F, Xie Y, Ning X, Wang J, Lin Z, et al. Nanoparticle-based antifungal therapies innovations mechanisms and future prospects. PeerJ. 2025;13:e19199.
309. Almehmady AM, El-Say KM, Mubarak MA, Alghamdi HA, Somali NA, Sirwi A, et al. Enhancing the antifungal activity and ophthalmic transport of fluconazole from PEGylated polycaprolactone loaded nanoparticles. Polymers. 2022;15(1).
310. Fernández de Ullivarri M, Arbulu S, Garcia-Gutierrez E, Cotter PD. Antifungal peptides as therapeutic agents. Front Cell Infect Microbiol. 2020;10:10.
311. Struyfs C, Cammue BPA, Thevissen K. Membrane-interacting antifungal peptides. Front Cell Dev Biol. 2021;9.
312. Ulrich S, Ebel F. Monoclonal antibodies as tools to combat fungal infections. J Fungi. 2020;6(1).
313. Rosario-Colon J, Eberle K, Xin H. Monoclonal antibodies targeting Candida disrupt biofilms and inhibit growth across global clinical isolates. iScience. 2025;28(5):112459.
314. Mendoza BJ, Zheng X, Clements JC, Cotter C, Trinh CT. Potency of CRISPR-Cas antifungals is enhanced by cotargeting DNA repair and growth regulatory machinery at the genetic level. ACS Infect Dis. 2023;9(12):2494–503.
315. Lightfoot JD, Fuller KK. CRISPR/Cas9-mediated gene replacement in the fungal keratitis pathogen Fusarium solani var. petroliphilum. Microorganisms. 2019;7(10)
316. Jacobowski AC, Boleti APA, Cruz MV, Santos KFDP, de Andrade LRM, Frihling BEF, et al. Combating antimicrobial resistance: innovative strategies using peptides, nanotechnology, phages, quorum sensing interference, and CRISPR-Cas systems. Pharmaceuticals. 2025;18(8):1119.

Fungal Infections of the Eyelids

4

Max Carlos Ramírez-Soto, Andrés Tirado-Sánchez, and Alexandro Bonifaz

4.1 Introduction

The eyelid is a complex anatomical structure, and its histological composition plays a critical role in its various functions, such as protecting the eye, maintaining the tear film, and facilitating blinking [1]. The eyelid skin is the thinnest in the body, making it more susceptible to damage and disease. The absence of subcutaneous fat in the eyelid skin distinguishes it from other skin areas. This layer contains the typical skin structures, including sweat glands and hair follicles, although the eyelids typically have fewer hair follicles. Orbicularis oculi muscle allows voluntary and involuntary closing of the eyelids. It plays an important role in blinking, which helps spread tears across the cornea, maintaining moisture and protecting against debris. It also contributes to facial expressions, especially those involving squinting or blinking. The tarsus is a firm, dense connective tissue structure that helps maintain the shape and structural integrity of the eyelid. It also houses the meibomian glands, which are critical for producing the lipid layer of the tear film, preventing evaporation of tears, and contributing to ocular comfort [2] (Fig. 4.1).

The palpebral conjunctiva is an important protective membrane. The epithelium of the conjunctiva is mostly cuboidal with goblet cells that produce mucin, a

M. C. Ramírez-Soto (✉)
Centro de Investigación en Salud Pública, Facultad de Medicina Humana, Universidad de San Martín de Porres, Lima, Peru

A. Tirado-Sánchez
Dermatology Service & Mycology Department, Hospital General de México "Dr. Eduardo Liceaga", Ciudad de México, Mexico

Internal Medicine Department, Hospital General de Zona 30, Instituto Mexicano del Seguro Social, Ciudad de México, Mexico

A. Bonifaz
Dermatology Service & Mycology Department, Hospital General de México, Ciudad de México, Mexico

M. C. Ramírez-Soto (ed.), *Fungal Eye Infections*,
https://doi.org/10.1007/978-3-032-19923-2_4

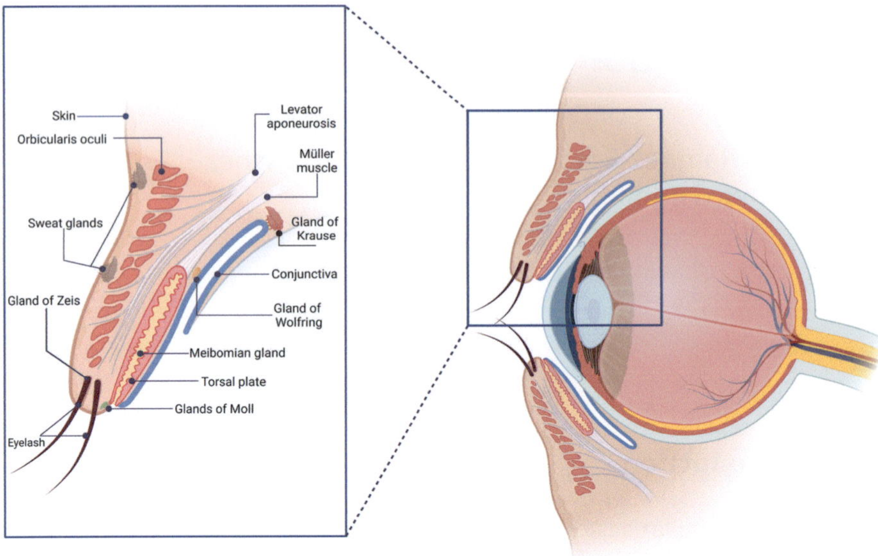

Fig. 4.1 Eyelid anatomy. Skin: the thinnest skin of the body, highly elastic. Orbicularis oculi muscle: a circular muscle responsible for blinking. Tarsal plate: provides shape and rigidity. Meibomian glands: secrete lipids to prevent evaporation of the tear film. Conjunctiva: a mucous membrane that lines the inside of the eyelid and covers the sclera. Orbicularis Oculi: closes the eyelid. Levator aponeurosis: raises the upper eyelid. Müller muscle: helping to raise the eyelid. Glands of Zeis: sebaceous glands at the base of the eyelashes. Glands of Moll: modified sweat glands near the lash follicles. Accessory Lacrimal Glands (Krause & Wolfring): contribute to tear production

component of the tear film that helps lubricate the eye and trap foreign particles [3, 4]. The substantia propria, or subepithelial stroma, consists of fibrovascular connective tissue that supports the conjunctival epithelium and harbors immune cells that help fight infection. The histologic structure of the eyelids is critical to both the diagnosis and treatment of disease. Each layer has a unique function, and changes within these layers—whether due to injury, disease, or tumor formation—can manifest as visible lesions on the eyelid.

The eyelid is the most exposed periocular structure to the surrounding environment and serves as the eye's first line of defense. Consequently, it is highly susceptible to pathogens, trauma, and noxious stimuli [5]. Eyelid infections may be confined to the anterior lamella, involve the full thickness of the eyelid, or extend to broader periocular or systemic infections. Given this broad spectrum, clinicians must be familiar with a wide range of infectious agents in order to accurately differentiate true eyelid infections from their mimics and to ensure effective treatment. This chapter discusses the epidemiological, clinical, diagnostic, and therapeutic features of eyelid mycoses.

4.2 Types of Eyelid Fungal Infections

Common eyelid conditions include marginal blepharitis (diffuse inflammation of the lid margins), hordeolum (localized acute infection of a meibomian gland), and chalazion, a non-tender inflammatory nodule that typically points toward the conjunctival surface [6–8]. Blepharitis and hordeolum are frequently associated with bacterial colonization by *Staphylococcus aureus* and are commonly managed by ophthalmologists, including those with oculoplastic expertise [6–8]. The subset of fungal infections involving the eyelids is a heterogeneous group of mycoses with diverse clinical presentations. This group includes superficial infections (dermatophytosis), subcutaneous infections (sporotrichosis), systemic infections (paracoccidioidomycosis, histoplasmosis, and cryptococcosis), and opportunistic infections (cryptococcosis, aspergillosis, candidiasis, and mucormycosis) [9–12]. These palpebral mycoses are difficult to diagnose and to differentiate from infectious and non-infectious conditions, potentially delaying accurate diagnosis, as no pathognomonic features have been consistently described. Therefore, a better understanding of their clinical characteristics is useful in the accurate recognition, differential diagnosis, and timely treatment of patients with these mycoses.

4.2.1 Superficial Infections

Fungal infections of the eyelid surface include blepharitis (chronic inflammation of the eyelid margins), tinea periocular (dermatophyte infection of the eyelid skin), including tinea blepharociliaris (dermatophyte infection involving the eyelid margins and eyelashes), and blepharoconjunctivitis (concurrent inflammation of the eyelids and conjunctiva). Preseptal cellulitis is an infection of the periorbital soft tissues located anterior to the orbital septum. Although it is not typically classified as a superficial mycosis, rare cases caused by dermatophytes have been reported and are discussed herein [9, 13–16].

4.2.1.1 Fungal Blepharitis

Blepharitis is an inflammation of the eyelid margins involving either the lash line (anterior blepharitis) or the meibomian glands (posterior blepharitis). Both forms are often associated with skin diseases such as seborrheic and atopic dermatitis and rosacea [13, 14].

Epidemiology Bacterial blepharitis is one of the most frequently encountered ocular surface disorders in clinical practice, whereas fungal blepharitis remains uncommon [13, 14]. The true prevalence of fungal blepharitis in the general population remains largely unknown due to limited epidemiological data. In a recent cross-sectional study conducted in Mexico among patients presenting with clinical signs of blepharitis, 33% had evidence of opportunistic fungal involvement, predominantly *Malassezia globosa* (31%), followed by *Candida albicans* (2%) [17]. Likewise, a study from Tunisia reported *Malassezia* spp. in 31.88% of patients with chronic blepharitis [18]. Although blepharitis may affect individuals across all age groups and ethnicities, it appears to be more frequently reported among young adults [17, 18].

Etiology and Pathogenesis Blepharitis is most commonly caused by bacteria such as *Staphylococcus aureus*, *S. epidermidis*, *Corynebacterium* spp., or among others. Fungal blepharitis is most commonly caused by opportunistic yeasts belonging to the species *M. globosa, M. furfur*, and *Candida albicans*; other species include *Penicillium* spp., *Cladosporium* spp., and dermatophytes such as *Trichophyton rubrum* [17–21]. *Malassezia* spp. are lipophilic yeasts that are part of the normal skin microbiota, especially in areas with sebaceous glands, such as the eyelids. These organisms depend on exogenous lipids for proliferation, and their enzymatic activity (particularly lipases and phospholipases) generates pro-inflammatory free fatty acids that have the potential to disrupt the tear film and irritate the eyelid margins. Overgrowth is often associated with conditions such as seborrheic dermatitis, chronic blepharitis, and meibomian gland dysfunction [22]. *Candida* species are commensal yeasts of mucocutaneous surfaces that can become pathogenic when local ocular defenses are compromised, for example, following prolonged topical corticosteroid or antibiotic use, contact lens wear, trauma, or in the presence of immunosuppression [19, 23].

Common Presenting Signs and Symptoms Based upon the etiological agent, blepharitis affects different structures in the eye [13, 14]. Regardless of etiology, the clinical manifestations of fungal blepharitis are often non-specific. Fungal blepharitis is a distinct etiology of anterior blepharitis, the clinical manifestations of which can mimic other more common forms of eyelid inflammation. Chronic symptoms are typically presented by patients, including pruritus, a burning sensation, and a foreign body sensation in the eyes. Upon clinical examination, the eyelids show classic signs of anterior blepharitis, characterized by erythema (redness), swelling, and tenderness of the eyelid margins. The inflammation caused by fungal pathogens, often *Malassezia* and *Candida* species, typically involves the eyelid skin, the base of the eyelashes, and the eyelash follicles (Fig. 4.2a, b). A key feature that distinguishes a fungal etiology is the chronic and recurrent nature of the condition, which typically demonstrates a poor or temporary response to conventional treatments for bacterial blepharitis, such as topical antibiotics and eyelid hygiene [17, 18, 22]. This limited therapeutic response frequently results in diagnostic delays and postponement of appropriate antifungal therapy. In advanced cases, fungal blepharitis may be associated with conjunctivitis, resulting in blepharoconjunctivitis or follicular conjunctivitis. Such presentations are uncommon but has been reported in infections caused by *Aspergillus* spp. [24] or *Trichophyton tonsurans* [25].

Diagnosis Blepharitis is generally diagnosed based on the patient's medical history and characteristic findings on slit-lamp examination. Common symptoms include redness, burning sensations, irritation, tearing, and eyelid crusting. Some

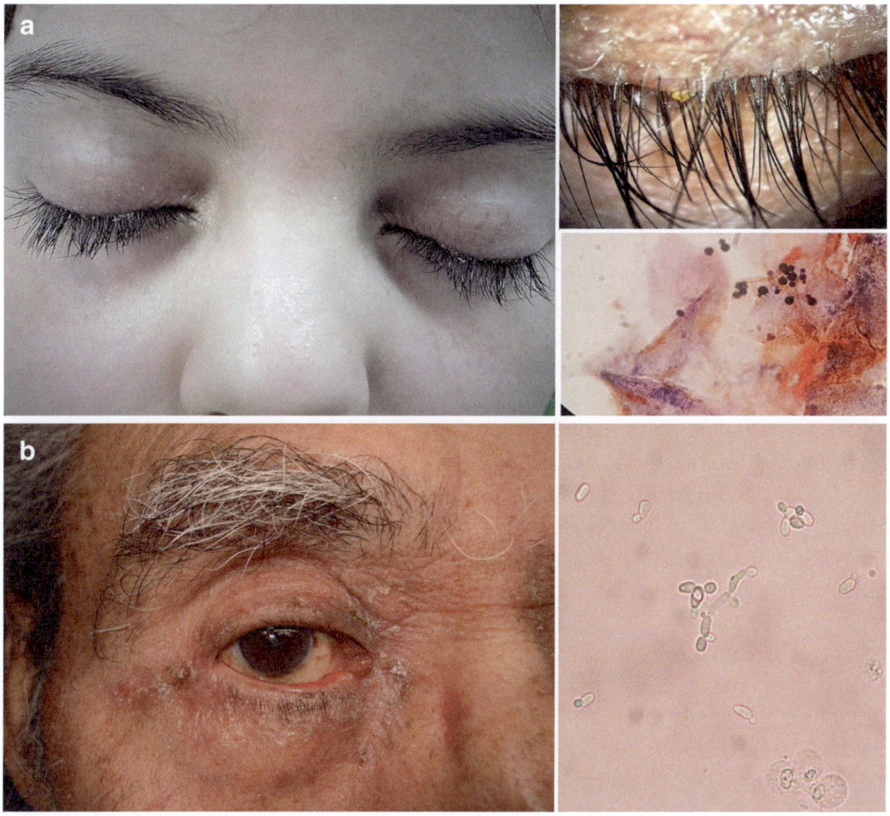

Fig. 4.2 Fungal blepharitis. (**a**) *Malassezia* sp. chronic blepharitis associated with severe seborrheic dermatitis (Courtesy of Jesús Heriberto Dávila-Alquisiras, Ophthalmology Service, Hospital General de México, "Dr. Eduardo Liceaga", Ciudad de México, Mexico). Multiple *Malassezia* sp. yeasts (Gram, 100×) (Courtesy of Sandra Miranda-Mauricio, Cd. Obregón México). (**b**) *Candida albicans* blepharitis. Direct examination with pseudohyphae and blastoconidia (KOH, 40×). (Courtesy of Prof. Alexandro Bonifaz)

patients may also report photophobia or blurred vision. Fungal blepharitis typically presents with erythema and swelling of the eyelid margins. In chronic or advanced cases, lash abnormalities such as madarosis or trichiasis may be observed. Long-standing or severe cases may be associated with eyelid ulceration and secondary corneal involvement, highlighting the importance of early recognition and appropriate management. To distinguish fungal blepharitis from bacterial or parasitic infections, the diagnosis relies primarily on characteristic clinical findings and may be confirmed by mycological testing. Direct microscopic examination of skin scrapings using potassium hydroxide (KOH) preparation may demonstrate fungal elements, including branched septate hyphae or yeast forms. Gram staining may also reveal fungal structures in selected cases. Fungal culture on Sabouraud dextrose agar enables isolation and definitive identification of the causative organism. Periodic acid–Schiff (PAS) staining can also demonstrate fungal elements in cases of chronic anterior blepharitis [26].

Differential Diagnosis In the differential diagnosis of fungal blepharitis, both infectious and non-infectious conditions must be considered. Infectious causes include bacterial diseases such as impetigo and erysipelas; viral infections due to herpes simplex virus, poxvirus, and varicella zoster virus; as well as parasitic infestations such as phthiriasis palpebrarum. Non-infectious etiologies encompass a broad range of immune-mediated disorders, including atopic and contact dermatitis, erythema multiforme, and pemphigus foliaceus, in addition to inflammatory dermatoses such as psoriasis, ichthyosis, exfoliative dermatitis, and erythroderma. Furthermore, benign eyelid tumors and traumatic lesions may mimic fungal blepharitis and should be carefully distinguished during clinical evaluation.

Treatment Fluconazole at a dose of 200 mg per day for 4 weeks, has demonstrated efficacy in patients with blepharitis caused by *Malassezia* spp. [27]. Topical ketoconazole has also shown favorable clinical outcomes [20]. In cases attributed to dermatophytes, oral itraconazole 100 mg daily for 2 weeks has been successfully [21].

4.2.1.2 Periocular Tinea

Dermatomycosis is a contagious fungal infection of the skin affecting both humans and animals. Dermatophytosis, also known as tinea, is a specific type of dermatomycosis caused by dermatophytes. These organisms are classified into three ecological groups, namely anthropophilic, geophilic, and zoophilic, according to their primary habitat and mode of transmission to humans [28]. In immunocompetent individuals, lesions are typically confined to the keratinized layers of the skin. Depending on the anatomical site involved, the infection is designated as tinea corporis, tinea pedis, tinea cruris, tinea capitis, or tinea faciei. In people with weakened immune systems, the infection may present as a more extensive or systemic disease [29, 30]. When the facial skin, including the periorbital area, is affected, the condition is referred to as periocular tinea, tinea palpebral or eyelid tinea [9]. Cases of tinea blepharo-ciliaris and tinea ciliaris have also been reported [15, 31–33].

Epidemiology Although periocular tinea is rare compared with tinea capitis or tinea faciei, cases have been reported in several countries. Most reports originate from tropical and subtropical areas where warm and humid climates favor dermatophytic infections including parts of Asia, Latin America, Africa, and Europe. In one study of 80 Indian patients with tinea incognita, eyelid involvement was documented in 48 cases, 40 of whom had positive KOH results [34]. Additional cases have been reported in the United States [9, 35, 36], Turkey [31], China [37, 38], Japan [39], Spain [40], Taiwan [41], Tunisia [42], Brazil [43], and Chile [44]. This condition primarily affects children (ages 3–16 years), young adults (ages 18–50 years), and older adults [9, 15, 31–44]. Among reported cases, contact with animal reservoirs such as dogs, cats, or rabbits was identified as the predominant mode of transmission.

Etiology and Pathogenesis The organisms responsible for periocular tinea vary by geographic region. Species of *Trichophyton* represent the predominant cause. Frequently reported species include *Trichophyton rubrum*, *T. verrucosum*, *T. mentagrophytes*, *T. tonsurans*, *T. interdigitale*, and *T. benhamiae*. Other reported dermatophytes include *Microsporum canis*, *Nannizzia gypsea (formerly M. gypseum)*, and *M. audouinii*. Rare cases caused by non dermatophyte molds, such as *Aspergillus fumigatus*, have also been described [15, 31–44]. Dermatophyte infections are typically confined to keratinized tissue; therefore, eyelid involvement usually represents extension from adjacent facial lesions. The eyebrows may also be affected [19]. Dermatophyte pathogenesis begins with conidial adhesion to keratinized tissues, followed by germination and production of keratinolytic enzymes. Fungal cell wall components modulate adhesion and host immune recognition, and clinical outcomes depend on the interplay between fungal virulence, host immune responses, and environmental factors. Anthropophilic species tend to cause chronic, less inflammatory infections, whereas zoophilic and geophilic species more often induce acute inflammatory responses. Immune evasion mechanisms contribute to persistence and recurrence [45–47].

Common Presenting Signs and Symptoms Periocular tinea presents with variable clinical manifestations. The incubation period ranges from 2 to 6 weeks following exposure. Eyelid tinea refers to a superficial fungal infection confined to the eyelid skin without involvement of the eyelashes and may elicit a significant inflammatory response. Periocular tinea is often bilateral and symmetrical and may also extend to adjacent facial areas. Clinical features include pruritus, erythema without pustules, scaling ranging from mild desquamation to hyperkeratosis, hyperpigmentation, and a burning sensation of the eyelids [9, 35–44] (Fig. 4.3a). In some cases, the infection may extend to the eyelid margin, resulting in eyelid tinea associated with blepharitis [31, 40]. Tinea blepharociliaris shares similar morphological features with eyelid tinea but involves both the eyelid and the eyelashes, leading to eyelid swelling and eyelash breakage. The condition most commonly presents as erythematous plaques with fine or prominent scales, small pustules, hyperkeratotic plaques, madarosis, and broken eyelashes or eyelash loss [15, 31–33, 48–50].

Although periocular tinea is generally benign, it is frequently misdiagnosed, particularly in cases with marked inflammatory responses. According to the published literature, several patients were initially treated for other condition, including eczema, herpes simplex, or cellulitis, before the correct diagnosis was established. These patients often received topical antibiotics and corticosteroids, including methylprednisolone, hydrocortisone, betamethasone, prednisolone acetate eye drops, or mometasone furoate. The inappropriate use of topical corticosteroids may alter the clinical presentation and delay accurate diagnosis.

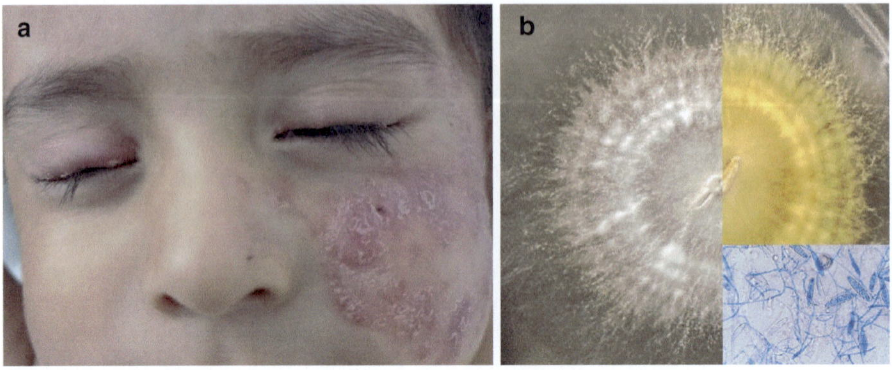

Fig. 4.3 Tinea palpebral. (**a**) Clinical presentation in a child showing an erythematous, scaly, annular plaque involving the periocular region and upper eyelid, associated with edema. The lesion exhibits the characteristic raised borders and central clearing typically seen in dermatophytosis. (**b**) Mycological culture on Sabouraud dextrose agar reveals the typical macroscopic morphology of *Microsporum canis*, with a white, cottony surface and a bright yellow reverse pigmentation. Inset: Lactophenol cotton blue preparation demonstrates the presence of spindle-shaped, thick-walled, rough macroconidia, a distinctive microscopic feature consistent with *M. canis*. (Courtesy of Prof. Alexandro Bonifaz)

Diagnosis Diagnosis is usually based on clinical findings and mycological examination. Direct microscopic examination of skin scrapings using KOH allows identification of fungal elements, such as branched septate hyphae or yeast forms. Fungal cultures on Sabouraud dextrose agar permits isolation and identification of the causative organism (Fig. 4.3b). Because culture results may require several days to weeks, empiric treatment may be initiated when the clinical presentation is consistent with periocular tinea.

Differential Diagnosis Atopic dermatitis, contact dermatitis, seborrheic dermatitis, periorbital cellulitis, ocular rosacea, angioedema, herpes zoster ophthalmicus, chalazion, demodicosis, and idiopathic orbital inflammation should be considered in the differential diagnosis of eyelid tinea and tinea blepharociliaris.

Treatment Topical antifungal therapy is the mainstay of treatment for localized eyelid tinea. More extensive disease or involvement of the eyelashes warrants antifungal therapy. Therapeutic options include systemic agents such as itraconazole, terbinafine, fluconazole, and griseofulvin, as well as topical agents including miconazole, ketoconazole, econazole, and clotrimazole for eyelid tinea and tinea blepharociliaris.

4.2.1.3 Preseptal Cellulitis

Preseptal cellulitis, also known as periorbital cellulitis, is an inflammation of the tissues located anterior to the orbital septum. It is typically a mild condition that rarely results in serious complications and is most commonly caused by bacterial infections, whereas fungal etiologies are extremely rare [51–53]. It typically presents with sudden onset of eyelid erythema, edema, warmth, and pain, while visual acuity and extraocular movements remain unaffected. Three cases of preseptal cellulitis due to dermatophytes have been reported. The first case involved a 10-year-old boy with a 15-day history of right eyelid pain, pruritus, photophobia, and vesicular lesions. Culture yielded *Trichophyton* spp., and the infection resolved after two courses of oral itraconazole [51]. The second case involved a 4-year-old girl presenting with a one week history of redness, swelling, and ulceration of the left upper eyelid, with vesicles beneath the eyebrow. Dermatophyte hyphae|were identified, and complete resolution followed treatment with griseofulvin [52]. The third case occurred in a 43-year-old man with erythematous lesions involving the right eyelids and cheek, associated with chemosis, conjunctival discharge, decreased vision, and vesicular ulcerative lesions on the hand. *T. mentagrophytes var. interdigitale* was isolated, and lesions resolved following treatment with topical miconazole and oral itraconazole [53].

4.2.2 Subcutaneous Infections

Subcutaneous mycoses are subacute or chronic infectious diseases of the skin and underlying structures, caused by a diverse group of fungi typically infect the host through traumatic implantation into the skin and subcutaneous tissue [54]. Several of these infections are classified as neglected tropical diseases. The most common subcutaneous mycoses include sporotrichosis, chromoblastomycosis, and eumycetoma. Eyelid involvement is uncommon and, when present, usually manifests as ulcerated lesions [10, 11].

Epidemiology Subcutaneous mycoses are endemic in tropical and subtropical regions due to the favorable environmental conditions particularly humidity and temperature, that support the growth and persistence of pathogenic fungi [54]. Palpebral sporotrichosis has been reported predominantly in tropical and subtropical areas [10, 55–58]. Most cases have been documented in hyperendemic regions, particularly in China and Peru [56–58], whereas Brazil, despite being recognized as a hyperendemic area, has accounted for comparatively fewer reported cases [59–61]. Sporadic cases have also been described in endemic areas such as the USA, Costa Rica, Japan, Argentina, Malaysia, and Australia [10, 55]. Transmission is typically associated with traumatic inoculation of contaminated plant material and contact with cats, particularly in Brazil, although a clear history of exposure is not identified in many cases [10, 55]. While palpebral sporotrichosis can affect individuals of all ages, children $\leq$15 years are most frequently affected, particularly in China and Peru [56–58]. To date, only three cases of palpebral eumycetoma have been reported: two pediatric cases in Sudan, a hyperendemic region, and one adult case in Canada [62, 63]. In these cases, the source of infection was not clearly identified. Additionally, only one case of chromoblastomycosis involving the eyelid in an older adult has been documented in Brazil [64].

Etiology and Pathogenesis The organisms that cause subcutaneous mycoses have distinct geographic distributions depending on the species [54]. Eyelid sporotrichosis is caused by species within the genus *Sporothrix*, particularly *S. brasiliensis* [10, 55, 61] and *S. globosa*. In most reported cases, *Sporothrix* has not been identified to the species level using molecular methods [10, 56–58]. The pathogenesis of sporotrichosis begins with traumatic inoculation of contaminated plant material containing *Sporothrix* species into the skin, followed by a thermally regulated dimorphic transition from the saprophytic hyphal form at 25 °C to the parasitic yeast form at 37 °C. This transition is essential for fungal growth, dissemination, and survival within mammalian tissue. Virulence factors, including adhesins, melanin, extracellular enzymes, and thermotolerance, contribute to colonization, persistence, and evasion of host defenses. The innate immune response involves macrophages, neutrophils, and activation of the inflammasome. The adaptive immune response is mediated by Th1 and Th17 pathways and is crucial for infection control. Among the species within the *Sporothrix* complex, *S. brasiliensis* is considered the most virulent [55]. The few reported cases of eyelid mycetoma have been caused by *Madurella mycetomatis* and *Scedosporium apiospermum* [62, 63].

Common Presenting Signs and Symptoms In eyelid sporotrichosis, the predominant clinical presentations are the lymphocutaneous and fixed cutaneous forms [56–58]. Eyelid involvement may occur as a primary localized lesion (fixed cutaneous) or as part of lymphocutaneous or disseminated cutaneous disease. Lymphocutaneous lesions typically begin as small subcutaneous nodules at the site of inoculation that subsequently ulcerate or spread along regional lymphatic channels [10, 56–58] (Fig. 4.4a–c). Fixed cutaneous lesions may present as nodular, papular, ulcerative, infiltrative, or mixed morphologies [10, 56–58] (Fig. 4.4d). Eyelid manifestations have also been described as granuloma annulare–like plaques, abscesses, and cyst-like lesions [10, 55]. In disseminated cutaneous infection, eyelid lesions may appear as clusters of papules and verrucous plaques. Clinical findings such as palpable lymphadenopathy or an ulcerated eyelid lesion in children or adults from hyperendemic or endemic regions for sporotrichosis are suggestive of palpebral sporotrichosis and may aid in differentiating it from other periocular infections [10, 55]. These lesions generally follow a less aggressive clinical course and can be cured with timely treatment.

In palpebral eumycetoma, eyelid sinuses with or without discharge and edematous swelling have been described, and in one reported case the patient was unable to close the eye [62, 63]. One reported case of chromoblastomycosis presented with severe ectropion and corneal exposure [64].

Diagnosis The diagnosis of sporotrichosis should be confirmed by isolation of *Sporothrix* species from clinical specimens, such as lesion aspirates or purulent discharge, on Sabouraud dextrose agar with or without antibiotics (Mycosel) agar.

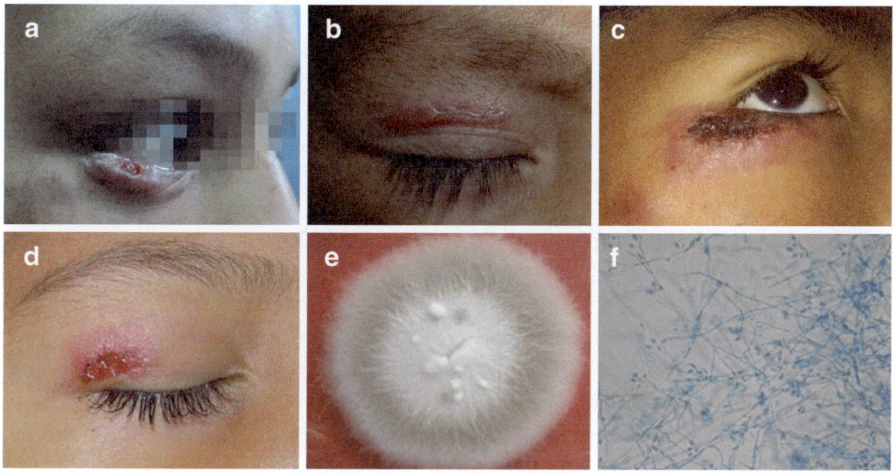

Fig. 4.4 Clinical forms of lesions observed in patients with eyelid sporotrichosis. (**a**) Lymphocutaneous form of the lower eyelid with indurated papule and adjacent nodules. (**b**) Fixed cutaneous form with granuloma-like plaque in the upper eyelid. (**c**) Lymphocutaneous form with ulceration in the right lower eyelid with palpable lymphadenopathy in the periocular region. (**d**) Fixed cutaneous form of the upper eyelid (reprinted from ref. 10 [published under a CC BY license]). (**e**) Macroscopic view shows a colony with filamentous growth on Sabouraud dextrose agar at 25 °C. (**f**) Microscopic view (lactophenol blue stain, ×40) shows hyaline hyphae and pyriform conidia in a flower-like arrangement

Cultures are incubated for 10–19 days at 25–28 °C, during which colonies initially appear white and progressively darken over time (Fig. 4.4e). Microscopic examination reveals septate, branched hyphae and characteristic sympoduloconidia (radulospores), typically arranged in a daisy-like or peach-blossom pattern [55, 65] (Fig. 4.4f). Fungal culture is the gold standard for diagnosis of eumycetoma. The causative fungus can be isolated on Sabouraud dextrose agar or Mycosel agar. The cultures are incubated at 25 °C–30 °C for 2–6 weeks. Colony morphology, including color and texture, together with microscopic characteristics, aids in species identification. Hematoxylin and eosin (H&E) staining reveals conidia embedded in tissue. Gomori methenamine silver (GMS) or periodic acid Schiff (PAS) stains highlight fungal hyphae. Polymerase chain reaction (PCR) assays can be used to identify the fungal species [66].

Differential Diagnosis Subcutaneous mycoses involving the eyelid can mimic a wide spectrum of infectious and non-infectious diseases. In endemic or hyperendemic areas, it is important to distinguish palpebral fungal infections from other endemic diseases including paracoccidioidomycosis, cutaneous blastomycosis, cutaneous coccidioidomycosis, cutaneous histoplasmosis, and cryptococcosis. Nonfungal conditions that should be considered in the differential diagnosis include chalazion, hordeolum, bacterial abscesses, and malignant eyelid tumors [10, 55].

Treatment In eyelid sporotrichosis, itraconazole is the drug of choice for lymphocutaneous and cutaneous fixed lesions. In cases of inadequate clinical response to itraconazole, terbinafine, fluconazole, or saturated solution of potassium iodide (SSKI) may be considered [10, 55–58]. Reported cases of eyelid eumycetoma have been successfully treated with ketoconazole and voriconazole [62, 63, 66].

4.2.3 Systemic Endemic and Opportunistic Infections Involving the Eyelid

Systemic mycoses are caused by primary and opportunistic fungal pathogens. Primary dimorphic pathogenic fungi can establish infection in immunocompetent hosts, whereas opportunistic fungi typically require an immunosuppressed host to cause disease. Primary deep fungal pathogens generally enter the body through the respiratory tract, while opportunistic fungi may gain access via the respiratory or gastrointestinal tract, or through intravascular devices [67, 68]. Among the primary dimorphic pathogenic fungi, *Paracoccidioides brasiliensis*, *Blastomyces dermatitidis*, *Coccidioides immitis,* and *C. posadasii* primarily affect the lungs, but may occasionally cause cutaneous infections, including involvement of the eyelid [69]. Of these, *P. brasiliensis* is the most frequently reported [70]. Among opportunistic fungi, *Mucor* spp., *Cryptococcus* spp., and *Aspergillus* spp. can also cause cutaneous infections with eyelid involvement, although such manifestations are rare [11, 69].

Epidemiology Most cases of paracoccidioidomycosis with eyelid involvement have been reported in Brazil, where the disease is endemic, with more than 50 cases documented since 1923 [70–76]. Additional cases have been described in Argentina, Venezuela, Mexico, Paraguay, and Colombia [70, 77, 78]. Eyelid blastomycosis has been reported in endemic regions of the US and Canada [79–86], whereas cases of eyelid coccidioidomycosis have been reported in the US, Mexico, and Guatemala [87–90]. Cutaneous mucormycosis involving the eyelid has been described in India, Spain, and the US [91–94]. Palpebral cryptococcosis has been reported in Brazil, China, and the Netherlands [95–97], and an ulcerated eyelid lesion caused by *Aspergillus* was described in the US [98]. These infections have been observed in both young and older adults, as well as in children; however, the specific risk factors associated with eyelid involvement remain incompletely understood.

Etiology The primary dimorphic fungi associated with eyelid infection include *P. brasiliensis*, *B. dermatitidis*, and *C. immitis/C. posadasii* [70–90]. Opportunistic pathogens implicated in eyelid involvement include *C. neoformans*, *Aspergillus* spp., and *Mucor* spp. [91–98].

Common Presenting Signs and Symptoms Although paracoccidioidomycosis, blastomycosis, and coccidioidomycosis are primarily pulmonary infections, all three may rarely manifest as primary cutaneous disease involving the eyelid. Their clinical presentations share several features, including indurated, verrucous, or ulcerated plaques often accompanied by crusting, erythema, and a chronic, slow-progressing course (Fig. 4.5a). Regional lymphadenopathy and conjunctivitis are more commonly described in paracoccidioidomycosis [70, 77, 78], whereas purulent or necrotic discharge and satellite lesions are more frequently associated with blastomycosis [79–86] (Fig. 4.5b). In contrast, coccidioidomycosis may present with draining sinuses and indurated nodules in addition to ulcerated or verrucous plaques [87–90] (Fig. 4.5c). Despite these differences, the overall chronicity and overlapping clinical features of these infections highlight the diagnostic challenge in distinguishing them from other eyelid pathologies.

Eyelid lesions due to *Cryptococcus* spp. are usually ulcerative. Necrotizing fasciitis of the eyelids and periorbital cellulitis due to *C. neoformans* have been reported [96, 97], while an eyelid nodule has been described as a sentinel lesion of disseminated cryptococcosis in a patient with AIDS [99]. Aspergillosis often involves the paranasal sinuses and predominantly presents in noninvasive forms, such as allergic sinusitis or aspergilloma. Eyelid aspergillosis has been observed to masquerade as invasive rino-orbital aspergillosis [100].

Diagnosis The diagnosis of primary cutaneous infections with eyelid involvement caused by dimorphic pathogenic fungi requires a high index of suspicion and is confirmed by direct microscopy, fungal culture, or histopathological examination. In histopathological analyses, granulomatous inflammation with broad-based budding yeast (hallmark of *Blastomyces*) is often reported. KOH preparation, PAS

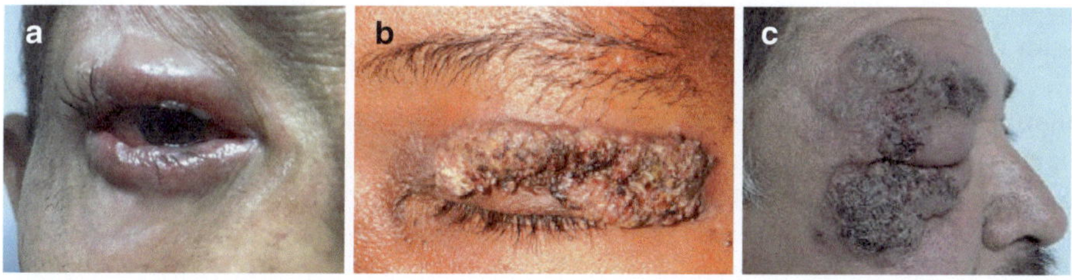

Fig. 4.5 Systemic endemic infections involving the eyelid. (**a**) Palpebral paracoccidioidomycosis. Severe right-eye edema and purulent secretion, consistent with blepharitis due to *Paracoccidioides brasiliensis*. Direct examination with lactophenol blue staining and culture from the eyelid biopsy were positive for *P. brasiliensis* (courtesy of Juan Cataño and Alexander Salinas, reproduced with permission; see also ref. 77). (**b**) Cutaneous blastomycosis of the eyelid. Progressive enlargement of a cutaneous lesion on the left upper eyelid over a 3-month period. Histopathological examination demonstrates fungal yeasts with thick walls and broad-based budding, highlighted by Periodic acid–Schiff and Gomori methenamine silver stains, consistent with blastomycosis (reprinted from Ophthalmology, 132/6, Levergood N, Miller Q, Klapper SR, A Rare Case of Cutaneous Blastomycosis of the Eyelid, Pages No. e111, Copyright (2024), with permission from Elsevier, ref. [79]). (**c**) Cutaneous coccidioidomycosis of the eyelid. Verrucous nodular plaques with edema and blood-crusted surfaces in the right periorbital (involvement of the upper and lower eyelid). Direct examination and culture were positive for *Coccidioides* spp. (reprinted from ref. 89 [published under a CC BY license])

stain, or GMS stain highlight yeast morphology (thick-walled fungal organisms with wide-based budding). Additionally, the fungus can grow in Sabouraud agar, however, this process takes several weeks. PCR and antigen detection (urine/serum) can assist diagnosis. *P. brasiliensis* is visible on H&E staining, but special stains such as PAS and GMS are useful in the diagnosis of the condition; gross and microscopic changes caused by *P. brasiliensis* are similar to those produced by the invasion of tissue blastomycosis and coccidioidomycosis organisms. The nonbudding yeast cells of *P. brasiliensis* may resemble *B. dermatitidis*; however, they show greater variation in size and shape, have thinner cell walls, and are not multinucleated [72]. Serologic tests indicate probable exposure to *C. immitis*, and elevated complement fixation titers suggesting dissemination [88].

Mucicarmine staining is a useful diagnostic tool in the diagnosis of cryptococcosis, as it allows for the identification of blastoconidia characterized by radiated capsules [96]. *Aspergillus* hyphae by their characteristic uniform size and dichotomous branching at approximately 45° can be seen on histopathological examination [100].

Differential Diagnosis Primary cutaneous eyelid infections caused by *P. brasiliensis*, *B. dermatitidis*, and *C. immitis* can mimic cutaneous tuberculosis, leishmaniasis, squamous cell carcinoma, other fungal infections, chalazion, or inflammatory lesions [72, 86, 88].

Treatment In mild cases of blastomycosis, itraconazole (200–400 mg/day) first-line therapy and should be administered for 6–12 months. In severe cases, induction therapy with amphotericin B is recommended, followed by step-down treatment with itraconazole or trimethoprim-sulfamethoxazole. Amphotericin B is also indicated for pregnant women or patients with central nervous system involvement. The mortality rate of untreated systemic disease approaches 60%, but decreases to approximately 10% with appropriate therapy [86]. In cases of paracoccidioidomycosis, the initial dose is 2.4 g sulfamethoxazole/480 mg trimethoprim daily (divided into three doses) for 6 months. Maintenance therapy includes 1.6 g of sulfamethoxazole plus 320 mg of trimethoprim daily (divided into two doses) for 2–3 years. Itraconazole (100 mg/day for 1 year) and ketoconazole (200–400 mg/day for 1 year) can also be used. Amphotericin B is reserved for severe cases resistant to the other drugs [70]. For eyelid coccidioidomycosis, oral azoles such as fluconazole or itraconazole with or without debridement may be necessary [88].

In immunocompromised patients, amphotericin B administered (1 mg/kg/day), followed by fluconazole (400 mg/day), is an effective treatment option. Eyelid lesions have been described in a patient with disseminated cryptococcosis [99]; the infection was controlled, with occasional recurrences, through a combination of surgical excision and intravenous amphotericin B and fluconazole. In cases of aspergillosis, surgical debridement combined with systemic antifungal therapy, such as intravenous amphotericin B or voriconazole, is recommended, followed by oral therapy with itraconazole or voriconazole [100].

4.3 Conclusion

Fungal infections of the eyelids are uncommon but clinically relevant conditions encompassing superficial, subcutaneous, and systemic mycoses with diverse presentations. Their rarity, overlapping manifestations with other periocular disorders, and lack of pathognomonic features frequently lead to misdiagnosis or delayed recognition. Therefore, familiarity with their epidemiological patterns, clinical spectrum, and diagnostic challenges is essential for clinicians involved in ocular care. Accurate diagnosis, ideally confirmed by mycological studies, is crucial for the timely initiation of antifungal therapy, which improves outcomes and prevents complications. Strengthening clinical awareness in endemic regions, enhancing diagnostic capabilities, and documenting additional case reports and series will further improve understanding and management of these rare but significant infections.

References

1. Ramesh S. Eyelid anatomy. In: Foundational papers in oculoplastics. Cham: Springer; 2022. https://doi.org/10.1007/978-3-030-92794-3_13.
2. Awh CA, Wilson MW. Basic histology of the eye and accessory structures [Internet]. EyeWiki; [citado 2025 Aug 8]. Disponible en: https://eyewiki.org/Basic_Histology_of_the_Eye_and_Accessory_Structures
3. Shumway CL, Motlagh M, Wade M. Anatomy, head and neck, eye conjunctiva. [Updated 2023 Aug 28]. In: StatPearls [Internet]. Treasure Island: StatPearls Publishing; 2025. Available from: https://www.ncbi.nlm.nih.gov/books/NBK519502/?utm_source=chatgpt.com
4. Leal SM Jr, Rodino KG, Fowler WC, Gilligan PH. Practical guidance for clinical microbiology laboratories: diagnosis of ocular infections. Clin Microbiol Rev. 2021;34(3):e0007019. https://doi.org/10.1128/CMR.00070-19.
5. Skalicky SE. Protective mechanisms of the eye and the eyelids. In: Ocular and visual physiology. Singapore: Springer; 2016. https://doi.org/10.1007/978-981-287-846-5_1.
6. Eberhardt M, Zeppieri M, Rammohan G. Blepharitis. [Updated 2025 Feb 3]. In: StatPearls [Internet]. Treasure Island: StatPearls Publishing; 2025 Jan. Available from: https://www.ncbi.nlm.nih.gov/books/NBK459305/?utm_source=chatgpt.com
7. Willmann D, Guier CP, Patel BC, et al. Hordeolum (Stye) [Updated 2024 Dec 11]. In: StatPearls [Internet]. Treasure Island: StatPearls Publishing; 2025. Available from: https://www.ncbi.nlm.nih.gov/books/NBK459349/?utm_source=chatgpt.com
8. Jordan GA, Beier K. Chalazion. [Updated 2023 July 31]. In: StatPearls [Internet]. Treasure Island: StatPearls Publishing; 2025. Available from: https://www.ncbi.nlm.nih.gov/books/NBK499889
9. Basak SA, Berk DR, Lueder GT, Bayliss SJ. Common features of periocular tinea. Arch Ophthalmol. 2011;129(3):306–9. https://doi.org/10.1001/archophthalmol.2011.14.
10. Ramírez-Soto MC, Tirado-Sánchez A, Bonifaz A. Ocular sporotrichosis. J Fungi (Basel). 2021;7(11):951. https://doi.org/10.3390/jof7110951.
11. Chang P, Moreno-Coutiño G. Periocular dermatoses. Int J Womens Dermatol. 2017;3(4):206–18. https://doi.org/10.1016/j.ijwd.2017.08.001.
12. Gervini RL, Vettorato G, Lecompte SM, Biasi TB, Ruthner FG, Kronbauer FL. Ocular paracoccidioidomycosis: report of two cases and review of literature. An Bras Dermatol. 2004;79:69–78.

13. Lin A, Ahmad S, Amescua G, Cheung AY, Choi DS, Jhanji V, et al. Blepharitis Preferred Practice Pattern®. Ophthalmology. 2024;131(4):P50–86. https://doi.org/10.1016/j.ophtha.2023.12.036.
14. Shtein RM, Jacobs DS. Blepharitis. UpToDate [Internet]. Waltham: UpToDate; [cited 2025 Sept 13]. Available from: https://www.uptodate.com/contents/blepharitis
15. Martínez-Ortega JI, Mut Quej JE, Medina Angulo TK. Tinea blepharociliaris: a case report and literature review. Cureus. 2024;16(12):e76308. https://doi.org/10.7759/cureus.76308.
16. Zeppieri M, Bourget D. Periorbital cellulitis. [Updated 2025 Feb 6]. In: StatPearls [Internet]. Treasure Island: StatPearls Publishing; 2025 Jan. Available from: https://www.ncbi.nlm.nih.gov/books/NBK470408/
17. Fierro-Arias L, Araiza J, Cortés D, Hernández MA, et al. Blepharitis associated to opportunistic fungi. Dermatol Rev Mex. 2014;58:134–41. [In Spanish]
18. Anane S, Anane Touzri R, Malouche N, El Aich F, Beltaief O, Zhioua R, et al. Which is the role of parasites and yeasts in the genesis of chronic blepharitis? Pathol Biol (Paris). 2007;55(7):323–7. [In French]. https://doi.org/10.1016/j.patbio.2007.03.005.
19. Klotz SA, Penn CC, Negvesky GJ, Butrus SI. Fungal and parasitic infections of the eye. Clin Microbiol Rev. 2000;13(4):662–85. https://doi.org/10.1128/CMR.13.4.662.
20. Derbel M, Benzina Z, Ghorbel I, Abdelmoula S, Makni F, Ayadi A, Feki J. Malassezia fungal blepharitis: a case report. J Fr Ophtalmol. 2005;28(8):862–5. https://doi.org/10.1016/s0181-5512(05)81007-1. French
21. Zhang C, Chen H. A case of blepharitis caused by Trichophyton rubrum. An Bras Dermatol. 2022;97(3):395–6. https://doi.org/10.1016/j.abd.2020.08.037.
22. Wang L, Deng Y. Malassezia species may play potential roles in the pathogenesis of meibomian gland dysfunction. Med Hypotheses. 2020;144:110137. https://doi.org/10.1016/j.mehy.2020.110137.
23. Mukai N, Takeichi Y, Yoshikawa Y, Tajiri K, Kida T. A case of a child with anterior blepharitis caused by Candida albicans: a case report. J Med Case Rep. 2025;19(1):94. https://doi.org/10.1186/s13256-025-05129-x.
24. Woldemariam M, Aklilu A, Manilal A, Mengistu M, Tadesse D, Siraj M, et al. Microbial profile and associated factors of external ocular bacterial and fungal infections in Arba Minch General Hospital: a cross-sectional study. Sci Rep. 2024;14(1):28744. https://doi.org/10.1038/s41598-024-77723-w.
25. Bothun CE, Decanini A, Bothun ED. Tinea blepharitis and follicular conjunctivitis in a child. J AAPOS. 2021;25(4):253–4. https://doi.org/10.1016/j.jaapos.2021.04.004.
26. Dadaci Z, Kılınç F, Ozer TT, Sahin GO, Acir NO, Borazan M. Periodic acid-Schiff staining demonstrates fungi in chronic anterior blepharitis. Eye (Lond). 2015;29(12):1522–7. https://doi.org/10.1038/eye.2015.144.
27. Zisova LG. Treatment of Malassezia species associated seborrheic blepharitis with fluconazole. Folia Med Plovdiv. 2009;51(3):57–9.
28. Chanyachailert P, Leeyaphan C, Bunyaratavej S. Cutaneous fungal infections caused by dermatophytes and non-dermatophytes: an updated comprehensive review of epidemiology, clinical presentations, and diagnostic testing. J Fungi (Basel). 2023;9(6):669. https://doi.org/10.3390/jof9060669.
29. Barac A, Stjepanovic M, Krajisnik S, Stevanovic G, Paglietti B, Milosevic B. Dermatophytes: update on clinical epidemiology and treatment. Mycopathologia. 2024;189(6):101. https://doi.org/10.1007/s11046-024-00909-3.
30. Li Q, Li J, Zhi H, Lv W, Sang B, Zhong Y, Chen X, et al. Epidemiological survey of 32,786 culture-positive dermatophytosis cases in Hangzhou from 2018 to 2023. Mycopathologia. 2024;189(6):98. https://doi.org/10.1007/s11046-024-00899-2.
31. Sahin GO, Dadaci Z, Ozer TT. Two cases of tinea ciliaris with blepharitis due to Microsporum audouinii and Trichophyton verrucosum and review of the literature. Mycoses. 2014;57(9):577–80.
32. Souissi A, Toukabri N, Jendoubi F, Jmour Y, Mokni M. Tinea ciliaris due to Microsporum canis. Presse Med. 2018;47(11–12 Pt 1):1030–2. https://doi.org/10.1016/j.lpm.2018.08.012.

33. Creach P, Auffret N, Buot G, Binet O. Teigne tondante ciliaire et blépharite à microsporum canis [Microsporum canis tinea ciliaris and blepharitis]. Ann Dermatol Venereol. 1995;122(11–12):773–4.
34. Ankad BS, Hurakadli SS, Chigurupati E. Dermoscopic distinction of tinea incognito on the face and topical steroid damaged face: a cross-sectional study in skin of color. Indian Dermatol Online J. 2024;15(6):949–54. https://doi.org/10.4103/idoj.idoj_57_24.
35. Amigo M, Milani-Nejad N, Mosser-Goldfarb J. Periocular tinea faciei. J Pediatr. 2020;221:255–6. https://doi.org/10.1016/j.jpeds.2020.02.031.
36. Huang WW, Tharp MD. A case of tinea versicolor of the eyelids. Pediatr Dermatol. 2013;30(6):e242–3. https://doi.org/10.1111/j.1525-1470.2012.01753.x.
37. Tian Y, Liao J, Luo S, Wang X, Zhang J, Zhang G, Long H. Image gallery: kerions involving the periorificial, perinasal regions, left upper eyelid and scalp: an unusual presentation of Trichophyton rubrum infection. Br J Dermatol. 2019;181(4):e89. https://doi.org/10.1111/bjd.18207.
38. Zhuang KW, Dai YL, Ran YP, Lama J, Fan YM. Tinea faciei on the right eyebrow caused by Trichophyton interdigitale. An Bras Dermatol. 2016;91(6):829–31. https://doi.org/10.1590/abd1806-4841.20165270.
39. Shimoyama H, Yo A, Makimura K, Sei Y, Kuwano Y. A case of tinea faciei due to Nannizzia gypsea: inflammatory eruption on the medial angle of the eyelid. Mycopathologia. 2020;185(4):699–703. https://doi.org/10.1007/s11046-020-00474-5.
40. Calles Monar PS, Juárez Martín A. Eyelid tinea with blepharitis due to Microsporum canis. Arch Soc Esp Oftalmol (Engl Ed). 2018;93(10):491–3. https://doi.org/10.1016/j.oftal.2018.04.005. English, Spanish.
41. Chen KL, Chien MM, Lu CY, Chiu HC. Zoophilic tinea faciei. J Pediatr. 2017;182:395–395.e1. https://doi.org/10.1016/j.jpeds.2016.12.040.
42. Amina A, Sana M. Tinea faciei incognito. Indian Pediatr. 2019;56(5):433. PMID: 31102391.
43. Machado AP, Hirata SH, Ogawa MM, Tomimori-Yamashita J, Fischman O. Dermatophytosis on the eyelid caused by Microsporum gypseum. Mycoses. 2005;48(1):73–5. https://doi.org/10.1111/j.1439-0507.2004.01053.x.
44. Urbina F, Sudy E. Tinea incognito. Piel. 2002;17(1):12–7. https://doi.org/10.1016/S0213-9251(02)72525-2.
45. Jartarkar SR, Patil A, Goldust Y, Cockerell CJ, Schwartz RA, Grabbe S, Goldust M. Pathogenesis, immunology and management of dermatophytosis. J Fungi (Basel). 2021;8(1):39. https://doi.org/10.3390/jof8010039.
46. Dubljanin E, Zunic J, Vujcic I, Colovic Calovski I, Sipetic Grujicic S, Mijatovic S, Dzamic A. Host-pathogen interaction and resistance mechanisms in dermatophytes. Pathogens. 2024;13(8):657. https://doi.org/10.3390/pathogens13080657.
47. Deng R, Wang X, Li R. Dermatophyte infection: from fungal pathogenicity to host immune responses. Front Immunol. 2023;14:1285887. https://doi.org/10.3389/fimmu.2023.1285887.
48. Buruiana AM, Mihali CV, Popescu C. Sequence-based identification of a zoophilic strain of Trichophyton interdigitale in a rare case of tinea blepharo-ciliaris associated with tinea barbae. Mycopathologia. 2015;180(5–6):403–6. https://doi.org/10.1007/s11046-015-9922-1.
49. Verzì AE, Lacarrubba F, Micali G. Trichoscopy of the eyelashes in tinea blepharo-ciliaris shows the full spectrum of tinea capitis features. JAAD Case Rep. 2020;6(7):661–2. https://doi.org/10.1016/j.jdcr.2020.05.009.
50. Wang FY, Sun PL. Tinea blepharo-ciliaris in a 13-year-old girl caused by Trichophyton benhamiae. J Mycol Med. 2018;28(3):542–6. https://doi.org/10.1016/j.mycmed.2018.05.002.
51. Velazquez AJ, Goldstein MH, Driebe WT. Preseptal cellulitis caused by trichophyton (ringworm). Cornea. 2002;21(3):312–4. https://doi.org/10.1097/00003226-200204000-00015.
52. Rajalekshmi PS, Evans SL, Morton CE, Williams RE, Ng CS. Ringworm causing childhood preseptal cellulitis. Ophthalmic Plast Reconstr Surg. 2003;19(3):244–6. https://doi.org/10.1097/01.iop.0000064989.80844.b8.
53. Kulkarni AR, Aggarwal SP. Preseptal cellulitis: an unusual presentation of Trichophyton interdigitale in an adult. Eye (Lond). 2006;20(3):381–2. https://doi.org/10.1038/sj.eye.6701848.

54. Queiroz-Telles F, Nucci M, Colombo AL, Tobón A, Restrepo A. Mycoses of implantation in Latin America: an overview of epidemiology, clinical manifestations, diagnosis and treatment. Med Mycol. 2011;49(3):225–36. https://doi.org/10.3109/13693786.2010.539631.
55. Ramírez-Soto MC. Extracutaneous sporotrichosis. Clin Microbiol Rev. 2025;38(1):e0014024. https://doi.org/10.1128/cmr.00140-24.
56. Zhang Y, Wang Y, Cong L, Yang H, Cong X. Eyelid sporotrichosis: unique clinical findings in 72 patients. Australas J Dermatol. 2016;57(1):44–7. https://doi.org/10.1111/ajd.12286.
57. Ramírez Soto MC. Sporotrichosis in the ocular adnexa: 21 cases in an endemic area in Peru and review of the literature. Am J Ophthalmol. 2016;162:173–9.e3. https://doi.org/10.1016/j.ajo.2015.11.015.
58. Fan B, Wang JF, Zheng B, Qi XZ, Song JY, Li GY. Clinical features of 10 cases of eyelid sporotrichosis in Jilin Province (Northeast China). Can J Ophthalmol. 2016;51(4):297–301. https://doi.org/10.1016/j.jcjo.2016.02.018.
59. Arinelli A, Aleixo A, Freitas DFS, do Valle ACF, Almeida-Paes R, Nobre Guimarães AL, Oliveira RVC, Gutierrez-Galhardo MC, Curi ALL. Ocular manifestations of sporotrichosis in a hyperendemic region in Brazil: description of a series of 120 cases. Ocul Immunol Inflamm. 2023;31:329–37. https://doi.org/10.1080/09273948.2022.2027465.
60. Ramírez-Oliveros JF, Casz Schechtman R, de Vries HJ, Lora L, Cardoso Arinelli A, da Costa Nery JA, Saraiva Freitas DF. Ocular adnexal sporotrichosis: a case series. JAAD Case Rep. 2021;13:52–6. https://doi.org/10.1016/j.jdcr.2021.04.019.
61. Gameiro Filho AR, Estacia CT, Gameiro RR, de Mattos Fonseca Vieira L, Socci da Costa D. Ocular and cutaneous sporotrichosis. Am J Ophthalmol Case Rep. 2020;20:100885. https://doi.org/10.1016/j.ajoc.2020.100885.
62. Ahmed-Hassan F, El Sheikh M, El Soura Mohamed EH, Ebtisam ET, Ahmed Mohamed EH. Eye eumycetoma: the mycetoma research centre case series. Infect Dis Clin Pract. 22(6):352–5. https://doi.org/10.1097/IPC.0000000000000157.
63. Zoroquiain P, Alghamdi S, Arthurs B, Levin L, Sheppard DC, Ralph B, et al. Eyelid mycetoma masquerading as sebaceous carcinoma. Ophthalmic Plast Reconstr Surg. 2017;33(3S Suppl 1):S101–4. https://doi.org/10.1097/IOP.0000000000000657.
64. Rios JE, Paiva CB, Paula GM, Figueiredo WR, Arantes JC, Almeida FM, et al. Chromomycosis, an unusual cause of cicatricial ectropion: a case report. Arq Bras Oftalmol. 2017;80(1):46–8. https://doi.org/10.5935/0004-2749.20170012.
65. Arenas R, Sánchez-Cardenas CD, Ramirez-Hobak L, Ruíz Arriaga LF, Vega Memije ME. Sporotrichosis: from KOH to molecular biology. J Fungi (Basel). 2018;4:62. https://doi.org/10.3390/jof4020062.
66. Zijlstra EE, van de Sande WWJ, Welsh O, Mahgoub ES, Goodfellow M, Fahal AH. Mycetoma: a unique neglected tropical disease. Lancet Infect Dis. 2016;16(1):100–12. https://doi.org/10.1016/S1473-3099(15)00359-X.
67. Bonifaz A, Vázquez-González D, Perusquía-Ortiz AM. Endemic systemic mycoses: coccidioidomycosis, histoplasmosis, paracoccidioidomycosis and blastomycosis. J Dtsch Dermatol Ges 2011;9(9):705–14; quiz 715. https://doi.org/10.1111/j.1610-0387.2011.07731.x. English, German.
68. Walsh TJ, Dixon DM. Chapter 75. Spectrum of mycoses. In: Baron S, editor. Medical microbiology. 4th ed. Galveston: University of Texas Medical Branch at Galveston; 1996. Available from: https://www.ncbi.nlm.nih.gov/books/NBK7902/.
69. Ramírez-Soto MC, Bonifaz A. Ocular fungal infections. J Fungi (Basel). 2022;8(10):1078. https://doi.org/10.3390/jof8101078.
70. Gervini R, Lecompte SM, Ruthner F, Vettorato G, Biasi T, Kronbauer F. Ocular paracoccidioidomycosis: report of two cases and review of literature. An Bras Dermatol. 2004;79(1):69–78.
71. Peruzzo J, Casagrande LC, Cartell AS, Maestri MK, Procianoy F, Procianoy PDC. Paracoccidioidomycosis simulating eyelid carcinoma. Arch Iran Med. 2022;25(3):194–5. https://doi.org/10.34172/aim.2022.33.

72. Odashiro AN, Odashiro PR, Fernandes PI, Leite LV, Odashiro M, Maloney S, Fernandes BF, Di Cesare S, Burnier MN Jr. Eyelid and conjunctival paracoccidioidomycosis simulating carcinoma. Int Ophthalmol. 2011;31(1):63–7. https://doi.org/10.1007/s10792-010-9407-7.
73. Cruz AA, Zenha F, Silva JT Jr, Martinez R. Eyelid involvement in paracoccidioidomycosis. Ophthalmic Plast Reconstr Surg. 2004;20(3):212–6.
74. Burnier SV, Sant'Anna AE. Palpebral paracoccidioidomycosis. Mycopathologia. 1997;140(1):29–33. https://doi.org/10.1023/a:1006803503033.
75. Belfort R Jr, Fischman O, de Camargo ZP, Almada A. Paracoccidioidomycosis with palpebral and conjunctival involvement. Mycopathologia. 1975;56(1):21–4. https://doi.org/10.1007/BF00493578.
76. Silva MR, Mendes RP, Lastória JC, Barraviera B, Marques SA, Kamegasawa A. Paracoccidioidomycosis: study of six cases with ocular involvement. Mycopathologia. 1988;102(2):87–96.
77. Cataño J, Salinas A. Ophthalmic Paracoccidioidomycosis. Am J Trop Med Hyg. 2017;97(6):1635. https://doi.org/10.4269/ajtmh.17-0613.
78. Zunino P, Arregui A, Fuentes M, Despouy E, Villgran E, Barciulli A. Ocular involvement in paracoccidioidomycosis. Optalmol Clin Exp. 2010;4(2):72–4.
79. Levergood N, Miller Q, Klapper SR. A rare case of cutaneous blastomycosis of the eyelid. Ophthalmology. 2025;132(6):e111. https://doi.org/10.1016/j.ophtha.2024.09.015.
80. Bartley GB. Blastomycosis of the eyelid. Ophthalmology. 1995;102(12):2020–3. https://doi.org/10.1016/s0161-6420(95)30760-9.
81. Pariseau B, Lucarelli MJ, Appen RE. A concise history of ophthalmic blastomycosis. Ophthalmology. 2007;114(11):e27–32. https://doi.org/10.1016/j.ophtha.2007.05.048.
82. Pemberton JD, Vidor I, Sivak-Callcott JA, Bailey NG, Sarwari AR. North American blastomycosis of the eyelid. Ophthalmic Plast Reconstr Surg. 2009;25(3):230–2. https://doi.org/10.1097/IOP.0b013e3181a3038d.
83. Phelps PO, Seagrave Z, Williams KM. Blastomycosis in the eyelid of a native Chicagoan. Ophthalmology. 2015;122(5):1015. https://doi.org/10.1016/j.ophtha.2014.12.021.
84. Schmutz JS, Ramey NA, Gauthier GM, Lucarelli MJ. Severe oculofacial sequelae of cutaneous Blastomyces dermatitidis. Ophthalmic Plast Reconstr Surg. 2016;32(3):e61–2. https://doi.org/10.1097/IOP.0000000000000245.
85. Safneck JR, Hogg GR, Napier LB. Endophthalmitis due to Blastomyces dermatitidis. Case report and review of the literature. Ophthalmology. 1990;97(2):212–6. https://doi.org/10.1016/s0161-6420(90)32604-0.
86. Rodriguez RC, Cornock E, White VA, Dolman PJ. Eyelid blastomycosis in British Columbia. Can J Ophthalmol. 2012;47(3):e1–2. https://doi.org/10.1016/j.jcjo.2012.03.008.
87. Faulkner RF. Ocular coccidioidomycosis. Report of a case of coccidioidal granuloma of the conjunctiva associated with cutaneous coccidioidomycosis. Am J Ophthalmol. 1962;53:822–7.
88. Ugurlu S, de Alba Campomanes AG, Naseri A, Blair JE, McLeish WM. Coccidioidomycosis of the eyelid. Ophthalmic Plast Reconstr Surg. 2005;21(2):157–9. https://doi.org/10.1097/01.iop.0000155854.21746.49.
89. Moreno-Coutiño G, Arce-Ramírez M, Medina A, Amarillas-Villalva A, Salas-Vargas V, Madrigal-Kazem R, et al. Cutaneous coccidioidomycoses: six Mexican cases report. Rev Chilena Infectol. 2015;32(3):339–43. https://doi.org/10.4067/S0716-10182015000400014. Spanish.
90. Dworak DP, Kapustiak J, Ehklassi TA, Patrianakos TD. Primary cutaneous coccidioidomycosis of the eyelid: a case report. Ophthalmic Plast Reconstr Surg. 2016;32(2):e40–1. https://doi.org/10.1097/IOP.0000000000000224.
91. Obón B, Zalba B, López C, Gutiérrez I, Villanueva B, González J. Exoftalmos y ptosis palpebral en paciente inmunodeprimido. An Med Interna (Madrid). 2003;20(6):309–11.
92. Chawla B, Sharma S, Kashyap S, Kabra SK, Pushker N, Bajaj MS. Primary orbital mycosis in immunocompetent infants. J AAPOS. 2011;15(2):211–3. https://doi.org/10.1016/j.jaapos.2010.12.016.

93. Zaman K, Kaur H, Rudramurthy SM, Singh M, Parashar A, Chakrabarti A. Cutaneous mucormycosis of scalp and eyelids in a child with type I diabetes mellitus. Indian J Dermatol Venereol Leprol. 2015;81(3):275–8. https://doi.org/10.4103/0378-6323.152740.
94. Smith LD, Ahmad M, Ashraf DC, Kersten RC, Winn BJ, Grob SR, et al. Cutaneous mucormycosis of the eyelid treated with subcutaneous liposomal amphotericin B injections. Ophthalmic Plast Reconstr Surg. 2024;40(2):e42–5. https://doi.org/10.1097/IOP.0000000000002545.
95. Doorenbos-Bot AC, Hooymans JM, Blanksma LJ. Periorbital necrotising fasciitis due to Cryptococcus neoformans in a healthy young man. Doc Ophthalmol. 1990;75(3–4):315–20. https://doi.org/10.1007/BF00164845.
96. Souza MB, Melo CS, Silva CS, Santo RM, Matayoshi S. Criptococose palpebral: relato de caso [Palpebral cryptococcosis: case report]. Arq Bras Oftalmol. 2006;69(2):265–7. Portuguese. https://doi.org/10.1590/s0004-27492006000200024.
97. Han G, Kwon SH, Song HJ, Jeon J. Disseminated cryptococcosis presenting as cellulitis. Indian J Dermatol Venereol Leprol. 2017;83(1):89–91. https://doi.org/10.4103/0378-6323.192959.
98. Gupta R, Hari P, Anandula V. Eyelid fungal infections are rare, and often associated with predisposing factors. We present the case of a child with an ulcerated lesion of fungal etiology on the eyelid. Can J Ophthalmol. 2017;52(1):e28–9. https://doi.org/10.1016/j.jcjo.2016.08.002.
99. Coccia L, Calista D, Boschini A. Eyelid nodule: a sentinel lesion of disseminated cryptococcosis in a patient with acquired immunodeficiency syndrome. Arch Ophthalmol. 1999;117(2):271–2. PMID: 10037581.
100. Rafizadeh SM, Mousavi A, Rajabi MT, Aghajani A, Nozarian Z, Zand A. Invasive bony destructive orbital aspergillosis in an immunocompetent child: a case report. J Ophthalmic Inflamm Infect. 2025;15(1):30. https://doi.org/10.1186/s12348-025-00485-7.

Fungal Infections of the Lacrimal System

5

Kun Shan and Jiaxu Hong

5.1 Introduction

The lacrimal apparatus is divided into the secretory portion (lacrimal gland, accessory lacrimal glands) and the excretory portion (puncta lacrimalia, lacrimal canal, lacrimal sac, nasolacrimal duct) (Fig. 5.1). The lacrimal system infections can be anatomically categorized into canaliculitis and dacryocystitis, with marked age-related epidemiological variations. The overall incidence in adults is approximately 0.02%, whereas pediatric populations exhibit a significantly higher prevalence of 5–10%, with nearly 95% of affected infants presenting symptoms within the first month of life, often attributable to neonatal dacryocystitis secondary to developmental anomalies of the nasolacrimal duct [1, 2]. Compared to bacterial infections, fungal lacrimal infections are exceedingly rare yet pose far greater clinical risks. Characterized by chronic, indolent progression, these infections frequently manifest with nonspecific symptoms (e.g., recurrent epiphora, discharge), leading to misdiagnosis as routine conjunctivitis or bacterial dacryocystitis and consequent diagnostic delays. Critically, fungal pathogens such as *Aspergillus* spp. and *Mucor* spp. exhibit unique tissue-invasive properties, capable of directly invading sinonasal mucosa, eroding osseous structures, or disseminating along skull base neurovascular pathways. This can precipitate catastrophic complications, including invasive sinusitis, orbital cellulitis, and intracranial infections [3, 4]. Early recognition and intervention are pivotal to improving outcomes. Clinicians must maintain a high index of suspicion for chronic lacrimal inflammation in high-risk populations (e.g., diabetes mellitus, immunocompromised states, prolonged corticosteroid use), integrating microbiological cultures, molecular diagnostics, and advanced imaging modalities for timely pathogen identification. Concurrent patient education is essential to mitigate the tendency to overlook symptoms due to their subtlety. This

K. Shan · J. Hong (✉)
Department of Ophthalmology, Eye and ENT Hospital, Fudan University, Shanghai, China
e-mail: Jiaxu.hong@fdeent.org

M. C. Ramírez-Soto (ed.), *Fungal Eye Infections*,
https://doi.org/10.1007/978-3-032-19923-2_5

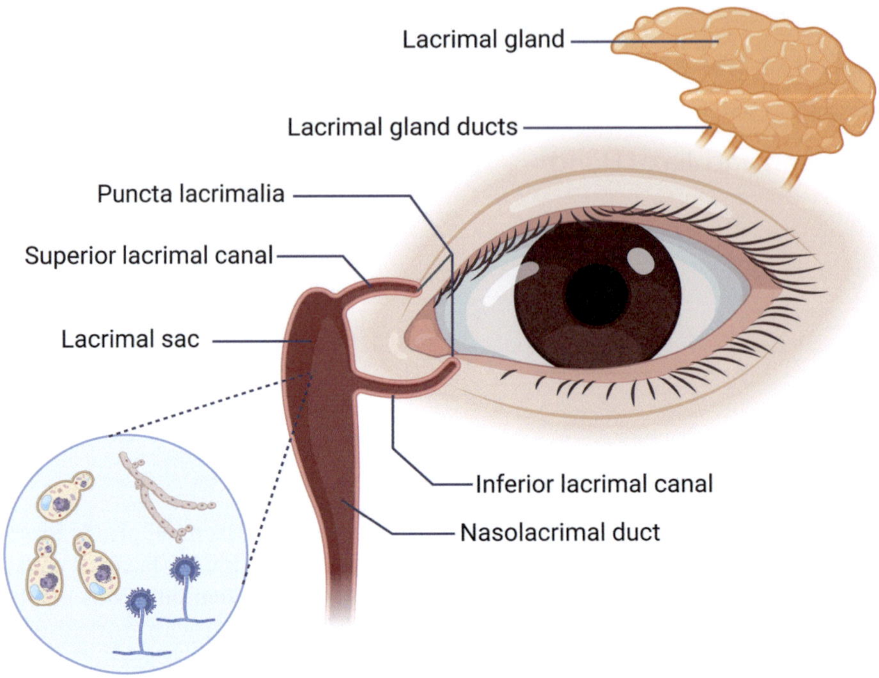

Fig. 5.1 The anatomy of the lacrimal apparatus

chapter systematically elucidates the pathogenesis, diagnostic algorithms, and therapeutic approaches in fungal lacrimal infections, aiming to establish evidence-based frameworks for reducing disability and mortality risks associated with these under-recognized yet potentially devastating infections.

5.2 Epidemiology, Etiology, and Risk Factors

Fungal canaliculitis and dacryocystitis represent rare subtypes of lacrimal infections, with their epidemiological profiles remaining poorly characterized due to limited systematic research. Current regional data suggest a higher incidence of fungal lacrimal infections in Asian countries (e.g., China, India) compared to Western populations, likely attributed to environmental exposures or geographic variations in pathogen distribution [5–7]. A large multicenter Chinese study (n = 15,452) reported a fungal infection rate of 4.7% in dacryocystitis patients, with *A. flavus* (1.8%), yeasts (1.5%), and *C. parapsilosis* (1.4%) as predominant pathogens [7]. In Northern China, a retrospective analysis of 477 lacrimal infections showed fungal involvement in 2.4% of cases, primarily presenting as chronic dacryocystitis (1.6%) and acute dacryocystitis (0.8%), with no fungal canaliculitis observed; *C. parapsilosis* and *C. albicans* were dominant isolates, accompanied by conditional pathogens including *Fusarium* spp. and *A. flavus* [8]. Central China data revealed fungal infection rates of 2.7% in adults versus 7.44% in children with dacryocystitis, with *C. parapsilosis* being the primary isolate in both groups; no significant gender-based pathogen distribution difference was noted despite higher overall dacryocystitis incidence in females [9]. Northwestern Iranian studies demonstrated a 10.4% fungal infection rate in dacryocystitis, predominantly *Candida* spp. (especially *C. albicans*) and *Aspergillus* spp. [6]. Indian research documented fungal colonization in 30% of congenital dacryocystitis cases, chiefly *C. albicans* and *A. niger* [10]. In view of this, current epidemiological insights are predominantly derived from regional, small-scale studies. Establishing global multicenter collaborations is imperative to refine disease burden estimates and elucidate pathogen diversity.

Despite heterogeneity across studies in sample size, geographic distribution, socioeconomic factors, and public health awareness, comprehensive analysis indicates that fungal dacryocystitis predominantly manifests as chronic dacryocystitis. Infection rates in adults are generally low (typically <5%), while pediatric cases show significantly higher prevalence, ranging from 7% to 30%. The mycological spectrum is dominated by *Candida* spp. and *Aspergillus* spp., with rare cases attributed to *Rhizopus* spp. and *Alternaria* spp. [11, 12]. Sporotrichotic dacryocystitis caused by *Sporothrix schenckii* has been exceptionally rarely reported, primarily in hyperendemic regions of Brazil [13, 14]. Notably, the conjunctival sac in healthy individuals harbors fungal carriage rates below 5%, with commensal colonization primarily by Ascomycota fungi including *Aspergillus* spp., *Rhodotorula* spp., and *Penicillium* spp. [10, 15]. *Cladosporium* spp., *Penicillium* spp., *Aspergillus* spp., and *Alternaria* spp. can also be isolated from the nasal passages of healthy subjects [16]. The mechanisms governing their transition to pathogenic states require further investigation.

Host immunocompetence is a critical determinant of infection risk, with advanced age, diabetes mellitus, immunosuppressant/corticosteroid use, prior lacrimal surgery, and neutropenia identified as established risk factors [12]. Additionally, hematologic malignancies, HIV infection, and organ transplant recipients are disproportionately vulnerable to invasive fungal disease. Exposure to animals infected with fungal diseases constitutes an independent risk factor. Contact with cats infected with sporotrichosis, for instance, can lead to *Sporothrix* dacryocystitis via nasal inhalation of pathogen-containing aerosols, with children demonstrating a significantly increased risk for this clinical manifestation [13].

5.3 Pathogenesis

The pathogenesis of fungal lacrimal infections encompasses three interrelated pathological pathways: direct colonization and invasion, obstruction-driven fungal proliferation, and immune dysregulation-mediated tissue destruction. Fungal spores initially penetrate the lacrimal punctum, breach anatomical barriers, and adhere to mucosal surfaces, where they establish persistent infection foci by triggering localized inflammatory cascades. Concurrently, mechanical obstruction (e.g., dacryolithiasis, stenosis, or atresia) induces tear stasis, altering the local microenvironment (pH, oxygen tension, and nutrient availability) to favor spore adhesion, hyphal differentiation, and biofilm formation, thereby accelerating fungal proliferation and dissemination. Furthermore, compromised host immunity (e.g., immunosuppression or immunodeficiency) disrupts mucosal defenses, enabling fungi to secrete extracellular proteases (e.g., elastase, phospholipases) that degrade host tissues while evading immune clearance through biofilm-mediated drug resistance, ultimately leading to invasive infections and structural damage [17]. Critically, biofilm formation not only enhances fungal adhesion to the lacrimal epithelium but also impedes antifungal drug penetration, exacerbating therapeutic challenges. These mechanisms synergistically drive the pathological transition from localized infection to invasive, tissue-destructive disease.

5.4 Clinical Presentation

Fungal infections of the lacrimal system are categorized into canaliculitis and dacryocystitis, characterized by distinct clinical presentations (Table 5.1). Fungal canaliculitis typically presents with a protracted clinical course, often manifesting insidiously over weeks to months. The cardinal symptom is mild to moderate epiphora, primarily resulting from canalicular obstruction. Characteristic signs include punctual erythema and swelling, palpable nodular swelling along the canaliculus with minimal tenderness, and expressible white, flocculent, or granular discharge that tends to adhere around the punctum and may form mycelial masses. Secondary conjunctivitis may develop, and prolonged infection can lead to canalicular stenosis or obliteration.

Fungal dacryocystitis is categorized into acute and chronic forms. The acute presentation is rare and clinically resembles bacterial dacryocystitis, while chronic fungal dacryocystitis represents the predominant reported form. Chronic fungal dacryocystitis manifests with insidious onset and persistent epiphora, with symptoms progressing gradually over weeks, months, or even years. Local signs include

Table 5.1 Differentiation between fungal canaliculitis and dacryocystitis

	Fungal canaliculitis	Fungal dacryocystitis
Onset	Chronic, insidious; duration weeks-months	Acute or chronic; acute mimics bacterial
Local signs	Punctal erythema/swelling; expressible discharge; palpable nodular canalicular swelling; mild tenderness	Lacrimal sac swelling; acute: erythema/pain; chronic: expressible copious discharge
Discharge character	White, flocculent/granular; adheres to punctum; may contain mycelial masses	Mucoid, purulent, or cheesy; copious; may contain fungal spores/hyphae
Epiphora	Mild to moderate (due to canalicular obstruction)	Persistent (more prominent in chronic phase)
Complications	Secondary conjunctivitis; chronic may cause canalicular stenosis/obliteration	Acute: abscess formation; chronic: keratitis, endophthalmitis, orbital cellulitis

Table 5.2 Differentiation between acute and chronic fungal dacryocystitis

	Acute dacryocystitis	Chronic dacryocystitis
Onset	Acute (symptoms evident within hours to 1–2 days)	Insidious; symptoms progress gradually over weeks, months, or even years
Local signs	Erythema, intense pain, and swelling over lacrimal sac; may form abscess; skin warmth and marked tenderness; severe cases may involve eyelid/facial swelling	No significant erythema/swelling or mild swelling only; copious discharge expressible from punctum upon sac compression
Epiphora	Marked tearing with increased discharge	Persistent, long-term epiphora
Systemic symptoms	May present with fever, malaise	Generally absent
Complications	May include orbital cellulitis, sepsis	Systemic complications rare; chronic inflammation may lead to keratitis, conjunctivitis, cutaneous fistula; invasive fungal infections may result in orbital cellulitis or even intracranial dissemination

minimal or mild swelling over the lacrimal sac area, with copious discharge expressible from the punctum upon sac compression. Systemic complications are infrequent; however, chronic inflammation may lead to keratitis, conjunctivitis, and in some cases, is accompanied by nasal mucosal bleeding (Table 5.2). Fungi such as *Alternaria* spp. may induce cutaneous fistula formation, particularly in predisposed populations like diabetics [11]. Patients with sporotrichosis can develop facial nodular ulcerated lesions, granulomatous conjunctivitis, and cutaneous fistulas along with dacryocystitis [13]. Notably, highly invasive pathogens such as *Aspergillus* spp. and *Mucor* spp. can cause local tissue destruction, exhibiting radiographic features mimicking malignancy with potential extension into the frontal sinus, ethmoid sinus, and periorbital structures. While such invasive forms predominantly affect immunocompromised individuals (e.g., diabetics, long-term immunosuppressant users), cases in immunocompetent hosts have also been documented [3, 4]. Uncontrolled infection may progress to orbital cellulitis, leading to irreversible vision loss or even fatal intracranial dissemination [18]. Consequently, enhanced monitoring in high-risk patients is crucial to detect potential transformation from chronic localized disease to invasive destructive forms.

Dacryocystitis-related orbital cellulitis, while relatively rare, poses a significant threat to vision. It occurs more frequently in non-immunosuppressed adults with lacrimal drainage obstruction, primarily due to primary acquired nasolacrimal duct obstruction (PANDO); other causes include lacrimal sac diverticulum, post-traumatic obstruction, leukemic infiltrate, and sinus-related obstruction. The condition can be polymicrobial, most commonly involving Gram-positive bacteria, but also encompassing Gram-negative organisms, filamentous fungi, and methicillin-resistant *Staphylococcus aureus*. Virtually all patients present with chemosis, severe periorbital edema, and erythema, with a subset exhibiting restricted ocular motility [19].

5.5 Diagnosis

The diagnostic framework for fungal lacrimal infections faces multifaceted challenges, primarily centered on balancing pathogen confirmation with clinical decision-making. In laboratory diagnosis, fungal culture and histopathological examination remain the gold standard. Pathogens can be identified by microscopic examination of hyphae/spores in lacrimal duct secretion smears, as well as through fungal culture of irrigation fluids or stone samples. However, underutilization of microbiological testing in clinical practice—exemplified by a mere 21.6% culture rate for dacryocystitis in Eastern China [7]—highlights the need to enhance clinician awareness of pathogen-driven diagnostic protocols.

Histopathological evaluation of lacrimal sac biopsies, while critical for diagnosing invasive infections (e.g., mucormycosis), remains contentious. Large-scale analyses reveal that only 3.9% of PANDO cases exhibit specific pathological alterations (e.g., sarcoidosis, lymphoma, papilloma), with malignancy detected in just 0.08% of unsuspected cases [20]. Consequently, some advocate for selective biopsy limited to scenarios with clinical/imaging suspicion of neoplasia or intraoperative tissue abnormalities to optimize cost-effectiveness. Nevertheless, missed diagnoses of rare but life-threatening infections (e.g., localized lacrimal sac mucormycosis in immunocompetent individuals) underscore the potential necessity of routine biopsy, particularly in rapidly progressive cases [21].

Imaging modalities (CT/MRI) aid in delineating infection extent (e.g., bony erosion, calcifications) but lack specificity. While intraluminal calcifications on CT may suggest *Aspergillus* spp. infection, their absence cannot exclude fungal colonization [3]. High-resolution techniques like ultrasound biomicroscopy (UBM) and anterior segment optical coherence tomography (OCT) excel in evaluating canaliculitis-related anatomical details. Molecular diagnostics, such as metagenomic next-generation sequencing (mNGS), revolutionize pathogen detection by rapidly identifying fungal lineages in polymicrobial infections, particularly in immunocompromised hosts with complex presentations.

5.6 Differential Diagnosis

Differential diagnosis encompasses bacterial lacrimal infections, dacryolithiasis, idiopathic orbital inflammation, and rhino-orbital malignancies. Systemic disorders such as sarcoidosis and granulomatosis with polyangiitis require exclusion through serological and histopathological correlation.

5.7 Treatment

Evidence-based studies emphasize that timely and standardized intervention in lacrimal system infections is critical for preventing severe complications such as endophthalmitis [22]. Current therapeutic strategies integrate dual pharmacological and

Table 5.3 Treatment approaches for fungal canaliculitis and dacryocystitis

Disease	Treatment approaches
Fungal canaliculitis	1. Topical antifungal therapy Eye drops: e.g., Natamycin, amphotericin B, Voriconazole Canalicular irrigation: With antifungal solutions (e.g., amphotericin B, fluconazole) to flush out fungal hyphae and debris 2. Surgical intervention Canalicular dilation and probing: dilate canaliculus; probe to remove fungal concretions; followed by topical therapy Canaliculotomy: if conservative measures fail, incise canaliculus to debride infected tissue; followed by sustained topical antifungals 3. Systemic therapy Oral Itraconazole or fluconazole; duration adjusted per clinical severity
Fungal dacryocystitis	1. Topical antifungal therapy Eye drops: as for canaliculitis, to control local infection Lacrimal sac irrigation: infuse antifungal solution via punctum to irrigate sac 2. Surgical management Dacryocystorhinostomy (DCR): primary procedure; creates drainage pathway to nose; removes fungal material; adjunctive post-op irrigation/medication Dacryocystectomy: reserved for severe disease, sac destruction, or failed DCR; excises infected sac to eradicate infection 3. Systemic antifungal therapy Oral or intravenous antifungals required in severe/systemic disease

surgical approaches (Table 5.3). For antifungal pharmacotherapy, targeted regimens are tailored to pathogen profiles and infection severity: localized infections may be managed with topical ophthalmic formulations (e.g., natamycin, amphotericin B, or voriconazole) combined with lacrimal irrigation using antifungal solutions (e.g., fluconazole) [23]. In contrast, invasive infections or immunocompromised patients require escalation to systemic antifungal therapy, including intravenous or oral administration of itraconazole, voriconazole, or amphotericin B. Treatment duration should extend until complete resolution of clinical signs and symptoms, with prolonged or indefinite maintenance therapy recommended for immunodeficient populations [3]. Notably, existing efficacy data for antifungal agents predominantly derive from clinical trials and retrospective case series, underscoring the necessity of integrating antifungal susceptibility testing to guide precision therapy.

For patients with inadequate responses to medical therapy, a stepwise surgical strategy is dictated by anatomical involvement. Focal canalicular infections may be addressed via canaliculotomy to excise fungal concretions and dacryoliths, while extensive lacrimal sac involvement warrants endoscopic dacryocystorhinostomy (DCR) or dacryocystectomy, accompanied by thorough intraoperative debridement and silicone stent placement to maintain lacrimal patency [10]. Postoperative adjunctive therapy with topical or systemic antifungals is considered the standard of care for invasive infections. Complex presentations, such as dacryocystitis with cutaneous fistulas, necessitate concurrent wound repair and symptom-specific

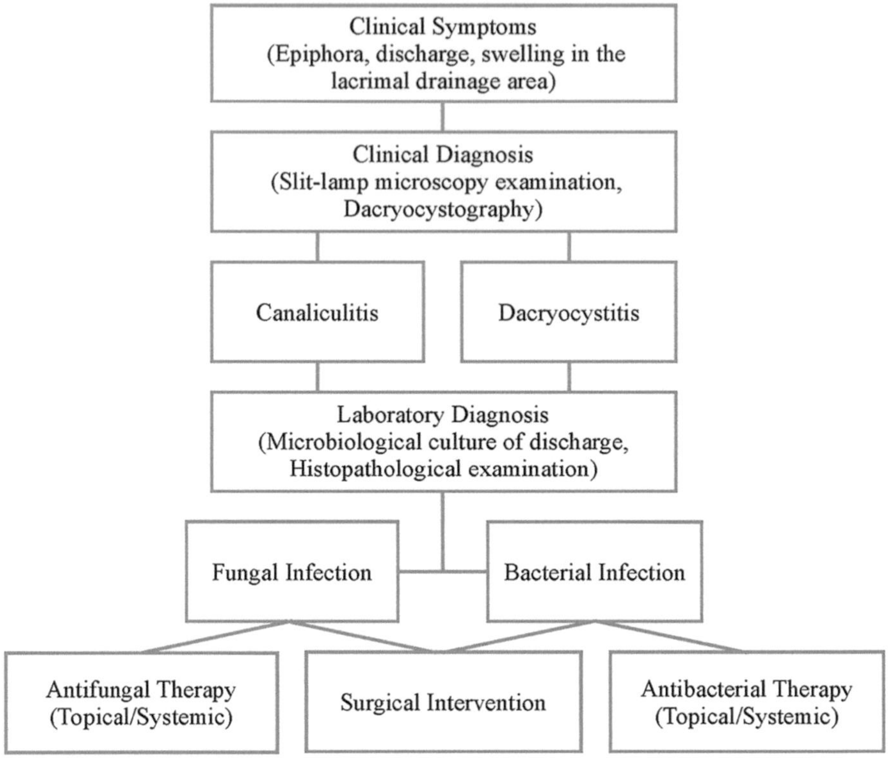

Fig. 5.2 Diagnostic and therapeutic pathway

interventions. This multimodal therapeutic paradigm aims to eradicate infection, restore lacrimal drainage function, and mitigate recurrence risks.

Microbial culture of silicone stents removed after DCR revealed fungal growth in 60% of cases, predominantly *Aspergillus* spp. (66.6%) followed by *Fusarium* spp. (26.6%); however, the isolated microorganisms did not impact surgical success rates [24]. The investigators propose that these fungi may represent commensal organisms from the patient's nasal cavity or that the stent could act as a breeding ground for environmental fungi inhaled via airflow. This finding underscores the need for regular postoperative follow-up (for at least 6 months) following stent removal to monitor for potential fungal recurrence. The diagnostic and therapeutic pathway is shown in Fig. 5.2.

5.8 Visual Prognosis and Complications

The prognosis of fungal lacrimal infections is closely linked to the invasiveness of the pathogen, host immune status, and timeliness of therapeutic intervention. Localized infections (e.g., canaliculitis, chronic dacryocystitis) managed with early and standardized treatment typically exhibit favorable visual outcomes, with rare severe sequelae. In contrast, invasive infections (e.g., rhinoorbitocranial spread by *Mucor* or *Aspergillus* spp.) may lead to catastrophic complications if inadequately controlled, including orbital cellulitis, optic nerve ischemia, cavernous sinus thrombosis, and intracranial dissemination, resulting in irreversible vision loss or mortality [4]. Immunocompromised patients (e.g., diabetics, transplant recipients) face significantly higher complication rates and mortality due to rapid tissue destruction compared to immunocompetent individuals. Chronic infections may also predispose to lacrimal duct stenosis, cutaneous fistulas, or recurrent dacryoliths, necessitating long-term surveillance. In general, visual outcomes hinge on early pathogen confirmation and multidisciplinary therapy, as delayed diagnosis and treatment significantly elevate the risk of irreversible blindness. Proactive screening of high-risk populations and vigilant recognition of invasive signs (e.g., progressive proptosis, cranial nerve palsies) are pivotal to optimizing prognosis.

5.9 Future Perspectives

To advance the management of fungal lacrimal infections, a systematic research agenda targeting four core domains is proposed. First, enhancing pathogen identification efficacy through optimized rapid molecular diagnostics—such as real-time quantitative PCR (qPCR) and metagenomic sequencing—is critical to achieve precise microbial characterization. Second, addressing drug-resistant fungi and biofilm-related challenges requires focused development of novel antifungal compounds (e.g., targeted small-molecule inhibitors) and nanoparticle-based drug delivery systems designed to penetrate biofilms and overcome conventional therapeutic limitations. Third, establishing evidence-based prevention protocols for high-risk populations (e.g., diabetics, immunocompromised individuals) is essential, including standardized lacrimal hygiene guidelines and early screening algorithms to mitigate infection risks. Fourth, a multidisciplinary care model integrating ophthalmic microsurgery, molecular diagnostics, and radiomics-driven imaging analysis should be implemented to formulate personalized treatment regimens. This integrative approach aims to suppress infection dissemination, reduce invasive complications (e.g., orbital cellulitis), and improve outcomes through synergistic collaboration among ophthalmologists, microbiologists, and radiologists. By prioritizing innovation in diagnostics, therapeutics, prevention, and interdisciplinary care, this framework seeks to redefine clinical standards for fungal lacrimal infections.

References

1. Woog JJ. The incidence of symptomatic acquired lacrimal outflow obstruction among residents of Olmsted County, Minnesota, 1976-2000 (an American Ophthalmological Society thesis). Trans Am Ophthalmol Soc. 2007;105:649–66.
2. Vagge A, Ferro Desideri L, Nucci P, Serafino M, Giannaccare G, Lembo A, et al. Congenital nasolacrimal duct obstruction (CNLDO): a review. Diseases. 2018;6(4):96.

3. Raguraman S, Kushwaha A, Penubarthi LK. Lacrimal sac Aspergillosis masquerading as malignancy: a rare case report. Indian J Otolaryngol Head Neck Surg. 2024;76(3):2833–6.
4. Ding JQ, Xie Y. A case report on clinical features, diagnosis, and treatment of rhino-orbito-cerebral mucormycosis. Immun Inflamm Dis. 2023;11(11):e1080.
5. Khatoon J, Rizvi SAR, Gupta Y, Alam MS. A prospective study on epidemiology of dacryocystitis at a tertiary eye care center in northern India. Oman J Ophthalmol. 2021;14(3):169–72.
6. Eslami F, Ghasemi Basir HR, Moradi A, Heidari Farah S. Microbiological study of dacryocystitis in northwest of Iran. Clin Ophthalmol. 2018;12:1859–64.
7. Chen L, Fu T, Gu H, Jie Y, Sun Z, Jiang D, et al. Trends in dacryocystitis in China: a STROBE-compliant article. Medicine (Baltimore). 2018;97(26):e11318.
8. Tian X, Sun H, Huang Y, Sui W, Zhang D, Sun Y, et al. Microbiological isolates and associated complications of dacryocystitis and canaliculitis in a prominent tertiary ophthalmic teaching hospital in northern China. BMC Ophthalmol. 2024;24(1):56.
9. Luo B, Li M, Xiang N, Hu W, Liu R, Yan X. The microbiologic spectrum of dacryocystitis. BMC Ophthalmol. 2021;21(1):29.
10. Ghose S, Mahajan VM. Fungal flora in congenital dacryocystitis. Indian J Ophthalmol. 1990;38(4):189–90.
11. Huang L, Dalzotto KF, Duffy MT, Gurwin J, van Landingham SW. Alternaria fungal dacryocystitis with cutaneous fistula: a case report. Orbit. 2024;43(6):747–50.
12. Slowik M, Biernat MM, Urbaniak-Kujda D, Kapelko-Slowik K, Misiuk-Hojlo M. Mycotic infections of the eye. Adv Clin Exp Med. 2015;24(6):1113–7.
13. Freitas DF, Lima IA, Curi CL, Jordao L, Zancope-Oliveira RM, Valle AC, et al. Acute dacryocystitis: another clinical manifestation of sporotrichosis. Mem Inst Oswaldo Cruz. 2014;109(2):262–4.
14. Ramirez-Soto MC, Tirado-Sanchez A, Bonifaz A. Ocular sporotrichosis. J Fungi (Basel). 2021;7(11):951.
15. Mohanty PK, Ambekar VA, Deodhar LP. Prevalence of mycotic infections of external eye. Indian J Ophthalmol. 1984;32(3):153–5.
16. Sellart-Altisent M, Torres-Rodriguez JM, Gomez de Ana S, Alvarado-Ramirez E. Nasal fungal microbiota in allergic and healthy subjects. Rev Iberoam Micol. 2007;24(2):125–30.
17. Horton MV, Holt AM, Nett JE. Mechanisms of pathogenicity for the emerging fungus Candida auris. PLoS Pathog. 2023;19(12):e1011843.
18. O'Rourke M, Tang YF, Pick Z, Tan JS, Tan PEZ, Athavale DD, et al. Orbital cellulitis secondary to dacryocystitis: a case series and literature review. Ophthalmic Plast Reconstr Surg. 2025;41(3):306–14.
19. Wladis EJ, Shinder R, LeFebvre DR, Sokol JA, Boyce M. Clinical and microbiologic features of dacryocystitis-related orbital cellulitis. Orbit. 2016;35(5):258–61.
20. Merkonidis C, Brewis C, Yung M, Nussbaumer M. Is routine biopsy of the lacrimal sac wall indicated at dacryocystorhinostomy? A prospective study and literature review. Br J Ophthalmol. 2005;89(12):1589–91.
21. Kapur R, Aakalu VK, August CZ, Weiss RA. Mucormycosis infection of the lacrimal sac. Ophthalmic Plast Reconstr Surg. 2009;25(6):494–6.
22. Shahraki K, Makateb A, Shirzadi K, Khosravifard K. Frequency of bacterial samples from patients with chronic acquired nasolacrimal duct obstruction. Med Arch. 2016;70(6):433–6.
23. Mycosis of the eye and its adnexa. Dev Ophthalmol 1999;32:i–ix, 1–201.
24. Ali MJ, Manderwad G, Naik MN. The microbiological spectrum and antibiotic sensitivity profile of extubated silicone stents following dacryocystorhinostomy. Orbit. 2013;32(5):298–303.

6 Fungal Conjunctivitis

Andrés Tirado-Sánchez, Alexandro Bonifaz,
Jesús Heriberto Dávila-Alquisiras,
and Max Carlos Ramírez-Soto

6.1 Introduction

The conjunctiva, defined as a mucous membrane that forms a clear outer layer around the eye, is both an exposed surface and a potential site of microbial contamination (Fig. 6.1). Consequently, this ocular surface harbors a distinct microflora, comprising bacteria that perpetually consume aeroplankton, yet are meticulously modified by the dynamic mechanisms of lacrimal flow and blinking [1]. The microbial flora present in the conjunctival region is primarily transient, a consequence of the cleansing effect of blinking and the antimicrobial effect of tear fluid. However, these processes are selective, resulting in the |relative stability of certain microbial communities that resist elimination. This phenomenon has been observed in the case of fungi. Fungal isolation from the conjunctival sac has been documented in 6–20% of healthy individuals [2, 3]. A seasonal increase in such cases has been observed, which may be related to the rise in allergic conjunctivitis cases, primarily attributed to the airborne transmission of *Candida* [4].

The original version of the chapter has been revised. A correction to this chapter can be found at https://doi.org/10.1007/978-3-032-19923-2_13

A. Tirado-Sánchez (✉)
Dermatology Service & Mycology Department, Hospital General de México "Dr. Eduardo Liceaga", Ciudad de México, Mexico

Internal Medicine Department, Hospital General de Zona 30, Instituto Mexicano del Seguro Social, Ciudad de México, Mexico

A. Bonifaz
Dermatology Service & Mycology Department, Hospital General de México, Ciudad de México "Dr. Eduardo Liceaga", Mexico

J. H. Dávila-Alquisiras
Oftalmology Service, Hospital General de México "Dr. Eduardo Liceaga", Ciudad de México, Mexico

M. C. Ramírez-Soto
Centro de Investigación en Salud Pública, Facultad de Medicina Humana, Universidad de San Martín de Porres, Lima, Peru

M. C. Ramírez-Soto (ed.), *Fungal Eye Infections*,
https://doi.org/10.1007/978-3-032-19923-2_6

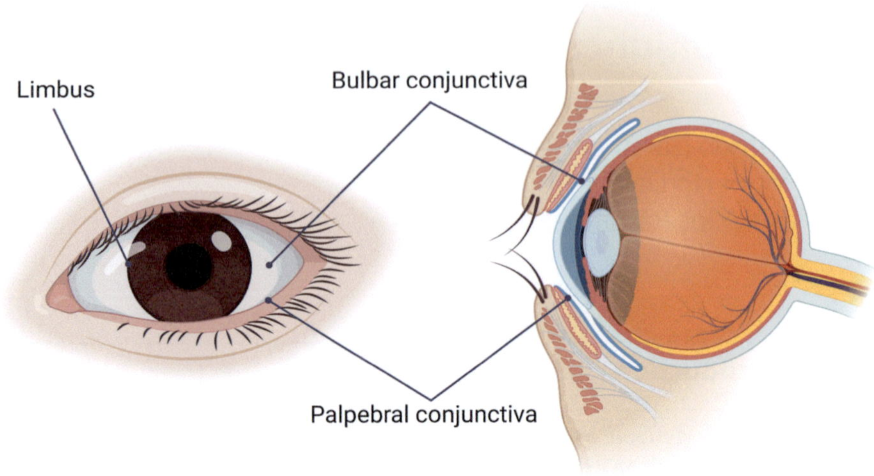

Fig. 6.1 Normal conjunctival anatomy

It is noteworthy that the presence of various microorganisms on the ocular surface does not necessarily lead to inflammation or infection, as they may coexist in a state of equilibrium that enables the proper functioning of the ocular ecosystem [5]. In a study involving 90 healthy volunteers, conjunctival samples were obtained and metagenomic sequencing was utilized to ascertain the relative composition of the conjunctival microbiome. The results indicated that the microbiome was predominantly bacterial (98.15%), with smaller percentages comprising fungi (0.94%) and viruses (0.91%) [6]. Another study, using next-generation sequencing technology to analyze the ocular surface fungal microbiome in 25 healthy individuals, detected the genera *Aspergillus*, *Setosphaeria*, *Malassezia*, and *Haematonectria* in tarsal conjunctiva samples. These findings suggest the potential for localized opportunistic fungal infections in the conjunctiva [7].

External eye infections, including conjunctivitis, and associated complications are significant problems that cause blindness if not treated promptly [8]. Conjunctivitis is characterized by inflammation and edema of the conjunctiva, accompanied by vascular congestion, ocular discharge, and pain [1]. This condition is primarily caused by bacterial and viral infections, whereas fungal conjunctivitis is rare and poses a diagnostic challenge [9]. Notably, more than 80% of acute cases of conjunctivitis are diagnosed by non-ophthalmologist health professionals, such as internists, family doctors, pediatricians, and nurses. Approximately 60% of patients diagnosed with acute conjunctivitis receive topical antibiotics, frequently in combination with a steroid. This figure undergoes a substantial change when cases of conjunctivitis are treated by an ophthalmologist, where only approximately 36% of cases receive topical antibiotics [10].

Conjunctival disease may progress to involve the surrounding tissue, such as the eyelid margins (e.g., blepharoconjunctivitis) and the cornea (as in keratoconjunctivitis) [8]. To distinguish infectious conjunctivitis from noninfectious conjunctivitis, it is essential to obtain the history of patients presenting with conjunctivitis in order to arrive at the correct diagnosis [11]. The specific ocular history should include the onset and duration of symptoms; laterality; visual impairment; presence of pruritus or pain; history of contact lens use; history of recent upper respiratory tract infection, sinusitis, and lymphadenopathy; previous episodes of conjunctivitis; systemic allergies and associated medication; and history of exposure to chemical agents [12]. In addition to a medical history of systemic diseases that may present as noninfectious conjunctivitis [11].

In this chapter, we present an overview of the epidemiology, clinical features, diagnosis and differential diagnosis, management, and visual prognosis of fungal conjunctivitis.

6.2 Epidemiology

Fungal conjunctivitis is frequently associated with keratitis, which is the most prevalent manifestation of fungal eye infections. Isolated fungal conjunctivitis, devoid of keratitis, is an exceedingly rare occurrence [13]. The spectrum of infectious conjunctivitis within a community or geographic region is shaped by a complex interplay of patient-related, microbial, and environmental factors. Key risk determinants include pathogen virulence and antimicrobial resistance, personal hygiene, socioeconomic status, nutrition, genetic predisposition, physiological characteristics, age, access to healthcare services, exposure to environmental pollutants, occupational hazards, and underlying comorbidities [11].

In a study conducted by Shah et al. [14], the highest proportions of fungal eye infections were reported from India and Nepal. In eastern India, fungi accounted for 67% of corneal infections. Among countries with a high prevalence of fungal ulcers, eastern India showed the highest proportion of *Aspergillus* species (60% of all fungal isolates), whereas a study from Hyderabad, India, reported the highest proportion of *Fusarium* species (73% of all fungal isolates). Most cases in these studies were diagnosed as fungal keratitis, with *Aspergillus* and *Fusarium* identified as the predominant etiological agents. These same pathogens may also contribute to the development of fungal conjunctivitis.

A correlation has been identified between specific geographic regions and a high frequency of fungal eye infections. Popular tourist destinations, such as countries in South Asia, have been associated with the highest rates of these infections [15]. Fungal conjunctivitis has also been identified as a prevalent condition in Western countries, with the potential to cause infections among the local population and among returning travelers. Furthermore, microsporidia have been associated with cases of conjunctivitis in healthy rugby players from Hong Kong, Malaysia, Australia, and the United Arab Emirates who returned from a tournament in Singapore in 2012. This entity should be included in the differential diagnosis of keratoconjunctivitis of unknown etiology in people returning from Asia, especially during the rainy season, as regional seasonal variations in infection have been described, with peaks in incidence during the monsoon period [15].

Candida infections have been reported to cause conjunctivitis, particularly following ocular trauma, which may facilitate fungal entry into the bloodstream and subsequent ocular involvement. The prevalence is highest among newborns and school-aged children [16]. *Candida* conjunctivitis has also been observed following the topical administration of corticosteroids and antibiotics in patients with ocular inflammation. Reported species include *C. albicans*, *C. parapsilosis*, and *C. tropicalis* [16]. The rising incidence of candidiasis is of particular concern due to the increased risk of complications, including conjunctivitis [17] (Table 6.1).

A study revealed that among the 259 patients diagnosed with external ocular infections in Ethiopia, 26.8% (42 cases) were attributed to fungal pathogens. Of these, 23% (n = 14) corresponded to cases of fungal conjunctivitis, in which *Aspergillus*, *Fusarium*, *Rhizopus* spp., and *Candida* spp. were identified as the etiological agents [18]. A recent study in India analyzed 38 cases of fungal conjunctivitis and found that filamentous fungi—particularly *Aspergillus* spp. (50%) and *Fusarium* spp. (13.15%)—were the most frequently isolated organisms. Dematiaceous fungi, such as *Curvularia* spp., were the second most common group [19]. The utilization of contact lenses has been proposed as a potential risk factor for fungal conjunctivitis particularly related with *Candida*, *Fusarium*, and *Aspergillus*. As indicated by the extant literature [20], several factors have been identified as contributing to fungal contamination of contact lenses. These factors include prolonged use, lens type [21], contaminated solutions, use of broad-spectrum antibiotics, steroids, warm and humid environments, and preexisting corneal diseases. Defects in the structural integrity of the lens surface resulting from the manufacturing process, cosmetic brushes, or repetitive handling facilitate the entry of fungi into the lens matrix, where they can generate biofilms, as has been seen with *Candida* and *Fusarium* [12] (Table 6.1).

Dimorphic fungi can also cause conjunctivitis. Conjunctival infections caused by *Sporothrix* species have been documented in hyperendemic regions of sporotrichosis, particularly in Brazil, where zoonotic transmission is highly prevalent [22, 23]. In addition, isolated cases have been reported in Malaysia, the United States, Japan, and Thailand. These infections are typically associated with the direct inoculation of fungal elements into the conjunctival tissue, with zoonotic transmission—especially from infected cats—now recognized as the predominant route of infection in most reported cases [24, 25] (Table 6.1). Ocular coccidioidomycosis presenting with conjunctivitis is rare and typically occurs as a manifestation of disseminated disease secondary to a primary pulmonary infection, which makes its true incidence difficult to establish [26–29]. Reported cases originate primarily from endemic regions such as southern Arizona, California, southern New Mexico, and western Texas [27]. Other species of dimorphic fungus identified as causative agents of fungal conjunctivitis include *Blastomyces dermatitidis* [30] and *Paracoccidioides brasiliensis* in Brazil [31, 32].

In immunocompromised patients, the cornea is often affected, resulting in keratitis, which can lead to secondary conjunctivitis. *Cryptococcus* and *Candida albicans* are the most commonly identified pathogens affecting both the cornea and conjunctiva in such cases [33].

Table 6.1 Epidemiology and etiology of fungal conjunctivitis

Type of fungus	Type of infection	Epidemiology	Patient type	Etiologic agent
Yeast	Candidiasis	Most frequent fungal conjunctivitis; often nosocomial or related to contaminated eye drops, prosthetics, or systemic candidemia	Mostly immunocompromised (HIV, ICU, etc.)	*Candida albicans, C. parapsilosis* and *C. glabrata*
Filamentous	Aspergillosis (hyaline)	Rare; may occur after trauma, surgery, or in immunosuppressed patients; often part of keratitis or endophthalmitis	Both immunocompetent and immunocompromised	*Aspergillus fumigatus, A. flavus* and *A. niger*
	Fusariosis (hyaline)	Associated with contact lens use, contaminated eyedrops, or ocular prostheses	Immunocompromised and hospitalized patients	*Fusarium* spp.
	Scedosporiosis (hyaline)	Extremely rare; ocular infection may occur after trauma, surgery, or from contiguous spread (keratitis, endophthalmitis)	Both immunocompetent and immunocompromised	*Scedosporium apiospermum*
	Cladosporiosis (dematiaceous)	Very rare cause of conjunctivitis; usually environmental contamination or post-trauma inoculation	Immunocompetent (mostly), occasionally immunocompromised	*Cladosporium* spp. (e.g., *C. cladosporioides*)

(continued)

Table 6.1 (continued)

Type of fungus	Type of infection	Epidemiology	Patient type	Etiologic agent
Dimorphic	Conjunctival sporotrichosis (primary conjunctivitis)	Hyperendemic (more common Brazil) and endemic areas (Thailand and Malaysia) Zoonotic (cats) or plant-related exposure; conjunctival cases may occur via trauma or hematogenous spread	Common in immunocompetent Rare in immunocompromised	*Sporothrix* spp. and *S. brasiliensis*
	Conjunctival coccidioidomycosis Secondary conjunctivitis (part of systemic or ocular mycosis)	Pacific northwest and southwestern United States, and parts of Mexico, Central America, and South America	Immunocompetent	*Coccidioides* spp.
	Paracoccidioidomycosis	Very rare conjunctival involvement; endemic in South America (especially Brazil, Colombia, and Venezuela); ocular cases occur in disseminated infection	Immunocompromised or debilitated patients	*Paracoccidioides brasiliensis* and *P. lutzii*
	Blastomycosis	Rare ocular involvement; endemic in North America (Great Lakes, Ohio and Mississippi River valleys); conjunctival lesions may occur in disseminated disease	Immunocompromised or immunocompetent	*Blastomyces dermatitidis*
Microsporidia	Conjunctival Microsporidiosis	Emerging infection, especially in tropical/subtropical regions; outbreaks associated with contaminated water or trauma	Mainly immunocompromised (HIV/AIDS), but also reported in immunocompetent individuals	*Encephalitozoon hellem*, *E. cuniculi*, and *Vittaforma corneae*

Recent studies have documented an upward trend in microsporidial conjunctivitis among non-HIV-infected patients, including travelers, children, elderly, and organ transplant recipients. This phenomenon can be attributed to heightened awareness and suspicion of this condition among immunocompetent individuals. In Singapore, a male predominance was observed, with a ratio of 8:1 between men and women. This phenomenon was frequently observed during periods of high rainfall. A subsequent study also noted an increase in cases during the monsoon season. It has been suggested that with increased rainfall, microsporidia will become more ubiquitous [34, 35]. The exact mechanism by which the pathogen reaches the ocular surface remains not completely understood. The most widely accepted hypothesis involves direct inoculation via the oro-fecal route, particularly through eye rubbing after exposure to contaminated mud or following ocular trauma. In immunocompetent individuals, risk factors include ocular trauma, prior refractive surgery, and exposure to rainwater, uncovered swimming pools, or stagnant water, as well as contact with soil or mud during activities such as soccer, golf, mountain biking, or military field exercises. A definitive association between contact lens wear and microsporidial conjunctivitis has not been established. Localized immunosuppression due to topical steroid use is considered a relevant risk factor, or may be part of systemic microsporidiosis. In addition to direct inoculation, one study suggested that ocular infection in immunocompromised patients could be acquired by reverse passage from a respiratory source through the lacrimal canaliculi and nasolacrimal ducts that drain secretions from the eyes into the sinuses [34]. *Encephalitozoon hellem* and *Vittaforma corneae* (formerly *Nosema corneum*) have been identified as causative agents of fungal conjunctivitis/keratoconjunctivitis in individuals with HIV-induced immunosuppression [36, 37] (Table 6.1).

Scedosporium apiospermum is a filamentous environmental fungus typically found in organically contaminated areas, including environments with bird or livestock excrement, swamps, and sewage. It has been implicated in a broad spectrum of localized and invasive infections, including those affecting the endocardium, lungs, joints, skin, and soft tissues. Ocular manifestations such as conjunctivitis, chorioretinitis, endophthalmitis, keratitis, and scleritis have also been documented [38–41]. The detection of this fungus in such anatomical sites reflects both its association with cutaneous infections and its ability to disseminate via conidia, allowing for potential involvement of the ocular and respiratory tracts [38]. The clinical variability of these infections is influenced by several factors, including the host immune status, disruption of the respiratory mucosa, cutaneous trauma, and previous surgical interventions [40].

Cladosporium species are ubiquitous environmental molds with the capacity to cause a range of infections, including those affecting the skin, toenails, eyes, sinuses, and lungs. Although *Cladosporium* is present as a commensal organism in the conjunctiva, cases of *Cladosporium*-associated conjunctivitis are exceedingly rare. *Cladosporium* spp. have been isolated from diverse environments, including soil, plant litter, leaf surfaces, and decaying vegetation. Their spores are efficiently dispersed by wind, making them prevalent in outdoor air, but they are also commonly found indoors, particularly on textiles, wood, and damp window sills.

Notably, these fungi can grow at low temperatures (as low as 0 °C) and have been isolated from refrigerated foods [42]. In a study investigating the fungal flora of the conjunctival sac in 919 eyes, *Cladosporium* and other airborne fungi were cultured from 6.6% (39 of 587 swabs) of healthy conjunctivae. The incidence of positive fungal cultures was significantly higher in diseased eyes. In total, 107 fungal isolates were identified, including *Cladosporium* spp. among others [2]. In a case involving a patient without a history of ocular trauma, the right conjunctiva presented with generalized chemosis and follicular reaction. After multiple unsuccessful treatments for suspected bacterial and mycobacterial infections, a fungal culture tested positive for *Cladosporium* sp. The patient reported a history of gardening activities and exposure to tree bark dust, which had entered the eye shortly before symptom onset—suggesting a possible predisposing environmental factor [43]. Predisposing factors for ocular involvement include the sharing of cosmetics, chronic use of broad-spectrum topical antibiotics, prolonged use of oral or topical corticosteroids, trauma from plant material, zoonotic transmission, and states of immunosuppression such as HIV infection, diabetes, or immunosuppressive therapy. Additionally, certain ocular surface diseases, such as dry eye syndrome, may also increase susceptibility [44, 45].

6.3 Clinical Manifestations

The clinical manifestations of fungal conjunctivitis depend on the specific fungal pathogen involved and the type of infection, although many cases present with overlapping symptoms [46]. Commonly reported findings include acute mucopurulent conjunctival inflammation, salmon-pink lesions resembling tumors on the bulbar conjunctiva, punctate epithelial keratoconjunctivitis, giant papillary conjunctivitis, and lesions mimicking squamous neoplasms [47]. The severity of these infections can range from mild, self-limiting conditions to severe presentations with potential systemic involvement. Diagnosis is based on a combination of factors, including the pattern and extent of conjunctival involvement, clinical presentation, associated systemic signs, and epidemiological context. Due to its low incidence and nonspecific clinical features, fungal conjunctivitis remains a rare and often underdiagnosed condition in ophthalmic practice [48]. It is imperative to distinguish between fungal conjunctivitis and other etiologies of red eye that may result in severe visual impairment or even fatal consequences, such as acute angle-closure glaucoma, uveitis, endophthalmitis, carotid-cavernous fistula, cellulitis, and anterior segment tumors [49].

The hallmark characteristics associated with fungal conjunctivitis include redness, itching, burning, discharge, and irritation. The severity of these symptoms is contingent upon the nature of the infectious agent, the extent of the infection, and the patient's immune status. Fungal infections are characterized by chronic inflammation and minimal ocular discharge.

Clinically, the following may be observed: conjunctival edema, tarsal and bulbar conjunctival hyperemia, and granulomas. The discharge may be mucopurulent or frankly purulent, yellow, or greenish in color [48].

6.3.1 Yeast Conjunctivitis

Candida conjunctivitis presents with acute or subacute purulent superficial epithelial lesions [46] (Fig. 6.2a). Chronic *Candida* conjunctivitis have been observed to activate the body's immune response, particularly the cellular type, resulting in a local granulomatous inflammatory response and potentially leading to proliferative conjunctival epithelial lesions [17]. Pina et al. [50] studied the morphological and pathological manifestations of chronic proliferative candidiasis of the oral and laryngeal mucosa, respectively, and both found that the histopathological changes were atypical squamous epithelial hyperplasia, which must be distinguished from squamous cell carcinoma. Consequently, it is proposed that chronic fungal infection may act as a predisposing factor for conjunctival squamous metaplasia. *Malassezia* has been observed to induce symptoms such as redness, irritation, and discharge (similar to catarrhal conjunctivitis) [51, 52].

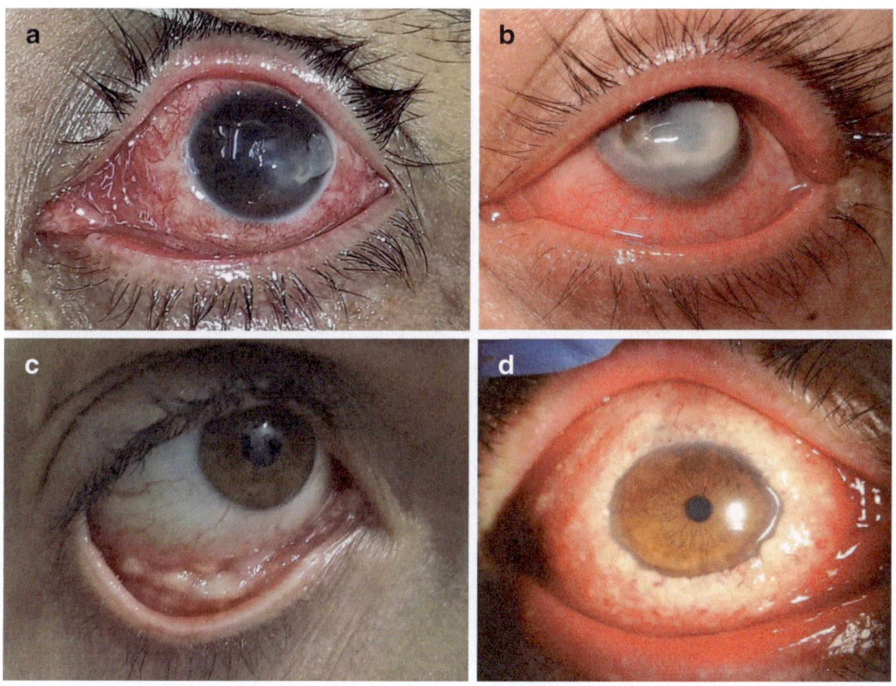

Fig. 6.2 Characteristic appearance of fungal conjunctivitis. (**a**) Keratoconjunctivitis due to *Candida* spp. [Courtesy of Prof. Alexandro Bonifaz]. (**b**) Keratoconjunctivitis due to *Fusarium* spp. [Courtesy of Prof. Alexandro Bonifaz]. (**c**) Granulomas in the right lower palpebral conjunctiva due to *Sporothrix* spp. (Reprinted from ref. 17 [published under a CC BY license and courtesy of Isabella D. Ferreira-Gremião, Fiocruz, Rio de Janeiro, Brazil]). (**d**) Primary unilateral bulbar conjunctival due to *Sporothrix globosa* (Reprinted from Ophthalmology, 130/12, Qi H, Huang Y, Wang L, Primary unilateral bulbar conjunctival sporotrichosis, Pages No. 1346, Copyright (2023), with permission from Elsevier)

6.3.2 Filamentous Fungal Conjunctivitis

Aspergillus conjunctivitis is typically secondary to inflammation of adjacent ocular structures, such as the cornea, lacrimal sac, or nasolacrimal duct. It presents with signs of acute conjunctival inflammation, often accompanied by mucopurulent or mucoid discharge [53, 54]. Reported cases describe conjunctival hyperemia, mass lesions, pronounced papillary or follicular reactions, and, in some instances, conjunctival edema or abscess formation [2, 55–57]. Conjunctival aspergillosis may also manifest as a polypoid lesion [58]. On the other hand, *A. niger* is the causative agent of follicular conjunctivitis with microhemorrhages [59, 60], in association with foreign body injuries and concomitant trachoma. *Fusarium* conjuntivitis is commonly related to trauma and further contamination-infection, developing severe, deep keratoconjunctivitis with rapidly progressing ulceration and necrosis [61] (Fig. 6.2b). These infections are not limited to the conjunctiva; in most cases, diagnosis occurs after progression to keratoconjunctivitis or even endophthalmitis [44].

6.3.3 Dimorphic Fungal Conjunctivitis

Conjunctival sporotrichosis is predominantly reported in young adults, with a higher incidence among females. *S. schenckii* is the most commonly isolated species, followed by *S. brasiliensis*. Clinically, it typically presents as a granulomatous lesion accompanied by conjunctival hyperemia, mucoid or purulent discharge, and eyelid edema, with or without regional lymphadenopathy. Four main clinical patterns have been described in ocular sporotrichosis: granulomatous conjunctivitis, dacryocystitis, Parinaud's oculoglandular syndrome, and bulbar conjunctivitis. The tarsal conjunctiva is more frequently affected than the bulbar conjunctiva (Figure 6.2c, d). Eyelid involvement is also commonly reported, with the lower eyelid being more frequently affected than the upper. Parinaud's oculoglandular syndrome is observed in approximately half of the cases, with preauricular lymphadenopathy being the most frequent form of lymph node involvement [22].

Conjunctivitis in coccidioidomycosis most commonly occurs in association with pulmonary or disseminated disease. *C. immitis* has been implicated in cases of severe necrotizing granulomatous conjunctivitis and follicular conjunctivitis [28, 29]. Although ocular involvement is often subclinical and incidentally discovered, conjunctivitis may, in rare cases, represent the initial or sole manifestation of systemic infection. Historical reports describe a range of presentations, including conjunctivitis with bulbar hyperemia, phlyctenular-like conjunctivitis, conjunctivitis occurring alongside systemic disease, and lesions affecting the palpebral conjunctiva [29]. Therefore, coccidioidomycosis should be included in the differential diagnosis of nodular or granulomatous conjunctivitis, particularly in immunocompromised individuals or those with a relevant travel history, as it may constitute an early or isolated sign of systemic fungal infection.

B. dermatitidis has been associated with contiguous spread and follicular and granulomatous conjunctivitis [30]. In cases of paracoccidioidomycosis, conjunctivitis usually occurs in association with eyelid lesions [32]. It may present with diplopia, ptosis, and persistent conjunctival inflammation, along with multiple flat,

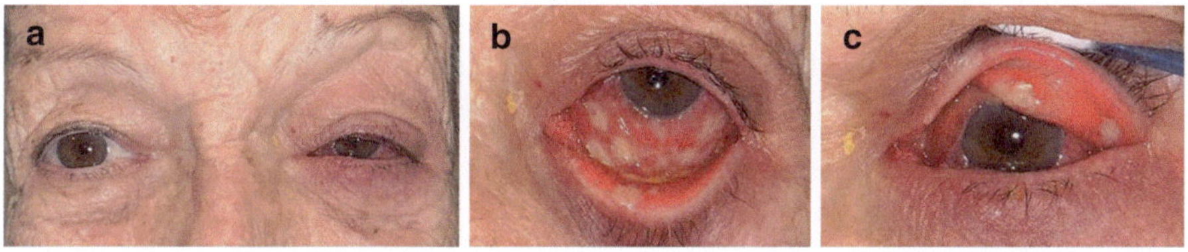

Fig. 6.3 Conjunctival Paracoccidioidomycosis. (**a**) Clinical photograph showing left ptosis and eyelid hyperemia. (**b**) and (**c**) Flat white lesions on the bulbar and tarsal conjunctiva (Adapted with permission from Wolters Kluwer Health, Inc.: [62])

white lesions disseminated over the bulbar, inferior fornix, and tarsal conjunctiva of the eyelids [62] (Figure 6.3a–c).

6.3.4 Microsporidial Conjunctivitis

The clinical manifestations of microsporidial conjunctivitis vary depending on the infecting species and the host's immune status, although this relationship has not been clearly established [63]. Common symptoms include ocular pain, redness, photophobia, tearing, and blurred vision, unilateral or bilateral. The majority of cases of microsporidial conjunctivitis present as keratoconjunctivitis. Slit-lamp biomicroscopy frequently reveals nonpurulent conjunctivitis with a papillary pattern in 60.5% of cases and a mixed papillary–follicular pattern in 39.5%. Characteristic corneal findings include multiple coarse, raised, punctate epithelial lesions with diffuse distribution, typical target-like lesions, and subepithelial infiltrates. Mild conjunctival hyperemia is commonly observed. In addition to keratoconjunctivitis, preauricular lymphadenopathy and periorbital edema have also been reported [34, 35]. *Encephalitozoon* is the causative agent of chronic superficial punctate keratoconjunctivitis, a condition most commonly observed in patients with acquired immunodeficiency syndrome (AIDS). In contrast, the genera *Vittaforma* and *Microsporidium* are associated with stromal keratitis in immunocompetent individuals, with and without a history of prior ocular trauma [34, 35].

6.4 Diagnosis

A high index of suspicion is essential for timely diagnosis, even in regions where fungal conjunctival infections are rare, as delayed recognition and poor response to empiric therapy are common. In such cases, the removal of infected tissue may be necessary to control the infection [64]. The diagnosis of fungal conjunctival infections remains challenging due to the lack of specific clinical features. However, recent advancements in laboratory and diagnostic techniques, coupled with greater awareness of the clinical presentation, have significantly improved the management of these infections [23, 65].

A thorough ophthalmological examination is essential to determine the nature of the discharge. A variety of clinical signs and symptoms are considered when diagnosing fungal conjunctivitis. These include eye discharge, conjunctival injection, redness of the eye, eyelashes that adhere together upon awakening, a gritty sensation in the eyes, eyelid or conjunctival edema, and a history of contact with individuals diagnosed with conjunctivitis [66] (Fig. 6.4).

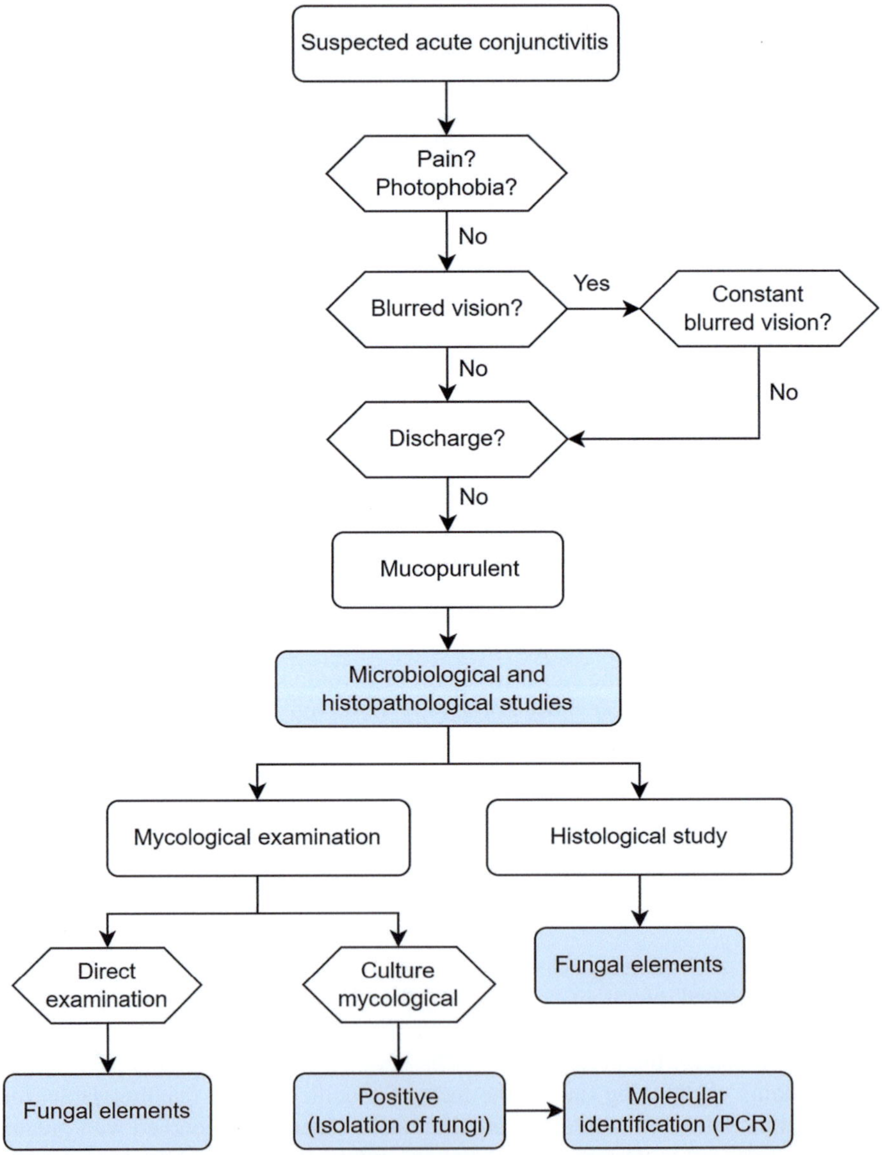

Fig. 6.4 Proposed algorithm for the diagnosis of fungal conjunctivitis

During the examination, under a slit lamp, the physician should also examine the eyelids for secretions on the eyelashes and the eyelid margin, as well as for irregularities on the margin and on the conjunctiva. The utilization of vital stains, such as fluorescein, facilitates the discernment of damage to the conjunctival or corneal epithelium. Furthermore, a thorough examination of the cornea is imperative for the identification of infiltrates, ulcers, edema, or clear indications of fungal infection, including feathery edges, lesions surrounding the primary lesion, an immune ring, retrocorneal plaque, hypopyon, or even corneal thinning or perforation. It is noteworthy that fungal conjunctivitis can be accompanied by fungal keratitis, underscoring the necessity for comprehensive evaluation and management [65].

Fungal conjunctivitis is often diagnosed by culturing samples from the patient's conjunctival sac. However, the sensitivity of culture is often reduced due to various factors, including the influence of the culture medium and the incubation temperature in the laboratory setting [67]. In the case of *Candida* conjunctivitis, Giemsa staining of a conjunctival scraping may reveal the presence of characteristic pseudohyphae and an inflammatory reaction of polymorphonuclear cells. In addition, these organisms demonstrate a proclivity for uncomplicated cultivation on blood or Sabouraud agar, and their identification as yeast (blastoconidia) or pseudohyphae is a relatively straightforward process [17]. Mucopurulent ocular discharge can be obtained using swabs or biopsies of the bulbar conjunctiva in cases of conjunctivitis caused by *Sporothrix* spp. [22, 68].

The invasive nature of the procedure and its potential sequelae, including scarring and conjunctivitis, complicate the diagnosis and management of this condition. The most frequently used stains for the histopathological diagnosis of fungal conjunctivitis include PAS, Giemsa, Gram stain, hexaammonium silver, and calcofluor white. In the case of *Candida*, the β-D-glucan test may be useful [17, 65].

In the case of *Candida* conjunctivitis, the presence of atypical granulomatous lesions necessitates laboratory identification. The diagnosis of candidiasis is typically suspected in patients with prolonged hospital stays or those suffering from diabetes mellitus. The identification of the causative organism can be obtained through culture or by polymerase chain reaction (PCR). In instances where the aforementioned tests yield inconclusive results, a conjunctival biopsy is recommended to facilitate histopathological evaluation and culture [17].

A variety of biopsy procedures can be performed on conjunctival lesions. Incisional biopsies involve the removal of a portion of the lesion, leaving a remnant on the ocular surface. Conversely, excisional biopsies entail the complete removal of the lesion using a no-touch technique, ensuring minimal damage to the surrounding tissue. The latter has the advantage of removing the entire lesion under study and being both diagnostic and therapeutic [17].

The identification of *Microsporidia* is typically performed through Gram staining on conjunctival and corneal scrapings, smears, and biopsies [35]. Alternatively, optical microscopy, accompanied by modified trichrome staining or polymerase chain reaction (PCR), is frequently utilized due to the time-consuming nature of transmission electron microscopy [35, 69]. The modified trichrome staining method is employed to identify microsporidia spores, which are stained pink on a blue-green background. The efficacy of other stains has also been evaluated; however, further research is necessary to determine their sensitivity and specificity. The following stains and their respective efficacies were observed: potassium hydroxide plus calcofluor white (96.7%), Gram (90%), Giemsa (73.3%), modified Ziehl-Neelsen (93.3%), and fluorescent techniques (calcofluor white). The sensitivity and specificity of these stains are comparable to those of modified trichrome staining [34].

A common finding in electron microscopy examinations of biopsy samples is the presence of organisms exhibiting morphological characteristics consistent with the genus *Encephalitozoon*. In immunocompetent individuals, the initial presentation includes an inflammatory infiltrate and stromal edema, a central area of epithelial irregularity, and iritis. In rare instances, a diagnosis is made following a corneal biopsy. Although keratoconjunctivitis is typically observed in patients with AIDS, this clinical picture has also been described in immunocompetent individuals. Although microsporidia are well known as opportunistic pathogens that cause infections in patients with AIDS, local immunosuppression from the use of topical corticosteroids is thought to predispose to microsporidian infection [34, 63].

More recently, deep metagenomic RNA sequencing has enabled the reliable detection and quantification of both common and rare pathogens causing conjunctivitis (e.g., *Candida*, *Microsporidia*), as well as strain identification. The unbiased nature of metagenomic RNA deep sequencing allows for the broadening of the scope of pathogen detection, including fungal species not usually associated with acute conjunctivitis. Furthermore, the identification of local host transcriptome signatures specific to the type of infection may facilitate the detection of pathogens even when the pathogen load is too low for direct identification [70].

6.5 Differential Diagnosis

The differential diagnosis encompasses infectious and noninfectious etiologies. The former category of etiologies includes bacterial conjunctivitis, which is typically caused by *Haemophilus influenzae*, *Streptococcus pneumoniae*, *Moraxella catarrhalis*, or *Pseudomonas aeruginosa*. Also, this category comprises viral conjunctivitis, often triggered by either the herpes simplex virus or the varicella-zoster virus, as well as Parinaud oculoglandular syndrome. A wide array of noninfectious etiologies has been identified, including allergic conjunctivitis, tumors, and toxic conjunctivitis resulting from the use of topical pharmaceuticals or systemic medications, such as chemotherapeutic agents or antihypertensive medications, which can lead to ocular surface damage and subsequent conjunctivitis. Additional noninfectious causes may include Sjögren's syndrome, which is characterized by the presence of conjunctivitis and scarring, as well as rare conditions such as ocular cicatricial pemphigoid and Stevens-Johnson syndrome (Table 6.2) [71].

However, the diagnostic complexity of fungal conjunctivitis is attributable to the causative species themselves. For example, ocular sporotrichosis has been observed to present with a wide range of clinical manifestations, mimicking a diverse

Table 6.2 Differential diagnoses of fungal conjunctivitis[13,23,33,59,62]

Characteristic	*Candida*	*Aspergillus*	*Fusarium*	*Sporothrix*	*Microsporidia*
Laterality	Commonly bilateral	Commonly unilateral	Commonly unilateral	Unilateral	Commonly unilateral
Morphology of conjunctival lesión	Erythematous conjunctiva, with mild mucopurulent discharge. Pseudomembranous exudates. Dense giant papillary hypertrophy	The superior tarsus with severe papillary and follicular reaction. Chronic, prominent mucous discharge	Edematous conjunctiva, with mild discharge, rapidly progressive ulceration	Granulomatous conjunctivitis with a salmon-pink appearance, with yellowish-white nodules, 'bread crumbs' appearance	Multifocal, elevated, coarse, round-oval epithelial/ sub-epithelial lesions, 'stuck-on' appearance
Biofilm	Yes	Yes	Yes	No	No
Site of infection	Mainly bulbar conjunctiva	Mainly tarsal conjunctiva	Satellite conjunctival (bulbar) infiltrates	Scattered in palpebral and bulbar conjunctiva	Diffuse, peripheral, paracentral
Progresión a keratitis	Elevated	Frequent, may develop subconjunctival fungus balls (aspergilloma).	Frequent, may develop keratoconjunctivitis simultaneously	No available	Appears gradually. Elevated
Severity and type of conjunctivitis	Mild to moderate	Moderate to severe	Moderate to severe	Mild to moderate granulomatous conjunctivitis with yellowish nodules	Mild to moderate conjunctival congestion Mixed follicular-papillary reaction
Symptom duration	Days to a few weeks	Days to a few weeks	Days to a few weeks	Days to weeks	Days to a few weeks
Sequelae	Fungemia. It may progress to endophthalmitis with irreversible visual loss	May develop scarring	In keratoconjunctivitis may develop scarring	Subepithelial fibrosis, symblepharon, and fornix shortening	Uncommonly, subepithelial scars
Associated systemic disease	Present rarely: Immunocompromised status	Frequently disseminated	Frequently disseminated	It may develop ipsilateral preauricular and submandibular adenomegaly (Parinaud's oculoglandular syndrome)	Present rarely: Immunocompromised status

spectrum of infectious and noninfectious diseases. In endemic and hyperendemic regions, it is imperative to differentiate ocular sporotrichosis from other endemic diseases. The diagnosis must be confirmed by mycological examination [23].

6.6 Treatment

The management of fungal conjunctivitis encompasses a significant challenge to healthcare providers. In the case of superficial conjunctivitis, empirical topical antifungal therapy may be adequate. However, systemic antifungal therapy may be necessary for deeper lesions [46].

The pharmaceutical agents employed in the treatment of fungal keratoconjunctivitis encompass natamycin, voriconazole, and amphotericin B. Among these, natamycin is regarded as a primary treatment option, with studies demonstrating its superior efficacy in patients afflicted with filamentous fungi when compared to voriconazole. Although sensitivity testing is not a customary practice, and data concerning sensitivity to region-specific antifungals is limited, such testing may be imperative in guiding treatment, given the recent emergence of drug resistance, particularly in cases of severe or recalcitrant infections [72].

In the case of *Candida* conjunctivitis, the infection responds to amphotericin B (3–8 mg/mL) in aqueous solution (not saline) or to the application of nystatin cream (100,000 U/g) four to six times daily [13]. The utility of miconazole drops has also been suggested [73].

In conjunctival sporotrichosis, treatment with itraconazole shows a favorable response, with reported cure rates of 79% in palpebral and 75% in bulbar conjunctival involvement. However, the itraconazole dosages used vary considerably depending on disease severity, and the limited number of patients and clinical studies precludes drawing more definitive conclusions [22]. Exceptionally, a case of conjunctival infection is resolved completely after surgical removal of the mass combined with oral itraconazole and topical fluconazole eye drops [24].

The management of microsporidial keratoconjunctivitis remains a significant challenge, as no definitive treatment has been established to date. This is further compounded by the intrinsic resistance of microsporidia to conventional antibiotics [35]. Albendazole, a benzimidazole that inhibits microtubule formation, has demonstrated efficacy against several *Microsporidia* species, including *Encephalitozoon*. In the treatment of microsporidial keratoconjunctivitis, the recommended dosage of the medication is 200–400 mg bid [25]. In clinical trials, itraconazole has demonstrated antifungal efficacy at a dose of 200 mg/day in cases of microsporidial conjunctivitis, even when administered as a monotherapy, particularly in cases of albendazole resistance [74]. A variety of topical treatment options exist, including fumagillin, fluoroquinolones, polyethylene biguanide, propamidine, and polyamines, which have demonstrated efficacy in the treatment of keratoconjunctivitis [36, 75]. Additionally, the use of topical voriconazole in conjunction with albendazole has been proposed, resulting in a favorable therapeutic response [76]. An isolated case of microsporidial keratoconjunctivitis in a woman with AIDS and severe immunosuppression was successfully managed with highly active antiretroviral therapy alone. This observation underscores the potential importance of immune reconstitution in the management of such patients [77].

In cases of microsporidial conjunctivitis with inadequate response to oral and/or topical antimicrobial therapy, surgical intervention may be required. The most effective procedures include therapeutic penetrating keratoplasty and deep anterior lamellar keratoplasty. Epithelial debridement has also proven beneficial, as it can reduce the microsporidial load. In patients with suspected microsporidial conjunctivitis and negative corneal scrapings, empirical treatment with topical fluoroquinolones has been used until disease resolution. The visual prognosis is generally favorable, with no loss of visual acuity. Additionally, confocal imaging has been proposed as a valuable tool to monitor treatment response [78].

There are several treatment options available, including the use of Argon laser to form cavitations in the cornea in cases of keratoconjunctivitis, direct damage to the infectious agent, and penetration of antimycotics. Another option, as previously mentioned, is the utilization of fluoroquinolones, particularly moxifloxacin, which has been documented to exert an effect on topoisomerase. Alternatively, toxicity can be induced by the use of preservatives, such as benzalkonium chloride. In instances where a patient does not respond to topical treatment, surgical procedures may be considered. If the cornea exhibits adequate thickness, a conjunctival lining may be performed. Conversely, if the cornea is not sufficiently thick, corneoscleral tissue may be placed to restore part of the thinning tissue. In advanced cases or when the size of the corneal perforation is substantial (greater than 4–5 mm), therapeutic penetrating keratoplasty may be indicated. In cases where the posterior segment of the eye has been infected and the vitreous cavity exhibits a poor response to intravitreal treatment, surgical removal of the eyeball is performed [78].

6.7 Visual Prognosis and Complications

Evolutionary complications of fungal conjunctivitis include progression to keratomycosis, which may progress to stromal lysis, descemetocele, corneal thinning and/or perforation, scleritis, endophthalmitis, purulent necrosis of the eyeball, and orbital cellulitis [79]. Conjunctival fibrosis, symblepharon, ectropion, paracentral leukoma, and limbal pannus are some complications in patients with conjunctival sporotrichosis [68, 80].

6.8 Conclusions

Fungal conjunctivitis is an uncommon but clinically significant ocular infection, often underdiagnosed due to its nonspecific presentation and rarity compared with bacterial and viral etiologies. Accurate diagnosis requires a high index of suspicion, particularly in chronic or recalcitrant follicular–papillary conjunctivitis unresponsive to topical antibiotics and must incorporate epidemiological, host-related, and environmental factors. Opportunistic species such as *Candida*, *Aspergillus*, *Fusarium*, and *Microsporidia*, as well as dimorphic fungi like *Sporothrix*, highlight the diverse etiological spectrum and the influence of immune status in disease expression and prognosis.

Management is complicated by the limited evidence base, as most available data derive from isolated case reports or cases series. Treatment strategies range from topical and systemic antifungals to surgical intervention in severe or refractory cases, with outcomes strongly dependent on early recognition and host immune competence. Continued research, including prospective studies and molecular diagnostic approaches, is essential to improve understanding, guide therapeutic protocols, and optimize visual outcomes in patients affected by this rare but challenging condition.

References

1. Mostafa F, Mahmoudabadi Z, Hosein R, Roja AZ. Conjunctival mycoflora in patients presenting to eye ward of Imam Khomeini Hospital, Ahvaz. Pak J Med Sci. 2010;26:935–7.
2. Ando N, Takatori K. Fungal flora of the conjunctival sac. Am J Ophthalmol. 1982;94:67–74. https://doi.org/10.1016/0002-9394(82)90193-3.
3. Segal E, Romano A, Eylan E, Stein R. Fungal flora of the normal conjunctival sac. Mykosen. 1977;20:9–14. https://doi.org/10.1111/j.1439-0507.1977.tb01475.x.
4. Bissinger I, Bareño J. Perfil clínico de sensibilización a hongos en Medellín, Colombia [Clinical profile of sensitization to fungi in Medellin, Colombia]. Rev Alerg Mex. 2016;63:123–34. https://doi.org/10.29262/ram.v63i2.108.
5. Aragona P, Baudouin C, Benitez Del Castillo JM, Messmer E, Barabino S, Merayo-Lloves J, Brignole-Baudouin F, Inferrera L, Rolando M, Mencucci R, Rescigno M, Bonini S, Labetoulle M. The ocular microbiome and microbiota and their effects on ocular surface pathophysiology and disorders. Surv Ophthalmol. 2021;66:907–25. https://doi.org/10.1016/j.survophthal.2021.03.010.
6. Wen X, Miao L, Deng Y, Bible PW, Hu X, Zou Y, Liu Y, Guo S, Liang J, Chen T, Peng GH, Chen W, Liang L, Wei L. The influence of age and sex on ocular surface microbiota in healthy adults. Invest Ophthalmol Vis Sci. 2017;58:6030–7. https://doi.org/10.1167/iovs.17-22957.
7. Shivaji S, Jayasudha R, Sai Prashanthi G, Kalyana Chakravarthy S, Sharma S. The human ocular surface fungal microbiome. Invest Ophthalmol Vis Sci. 2019;60:451–9. https://doi.org/10.1167/iovs.18-26076.
8. Reginatto P, Agostinetto GJ, Fuentefria RDN, Marinho DR, Pizzol MD, Fuentefria AM. Eye fungal infections: a mini review. Arch Microbiol. 2023;205:236. https://doi.org/10.1007/s00203-023-03536-6.
9. Woodland RM, Darougar S, Thaker U, Cornell L, Siddique M, Wania J, Shah M. Causes of conjunctivitis and keratoconjunctivitis in Karachi, Pakistan. Trans R Soc Trop Med Hyg. 1992;86:317–20. https://doi.org/10.1016/0035-9203(92)90328-a.
10. Shekhawat NS, Shtein RM, Blachley TS, Stein JD. Antibiotic prescription fills for acute conjunctivitis among enrollees in a large United States managed care network. Ophthalmology. 2017;124:1099–107. https://doi.org/10.1016/j.ophtha.2017.04.034.
11. Gin C, Crock C, Wells K. Conjunctivitis: a review. Aust J Gen Pract. 2024;53:847–52. https://doi.org/10.31128/AJGP-09-23-6960.
12. Lalitha CS, Nayak B, Hallur V, Kharolia A. Invasion of the therapeutic contact lens by a rare fungal species presenting as the acute red eye: a case report. Indian J Ophthalmol. 2020;68:2548–50. https://doi.org/10.4103/ijo.IJO_1634_20.

13. Nivenius E, Montan P. Candida albicans should be considered when managing keratitis in atopic keratoconjunctivitis. Acta Ophthalmol. 2015;93:579–80. https://doi.org/10.1111/aos.12708.
14. Shah A, Sachdev A, Coggon D, Hossain P. Geographic variations in microbial keratitis: an analysis of the peer-reviewed literature. Br J Ophthalmol. 2011;95:762–7. https://doi.org/10.1136/bjo.2009.169607.
15. Norman FF, González-López JJ, Gayoso-Cantero D, Vicente-Antolin M, Corbacho-Loarte MD, López-Vélez R, González-Sanz M. Ocular infections in international travelers. Travel Med Infect Dis. 2025;63:102789. https://doi.org/10.1016/j.tmaid.2024.102789.
16. Lupetti A, Tavanti A, Davini P, Ghelardi E, Corsini V, Merusi I, Boldrini A, Campa M, Senesi S. Horizontal transmission of Candida parapsilosis candidemia in a neonatal intensive care unit. J Clin Microbiol. 2002;40:2363–9. https://doi.org/10.1128/JCM.40.7.2363-2369.2002.
17. Peng ZY, Qian J, Han YN. A case of fungal conjunctivitis manifested by a conjunctival mass. Zhonghua Yan Ke Za Zhi. 2022;58:1075–8. https://doi.org/10.3760/cma.j.cn112142-20211210-00582.
18. Woldemariam M, Aklilu A, Manilal A, Mengistu M, Tadesse D, Siraj M, Hatamleh AA, Alnafisi BK, Idhayadhulla A. Microbial profile and associated factors of external ocular bacterial and fungal infections in Arba Minch General Hospital: a cross-sectional study. Sci Rep. 2024;14:28744. https://doi.org/10.1038/s41598-024-77723-w.
19. Maiti S, Gandhi J, Joseph J. Microbiological spectrum and antibiotic susceptibility patterns of non-viral conjunctivitis over 16 years at a tertiary eye care center in southern India. Int Ophthalmol. 2023;43:3717–24. https://doi.org/10.1007/s10792-023-02781-4.
20. Gray TB, Cursons RT, Sherwan JF, Rose PR. Acanthamoeba, bacterial, and fungal contamination of contact lens storage cases. Br J Ophthalmol. 1995;79:601–5. https://doi.org/10.1136/bjo.79.6.601.
21. Radhakrishnan N, Panigrahi AK, Balasubramanium A, Das M, Prajna NV. Colonization of therapeutic contact lens by dematiaceous fungi. Cont Lens Anterior Eye. 2019;42:470–2. https://doi.org/10.1016/j.clae.2019.04.008.
22. Ramírez-Soto MC, Tirado-Sánchez A, Bonifaz A. Ocular sporotrichosis. J Fungi (Basel). 2021;7:951. https://doi.org/10.3390/jof7110951.
23. Ramírez-Soto MC, Bonifaz A. Ocular fungal infections. J Fungi (Basel). 2022;8:1078. https://doi.org/10.3390/jof8101078.
24. Hampton DE, Adesina A, Chodosh J. Conjunctival sporotrichosis in the absence of antecedent trauma. Cornea. 2002;21:831–3. https://doi.org/10.1097/00003226-200211000-00021.
25. Ferreira TA, Sodré CT, Costa JM, Setta CRP, Ramos-E-Silva M. Primary conjunctival sporotrichosis: an atypical presentation of the disease. JAAD Case Rep. 2018;4:497–9. https://doi.org/10.1016/j.jdcr.2018.01.022. PMID: 29984295; PMCID: PMC6031559.
26. Quinlan EJ, Gill V. Initial presentation of disseminated coccidioidomycosis with ocular lesions. Case Rep Infect Dis. 2020;2020:1305193. https://doi.org/10.1155/2020/1305193.
27. Donovan FM, Ampel NM, Thompson GR 3rd. Coccidioidomycosis. Infect Dis Clin N Am. 2025;39:183–97. https://doi.org/10.1016/j.idc.2024.11.012.
28. Maguire LJ, Campbell RJ, Edson RS. Coccidioidomycosis with necrotizing granulomatous conjunctivitis. Cornea. 1994;13:539–42.
29. Faulkner RF. Ocular coccidioidomycosis. Report of a case of coccidioidal granuloma of the conjunctiva associated with cutaneous coccidioidomycosis. Am J Ophthalmol. 1962;53:822–7.
30. Slack JW, Hyndiuk RA, Harris GJ, Simons KB. Blastomycosis of the eyelid and conjunctiva. Ophthalmic Plast Reconstr Surg. 1992;8:143–9. https://doi.org/10.1097/00002341-199206000-00011.
31. Costa PS, Hollanda BV, Assis RV, Costa SM, Valle LM. Parinaud's oculoglandular syndrome associated with paracoccidioidomycosis. Rev Inst Med Trop Sao Paulo. 2002;44:49–52. https://doi.org/10.1590/s0036-46652002000100008.
32. Gervini RL, Vettorato G, Lecompte SM, Biasi TB, Ruthner FG, Kronbauer FL. Ocular paracoccidioidomycosis: report of two cases and review of literature. An Bras Dermatol. 2004;79:69–78. https://doi.org/10.1590/S0365-05962004000100008.

33. Haq A, Wardak H, Kraski N. Infective conjunctivitis—its pathogenesis, management and complications [Internet]. In: Common eye infections. InTech; 2013. Available from: https://doi.org/10.5772/52462.
34. Tham AC, Sanjay S. Clinical spectrum of microsporidial keratoconjunctivitis. Clin Experiment Ophthalmol. 2012;40:512–8. https://doi.org/10.1111/j.1442-9071.2011.02712.x.
35. Lekskul M, Sasiprapha N, Mungthin M, Ruang-Areerate T, Rangsin R, Thongruay R. Clinical characteristics, progression patterns and treatment outcomes in microsporidial keratoconjunctivitis: a prospective study in Thailand. Int Ophthalmol. 2024;44:432. https://doi.org/10.1007/s10792-024-03340-1.
36. Zhang Y, Xu S, Xu Y. Clinical analyses of 4 cases of microsporidial keratoconjunctivitis. Acta Parasitol. 2025;70:71. https://doi.org/10.1007/s11686-025-01010-5.
37. Mandal S, Sucharita S, Deshmukh V, Priyadarshini SR, Sahu SK, Das S. Histopathological evaluation of corneal tissues in microsporidia stromal keratitis. Invest Ophthalmol Vis Sci. 2025;66:9. https://doi.org/10.1167/iovs.66.4.9.
38. Iskandar E, Ferraro N, Secchi FG, Ferrari G, Pitrolo AMG, Rama P, Baldanti F, Cavanna C. Fungal keratitis caused by Scedosporium apiospermum in an immunocompetent patient: how challenging can treatment get? New Microbiol. 2025;48:89–94.
39. Czech MM, Cuellar-Rodriguez J, Kwon-Chung KJ, Stock F, Aneke CI, Olivier KN, Fennelly KP, Gea-Banacloche J, Zerbe CS, Freeman AF, Holland SM, Lionakis MS, Seyedmousavi A. Clinical significance and antifungal susceptibility profile of 103 clinical isolates of Scedosporium species complex and Lomentospora prolificans obtained from NIH patients. J Clin Microbiol. 2025;63:e0155024. https://doi.org/10.1128/jcm.01550-24.
40. Cortez KJ, Roilides E, Quiroz-Telles F, Meletiadis J, Antachopoulos C, Knudsen T, Buchanan W, Milanovich J, Sutton DA, Fothergill A, Rinaldi MG, Shea YR, Zaoutis T, Kottilil S, Walsh TJ. Infections caused by Scedosporium spp. Clin Microbiol Rev. 2008;21:157–97. https://doi.org/10.1128/CMR.00039-07.
41. Fernandez-Flores A, Lopez-Medrano R, Fuster-Foz C. Histopathological clues in the diagnosis of fungal infection by Scedosporium in a case of endophthalmitis starting as conjunctivitis. J Cutan Pathol. 2016;43:461–7. https://doi.org/10.1111/cup.12689.
42. Cheng SC, Lin YY, Kuo CN, Lai LJ. Cladosporium keratitis – a case report and literature review. BMC Ophthalmol. 2015;15:106. https://doi.org/10.1186/s12886-015-0092-1.
43. Sinnappan S, Che-Hamzah J, Santhirathelagan CT. Cladosporium conjunctivitis – a rare entity. Int J Med Sci. 2019;4:33–6.
44. Behrens-Baumann W. Mycoses of the eye and its adnexa. Dev Ophthalmol. 1999;32:68–94.
45. Müller G, Schlecht KA, Schlecht C, Voth JA. Zur Bedeutung der Candida albicans-Infektion der Konjunktiva [The significance of candida albicans conjunctivitis (author's transl)]. Klin Monatsbl Augenheilkd. 1981;178:69–71. https://doi.org/10.1055/s-2008-1055299.
46. Thomas PA. Current perspectives on ophthalmic mycoses. Clin Microbiol Rev. 2003;16:730–97. https://doi.org/10.1128/CMR.16.4.730-797.2003.
47. Aboutalebian S, Charsizadeh A, Eshaghi H, Nikmaesh B, Mirhendi H. A case of Candida metapsilosis conjunctivitis in a neonate admitted to the cardiac heart intensive care unit. Clin Case Rep. 2023;11:e6870. https://doi.org/10.1002/ccr3.6870.
48. Sehgal SC, Dhawan S, Chhiber S, Sharma M, Talwar P. Frequency and significance of fungal isolations from conjunctival sac and their role in ocular infections. Mycopathologia. 1981;73:17–9. https://doi.org/10.1007/BF00443007.
49. Watkinson S. Assessment and management of patients with acute red eye. Nurs Older People. 2013;25:27–34. https://doi.org/10.7748/nop2013.06.25.5.27.e442r1.
50. Pina PSS, Custódio M, Sugaya NN, de Sousa SCOM. Histopathologic aspects of the so-called chronic hyperplastic candidiasis: an analysis of 36 cases. J Cutan Pathol. 2021;48:66–71. https://doi.org/10.1111/cup.13875.
51. Alofi RM, Alrohaily LS, Alharthi NN, Almouteri MM. Ocular manifestations in seborrheic dermatitis epidemiology, clinical features, and management: a comprehensive review. Cureus. 2024;16:e70335. https://doi.org/10.7759/cureus.70335.

52. Karalezli A, Borazan M, Dursun R, Kiyici H, Kucukerdonmez C, Akova YA. Impression cytology and ocular surface characteristics in patients with seborrhoeic dermatitis. Acta Ophthalmol. 2011;89:e137–41.
53. Słowik M, Biernat MM, Urbaniak-Kujda D, Kapelko-Słowik K, Misiuk-Hojło M. Mycotic infections of the eye. Adv Clin Exp Med. 2015;24:1113–7. https://doi.org/10.17219/acem/50572.
54. Spadea L, Giannico MI. Diagnostic and management strategies of Aspergillus endophthalmitis: current insights. Clin Ophthalmol. 2019;13:2573–82. https://doi.org/10.2147/OPTH.S219264.
55. Perry HD, Donnenfeld ED, Grossman GA, Stein M, Epstein AB. Retained Aspergillus-contaminated contact lens inducing conjunctival mass and keratoconjunctivitis in an immunocompetent patient. CLAO J. 1998;24:57–8.
56. Chen JL, Wang CC, Sheu SJ, Yeh TI. Conjunctival aspergilloma with multiple mulberry nodules: a case report. Kaohsiung J Med Sci. 2005;21:286–90. https://doi.org/10.1016/S1607-551X(09)70203-7.
57. Gus PI, Bayer MC, Matos GH, Baes CV, Martins MF, Vargas Neto J, Onsten TG. Aspergilose orbitária: relato de caso [Ocular aspergillosis—case report]. Arq Bras Oftalmol. 2005;68:133–5. https://doi.org/10.1590/s0004-27492005000100025.
58. Yadav S, Lomi N, Mukhija R, Kashyap S, Tandon R. An unusual presentation of conjunctival aspergillosis as a polyp in an immunocompetent child. Natl Med J India. 2021;34:279–80. https://doi.org/10.25259/NMJI_251_20.
59. Segal E, Eylan E, Bentovim T, Stein R, Romano A. Mycotic keratoconjunctivitis due to Aspergillus niger. Mykosen. 1974;17:147–52. https://doi.org/10.1111/j.1439-0507.1974.tb04306.x.
60. Romano A, Segal E, Ben-Tovim T. Aspergillus niger keratoconjunctivitis. Ophthalmologica. 1973;166:81–7. https://doi.org/10.1159/000306798.
61. Chacon-Cruz E, Male-Valle F, Rivas-Landeros RM, Lopatynsky-Reyes EZ, Almada-Salazar LA, Becka CM. Severe mycotic keratoconjunctivitis caused by Fusarium sp. in an immunocompetent child successfully treated with intravenous voriconazole and keratoplasty: case report and short review of the literature. Ther Adv Infect Dis. 2018;6:2049936118811213. https://doi.org/10.1177/2049936118811213.
62. Cunha BSA, Grecca LS Jr, Chahud F, Cruz AAV. Disseminated conjunctival paracoccidioidomycosis. Ophthalmic Plast Reconstr Surg. 2021;37:e153. https://doi.org/10.1097/IOP.0000000000001844.
63. Sridhar MS, Sharma S. Microsporidial keratoconjunctivitis in a HIV-seronegative patient treated with debridement and oral itraconazole. Am J Ophthalmol. 2003;136:745–6. https://doi.org/10.1016/s0002-9394(03)00391-x.
64. Keay LJ, Gower EW, Iovieno A, Oechsler RA, Alfonso EC, Matoba A, Colby K, Tuli SS, Hammersmith K, Cavanagh D, Lee SM, Irvine J, Stulting RD, Mauger TF, Schein OD. Clinical and microbiological characteristics of fungal keratitis in the United States, 2001–2007: a multicenter study. Ophthalmology. 2011;118:920–6. https://doi.org/10.1016/j.ophtha.2010.09.011.
65. Shimokawa A, Kobayashi A, Saeki Y, Uchio E. A case of fungal conjunctivitis with giant papillae treated surgically. Taiwan J Ophthalmol. 2020;11:417–20. https://doi.org/10.4103/tjo.tjo_46_20.
66. Everitt H, Little P. How do GPs diagnose and manage acute infective conjunctivitis? A GP survey. Fam Pract. 2002;19:658–60. https://doi.org/10.1093/fampra/19.6.658.
67. Azari AA, Barney NP. Conjunctivitis: a systematic review of diagnosis and treatment. JAMA. 2013;310:1721–9. https://doi.org/10.1001/jama.2013.280318.
68. Ramírez-Soto MC. Extracutaneous sporotrichosis. Clin Microbiol Rev. 2025;38(1):e0014024. https://doi.org/10.1128/cmr.00140-24.
69. Conners MS, Gibler TS, Van Gelder RN. Diagnosis of microsporidia keratitis by polymerase chain reaction. Arch Ophthalmol. 2004;122:283–4. https://doi.org/10.1001/archopht.122.2.283.

70. Lalitha P, Seitzman GD, Kotecha R, Hinterwirth A, Chen C, Zhong L, Cummings ME, Lebas E, Sahoo MK, Pinsky BA, Lietman TM, Doan T. Unbiased pathogen detection and host gene profiling for conjunctivitis. Ophthalmology. 2019;126:1090–4. https://doi.org/10.1016/j.ophtha.2019.03.039.
71. Simmons BA, Kupcha AC, Law JJ, Wang K, Carter KD, Mawn LA, Shriver EM. Misdiagnosis of fungal infections of the orbit. Can J Ophthalmol. 2023;58:449–54. https://doi.org/10.1016/j.jcjo.2022.04.007.
72. Ansari Z, Miller D, Galor A. Current thoughts in fungal keratitis: diagnosis and treatment. Curr Fungal Infect Rep. 2013;7:209–18. https://doi.org/10.1007/s12281-013-0150-110.1007/s12281-013-0150-1.
73. Gyanfosu L, Koffuor GA, Kyei S, Ababio-Danso B, Peprah-Donkor K, Nyansah WB, Asare F. Efficacy and safety of extemporaneously prepared miconazole eye drops in Candida albicans-induced keratomycosis. Int Ophthalmol. 2018;38:2089–100. https://doi.org/10.1007/s10792-017-0707-z.
74. Rossi P, Urbani C, Donelli G, Pozio E. Resolution of microsporidial sinusitis and keratoconjunctivitis by itraconazole treatment. Am J Ophthalmol. 1999;127:210–2. https://doi.org/10.1016/s0002-9394(98)00352-3.
75. Tung-Lien Quek D, Pan JC, Krishnan PU, Zhao PS, Teoh SC. Microsporidial keratoconjunctivitis in the tropics: a case series. Open Ophthalmol J. 2011;5:42–7. https://doi.org/10.2174/1874364101105010042.
76. Donovan CP, Margo CE, Espana EM. Stromal microsporidial keratitis successfully treated with medical therapy. Am J Ophthalmol Case Rep. 2021;23:101178. https://doi.org/10.1016/j.ajoc.2021.101178.
77. Martins SA, Muccioli C, Belfort R Jr, Castelo A. Resolution of microsporidial keratoconjunctivitis in an AIDS patient treated with highly active antiretroviral therapy. Am J Ophthalmol. 2001;131:378–9. https://doi.org/10.1016/s0002-9394(00)00810-2.
78. Guo F, Liang QF. Advances in clinical diagnosis and treatment of microsporidial keratitis. Zhonghua Yan Ke Za Zhi. 2024;60:854–9. https://doi.org/10.3760/cma.j.issn.0412-4081-20240329-00149.
79. Bourcier T, Sauer A, Dory A, Denis J, Sabou M. Kératites fongiques [Fungal keratitis]. J Fr Ophtalmol. 2017;40:882–8. https://doi.org/10.1016/j.jfo.2017.05.013.
80. Arinelli A, Aleixo A d C, Freitas DFS, do Valle ACF, Almeida-Paes R, Gutierrez-Galhardo MC, Curi ALL. Ocular sporotrichosis: 26 cases with bulbar involvement in a hyperendemic area of zoonotic transmission. Ocul Immunol Inflamm. 2020;28:764–71. https://doi.org/10.1080/09273948.2019.1624779.

Fungal Keratitis: Epidemiology, Diagnosis and Therapy

7

Alejandro Rodriguez-Garcia and Guillermo Amescua

7.1 Introduction

Infectious keratitis remains among the most challenging ocular disorders, representing the fifth leading cause of blindness worldwide with approximately 36 million (3.5%) blind individuals up to 2015 [1]. Furthermore, a nationwide study in China found that infectious keratitis is the leading cause of corneal blindness in that country. This condition is primarily driven by an increased risk of agriculture/construction related trauma, along with low socioeconomic status and widespread illiteracy [2, 3].

Corneal infections can be divided according to microorganism class into bacterial, viral, fungal, and protozoan keratitis. The most common pathogens responsible for infectious keratitis include *Staphylococcus aureus*, *Pseudomonas aeruginosa*, *Streptococcus pneumonia,* and *Serratia* spp. Fungal agents include filamentous (*Fusarium* spp., *Aspergillus* spp., and *Curvularia* spp.) and yeasts (*Candida* spp.), while *Acanthamoeba* spp. is the most prevalent protist, causing significant ocular morbidity [4]. The most common microbe genera infecting the cornea are bacteria and fungi, with the latter carrying the worst prognosis, reflected in a 5–6 times more corneal perforation possibilities than bacterial infection [5, 6].

The main predisposing factors for infectious keratitis include ocular trauma, soft contact lens wear, especially overnight and extended wear lenses, poor hygiene, and inadequate disinfecting solutions. Other risk factors include corneal and ocular surface surgery, chronic inflammatory ocular surface disease, including severe dry eye, autoimmune and metabolic diseases, along with immunodeficiency, and extended topical corticosteroid use [4, 7].

A. Rodriguez-Garcia (✉)
Institute of Ophthalmology and Visual Sciences, School of Medicine and Health Sciences, Tecnologico de Monterrey, Monterrey, Mexico

G. Amescua
Bascom Palmer Eye Institute, University of Miami, Miami, FL, USA

M. C. Ramírez-Soto (ed.), *Fungal Eye Infections*,
https://doi.org/10.1007/978-3-032-19923-2_7

Fungal or mycotic keratitis is the corneal infection by filamentous and/or yeast-like fungi, accounting for more than 50% of all culture-positive microbial keratitis, mainly in tropical and subtropical countries [8]. Furthermore, the types of pathogens involved in specific keratomycosis tend to correlate with certain geographic zones. An example is the larger proportion of yeast-like fungal keratitis seen in temperate climates, whereas filamentous fungi keratitis is more common in tropical latitudes [9].

Fungal keratitis is a diagnostic challenge due to several factors, including its non-specific clinical appearance, prolonged isolation time, and negative culture results. To address this, direct microscopic observation of stained corneal scrapings is a key technique in the preliminary diagnosis [10, 11]. This is followed by the high-specific but low-sensitive isolation on Sabouraud's dextrose and blood agars, which is the gold standard diagnostic technique [12]. The combination of a serious disease prognosis, limited access to specialized medical facilities provided with advanced molecular and imaging diagnostic technologies, and restricted treatment options contributes to the progression of mild fungal keratitis into severe corneal disease [9, 13–15].

Medical treatment for fungal keratitis currently involves partially effective antifungal agents, including topical natamycin, amphotericin B, fluconazole, and voriconazole [16, 17]. However, severe inflammation caused by the fungus and a strong adaptive immune response can lead to corneal ulceration and stromal meltdown. This ultimately results in corneal scarring and vision impairment [18, 19]. Therefore, under such clinical circumstances, interventional therapies, from photodynamic-collagen cross-linking (CXL) to opportune tectonic or penetrating keratoplasty, are necessary to overcome the pathogen invasiveness and corneal destruction capacity and for visual rehabilitation [20–22].

This chapter is intended to bring clinicians a comprehensive overview of the impact of fungal keratitis. It offers accurate and current information on the most effective diagnostic techniques and treatment strategies for managing this serious and often devastating infectious eye disease.

7.2 Epidemiologic Features and Risk Factors

1. *Overview.* The epidemiological features of fungal keratitis vary based on geographic location, season, ethnicity, socioeconomic status, occupation, and various other demographic and risk factors [23]. A systematic literature review published in 2021 analyzed 118 studies, which provided the incidence of fungal keratitis as a proportion of microbial keratitis. Data from 72 years estimated the minimum annual incidence of fungal keratitis to be between 736,251 and 1,367,323 cases, with the highest rates seen in Asia and Africa, and an annual loss of 84,143–115,697 eyes due to the infection [24].
2. *Epidemiologic and demographic reports.* A multicentric study performed in 11 tertiary eye centers across the United States between 2001 and 2007 found 733 fungal keratitis cases, most of them culture (94.7%) or biopsy (2.6%) proven.

The most frequently associated risk factor for fungal keratitis was contact lens wear (37% of cases), followed by ocular surface disease (29%) and ocular trauma (25%). Most contact lens-associated infections (86% of cases) and those of ocular trauma (78%) were caused by a filamentous fungus, while yeast (most commonly *Candida* spp.) was the causative microorganism in 53% of ocular surface disease cases [25]. The youngest mean age (38.9 ± 16.5 years) was found in females (63.1% of cases) wearing contact lenses, and the oldest (60.3 ± 18.5 years) was also found in females (50.7%) with ocular surface disease-associated infection. Contrarywise, males (77.8%) predominated in the ocular trauma-associated infection (mean age, 46.2 ± 16.5 years) [25].

An epidemiologic report on fungal keratitis performed in the United Kingdom (temperate climate) from 2003 to 2005 found a minimum average annualized incidence of 0.32 (95% CI, 0.24–0.44) cases per million individuals. *Candida* spp. represented 56% of the cases; of these, 63% were associated with long-term topical corticosteroid therapy for ocular surface disease. On the other hand, filamentary fungus infection was significantly more common in male patients, particularly those suffering from ocular trauma [26].

A study conducted at a tertiary eye care center in Hyderabad, India, from 1991 to 2001, identified fungal keratitis as the second leading cause of corneal infections, accounting for 38.2% of cases ($n = 1360$). The primary cause of these infections was found to be *Fusarium* spp., which represented 36.6% of the cases. Notably, the study revealed that a higher percentage of patients with fungal keratitis (50.8%) required surgical intervention compared to those with bacterial infections, indicating a poorer outcome for these cases [27].

A much larger microbial keratitis analysis performed at Aravind eye hospital in Madurai, India, from 2002 to 2012 found 34.3% ($n = 8206$) fungi-confirmed isolations from a total of 14,738 of 23,897 (61.7%) smears performed on presumed infectious keratitis patients. Furthermore, the number of fungal smears increased from 609 to 863 per year during the study period. The most common pathogens were *Fusarium* spp. ($N = 2274$; 14.5% of cultures) and *Aspergillus* spp. ($N = 1390$; 8.8%) [28].

Another comprehensive fungal keratitis epidemiologic study from central China included 2064 culture-proven eyes diagnosed between 2000 and 2009. The predominant fungal species isolated were *Fusarium* spp. (56.93%, $n = 1175$) followed by *Aspergillus* spp. (15.26%, $n = 315$) and *Alternaria* spp. (7.32%, $n = 151$). Of the 2064 patients, 1297 (62.84%) were men, and 767 (37.16%) were women (male-to-female ratio = 1.6:1). Patients aged 41–50 were most frequent (26.79%), followed by 51–60 (25.58%). Among these patients, the great majority were farmers (92.39%, $n = 1907$), 82 (3.97%) students, and 39 (1.89%) physical laborers [29]. Considering risk factors, corneal trauma was recorded in 656 eyes (31.78%), with plants (16.86%) being the major agent involved. However, 1292 patients (62.60%) had no risk factors record. Regarding seasonal variation, fungal keratitis was reported more often from October to December, followed by July to September [29] (Table 7.1).

Table 7.1 Worldwide epidemiologic features of the most important infectious keratitis epidemiologic studies (N ≥500) from 1975 to 2023, highlighting fungal causalities

Author/year	Study period	Geographic region	Total no. of cases	Mean age (years)	Males (%)	Positive culture (%)	Fungus proportion (%)	Fungus species (%)
Cariello et al. [365] 2011	1975–2007	Brazil	6804	42.1 ± 21.4	60.0	48.6	11.0	NA
Rautaraya et al. [366] 2011	2006–2009	India	997	NA	71.1	74.6	26.4	*Aspergillus* spp. (23.1); *fusarium* spp. (19.2)
Lin et al. [367] 2012	2006–2009	India	5221	NA	NA	58.0	63.0	*Fusarium* spp. (15.5)
Marujo et al. [368] 2013	2005–2009	Brazil	2049	45.0	55.0	71.6	7.0	NA
Kaliamurthy et al. [369] 2013	2005–2012	India	2170	45.7 ± 16.6	58.7	77.0	22.7	NA
Hernandez-Camarena et al. [370] 2015	2002–2011	Mexico City, Mexico	1638	45.0	48.6	38.0	12.0	NA
Lalitha et al. [28] 2015	2002–2012	India	23,897	NA	NA	59.0	34.3	*Fusarium* spp. (14.5); *aspergillus* spp. (8.8)
Wang et al. [30] 2015	2013–2014	China	1000	NA	68.2	53.5	100.0	*Aspergillus* spp. (53.8); *fusarium* spp. (19.3)
Hsiao et al. [371] 2016	2003–2012	Taiwan	2012	NA	NA	49.3	16.0	NA
Politis et al. [372] 2016	2002–2014	Israel	943	47.0 ± 25.2	53.0	47.9	8.2	NA
Tan et al. [373] 2017	2004–2015	Manchester, UK	4229	45.9	NA	32.6	7.1	NA
Tam et al. [374] 2017	2000–2015	Toronto, Canada	2330	41.6 ± 24.0	47.0	57.3	4.9	NA
Ting et al. [5] 2018	2008–2017	Sunderland, UK	914	55.9 ± 21.0	47.9	46.1	4.2	NA
Khor et al. [375] 2018	2012–2014	Asia	6626	46.0	60.8	70.7	32.7	*Fusarium* spp. (18.3); *aspergillus flavus* (8.3)

Tavassoli et al. [376] 2019	2006–2017	Bristol, Bath, UK	2614	47.7 ± 21.2	49.9	38.1	6.9	NA
Kowalski et al. [377] 2019	1993–2018	Pittsburgh, USA	1387	NA	NA	100.0	6.7	NA
Lin et al. [378] 2019	2010–2018	China	7229	NA	NA	42.8	57.6	*Fusarium* spp. (23.5); *aspergillus* spp. (12.2)
Green et al. [379] 2019	2005–2015	Queensland, Australia	3182	53 ± 22.6	52.4	73.6	6.3	NA
Ting et al. [380] 2020	2007–2019	Nottingham, UK	1333	49.9 ± 22.2	50.4	37.7	3.0	NA
Khoo et al. [381] 2020	2012–2016	Sydney, Australia	979	54.7 ± 21.5	NA	69.0	2.3	NA
Bajracharya L et al. [382] 2020	2013–2015	Nepal	598	47.9	53.8	49.6	53.9	*Aspergillus* spp. (28.3) *Fusarium* spp. (28.3)
Soleimani M et al. [383] 2021	2012–2018	Tehran, Iran	6282	54.6 ± 23.3	63.0	39.5	15.4	*Fusarium* spp. (8.0) Aspergillus spp. (4.0) *Candida* spp. (3.0)
Hoffman JJ et al. [384] 2022	2019–2020	Nepal	642	45.9	39.0	75.1	75.1	*Dematiaceous* (50.6) *Curvularia* spp.
Shekhawat et al. [385] 2023	2016–2020	Mid-Atlantic USA	NA	NA	NA	NA	10.1	*Candida* spp. (45.4) *Fusarium* spp. (10.9) *Aspergillus* spp. (10.9)
Rakhi K et al. [386] 2023	2019–2022	Eastern India	2303	48.4 ± 16.5	65.0	75.4	34.6	*Aspergillus* spp. (41.6) *Fusarium* spp. (19.7) *Dematiaceous* (8.5)
Kang L et al. [387] 2023	2012–2021	Midwestern USA	1012	NA	NA	49.3	7.8	NA

(continued)

Table 7.1 (continued)

Author/year	Study period	Geographic region	Total no. of cases	Mean age (years)	Males (%)	Positive culture (%)	Fungus proportion (%)	Fungus species (%)
Ngarmsom R et al. [388] 2024	2012–2019	Thailand	638	50.2 ± 19.8	68.3	53.6	46.5	*Fusarium* spp. (17.4) *Aspergillus* spp. (4.1)
Kase C et al. [389] 2024	2010–2019	Sao Paulo, Brazil	4047	47.7 ± 20.6	53.2	75.3	7.31	*Fusarium* spp. (35.4) *Candida parapsilosis* (16.0)
Sharma P et al. [390] 2025	2018–2022	Southwest England	872	56.8 (4–97)	47.2	39.5	2.5	Yeast (1.7) Filamentous (0.8)
Xu et al. [391] 2025	2016–2023	Zhejiang, China	1382	58.6 ± 14.7	70.8	38.7	58.3	*Fusarium* spp. (21.3) *aspergillus* spp. (6.6) *Alternaria* spp. (4.3)
Yamada N et al. [392] 2025	2009–2021	Japan	500	63.0 ± 22.0	54.0	100%	10.2	*Candida* spp. (8.9)

NA not available

3. *Relation to geographic and climate conditions.* At least 100 species of yeasts and filamentous fungi have been reported to cause infectious keratitis in humans. The prevalence is particularly high in regions with warmer and humid climates, such as India and central China. Under these conditions, non-dermatophyte mold species, like *Fusarium* spp. and *Aspergillus* spp., are more common, accounting for up to 60% of the extensive reports of microbial keratitis [28, 30]. Conversely, yeasts such as *Candida* spp. are more common in developed countries and regions with colder climates (e.g., United Kingdom), where corticosteroid use and contact lens wear are more significant risk factors [31].

   Thus, the highest annual incidence of fungal keratitis occurs in subtropical and tropical regions, primarily affecting healthy males between 20 and 50 years and agricultural or outdoor workers who often sustain minor eye injuries from organic materials [32, 33]. However, the rapid pace of human progress, modernization, and urbanization has significantly increased the prevalence of fungal keratitis in urban regions compared to rural areas, with one specific contributor to this trend being excessive contact lens wear [25, 34].
4. *Risk factors.* Factors that predispose individuals to filamentous fungal keratitis include farming and factory (silica, granite, and marbles) ocular trauma, contact lens usage, ocular surface diseases and dry eye, previous ocular surgery, topical or systemic corticosteroids, and immunosuppressive conditions such as diabetes or HIV/AIDS [32, 35]. A 14-year population-based study performed in Taiwan identified the following risk factors for microbial keratitis: contact lens wear, eye trauma, prior eye surgery, ocular surface diseases such as blepharitis, dry eye, dacryocystitis, dacryoadenitis, and neurotrophic keratopathy; topical/systemic corticosteroid use; topical antiglaucoma medication use; autoimmune diseases, diabetes mellitus (DM), malignancy, and malnutrition [36].

   In temperate regions, ocular surface diseases, such as hyposecretory dry eye and impaired eyelid closure, can make individuals more susceptible to infections from *Candida* spp. Such fungal infections may occur alongside pre-existing conditions like herpes simplex keratitis or corneal damage resulting from inadequate contact lens use, particularly in low socioeconomic status wearers at increased risk of developing the condition [37]. A recent study performed in Galicia, Spain, a geographic area with a temperate climate, found *Candida* spp. infections as the most frequent type (55.8%), with primary risk factors including corticosteroid eyedrops use (29.9%), recent keratoplasty (18.2%), ocular trauma (19.5%), and contact with vegetable matter (11.7%) [38].

7.3 Etiologic Agents

1. *Taxonomic classification of fungi infecting the cornea.* The kingdom fungi are currently divided into seven phyla based on their reproductive structures and life cycles, of which Ascomycota, Basidiomycota, Zygomycota (Mucorales), and

Entomophthoromycota may infect humans [39, 40]. All fungal pathogens responsible for keratitis are ubiquitous saprophytic microorganisms. From the phylum Ascomycota, *Fusarium* spp., *Aspergillus* spp., and *Candida* spp. (order Saccharomycotina), are the three most common fungi infecting the cornea, particularly in immunocompromised hosts [41]. Other opportunistic filamentous ascomycetes, include *Scedosporium* spp., *and common* pigmented filamentous ascomycetes, also called dematiaceous fungi, infect immunocompromised and, rarely, immunocompetent individuals capable of infecting the cornea are *Curvularia* spp., *Bipolaris* spp., *Alternaria* spp., *Cladosporium* spp., *and Ramichloridium* spp. [40, 41]. In the same phylum, from the *Ajellomycetaceae* family, the corneal pathogens, *Histoplasma* spp., *Blastomyces* spp., *Coccidioides* spp., *Paracoccidioides* spp., and *Sporothrix* spp. (order *Ophiostomatale*), are less common causes of fungal keratitis [39–41].

From the phylum Basidiomycota, *Cryptococcus* spp. a non-filamentous species is the most prominent corneal pathogen [41]. And, in the Zygomycota (Mucorales) Phylum, *Mucor* spp. *and Rhizopus* spp. are ubiquitous, ancient group mostly of saprotrophs that might infect the cornea, which, unlike the Ascomycota and Basidiomycota (the Dikarya), do not manifest sophisticated adaptations to diverse substrates, but rapidly use up available sugars to move via their sporangiospores [39–41]. (Table 7.2)

2. *Corneal infectious fungi properties.* Out of the estimated 1.5–5.0 million fungal species on Earth, only several hundred from the four phyla described above are known to cause human disease [42]. This is because they are required to meet four basic conditions necessary to infect humans: (1) fungi need to tolerate the high temperature of the human body (≥37°C), (2) they must have the ability to invade their host by penetrating or circumventing host barriers, (3) possess capability to induce tissue lysis by digesting and absorbing the host's components, and (4) be able to resist or evade the immune system [40]. This is why only very few, approximately 105 species in 35 genera of fungi, have been reported to cause keratitis, with over 95% of them attributed to the filamentous fungi *Fusarium* spp. and *Aspergillus* spp., and the yeast *Candida* spp. [31, 43]. Other filamentous fungi, like *Cryptococcus* spp., *Phaeohyphomycetes* spp., *Curvularia* spp., *Alternaria* spp., *Clodosporidium* spp., *Paecilomyces* spp., *and Scedosporium apiospermum* are also frequent causes of fungal keratitis. Filamentous fungi tend to have a worse prognosis and are responsible for most fungal infections in tropical and subtropical climates, while yeast infection are more frequent causes in temperate climates [44].

Table 7.2 Fungus species by infective prevalence in the human cornea [393]

Fungus species by infective prevalence	Type
High morbidity	
Fusarium spp. *Aspergillus* spp.	Filamentous
Candida spp.	Yeast, dimorphic
Yeast *Cryptococcus* spp.	No filamentous
Moderate to high morbidity	
Mucor spp.	Filamentous
Moderate morbidity	
Curvularia spp. *Alternaria* spp. *Cladosporium* spp. *Acremonium* spp. *Penicillium* spp. *Bipolaris* spp. *Scedosporium* spp. *Paecilomyces* spp. *Botryodiplodia* spp. *Exserohilum* spp. *Helminthosporium* spp.	Filamentous
Rare	
Blastomyces spp. *Coccidioides* spp. *Paracoccidioides* spp. *Sporothrix* spp. *Histoplasma* spp.	Dimorphic
Mycelia sterilia *Phialophora* spp. *Cephalosporium* spp.	Unspecified
Other rare species reported	
Trichoderma spp., *Sepedonium* spp., *Phoma* spp., *Chaetomium* spp., *Brachysporium* spp., *Rhizopus* spp., *Verticillium* spp., *Paecilomyces* spp., *Helminthosporium* spp., *Periconia*, spp., *Geotrichum* spp., *Doratomyces* spp., *Gliocladium* spp., *Stachybotrys* spp., *Sporotrichum* spp., *Monotospora* spp., *Trichothecium* spp., *Rhizoctonia* spp., *Hormiscium* spp., *Cunninghamella* spp., *Pythium* spp., *Beauveria* spp., *Gongromeriza* spp., *Eremothecium* spp., *Corynespora* spp., *Pyrenochaeta* spp., *Fusoma* spp., *Fusicladium* spp., *Cephaliophora* spp., *Saccharomyces* spp., *Heerosporium* spp., *Syncephalastrum* spp., *Scopulariopsis* spp., *Cercospora* spp., *Exserohilum* spp., *Bactridium* spp., *Stemphylium* spp., *Zygorhynchus* spp., *Colletotrichum* spp.	

7.4 Pathogenesis

1. *Corneal and ocular surface defense properties.* The host's corneal and ocular surface defense mechanisms are vast. They range from the eyelids and their blinking reflex, corneal epithelium integrity, and the tear film innate immune system components to specific and complex adaptive immune responses [45, 46]. The corneal epithelium is a physical barrier that protects the cornea from commensal flora and opportunistic pathogens invasion [47, 48]. Additionally,

the epithelial cells can generate and secrete antimicrobial and immune-modulating molecules during corneal infection [48].

Tear film proteins have diverse mechanisms to protect the cornea from invading microorganisms. Pathogen aggregation and washout, direct killing, decoy receptors, nutrient scavenging, and immune cell recruitment are the most relevant. The over or under-expression of these proteins occurs during fungal keratitis [49, 50]. Lysozyme, lactoferrin, and lipocalin are the most abundant proteins within the tear film, making 80% of the total protein. Lysozyme acts on fungi by hydrolyzing N-glycosidic linkages within their cell wall, and it can also disrupt their cell membrane through cationic–protein interactions, leading to cell death [51]. Lactoferrin also has a direct antifungal action similar to lysozyme, interacting with the fungal cell surface, resulting in damage to the cell membrane and a fungal apoptosis-like process [52]. Furthermore, lactoferrin and lipocalin act as fungistatic agents by interfering with iron availability, essential for redox reactions of fungal antioxidants, preventing conidia from germinating [53, 54]. Secretory immunoglobulin-A (sIgA), the primary antibody present in tears, binds to lectin-type adhesion molecules on the fungal cell surface, thus preventing their binding to the corneal epithelium and promoting pathogen aggregation, resulting in direct removal by the tear film [55]. Complement component-3 (C3), the most abundant complement protein in tears, plays an essential role in the control of opportunistic fungal infections via opsonization and, ultimately, fungal clearance mainly through the alternative pathway triggered by lectin [56].

Other tear film proteins that have anti-fungal activity include α and β-defensins, which are small, cysteine-rich, non-glycosylated cationic and amphipathic peptides present in closed-eye tears or recruited during fungal keratitis where they block *Candida* adhesion to the human epithelium, preventing biofilm formation [57]. Histatins are histidine-rich small peptides with fungicidal activity against *Candida*, which is related to decreasing mitochondrial ATP synthesis and promoting the generation of ROS [58]. C-type lectins are proteins that moderate inflammatory responses and thus limit infections on the ocular surface. The most abundant in tears are mannose-binding proteins (MBP) and surfactant proteins (SP-A and SP-D), which recognize pathogen-associated molecular patterns (PAMPs) on the yeast-like and filamentous fungi cell surface, eliciting a wide range of responses, including aggregation and opsonization, increasing killing efficacy during phagocytosis and complement activation [59]. Secretory leukocyte protease inhibitor (SLIPI) and Elafin control the enzymatic activity of neutrophil serine proteases, specifically, neutrophil elastase and cathepsin-G, whereas Elafin inhibits neutrophil elastase and proteinase 3 [60]. While such inhibitory activities protect the ocular surface by dampening these hydrolytic, tissue destructive proteases, SLIPI and Elafin also have direct anti-fungal roles via cationic disruption of the fungal membrane [61].

On the other hand, corneal avascularity, its immune privilege, including the anterior chamber immune deviation phenomenon may contribute to its susceptibility to fungal infection and colonization. Such microstructural and functional conditions significantly limit immune defense capabilities, including a scarcity of antigen-presenting cells (Langerhans and dendritic interdigitating cells), restricted access for effector immune cells (neutrophils, macrophages, cytotoxic lymphocytes), and a low concentration of immunoglobulins and complement components [20, 62, 63].

2. *Fungal infective properties and immune evasion.* In order to infect the human cornea, a fungus species is required to survive and grow in the cornea, beginning with its capacity to adhere to its surface epithelium, which has an approximate central temperature of 32.6 ± 0.70°C, an environment suitable for the growth and toxigenicity of *Fusarium* spp. and *Aspergillus* spp., the most common pathogens observed in human fungal keratitis [36, 39, 64]. Then, fungi require specific abilities to penetrate the corneal stroma despite its structure barriers and immune defenses, digest and absorb the host's corneal nutrients, and resist the immune system's actions to destroy it [20, 63]. Hence, fungal corneal infection develops progressively, starting with bio-adhesion, then invasion, morphogenesis, mycotic viability, replication within phagocytes, and favorable conditions for fungal budding infection [41].
3. *Fungal surface bio-adhesion.* As mentioned, the initial pathogenic part of fungal keratitis and growth begins with the surface adherence capacity of the fungus, which is mediated by interactions between adhesins (mainly mannoproteins) and the epithelial surface. Bio-adhesion occurs through potential fungal binding sites (laminins, fibronectins, and collagens) [65]. Additionally, many hydrophobins and conidia cell-surface proteins mediate host cell adherence. The outer fibril layer of yeast and filamentous fungal conidia comprises the lectin-like proteins mannan and galactomannan, which recognize corneal epithelial cell membrane glycoproteins [66]. Moreover, traumatic abrasion of the corneal epithelium induces overexpression of cell-surface mannose glycoproteins during the wound healing process, further enhancing the availability of these cell-surface receptors for bio-adhesion [41]. Upon initial contact with the host, fungi interact not only with pattern recognition receptors (PRRs), including the Toll-like receptors (TLRs) TLR2 and TLR4, but also by the C-type Lectin receptors (CLRs) Dectin-1, Dectin-2, and Mincle (Macrophage-inducible C-type lectin) expressed on host epithelial and immune cells [67].
4. *Morphogenesis and fungal invasion.* Morphogenesis is the ability of the fungal pathogens to transform from yeast to hyphal form. While fungi can disseminate more efficiently at the yeast stage, the hyphal forms are more capable of invading and damaging tissues [68]. Once bio-adhesion occurs under a favorable microenvironment (nutrient availability and temperature), conidia swell and begin germination, producing fungal hyphae, which are capable of growing and penetrating the corneal epithelium to reach the stroma and even the anterior chamber under a favorable immune condition. Fungi may also invade de corneal epithelium via endocytosis, accomplished with the help of invasion proteins and through epithelial cell tight-junctions disruption by proteolytic digestion [69]. However, the activation of TLRs in the corneal epithelium induces the production of CXC chemokines and the recruitment of neutrophils, which are the key players in the immune response, accounting for more than 90% of the infiltrating

cells. They are the predominant source of mature interleukin-1β (IL-1β) and acidic mammalian chitinase (AMCase) in corneas, which can inhibit hyphal growth [30, 70]. Additionally, the overexpression and activation of these PPRs by fungi result in increased secretion of inflammatory cytokines (IL-1β, IL-6, IL-8, IL-17, and IL-23) in corneal epithelial cells and neutrophils, and elevated levels of IL-1β, TLR4, Dectin-1, and LOX-1, which increase the production of reactive oxygen species (ROS), facilitating fungal killing [71, 72]. During oxidative stress, the transcription factor Skn7, which regulates the expression of protein phosphatase PhzA, also contributes to the resistance to host defense [73]. Therefore, fungal invasiveness capacity is related to fungal load and inversely proportional to the host immune response [74].

5. *Mycotic viability, replication, and favorable conditions for infection.* Despite the host adaptive immune response mediated by epithelial cells, macrophages, neutrophils, and dendritic cells, fungal pathogens may overcome such defense mechanisms described above by their capacity to degrade physical barriers efficiently and the production of microbial proteins. Apart from physical disruption of the corneal epithelium, stroma, and endothelium caused by the hyphal growth, fungi can produce extracellular enzymes and secondary metabolites with a broad range of roles, which contribute to their invasiveness [75, 76]. Mycotoxins produced by *Aspergillus* (aflatoxin B1, gliotoxin A, fumagillin, helvolic acid) and *Fusarium* (nivalenol, T-2 toxin, deoxynivalenol, diacetoxyscirpenol, fusaric acid, zearalenone) have a profound impact on immune function. They can inhibit phagocytosis, intracellular killing, cytokine production, antigen presentation, and the production of ROS by macrophages. In addition, they may play a role in inhibiting T-cell function and breaking down tissues [77–81]. Mycotoxins work in conjunction with fungal cytosolic proteins and peptide toxins, leading to the release of a destructive biological mixed inflammatory storm of cytokines (IL-1α and IL-6), tumor necrosis factor-alpha (TNF-α), and platelet-derived growth factor (PDGF), among others. This cytokine storm significantly contributes to the destruction of corneal epithelial cells [82]. The great diversity of fungal proteolytic enzymes (serine and cysteine proteases, collagenolytic matrix metalloproteinases, and collagenases), phospholipase activity, and other extracellular enzymes, including nucleases, oxidases, catalases, phosphatases, and peptidases may cause corneal-ulceration, among other fungal-specific species immune evasive activities [63, 83–88]. Together, these enzymes degrade complex macromolecules and provide nutrients (amino acids, lipids) and metals (iron, zinc, manganese, copper) for fungal growth, which are sequestered through siderophores (high-affinity metal-binding compounds) secreted by the fungi [89]. Furthermore, the continuous flow of the tear film over the ulcer enriched with cytokines, proteolytic enzymes, and neutrophils tend to worsen the condition, progressing to severe corneal stromal melt [20, 82].
6. *Role of biofilm in corneal fungal infection.* Single or multiple microbial florae can form a biofilm on biotic or abiotic surfaces. Biofilms are three-dimensional extracellular polymer matrix structures composed of complex and heterogeneous mixtures of proteins, carbohydrates, lipids, and nucleic acids [90, 91].

Biofilms play diverse roles during fungal infection on the ocular surface. They promote fungal adhesion and structural stability while protecting the fungi from external threats [90, 92, 93]. Compared to free-living cells, biofilms exhibit different phenotypic behaviors in growth rate and changes in gene expression [94]. They are often highly resistant to antifungal treatment and the host's adaptive immune response [93]. Several genera of fungi can form biofilms, including *Candida* spp., *Aspergillus* spp., and *Fusarium* spp. [95–98]. Biofilm is also formed on the surface of a soft contact lens from a contaminated solution, creating a massive outbreak of contact lens-associated fungal keratitis [99].

7. *Host's fungal keratitis immune response and inflammation.* The inflammatory component of the fungal keratitis pathogenesis initiates when the pathogen gets in contact with the cornea, inducing overexpression of PPRs, which promote the production of pro-inflammatory cytokines through MyD88/NF-kB or Syk/PKCδ/Card9-Bcl-10-MALT1/NF-kB signaling, and a large number of neutrophils recruited [67, 72, 100]. Moreover, even though neutrophils are the mainstay to fight fungi, they also contribute to additional severe inflammatory corneal damage through innocent bystander response (respiratory burst-ROS generation, myeloperoxidases, elastases, cathepsins, collagenases, and antimicrobial defensins, and acid hydrolases), including ulceration, stromal melting, opacification, and scarring (fibrosis) [101–103]. As mentioned before, the inflammatory response in fungal keratitis induces overexpression of various cytokines, including IL-1β, IL-6, IL-8, IL-17, IL-23, and IFN-γ in the aqueous humor compared to healthy controls [63, 70, 104, 105]. Among these, IL-1β is recognized as a marker for the severity of inflammation. Additionally, IL-1β, IL-6, and IL-23 play a role in promoting the differentiation of Th17 cells, which in turn stimulate the secretion of IL-17 and IL-22 [67, 71, 104]. Furthermore, both IL-6 and IL-23 are necessary for the production of IL-17 in neutrophils, and IL-17 itself may induce the production of ROS [70, 104].
8. *Fungal keratitis progressive pathway.* Fungi infiltrating the corneal stroma through epithelial defects is the most common invasive pathway. Such a mechanism explains the increased risk associated with factors affecting the epithelium integrity, like trauma involving vegetative matter, soil or dust, contact lens wear, prior ocular surgery, and retained foreign bodies [106]. Trauma involving vegetable material can directly introduce fungal conidia onto the corneal surface, resulting in infection or damage to the overlying corneal epithelium and facilitating fungal invasion. The rapid growth of fungi then triggers heightened inflammatory reactions and tissue necrosis [27, 107]. Once inside the cornea, fungi initiate replication within the stroma, exhibiting circumferential expansion with satellite lesions. Progressively, they penetrate deeper into the stroma, breaching Descemet's membrane and gaining access to the anterior chamber (AC), forming AC vegetations. This progression may culminate in corneal perforation and endophthalmitis unless the innate and adaptive immune defenses or appropriate treatment intervene effectively [106]. Fungal infiltration can extend beyond the cornea, including the sclera and surrounding structures; hence, precipitating severe infectious scleritis and even panophthalmitis [108, 109]. Fungal keratitis

can also be a sequela of fungal endophthalmitis, in which the fungus retraces its course, spreading reverse from the posterior segment to Descemet's membrane, then permeating to the corneal stroma or infiltrating the corneoscleral trabeculae to reach the cornea [110].

9. *Specific fungal genera virulence mechanisms.* The virulence of fungal infections depends on the fungal-produced substances and the host's immune response. *Candida* primarily invades pre-existing epithelial defects, while filamentous fungi are commonly implicated in post-traumatic infections. Some fungi can thrive within the corneal stroma by delaying the release of chemotactic substances, evading the host's immune and inflammatory reactions. Proteases from *Candida* can degrade C3 from human serum *in vitro* [111]. Moreover, *Candida albicans* produces phospholipase-A and lysophospholipase on blastospores surfaces, aiding tissue penetration. *Fusarium* is also known to penetrate the corneal stroma and Descemet's membrane [20, 63]. Aflatoxin B1, an important mycotoxin produced by *Aspergillus*, is acutely and chronically toxic to humans. Its production by *A. flavus* isolates obtained from fungal keratitis patients is highly variable but increased compared to that collected when grown *in vitro* [112]. Furthermore, fungal serine proteases may cleave Dectin-1, an important immune cell surface receptor that recognizes β-glucan, a component that is abundant in the fungal cell wall [113].

7.5 Clinical Manifestations

1. *Initial presentation and symptoms.* Contrary to bacterial keratitis, the symptoms of fungal keratitis are often disproportionately less severe than might be expected considering the ulcer extension, and this is probably the main reason that patients present late to the clinic with an advanced fungal ulcer for treatment. Also, when dealing with any case of keratitis, it is essential to consider the possibility of fungal infection [114, 115]. This condition generally has an insidious onset, and the symptoms progress gradually. They include eye pain, redness, blurred vision, excessive watery discharge, photophobia, blepharospasm, and foreign body sensation [114]. As mentioned above, unlike bacterial keratitis, signs often surpass symptoms in fungal keratitis. Also, symptoms persist for a longer duration compared to bacterial keratitis [116]. Finally, the degree of visual impairment is directly related to the location of the corneal lesion, which can be central (within 4 mm), paracentral (4–8 mm), or peripheral (beyond 8 mm) [115, 117].
2. *Signs.* Like symptoms, signs, including lid edema and erythema, conjunctival injection, chemosis, and mucopurulent discharge, corneal epithelial defect, and underlying stromal infiltrate are less severe compared to bacterial keratitis. The fungal corneal ulcer is typically described as a dry-base ulcer with a gray-white infiltrate and feathery margins (70% of cases), satellite lesions (10% of cases), and creamy exudates at its base. Feathery ulcer margins are the most characteristic clinical feature of fungal keratitis and they appear in the early stages of the infiltration [41]. The presence of a fixed or immobile hypopyon is also a

common feature, seen in about 45–66% of cases [118] (Fig. 7.1a–c). However, as an exception to the rule, not all fungal ulcers demonstrate these characteristic signs. Even acknowledging above more commonly clinical manifestations, the overall clinical diagnostic accuracy is less than 70%, even in the hands of a corneal specialist [119]. Other less usual features include an immune ring, deep stromal abscess, and an extending endothelial plaque (Fig. 7.2a–c). While ring infiltrates can occur in fungal and bacterial keratitis, it is ten times more likely to indicate *Acanthamoeba* keratitis. Also, multifocal lesions are more commonly seen in *Acanthamoeba* infection than fungal keratitis [41].

The corneal epithelium over the deep-seated stromal infiltrates might be intact; however, corneal perforation is far more common (5–6 times) than in bacterial keratitis (Fig. 7.3a). The final consequences may range from severe visual impairment and blindness to loss of the globe and disfiguration.

3. *Distinctive corneal manifestations features* may be linked to the type of fungi invading the cornea. For instance, *Candida* keratitis often presents with a yellow whitish densely suppurative "collar button" infiltrate [120]. *Dematiaceous* fungi can present with superficial and deep-seated ulcers characterized by gray or brown pigmentation. This pigmented appearance is due to the alteration in

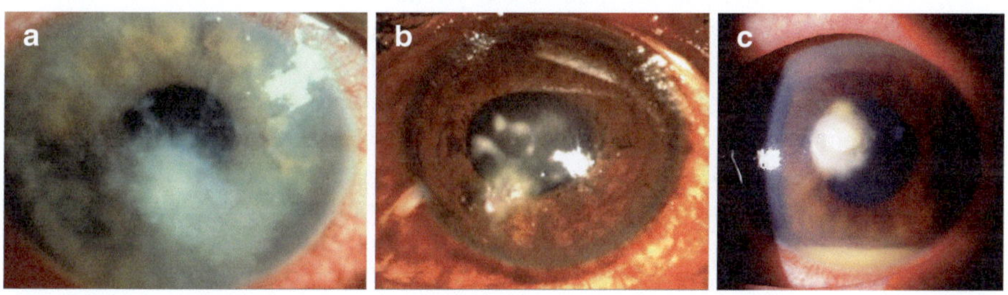

Fig. 7.1 Typical signs of fungal keratitis. (**a**) Active Fusarium corneal infiltrate with classic feathery margins. (**b**) Multiple focal and satellite fungal infiltrates. (**c**) Central and deep stromal fungal infiltrate with a fixed hypopyon. (Figures **a** and **b**, courtesy of Bascom-Palmer Eye Institute photography department)

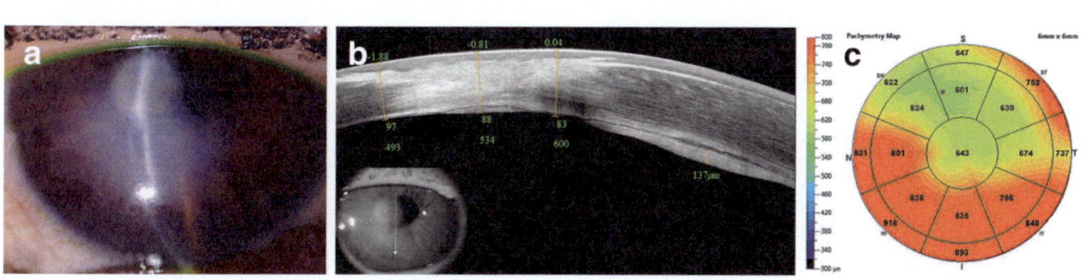

Fig. 7.2 *Fusarium* spp. reactivated as endothelial plaque keratitis. (**a**) Central rounded and dense stromal infiltrate with an inferior extension in the form of a growing endothelial plaque. (**b**) AS-OCT showing both lesions, particularly the dense endothelial plaque extended inferiorly to the infiltrate, causing endothelial cell dysfunction and subtle stromal edema. (**c**) Tomographic pachymetry showing a significant increase in stromal thickness (796–916 m) above the fungal endothelial plaque

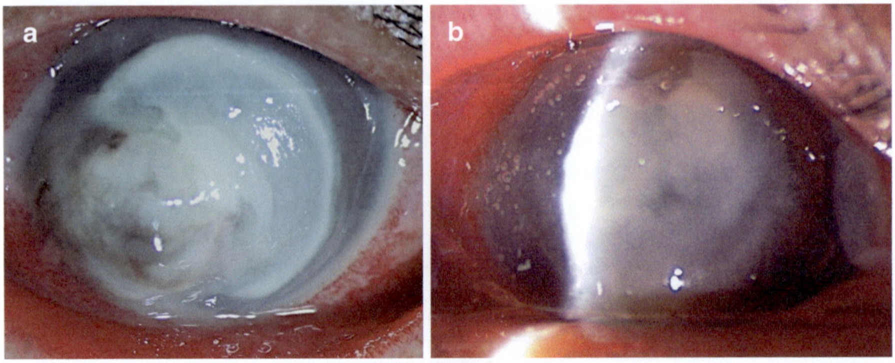

Fig. 7.3 Severe fungal keratitis. (**a**) Large area of stromal melting inferior-nasal with dark pigmentation corresponding with a perforation with uveal plugging. (**b**) *Fusarium* spp. recalcitrant contact lens-associated keratitis showing a large and deep infiltrate with deep stromal melting and a central descemetocele. (Figure **a**, courtesy of Bascom-Palmer Eye Institute photography department)

melanin metabolism, indicating a superficial infection caused by a less virulent organism that incites a lesser inflammatory reaction. These initial signs typically take several hours or days to develop. In contrast, virulent fungi such as *Aspergillus* or *Fusarium* species exhibit a rapidly progressive grey or yellow-white stromal infiltrates with indistinct fluffy margins, leading to potentially severe complications such as corneal perforation and endophthalmitis. Other complications include stromal melt, descemetocele formation, scleritis, ocular hypertension or hypotony, endophthalmitis, panophthalmitis, and orbital cellulitis (Fig. 7.3b).

7.6 Diagnosis

1. *Clinical history.* Obtaining a thorough clinical history is essential in identifying potential predisposing factors and sources of fungal exposure. It is important to ask detailed questions about the patient's occupation, any eye trauma involving plant material or organic debris, and their contact lens habits, including hygiene practices, whether they engage in extended wear and improper usage [114]. Other important factors to consider that may predispose individuals to fungal keratitis include older age, immunosuppression (HIV/AIDS or diabetes), pre-existing chronic inflammatory ocular surface disorders, prolonged use of topical corticosteroids, and any previous ocular surgeries [31].

   Diagnosing fungal keratitis requires a comprehensive approach once the patient's demographic background and risk factors are recorded. It is based on its clinical manifestations supported by microbiology laboratory tests, digital imaging techniques, and more sophisticated molecular diagnostic techniques [12, 13, 20, 114].

2. *Smear and staining.* Detecting a corneal fungal infection is a meticulous process that begins by collecting an appropriate corneal sample from the suspicious lesion for stain and culture. The smears permit direct microscopic examination utilizing various stains such as 10–20% potassium hydroxide (KOH), Gram, Giemsa, Gomori/Grocott's Methenamine Silver stains, 0.06% Trypan blue, Periodic Acid-Schiff (PAS), Lactophenol cotton blue, Calcofluor white, and methylthioninium chloride [10, 11, 120, 121] (Fig. 7.4a–d). While the KOH preparation is a highly effective and quick diagnostic tool, with a high sensitivity (80–99.3%) and specificity (83.8–99.1%) in detecting fungal elements, its specificity may vary mainly depending on the microscopist's experience, the corneal ulcer size, and the amount of sampling material [12, 13, 122, 123]. Gram and Giemsa staining are less sensitive staining techniques (approx. 50%). On the other hand, considering fungi's tendency to penetrate deep into the cornea, tissue swabbing is inadequate for confirming infection, and deep corneal scrapings are preferably required for accurate diagnosis [13].
3. *Fungal culture.* Currently, the definitive diagnosis of fungal keratitis relies on fungal culture (Fig. 7.5a). The most common fungi culture media used include Sabouraud's dextrose agar, blood agar, thioglycolate broth, and brain-heart infusion, each designed to isolate different types of fungi [13,

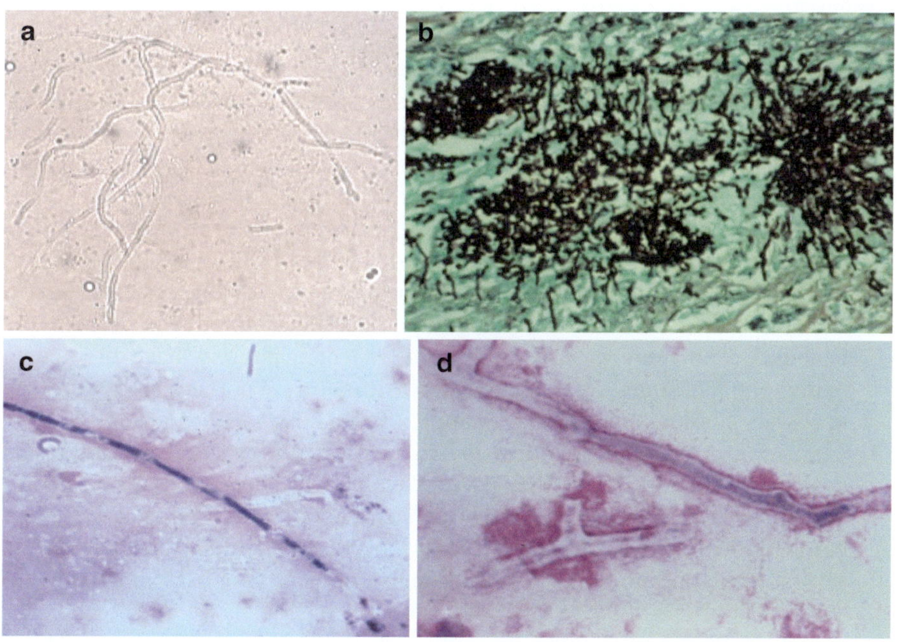

Fig. 7.4 Smear staining for fungal keratitis. (**a**) 10–20% potassium hydroxide (KOH). (**b**) Gomori Methenamine Silver (GMS). (**c**) Gram (crystal violet-iodine complex). (**d**) Giemsa (methylene blue/azure) and acidic (eosin) dyes. (Figures, courtesy of Bascom-Palmer Eye Institute photography department)

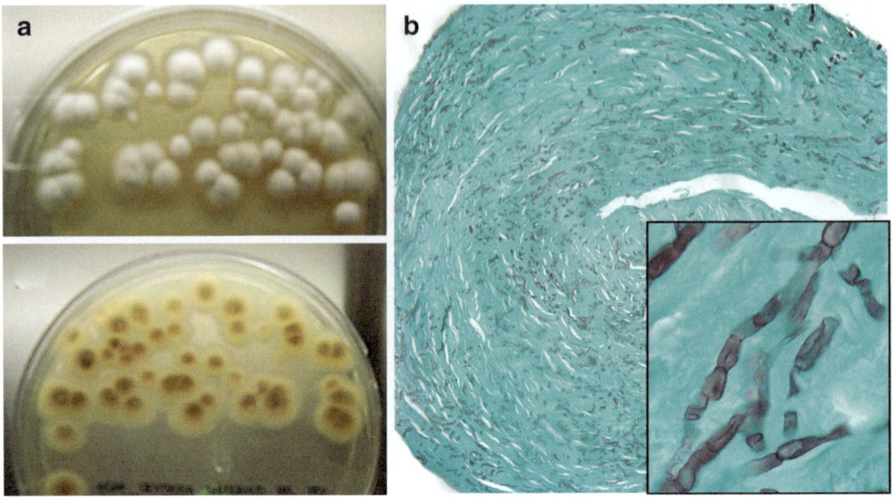

Fig. 7.5 Fungal culture and corneal biopsy for definitive diagnosis of fungal keratitis. (**a**) Sabouraud dextrose *Fusarium* spp. growth from a diabetic patient with severe fungal keratitis. (**b**) Corneal biopsy specimen showing Gomori methenamine silver stain (GMS) demonstrating septate fungal elements present throughout the tissue with extension to multiple margins. The inset highlights the fungal septae. (Figure **b**, courtesy of Bascom-Palmer Eye Institute photography department)

120]. However, fungal culture has several disadvantages. These include the risk of complications from invasive tissue sampling and its relatively low sensitivity, which can lead to false-negative results, especially with small inoculum. Additionally, identifying pathogens can take a significant amount of time. Initial fungal growth is observed within 72 h in 83% of cultures and within 1 week in 97% of cases [124]. However, some culture media may require incubation for an extended period, sometimes lasting 4–6 weeks [12, 13, 120, 122]. As a result, the speed and accuracy of diagnoses are often limited, which can delay appropriate antifungal treatment. This issue becomes even more pronounced in cases where patients have previously undergone antifungal treatment. In such situations, a corneal biopsy may be necessary to obtain an adequate sample (Table 7.3).

4. *Corneal biopsy.* A corneal biopsy is indicated when fungal keratitis progresses despite intensive antifungal therapy, especially in the absence of positive microbiological results. All antimicrobial treatments are usually withheld for 24–48 h before corneal biopsies are performed to increase the culture yield. There are several techniques to obtain a representative corneal sample from the edge of the infectious lesion for biopsy and histopathologic analysis. Such techniques include a 10–0 Nylon suture pass through the stroma, a mid-depth corneal trephination with a 3–4 mm skin punch, a freehand blade lamellar dissection, a lamellar flap, and reverse-cutting blade to a femtosecond and/or anterior segment optical coherence tomography (AS-OCT) assisted biopsy [125]. Once the

Table 7.3 Advantages and disadvantages of the most significant diagnostic methodologies for fungal keratitis, along with their sensitivities and specificities

Diagnostic methodology	Advantages	Disadvantages	Sensitivity/Specificity	References
Traditional				
Smear (KOH, fluorescent brightener 85)	Direct detection method, relatively simple, fast, and inexpensive.	Corneal ulcer size and amount of sampling material affect its sensitivity.	Both >98% KOH = 85.3%/99.1%	[12, 123, 394]
Culture (Sabouraud dextrose)	Makes the definitive diagnosis. More accurate for identifying the fungal pathogen.	Invasive tissue sampling risks Longer time to identify pathogens (1–2 weeks to a month). Low diagnostic accuracy (contamination).	75.7%/100%	[8, 120, 395]
Corneal biopsy	High diagnostic yield (39–82%). Samples obtained from deeper corneal layers and/or debulking the infection.	Invasive and risky procedure (inadvertent corneal perforation). Requires stopping antifungal medications.	82%/100%	[396–398]
Molecular				
Conventional PCR	Rapid detection with high sensitivity and specificity. Cost-effective when used selectively for a targeted approach.	Possible cross-contamination. Over-diagnosis by non-pathogenic bacteria.	57–91%/79%	[144, 399]
Multiplex PCR	Rapid and specific identification method. Simultaneously identifies various pathogens in one reaction, reducing misdiagnosis. High specificity and isolation rate, rapid response, and easy operation.	Potential for false positives due to amplification of normal flora. Challenges in optimizing conditions for different pathogens. Risk of qualitative rather than quantitative results.	60–95%/74–99%	[140, 146, 149]

(continued)

Table 7.3 (continued)

Diagnostic methodology	Advantages	Disadvantages	Sensitivity/Specificity	References
q-PCR	Faster results, increased sensitivity, and ability to detect fungal DNA in negative cultures. Quantitative measures. Low risk of contamination.	Non-specific binding potential for overdiagnosis due to artifactual amplification of non-pathogenic DNA. High cost and limited availability, and need for specialized equipment and trained personnel.	18S RNA & ITS = 98.2%/100% ITS = 74.3%	[140, 146, 149]
LAMP	High specificity, sensitivity, and efficiency. Low requirements and cost.	Contamination prone. Amplification of short-stranded DNA with small samples.	88%/98%	[131, 150, 400]
DNA sequencing	Distinguishes species more rapidly and identify rare species. Help predict/identify antifungal drug sensitivity and treatment outcomes.	Is time-consuming, requires skilled technicians and expensive laboratory equipment. Now mostly used for research and not used in clinical practice.	90.9–98.0%/81.8–94.7%	[131, 153, 157, 158, 401]
DHA	Rapid diagnosis from corneal scraping samples. Higher sensitivity than culture. Differentiates *Fusarium* and *Aspergillus* and identifies *F. solani*.	Low sensitivity for certain fungal species. Slow turnaround time, labor-intensive nature, and the need for invasive sample collection.	Overall, 93.5%/97.4%	[132, 402]

(continued)

Table 7.3 (continued)

Diagnostic methodology	Advantages	Disadvantages	Sensitivity/Specificity	References
NGS PCR target amplicon sequencing	Amplicon sequencing (18 s rDNA and ITS) is targeted, somewhat less expensive and faster than metagenomic sequencing.	The high detection sensitivity makes it prone to a high false-positive rate due to microbial contamination in any step of the procedure Requires a −80°C freezer for sample storage and expert/experienced lab personal	57–91%/79%	[403, 404]
Imagenology				
UBM/US-B	Adjuvant for indirect visualization of the extension and anatomic characteristics of the eyes anterior and posterior segments in severe fungal infections. Allows evaluating the extent of invasiveness and tissue damage. Specific value in trauma-related fungal keratitis with intraocular extension.	Expensive equipment, requiring an expert operator and examiner to interpret the images Limited use in perforated fungal ulceration. Does not recognize type of fungi infecting the eye.	NA	[405–407]

(continued)

Table 7.3 (continued)

Diagnostic methodology	Advantages	Disadvantages	Sensitivity/Specificity	References
AS-OCT (spectral domain and swept source)	Accurately determine and delineate depth and extent of ulceration, infiltrates, haze, and endothelial plaques. Characterize, quantify, and monitor disease progress. Objectively measure corneal thickness, determine the risk of corneal perforation, and predict response to PACK-CXL.	Expensive equipment, particularly ultra-high-resolution devices. Does not identify the type of fungi (yeast/ filamentous). Poor definition in significantly opaque corneas.	NA	[320, 408–410]
IVCM	Fast, non-invasive, direct fungus observation (characteristics). Consistent sensitivity/ specificity with traditional methods. Detection of deep fungal infection.	Almost impossible to distinguish *Fusarium* from *Aspergillus* spp. Costly equipment, requiring a skilled operator/ experienced viewer. Requires patient cooperation Limited view in scarred tissue.	66.7–85.7%/81.4–100%	[14, 172, 173, 176, 411, 412]

(continued)

Table 7.3 (continued)

Diagnostic methodology	Advantages	Disadvantages	Sensitivity/Specificity	References
TPM	Intravital high-resolution functional microscopy techniques that image dynamic molecular processes. Minimally invasive, allowing for deep levels of tissue penetration and high resolution.	Suboptimal image quality due to poor image stability. Signal attenuation with depth results from scattering and absorbance of the laser. Rapid image collection is required for *in vivo* microscopy to minimize the effects of movement that compromise image quality.	NA	[190, 191, 194]

KOH Potassium hydroxide, *PCR* polymerase chain reaction, *q-PCR* quantitative polymerase chain reaction, *LAMP* loop-mediated isothermal amplification, *DNA* deoxynucleic acid, *DHA* dot hybridization array, *NGS* next generation sequencing, *UBM* ultrasound biomicroscopy, *US-B* ultrasound-B, *AS-OCT* anterior segment optical coherence tomography, *IVCM in vivo* confocal microscopy, *TPM* two-photon excitation microscopy, *NA* not available

tissue is harvested, it must be handled carefully and placed in a Petri dish with balanced saline solution (BSS) for immediate processing. Alternatively, it can be put in a small container for easy visualization by an experienced technician or pathologist for further processing. The sample can be stained using various techniques, with the most common being an ink-potassium hydroxide combination, Gomori's Methenamine Silver (GMS), and Periodic Acid-Schiff (PAS) stains [126–128] (Fig. 7.5b). Ideally, each specimen should undergo histopathologic analysis, culture, and polymerase chain reaction (PCR) testing, especially if the initial smear is negative [13, 122]. Traditional methods such as smears, cultures, and morphology-based fungal identification may not always yield sufficient resolution for accurately identifying fungal species. Therefore, molecular detection techniques can be advantageous in these situations, as they provide reliable results more quickly.

5. *Polymerase chain reaction (PCR).* Polymerase Chain Reaction has proven useful for detecting many difficult-to-cultivate organisms, including *Mycobacteria, Microsporidia, Acanthamoeba,* and various fungi species [129]. Several molecular techniques based on amplification, such as nested PCR [13], real-time PCR [130], loop-mediated isothermal amplification [131], and dot hybridization [132], have been developed specifically for fungi. These methods are faster and more sensitive than conventional PCR; however, they all require the extraction of template DNA. This process is not only time-consuming but can also be limited by the small amount of specimen available from pathogenic corneas, as

some template DNA may be lost during extraction. A direct PCR assay using a specialized polymerase (MightyAmp DNA Polymerase Ver. 2) circumvents these disadvantages, yielding a total positive detection rate of 82.5% (66/80) in cases of fungal keratitis. For patients with a high suspicion, the positive detection rate was 84.8%, and it increased to 91.2% when repeated scrapings were excluded. The direct PCR assay is also rapid, requiring only 3 h for the entire process [133]. However, PCR techniques still have significant limitations, including sample contamination from the environment, non-pathogenic bystanders, or colonizers and commensals, which can result in false-positive results [134, 135]. A study comparing the microbial culture and sequenced PCR found that PCR matched the culture results in 29 out of 31 culture-proven cases of fungal keratitis [135]. Other studies found that 93.6% of culture-proven fungal keratitis yielded a positive PCR, matching the pathogen to that identified by culture [136]. A dot hybridization assay demonstrated twice the sensitivity and similar specificity to culture. As a result of high sensitivity, the number of false-negative cultures outnumbered the false-positive by dot hybridization, which had a negative culture result [132]. While data on the potential false positive rates of investigations like cultures and PCR are helpful, more information is needed to fully evaluate their relevance in the context of fungal keratitis. In contrast to specialized institutional practices, countries where fungal keratitis is more common, such as India and China, often rely on expert interpretation of KOH smears for fungus identification. This method offers a rapid, inexpensive, sensitive, and specific diagnosis [137, 138]. PCR may not be easily accessible in all healthcare facilities, as it requires a specialized diagnostic laboratory and can be relatively expensive. Consequently, it is typically limited to large-scale, specialized, and tertiary institutions worldwide, making it unsuitable for routine clinical use at present [114, 139] (Table 7.3).

6. *Omics approach for diagnosing fungal keratitis.* Applying genome-based tests to the diagnosis of fungal keratitis represents huge advantages over traditional cultures since these molecular techniques are highly sensitive and more rapid to perform; therefore, they are ideal for small and low inoculum corneal samples, such as those obtained in fungal keratitis. The target DNA detection include highly conserved ribosomal RNA (rRNA) genes (18S, 5.8S, and 28S rRNA genes), internal transcribed spacers (ITSs 1 and 2), elongation factor 1-alpha gene, and the mitochondrial cytochrome b gene [130, 140]. Among the target DNA, the amplicons of the PCR amplified from the 18S and 28S rRNA genes are most commonly used for detecting fungal infection. ITSs 1 and 2 have a high copy number, the same as rRNA genes, but vary among species [130]. Therefore, amplicons with ITS regions can identify fungal species through the versatile methods of DNA sequencing [141], multiplex PCR [142], or hybridization [143].
7. *Genomic assays.* The diagnosis of fungal keratitis by PCR is a process that involves the amplification of fungal DNA sequences obtained from tiny corneal samples and other ocular tissues, including tears and aqueous humor. This method allows for a more sensitive identification of precise fungal species. PCR

is known for its remarkable speed, providing results within 2.5–8 h, which reassures medical professionals about its efficiency in diagnosing fungal keratitis, even in cases with negative cultures [130, 144]. The high-resolution melting analysis (PCR-HRM) technique can detect fungi, differentiate yeasts from filamentous fungi, and simultaneously discriminate among relevant species of yeasts [139]. Despite its diagnostic efficiency, such techniques require specialized and costly equipment with limited availability [8, 13, 120]. Other PCR testing disadvantages include a reduced specificity, leading to false-positive results due to cross-contamination with conjunctiva pathogen flora, overdiagnosis by non-pathogenic bacteria, and the requirement for suspicion of targeted pathogens due to the lack of a panfungal discrimination [144, 145]. Also, PCR has shown different sensitivities depending on the fungal flora. The amount of DNA required for *Fusarium spp.* (10 fg/μL) differs from *Aspergillus flavus* (1 pg/μL) and A*spergillus fumigatus* (300 pg/μL) [142]. Given the challenges in detecting fungal DNA, particularly the low amount obtained in clinical samples compared to bacterial and viral pathogens, there is a need for strategies to enhance its sensitivity. These strategies include several types of PCR, such as real-time quantitative PCR (qPCR), multiplex PCR, loop-mediated isothermal amplification (LAMP), and others, each with unique benefits and applications [146–150].

The dot hybridization assay (DHA) is a highly sensitive and specific technique that enables the development of an oligonucleotide array for the rapid identification of fungal pathogens at the species level within a day. DHA offers significantly higher sensitivity—100%—compared to conventional culture methods, which have a sensitivity of only 50% [132]. When designing oligonucleotide probes for DHA, it is important to target common fungal species, particularly those that are often resistant to antifungal agents [50]. Finally, although, most genome-based tests for diagnosing the cause of fungal keratitis have sensitivities of 90% or higher, their specificities vary significantly, ranging from 17% to 97%. The lower specificities reported in some studies may be due to the assumption that samples that test positive through PCR but yield negative culture results are false positives. This issue could also arise from environmental contamination during either the sampling process or laboratory analysis [50] (Table 7.3).

8. *Metagenomic deep sequencing (MDS).* Metagenomic analysis through DNA sequencing performed in tiny corneal scrapings and aqueous fluid samples is the gold standard applied technique for more rapid identification of unculturable, slow-growing, and clinically rare species, outperforming genomics-based tests [151, 152]. Furthermore, it can also help predict/identify antifungal drug sensitivity and treatment outcomes, thus benefiting from the treatment and improving the prognosis [153]. However, it is time-consuming and requires skilled technicians and expensive laboratory equipment. Moreover, data processing is too heavy to be routinely performed [50].

A standardized metagenomic analysis pipeline that removes ambiguous and host-derived short reads can swiftly identify disease-causing pathogens in fungal keratitis patients. Additionally, target enrichment next-generation sequencing for the fungal internal transcribed spacer (ITS) region can significantly enhance the reliability of results by capturing the target genes and excluding non-target genes before sequencing [154]. Hence, more complex molecular sequencing methodologies, including the ITS and the intergenic spacer (IGS), can provide a classification basis for higher ranks (such as species, subspecies, varieties, and even strains), showcasing the versatility of rDNA sequencing [155, 156]. ITS is a universal DNA barcode marker for fungi with high sensitivity and specificity in identifying phylogenetically similar species [157]. At present, these fragments are used to identify the fungi of several genera to the species, such as in the genus *Trichosporon*, *Candida,* and *Aspergillus* [158, 159]. Although ITS sequence can reach species-level identification, high length, and sequence differences weaken the distinguishing power for classification at high taxonomic ranks [160]. The IGS region is more variable than other existing loci of interest, allowing the separation of clinical *Cryptococcus neoformans* isolates, as well as other rare strain types [161]. So, the interspecies variability of IGS sequences is useful for epidemiological analysis but not for discriminating some fungal pathogens [157].

9. *Proteomic assays.* The collection of tear samples for protein analysis to identify or differentiate different expressions in fungal keratitis by matrix-assisted laser desorption/ionization-time of flight mass spectrometry (MALDI-TOF MS) is a significant technique for diagnosing fungal keratitis. The detection of glutaredoxin-related protein, a protein only produced by *Aspergillus* under oxidative stress conditions during fungal keratitis, in the tears of convalescent patients, indicates the presence of the fungus. Moreover, the upregulation of prolactin inducible protein and serum albumin precursor and the downregulation of cystatin S precursor, cystatin SN precursor, cystatin, and lipocalin in patients with keratomycosis provide additional markers for the disease. The tear proteins mentioned above, serving as biomarkers, play a crucial role in diagnosing and monitoring patients [162].

   Addressing the main limitations of conventional 2D-PAGE, including low sensitivity, limited dynamic range, and variability between gels, a two-dimensional difference gel electrophoresis (2D-DIGE) in conjunction with liquid chromatography-tandem mass spectrometry (LC-MS/MS) has been instrumental in analyzing tear samples from patients with *Fusarium* keratitis. These advanced protein analysis techniques enable more accurate and sensitive segmenting of proteins, thereby revealing the differential regulation of tear proteins at various stages of the disease. As *Fusarium* keratitis progresses, several key proteins are found to be progressively upregulated, including α-1-antitrypsin, haptoglobin α2 chain, zinc-α-2-glycoprotein, apolipoprotein, albumin, haptoglobin precursor (β chain), and lactoferrin. In contrast, the expression of lacritin is significantly reduced in the early stages compared to control samples. Additionally, during the late stages of *Fusarium* keratitis, cystatin SA III and lipocalin levels are downregulated. The use of Western blot analysis further confirms the observed upregulation or downregulation of three specific proteins: haptoglobin, lacritin, and lipocalin [163].

Finally, the separation of tear proteins by glycosylation, 1D-PAGE, and in-gel digestion for LC-MS/MS tear protein identification from an early *Aspergillus* keratitis pooled tears sample identified complement system proteins, proteins specific for neutrophil extracellular traps, and proteins involved in wound healing. Such findings indicate that the early appearance of host defense proteins and a wound-healing response in *Aspergillus* keratitis tears can be used as markers for monitoring the progression of the corneal fungal infection [164]. This evidence not only indicates that tear proteomic analysis is a promising approach for investigating fungal keratitis clinical course but also holds great potential for future research. However, a personalized tear proteomic approach is required for diagnosing fungal keratitis and monitoring disease progression, offering hope for more effective and personalized treatments in the future [165].

10. *Beta-D-glucan detection.* Beta-D-glucan is a component of the cell wall found in many fungal species, which can be used as a reliable alternative to identify fungal pathogens in the bloodstream of patients with invasive fungal infections [166]. Previous research has demonstrated that beta-D-glucan testing outperforms fungal cultures regarding diagnostic quickness and sensitivity in systemic fungal infections, mainly when organisms do not thrive in blood cultures, such as *Aspergillosis* [167]. Moreover, beta-D-glucan has the potential to be detected in tear samples from individuals affected by fungal keratitis and in intraocular fluids from fungal endophthalmitis, expediting early and prompt diagnosis [168, 169]. Anterior chamber tap is recommended in resistant cases, particularly when endothelial plaques are present, as fungal infiltration is often observed to penetrate the endothelium [12].

7.7 Non-invasive Imaging Techniques

In recent years, ophthalmic imaging techniques have advanced significantly, offering high sensitivity and accuracy in detecting microorganisms responsible for fungal keratitis. These techniques also provide quick acquisition time, high resolution, multimodality, image storage management and sharing, and the incorporation of artificial intelligence for image processing. Different strategies and equipment are now available in the diagnostic armamentarium that may be applied to fungal keratitis, including *in vivo* confocal microscopy (IVCM), anterior segment optical coherence tomography (AS-OCT), two-photon microscopy (TPM), high-resolution UBM and B-scan ultrasonography, and other imaging modalities [114, 170] (Table 7.3).

1. *In vivo confocal microscopy.* Three IVCM microscopes have been used clinically to analyze the structure and morphology of corneal pathology, the tandem (TSCM), the slit (SSCM), and the laser scanning confocal microscope (LSCM).

The latter, known as the Heidelberg Retinal Tomograph 3 (HRT3) with the Rostock Cornea Module (RCM) uses a 670 nm red wavelength diode laser and offers up to 400 times magnification with an axial resolution of approximately 1 μm [15, 171].

IVCM is a non-invasive imaging technique widely used in clinical practice to observe fungi morphology dynamically and the depth of fungal infection in the cornea [14, 172, 173]. Recognition of filamentous fungal hyphae is the key to the utility of IVCM in assessing potential cases of fungal keratitis [174, 175]. The morphological features of different fungi species, such as hyphal branching angles along spore formation or hyphae dipartites, may be characterized by IVCM to a 1 m resolution [15, 172].

Relevant morphological features of common fungi infecting the cornea seen under the IVCM are the mycelium length of *Aspergillus* and *Fusarium* (200–400 μm), the branching angle (*Aspergillus* = 45° and *Fusarium* = 90°). A difference in hyphae diameter permits distinguishing fungal from basal corneal epithelial nerves (Fig. 7.6a). Also, basal corneal epithelial nerves are much larger than fungal hyphae (i.e., nerve diameter is 5–10 times larger than the Aspergillus mycelium's). However, despite significant differences in branching angle, it is almost impossible to distinguish *Fusarium* from *Aspergillus* because the fungal branches are not common. Therefore, culture is still crucial in identifying fungal pathogens in keratitis [172]. On the other hand, IVCM provides reasonable diagnostic sensitivity and specificity compared to smear microscopy. However, such parameters can vary significantly based on the performance of examiners and assessors, as well as the application of artificial intelligence (AI) in the diagnostic analysis. One study focusing on fungal culture-positive keratitis using IVCM reported a sensitivity of 94% and a specificity of 78% in leading to correct diagnoses [176]. However, using masked clinical and non-clinically trained assessors with varying degrees of IVCM experience to analyze fungal keratitis' diagnostic accuracy yielded a low percentage (8.3–41.2%) of correct diagnosis considering

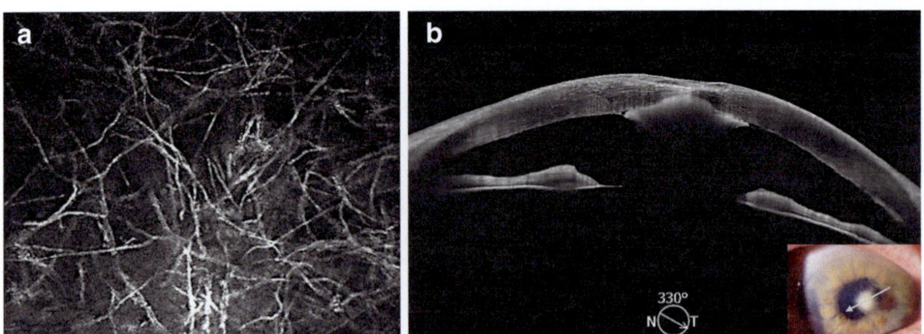

Fig. 7.6 (**a**) *In vivo* confocal microscopy (IVCM) demonstrating numerous fungal hyphae elements from a scrape sample corresponding to *Fusarium* spp. (**b**) Anterior segment optical coherence tomography (AS-OCT) showing a full-depth central stromal fungal infiltrate and an endothelial plaque. (Figure **a**, courtesy of Bascom-Palmer Eye Institute photography department)

all assessors. Nevertheless, on subgroup analysis, high sensitivity and specificity for IVCM detection of fungi, 89.2% and 92.7%, respectively, were found [177]. Another IVCM diagnostic accuracy study for the diagnosis of moderate to severe fungal keratitis using five masked experienced confocal assessors with a positive culture result or presence of fungal hyphae on light microscopy as the reference diagnosis method reported a pooled sensitivity of 85.7% and a specificity of 81.4% for all assessors [178]. Such differences in diagnostic sensitivity and specificity depend partly on the examiner's experience in recognizing morphologic features and interpreting IVCM images. This human limitation led to the application of AI-based techniques for image classification. An intelligent system based on automated image recognition employs adaptive robust binary pattern (ARBP) analysis and support vector machine (SVM) algorithms coupled with a line segment detector (LSD) for hyphal quantification and classification [179]. This system, in a promising demonstration of its potential, identified fungi hyphae in a significantly greater proportion of cases than corneal smear, achieving a sensitivity of 89.29% and a specificity of 95.65% [179]. Notably, there was no statistically significant difference between the automatic hyphae detection system and manual detection by the experienced ophthalmologist. This finding reminds us that AI technologies are especially useful in cases of insufficient human experience in IVCM image assessment [15, 179]. Furthermore, despite the advantages of IVCM for diagnosing fungal keratitis, it is not exempt from limitations, including high cost, skilled and experienced operator, patient cooperation, and view limitation under scars [175].

2. *Anterior segment optical coherence tomography.* AS-OCT is a precise non-contact *in vivo* ocular imaging technology that uses low coherence interferometry to measure the echo time delay of light backscattered from tissue structures [180]. This precision allows for producing two- and three-dimensional cross-sectional imaging of tissue, making it faster, less invasive, and more patient-friendly than other anterior segment imaging devices such as ultrasonic biomicroscopy (UBM) [181]. Spectral-domain OCT (SD-OCT) generates varying wavelengths of light with a higher acquisition speed [180, 182]. Other SD-OCT variations are custom-built designs with improved axial resolution, termed "ultrahigh-resolution OCT" (UHD-OCT) reach an axial resolution of 14 μm, with scan widths of 5–12 mm. Such a degree of image resolution and definition enables visualization of each layer of the cornea [183].

   Therefore, AS-OCT provides quantitative, cross-sectional examination of various corneal parameters, allowing for precise assessment and monitoring of the progression of corneal infectious diseases caused by different pathogens. Fungal keratitis, in particular, can be diagnosed and monitored with precision, as AS-OCT can identify unique patterns such as localized small or large full-thickness cystic spaces within the stroma, evidencing stromal necrosis, mainly in *Aspergillus spp*, and endothelial plaques denoting hyphal spread [184, 185] (Fig. 7.6b). The main advantages of AS-OCT lie in its ability to accurately determine and delineate the depth and extent of corneal ulceration, infiltrates, and haze. AS-OCT may help confirm the exact location of the keratitis, as shown in cases of multiple high-reflective whitish infiltrates with less defined margins [186, 187]. It might also help demonstrate the exact location and the extension of a fungal endothelial plaque. Certainly, most cases of fungal keratitis show an indistinct and irregular boundary between the endothelial plaque and the cornea [187]. This finding implies that the fungal damage to the endothelium expands from the stroma into the anterior chamber. AS-OCT can also be used to objectively measure corneal thickness, determine the risk of corneal perforation, and predict the treatment response according to the infiltrate size and inflammation area following therapeutic corneal cross-linking (PACK-CXL), which has been shown to be less effective for deep-seated fungal keratitis [188, 189].

3. *Two-photon microscopy (TPM).* TPM is a highly precise three-dimensional microscopic technique based on nonlinear two-photon fluorescence. It allows for the separate imaging of cells and corneal collagen through the intrinsic contrast of autofluorescence (AF) and second harmonic generation (SHG) [190]. Compared with IVCM, TPM reduces light damage and the scattering of infrared light as it penetrates living tissues, enabling the imaging of deeper structures with utmost reliability [191]. Compared to reflectance confocal microscopy, TPM can be used to observe deeper tissues with longer-wavelength light, and it is less affected by corneal opacity, albeit with longer imaging times [192, 193]. The use of moxifloxacin as a cell marker for TPM imaging further enhances its precision. A TPM imaging *in vitro* study of fungal keratitis in rabbit corneas caused by *Aspergillus fumigatus* and *Candida albicans* found a ten-fold increase in visibility in the fluorescence signal of fungal cells labeled with moxifloxacin [194].
4. *High-resolution UBM and B-scan ultrasonography.* These imaging techniques are not just valuable but crucial tools for diagnosing and monitoring cases suspected of fungal infection with large, dense, and obstructing corneal stromal infiltrates progressing toward the anterior chamber (vegetations). UBM permits the structural analysis on the status of the anterior chamber, its angle, the iris, lens, and anterior vitreous in a severe case of fungal keratitis. The B-scan ultrasound allows the structural evaluation of the vitreous cavity and posterior pole (retina and optic nerve), particularly if a surgical reconstructive intervention deems necessary or when endophthalmitis is suspected and extensive corneal fungal infiltration precludes anterior segment and fundus examination [195].
5. *Smartphones-based imaging and diagnosis.* With the rapid development of smartphone imaging technologies, the ability to rapidly, economically, and reliably diagnose fungal keratitis on the spot through smartphones equipped with simple lens systems, microsensors, micro-processing, and digital display systems is a significant leap forward. When combined with fluorescent labeling, smartphones can even detect microorganisms' subcellular proteins and nucleic acids *in vitro* [196, 197]. A case report on smartphone-based digital imaging for diagnosing fungal keratitis showed that corneal lesions can be photographed and enlarged on screens to help detect fungal hyphae. This method combines the use

of the smartphone and a microscope with an integrated light-emitting diode assembly. Compared to traditional corneal scraping and staining, smartphone-based imaging offers greater portability and accessibility, making diagnosis quicker and easier, particularly when experienced physicians and specialized microbiology facilities are not available [198]. Furthermore, smartphones incorporate AI for increasing diagnostic performance. However, this technology is still in its early stages, and likely there will be more emphasis on its development due to the benefits it provides.

7.8 Differential Diagnosis

The differential diagnosis of fungal keratitis includes bacterial, amoebic, oomycete, parasitic, or viral causes [24]. Recognizing the specific clinical features of fungal keratitis is crucial in its differential diagnosis. The patient's history of corneal trauma, contact lens misuse, an immunosuppressive state, a firm or dry elevated corneal slough, an irregular or feathery stromal infiltrate edge, satellite infiltrates, an immune ring, and endothelial plaques all point to a potential fungal infection [20, 32, 114, 124, 184]. A hypopyon might also be present; however, its overlap with other etiologies and similarities in the clinical signs at presentation from a wide variety of pathogens make it almost impossible to distinguish fungal keratitis from different types of corneal infection clinically. Moreover, in most cases, hypopyon ulcers are diagnosed primarily as bacterial infections and treated empirically with broad-spectrum antibiotics [32, 63, 115]. Then, misdiagnosis of fungal keratitis is mainly due to ophthalmologists' inexperience in differentiating clinical signs between different types of microbial keratitis or due to close similarities in clinical manifestations of different corneal pathogens. Other common causes for misdiagnosis are a deficiency in the complete diagnostic equipment at medical facilities or primary care units and a lack of qualified personnel for the handling and processing samples [63, 116, 123, 199].

Furthermore, corneal scraping for smear and culture is not performed routinely, and noninvasive imaging equipment like IVCM is not regularly available. Due to these inconveniences and a tiny inoculum harvested, negative cultures frequently occur. Therefore, referral to a tertiary eye care center facility is considered late after treatment failure and the ulcer progresses with severe complications [200].

A study on the diagnosis of microbial keratitis highlighted that fungal keratitis poses significant diagnostic challenges, with a sensitivity of only 38% and a specificity of 45% [116]. Even cornea specialists, despite their expertise, succeed in distinguishing between fungal and bacterial keratitis in only about two-thirds of cases [201]. Among the more difficult infections is *Pythium* keratitis, which can often be misdiagnosed as fungal keratitis. Research has shown that most culture-confirmed cases of *Pythium* keratitis were initially misidentified as suspected or unidentified fungi due to their similar clinical presentations [202].

7.9 Medical Management

Managing fungal keratitis poses significant challenges even in specialized medical facilities. A clear understanding of the disease's pathogenesis, combined with timely diagnosis and effective prevention strategies, is crucial for successfully managing fungal keratitis [63]. The complexity of the condition, particularly when delayed adequate attention and diagnosis or untimely and inadequate therapy is applied, allows fungal growth deep into the cornea. Once fungi penetrate the Descemet membrane, they become very difficult to eliminate, increasing the risk of endophthalmitis [20, 117, 203]. Low topical antifungal drug bioavailability into and beyond the cornea and the ease of developing antifungal resistance are the two major drawbacks of antifungal drug therapies. Antifungal drug resistance may result from reduced intracellular drug accumulation, changes in drug targets and membrane sterol synthesis pathways, changes in fungal cell wall component alterations, biofilm formation, and fungi morphogenesis [204, 205]. Due to these challenges, there has been an increased focus on antifungal susceptibility testing (AFST) in recent times [206]. Such clinical circumstances have also led physicians to consider an earlier therapeutic keratoplasty (TKP) to eliminate fungal infections. However, in addition to the surgical risks and potential complications, the availability of fresh donor tissue and the high rates of infection recurrence associated with this procedure do not bode well for achieving satisfactory therapeutic outcomes [22, 207, 208]. More recently, other interventional therapeutic modalities, including photodynamic therapy, have emerged to try to overcome the challenge that fungal keratitis represent [21, 209] (Table 7.4).

Finally, an established or recurrent fungal corneal ulceration represents a significant economic burden for the patient, family, or insurance agency. Once the keratitis is finally resolved, the visual outcome will frequently be limited, necessitating a costly visual rehabilitation surgical procedure [63]. It is estimated that at least one-third of the patients will eventually suffer from impaired eyesight [210].

1. *Medical therapy.* Topical antifungal medications are the main treatment for fungal keratitis. Treatment should start immediately after a high clinical suspicion (empirical) and, mostly, after confirmation of the clinical diagnosis with a smear or positive culture. However, it is important to note that intra-stromal and intracameral injections and oral routes could be considered in individual cases, and according to the severity, corneal invasiveness and extension of the infectious process [20, 170, 211–213]. Topical broad-spectrum antibiotics, usually a fourth-generation fluoroquinolone, should be added prophylactically to avoid an opportunistic bacterial superinfection. Additionally, a cycloplegic agent may decrease pain and relieve associated iridocyclitis. In case of high intraocular pressure, anti-glaucoma medications should be considered [16, 115, 170, 211, 213, 214]. Topical corticosteroids should be avoided in fungal keratitis. They decrease the efficacy of antifungal medication when given together, and when given alone, they worsen the condition. Furthermore, corticosteroids predispose to opportunistic bacterial superinfection, hinder epithelial healing, and increase the risk of further stromal melting [16, 170, 213, 215, 216].

Table 7.4 Types by antifungal agents, routes, and dosage of administration, along with their indications, limitations, and side effects

Class/Agent	Route of administration dose	Indications	Limitations/side effects
Polyenes			
Natamycin	Topical 5% (50 mg/ml) IS 10 µm/0.1 ml	First choice for filamentous fungi, particularly *Fusarium* spp.Good activity against *Aspergillus* spp., less effective against *Candida* spp.	Low corneal penetration Superior to topical voriconazole and fluconazole in *Fusarium* spp. [211] IS injection beneficial in patient's refractory to topical administration [413].
Amphotericin B	Topical 0.15–0.5% (1.5-5 mg/ml) SC 1.5 mg/0.1 ml IS 5–10 µg/0.1 ml IC 5–10 µg/0.1 ml IV 600–1200 mg/day	First line therapy for *Candida* spp. Good to moderate activity against filamentous fungi [307]. Deep keratitis with partial response to topical therapy.	Not commercially available. Side effects: conjunctival necrosis (SC), cataract, iritis, and corneal edema (IC).
Azoles			
Imidazoles			
Miconazole	Topical 10 mg/ml SC 1.2–10 mg/ml IV 600–1200 mg/day	Effective against *Candida* spp. adjuvant with topical therapy in patients with low compliance	Less effective than polyenes. It is fungistatic, not fungicidal [17].
Ketoconazole	Topical 1–2% Oral 200–400 mg/day	Broad spectrum as an adjuvant in deep keratitis [247]	Less effective, systemic toxicity (gastric intolerance and hepatotoxicity).
Econazole	Topical ointment/hydrogels 1–2% (10–20 mg/ml)	Effective against *Fusarium*, *Aspergillus*, and *Candida* species. Therapeutic efficacy comparable to natamycin 5% [274]	Not commercially available for ophthalmic use.
Clotrimazole	Topical 0.5% (5 mg/ml)	Effective against *Aspergillus* spp. but not *Fusarium* keratitis [281].	Fungistatic activity. Generally, well tolerated but induces corneal toxicity with long-term use.
Luliconazole	Topical 1% suspension	Broad-spectrum antifungal activity. Therapeutic efficacy comparable to natamycin in filamentous keratitis [273].	Poor solubility. Further studies are required to elucidate its antifungal efficacy.

(continued)

Table 7.4 (continued)

Class/Agent	Route of administration dose	Indications	Limitations/side effects
Triazoles			
Itraconazole	Topical 1% (10 mg/ml) Oral 200–400 mg/day	Effective against *Aspergillus*, *Curvularia*, and *Candida*. Less effective against *Fusarium* species [414]. Adjuvant therapy in deep keratitis/intraocular involvement by yeasts.	Less effective than Natamycin. Lower bioavailability, and penetration into ocular tissues than other azoles.
Fluconazole	Topical 0.2% (2 mg/ml) SC 2 mg/ml Oral 100–400 mg/day oral	Effective against *Candida* spp., less effective against filamentous fungi [268]. Good intraocular penetration, used as adjuvant with topical agents.	Orally has excellent ocular tissue bioavailability. Filamentous fungi exhibit resistance. Requires liver enzyme monitoring.
Voriconazole	Topical 1–2% (10–20 mg/ml) SC 10 mg/0.1 ml IS 50 μg/0.1 ml IC 50 μg/0.1 ml Oral 400 mg/day	Broad spectrum, fungal keratitis resistant to polyenes/first-line triazoles. Deep keratitis and intraocular involvement.	Less effective than natamycin. Side effects – blurred vision change in color perception; liver enzyme monitoring during oral use [226].
Posaconazole	Topical 4–10% (40–100 mg/ml) Oral 800 mg/day	Broad spectrum with proved effectiveness in rare fungal infections and recalcitrant keratitis resistant to polyenes/first-line triazoles [17].	Orally well-tolerated with minor side effects: nausea, vomiting, diarrhea, abdominal pain, rare hepatotoxicity. RCTs are necessary to optimize dosage.
Fluorinated Pyrimidines			
Flucytosine	Topical 1% (10 mg/ml) Oral 25 mg/kg/day	Synergistic effect with topical Amphotericin B in *Candida* keratitis [415].	Narrow antifungal spectrum, particularly against filamentous fungi. Good penetration into the cornea and anterior chamber. Rapid emergence of resistance if used alone.
Echinocandins			
Caspofungin	Topical 0.5% (5 mg/ml IS 5 mg/0.1 ml IC 50–250 μg/0.1 ml	Excellent *in vitro* activity against *Aspergillus*, and *Candida* spp. Used against yeasts resistant to polyenes and first-line triazoles.	No significant corneal endothelial toxicity has been found *in vitro* at concentrations up to 75 μg/0.1 ml [416].

(continued)

Table 7.4 (continued)

Class/Agent	Route of administration dose	Indications	Limitations/side effects
Micafungin	Topical 0.1% (1 mg/ml) SC 1 mg/0.1 ml IS 1 mg/ml (0.05 ml)	Used against yeasts resistant to polyenes and first-line triazoles [293]. Reported as effective as topical fluconazole 0.2% for *Candida* keratitis. Can be used as an adjunctive treatment for refractory *Beauveria* keratitis.	No serious side effects have been shown. Further studies are necessary to elucidate its effectiveness and safety.
Allyamine			
Terbinafine	Topical 0.2–0.5% (2–5 mg/ml) Oral 250 mg/day	Active against *Aspergillus*, *Fusarium*, *Scedosporium* and *Candida*. Valuable adjunctive agent for *Fusarium* keratitis combined with Amphotericin B [417].	Generally, well tolerated. Poor corneal penetration following topical administration in intact eyes.

IC intracameral, *IS* intrastromal, *SC* subconjunctival injections, *IV* intravenous infusion, *RCT* randomized controlled trial

Other prognostic factors that indicate the severity of infection and a poor response to topical antifungal therapy include the size of the ulcer and the extent of stromal necrosis. Ulcers larger than 4 mm in diameter are more likely to fail medical treatment compared to those smaller than 4 mm. Additionally, superficial ulcers tend to have better outcomes than deeper ones. In deeper ulcers, antifungal agents may struggle to penetrate to the level of infection, making it difficult to achieve the necessary therapeutic concentrations [217]. Other risk factors for poor prognosis include the fungus load, hypopyon, treatment delay, and *Fusarium* species as the causative organism [74, 218] (Table 7.4).

2. *Antifungal susceptibility testing (AFST).* Due to increased antifungal resistance, AFST and minimum inhibitory concentration (MIC) determination are crucial for effectively treating fungal keratitis and optimizing patient outcomes. The primary objective of AFST is to provide clinicians with the susceptibility and resistance profile of a fungal pathogen before and during treatment. Although initial antifungal treatment is determined by the pathogen identification and previous therapeutic experience, AFST is crucial in severe invasive fungal infections, when drug resistance is suspected, or in patients unresponsive to treatment [216]. MIC values have already been set for *Aspergillus* and *Candida* but not for other species [219]. A recent study that determined the MICs of natamycin and voriconazole on isolates from fungal keratitis demonstrated that natamycin had greater breakpoint values against all specimens except for *Fusarium* spp. In contrast, voriconazole had the lowest breakpoint value targeting *Aspergillus* spp. They also showed that the greater the MIC breakpoint value, the greater the odds of developing corneal perforation [220]. AFST performed using the disk

diffusion method found that *Aspergillus* spp. and *Fusarium* spp. had a higher sensitivity to voriconazole than natamycin, while amphotericin B showed effectiveness against yeasts [221]. Another study found a potent Natamycin antifungal activity against *Candida albicans* with a MIC range from 1 to 2 μg/mL [222] and others reported a low Natamycin activity against *C. parapsilopsis* with a high MIC = 150 μg/mL [223]. Such wide MIC variations remind us that when dealing with a fungal corneal infection, it is ideal to obtain AFST and MICs for each case, albeit of the availability limitations and the need for a specialized microbiology lab, which in many cases may not be available.

3. *Topical and systemic antifungal agents.*
   Natamycin 5% is a polyene macrolide that is considered the first-line treatment for filamentous fungal keratitis and is the first antifungal medication to receive approval. It works by binding to sterols, primarily ergosterol, in the fungal cell membrane, resulting in membrane instability and ultimately leading to fungal cell death. Natamycin has a broad spectrum of activity, particularly against species of *Fusarium* and *Aspergillus*, but it is also effective against *Alternaria, Candida, Cephalosporium, Colletotrichum, Curvularia, Lasiodiplodia, Scedosporium, Trichophyton*, and *Penicillium* [222, 224]. Initially, it should be administered hourly until improvement is observed, indicated by partial resolution of infiltration. Once improvement is noted, the frequency can be reduced accordingly. After the infection resolves, natamycin should be continued for an additional 2 weeks [225]. However, a significant limitation of natamycin is its poor ocular penetration, which can prolong the resolution of keratitis. The mycotic ulcer treatment trial (MUTT), a double-masked multicentric randomized controlled trial involving 323 participants, compared topical natamycin 5% with voriconazole 1%. The results showed that natamycin was associated with better clinical and microbiological outcomes in smear-positive filamentous fungal keratitis, especially in cases of *Fusarium* keratitis. Additionally, the rates of corneal perforation and the need for penetrating keratoplasty were higher in the voriconazole group compared to the natamycin cohort [226]. Similar findings were reported in another randomized controlled trial with 118 participants, where the natamycin group demonstrated faster healing and better final visual acuity than the voriconazole group for filamentous fungal keratitis, particularly in cases involving *Fusarium* [227]. A Cochrane review of the efficacy of various antifungal medications also indicated that natamycin yielded better clinical outcomes than voriconazole [228].

   Intrastromal natamycin is not commonly used due to its poor water solubility and limited ocular bioavailability. To address the need for a natamycin formulation that offers greater ocular bioavailability and requires a lower dosage, researchers developed a 1% natamycin solution by combining it with hydroxylpropyl-beta-cyclodextrin (HPβCD). This formulation resulted in improved ocular bioavailability [229]. A clinical trial comparing the intrastromal use of this 0.01% natamycin solution with other agents, such as voriconazole and amphotericin B, demonstrated that the new formulation had a significantly shorter mean healing time compared to the other two agents [230].

Amphotericin B is a broad-spectrum antifungal agent classified as a polyene macrolide, produced by *Actinomyces Streptomyces nodusus*. It was the first antifungal agent used clinically. Amphotericin B is fungicidal due to its interaction with ergosterol in the fungal cell membrane, which results in cell death by forming pores and causing lethal changes in membrane permeability. Amphotericin B 0.15% is frequently used in cases not responding to natamycin 5%. It is also considered a first-line treatment in cases of fungal keratitis caused *by Candida* spp. [12]. Its spectrum of activity mainly includes *Candida* spp., *Aspergillus* spp., and *Cryptococcus* spp., but it is less effective against *Fusarium* spp. and other *Mucorales*, which have higher MIC values [231]. Amphotericin B is commonly used as a topical solution at concentrations ranging from 0.15 to 0.5%, requiring preparation by a pharmacy. However, it has poor ocular penetration and is associated with frequent side effects, such as cytotoxicity at high concentrations, which can lead to punctate corneal erosions, epithelial defects, stromal edema, and occasionally, iritis [232, 233]. Because oral amphotericin B is associated with many side effects, including nephrotoxicity, hepatotoxicity, and skin erythema and hyperemia, it is not a preferred systemic antifungal agent [232]. Recent studies have explored the intrastromal, intracameral, and intravitreal routes for delivering amphotericin B, primarily due to concerns about its bioavailability limitations and potential negative side effects [212, 234–236]. Intrastromal injection of amphotericin B has shown promise in treating indolent keratitis caused by *Candida* spp. and other fungi. However, the relatively small number of patients treated, along with the concurrent use of other topical or systemic antifungal agents, makes it difficult to draw strong conclusions about its effectiveness. Notably, there has been a higher rate of deep vascularization during healing with intrastromal amphotericin B compared to treatments with natamycin and voriconazole [230, 235, 237]. Regarding intracameral amphotericin B injections, there are conflicting results between a study reporting benefit with faster therapeutic response and a more recent randomized control trial showing no added advantage of intracameral amphotericin B over topical antifungal therapy [234, 238]. Conversely, a combination of intracameral with intrastromal amphotericin B injections in severe recalcitrant fungal keratitis showed a satisfactory response [212]. Finally, subconjunctival amphotericin B injection is not favored due to serious complications, including conjunctival granuloma formation, necrosis, and scleritis [236, 239].

Voriconazole 1% is a newer generation antifungal agent derived from fluconazole. It works by inhibiting the enzyme 14α-lanosterol demethylase, which affects the synthesis of ergosterol, a crucial component of fungal cell walls. Voriconazole is FDA-approved for the treatment of invasive aspergillosis and can be used "off label" topically for ophthalmic fungal infections. This drug is effective against a broad spectrum of fungi, including filamentous and yeast forms such as *Aspergillus* spp., *Fusarium* spp., *Candida* spp., *Scedosporium* spp., and *Cryptococcus* spp. However, it has minimal efficacy against Mucorales [228, 240]. Topical and intrastromal administration are the two common routes for using voriconazole in cases of fungal keratitis. Although topical voriconazole 1% is not commercially available as an ophthalmic formulation, it can be prepared in pharmacies from the parenteral form.

The voriconazole MIC is 0.5 μg/mL, which is lower than that of other imidazole drugs [17, 241]. Although the MUTT-1 trail, which compared topical 1% voriconazole to natamycin 5%, failed to demonstrate superiority over commercially available natamycin drops, it is considered a good alternative to natamycin and amphotericin B in resistant cases, and also as an adjunctive therapy in severe fungal keratitis [214, 226, 240]. Furthermore, despite a RCT evaluating the effectiveness of intrastromal voriconazole showing no significant benefit, it remains the most commonly used intrastromal antifungal agent, with many reports indicating positive treatment outcomes with intrastromal injections of voriconazole at doses of 50–100 μg/0.1 mL [230, 242–244].

Oral voriconazole is used to treat keratitis associated with scleritis or endophthalmitis, especially when conventional therapies have failed. Although the MUTT-2 trial did not demonstrate any significant advantage of oral voriconazole in the treatment regimen, a secondary data analysis indicated a non-statistically significant beneficial role as an adjunct treatment for *Fusarium* keratitis [245, 246]. Additionally, a comparative study showed that oral voriconazole is more therapeutically effective than oral ketoconazole in treating fungal keratitis [247]. A recent study has also shown promising results for oral voriconazole (400 mg/day) as an alternative for the prophylaxis and treatment of fungal keratitis [248].

Itraconazole is a synthetic antifungal agent belonging to the dioxolane triazole class. Its mechanism of action is like that of other triazoles. Itraconazole is effective against various fungi, including *Candida* spp. and *Aspergillus* spp. Notably, it shows synergistic effects when combined with 5% natamycin in treating *Fusarium* keratitis [249, 250]. Itraconazole is available in ophthalmic solution and ointment at a concentration of 1% (10 mg/mL). However, the lipophilic nature of the drug limits the effectiveness of topical formulations due to poor ocular bioavailability. Multiple experimental assays designed to overcome such limitations incorporate itraconazole into nanosized carriers, like niosomes [251], microemulsions [252], nanosuspensions [253], solid–lipid nanoparticles [254], nanovesicles-spanlastics [255], and nanocrystals (ITZ-NC) [256]. Such formulations, enhanced the antifungal activity by improving its absorption. For oral administration, the recommended dose of itraconazole is between 200 and 400 mg per day. However, systemic use can lead to side effects, including headaches, gastrointestinal upset, transient skin reactions, and, in rare cases, hepatitis [257].

Posaconazole, a second-generation synthetic triazole agent and an analog of itraconazole, is a key anti-fungal agent of the future due to its broad-spectrum activity against most pathogenic fungal species at low MIC values. This unique characteristic allows its use in natamycin and voriconazole-resistant cases [258, 259]. Posaconazole is administered at a dosage of 800 mg/day oral suspension systemically, hourly, or two-hourly at a concentration of 10 mg/0.1 mL or 4 mg/0.1 mL topically [260]. It is a well-tolerated drug with minor side effects like nausea, vomiting, diarrhea, abdominal pain, and rarely liver function test alteration, providing a balanced view of its tolerability [261]. Several case reports have shown the effectiveness of posaconazole with rare pathogens and recalcitrant keratitis previously treated with voriconazole, amphotericin, fluconazole, and natamycin [262–265].

Two *Fusarium* keratitis cases resistant to oral and topical voriconazole and fluconazole, responded rapidly to oral (200 mg/day) and topical posaconazole (4 mg/0.1 mL) [264]. Thus, the spectrum of activity of posaconazole includes common fungi causing keratitis like *Fusarium* spp., *Aspergillus* spp., *Candida* spp., and rare fungi like *Paecilomyces* spp. and *Beauveria* spp. [260, 264, 265]. Experimental nanoparticle drug delivery studies in the form of posaconazole micelles have shown a better ocular permeation profile than the diluted oral suspension formulation [266].

Fluconazole 2% is a fungistatic bis-triazole antifungal agent commonly used in combination with other antifungal medications, such as amphotericin B, to treat fungal keratitis caused by *Candida* or *Aspergillus* species [267]. A comparative study examined the effectiveness of topical fluconazole 0.2% administered alone or in combination with oral ketoconazole (200 mg twice daily) over a period of 4–12 weeks for culture-positive filamentous fungal keratitis. The results showed that 70% of patients achieved a satisfactory clinical outcome, while 30% required surgical intervention to control the infection [268]. These results are comparable to those observed with 5% natamycin in the treatment of fungal keratitis [269]. Another clinical study analyzed the effectiveness of daily subconjunctival fluconazole (0.5 ml of fluconazole 2% IV preparation) as an adjunct therapy in recalcitrant fungal keratitis unresponsive to conventional therapy (combination of topical natamycin 5% with econazole 2% or clotrimazole 1%, and itraconazole 1% ointment) and oral ketoconazole (200 mg two times a day), progressing to deep stromal and endothelial involvement [270]. A total of 33 culture-proven filamentous fungal keratitis cases with documented failure were included. Infection was eradicated without recurrence in 54.6% of eyes. However, in 45.4% of them, the infection progressed, requiring a therapeutic penetrating keratoplasty. Importantly, no toxicity, such as conjunctival ischemia, necrosis, or fibrosis was observed during the treatment [270]. Similar to the case of econazole, fluconazole has been incorporated into a Spanlastic vesicular system to achieve a prolonged and enhanced therapeutic effect in a porcine corneal model [271]. Spanlastics were three times smaller in size and showed a better permeation in comparison to a corresponding niosomal formulation. The system exhibited a threefold increase in the apparent permeability coefficient compared to the marketed formulation, attributed to its elastic nature. Finally, the developed system was found to be stable for 2 months under both refrigerated and extreme storage conditions [271]. Further clinical trials are needed to test the efficacy and safety of these pharmaceutical preparations in humans.

7.9.1 Other Azoles

Luliconazole is a new imidazole antifungal agent with broad-spectrum activity. It is currently available in topical formulations as a 1% cream, 1% ointment, and 1% solution for treating dermatomycoses and onychomycoses [272]. An *in vitro* study analyzed the MIC of luliconazole against keratitis-derived *Fusarium* spp., and other reference strains. The results showed that luliconazole had the lowest MIC value against all tested filamentous fungi, with an MIC-90 of 0.06 μg/mL against *Fusarium* spp. [273] Therefore, further experimental and clinical studies are needed to evaluate this promising antifungal agent as a topical treatment option for filamentous fungal keratitis.

Econazole 1% is an azole antifungal agent that has been shown to be as effective as natamycin 5% for treating fungal keratitis caused by *Aspergillus* spp. and *Fusarium* spp. [274]. However, like many topical antifungal agents, econazole 1% has poor aqueous solubility, which results in limited tissue penetration and reduced availability at the site of infection [17, 124]. To overcome this disadvantage, econazole nitrate has been solubilized with cyclodextrins and incorporated into two types of ophthalmic hydrogels: an *in situ* ion-sensitive hydrogel [275] and a mucoadhesive hydrogel based on hyaluronic acid [276]. These formulations provide prolonged retention time on the ocular surface, controlled release of econazole nitrate, and safety [277]. Another innovative delivery strategy for econazole 1% nitrate utilizes a novel nano system for ocular drug delivery. This approach employs a surfactant-based elastic vesicular system called Spanlastics, which enhances the ocular permeability and bioavailability of antifungal drugs [278]. Spanlastics are highly deformable and elastic carriers, like transferosomes, and can reach the posterior segment of the eye when administered topically in the form of eye drops [271]. The optimized Econazole-loaded nano vesicular carriers had a greater antifungal activity, and a longer mean residence time of the drug on the ocular surface compared to pharmacy compound drug suspensions [278]. Further randomized controlled clinical trials are needed to prove the safety and efficacy of these novel antifungal formulations.

Clotrimazole 1% is a synthetic imidazole derivative available as a pharmaceutical compound for topical treatment of fungal keratitis [279]. A retrospective study of 32 eyes with lab-proven fungal keratitis (mainly *Aspergillus* and *Fusarium* species), 62.5% severe and 37.5% mild to moderate keratitis, analyzed the efficacy of 1% clotrimazole as monotherapy, or sequentially with topical amphotericin-B [280]. The study found no initial therapeutic response with clotrimazole as monotherapy, but 79.1% of eyes treated initially with amphotericin-B (induction phase) showed a favorable response (nine with non-severe and ten with severe keratitis). After 2 and 3 weeks in non-severe and severe cases, respectively, the regimen was changed to maintenance with 1% clotrimazole monotherapy, resulting in a continued favorable response in all eyes. The keratitis healed after 4–10 weeks from the initial treatment [280]. In conclusion, a combination with a polyene derivative should be considered in the treatment of fungal keratitis with clotrimazole, mainly due to *Fusarium* spp. [281].

Echinocandins are a group of antifungal drugs that induce fungal cell lysis by inhibiting (1,3)-D-glucan synthesis, a crucial component of fungal cell walls, thereby causing apoptosis and the death of the fungus [282]. The selective action of echinocandins helps limit toxic side effects and enhances their therapeutic efficacy against strains that are resistant to azole and polyene antifungal agents [282].

Caspofungin, micafungin, and anidulafungin are the three FDA-approved commercially available echinocandins for the management of invasive systemic fungal infections. Several studies have demonstrated the clinical efficacy of echinocandins in treating refractory fungal keratitis. Their spectrum of activity includes mainly *Candida* (fungicidal due to the high glucan content) and *Aspergillus* (fungistatic) and is less effective against *Fusarium* spp. [282–284]. Several *in vitro* and *in vivo* studies have shown promising results regarding the safety, efficacy, and dosage of these agents [285, 286]. Caspofungin ocular penetration studies in an animal model and human volunteers found better corneal penetration in the presence of an epithelial defect or an inflamed cornea [287, 288]. Caspofungin available in concentrations of 1–0.5% for topical use and intravenous formulation for systemic use have an adjunctive role in the management of ocular fungal infections caused by *Alternaria* [289, 290] voriconazole-refractory *Candida albicans* [291] and recurrent *Candida parapsilosis* keratitis [292]. Micafungin is the second drug in this category that has been investigated for ophthalmic use. A topical ophthalmic solution at a concentration of 0.1% has proven effective for treating persistent yeast-related corneal ulcers, showing comparable efficacy to fluconazole 0.2% drops in cases of *Candida* keratitis [293, 294] (Table 7.4).

Antiseptic agents. Commonly used surface antiseptics and disinfecting solutions in general ophthalmology practice have demonstrated broad-spectrum activity against bacteria, yeasts, molds, and certain viruses [295]. Chlorhexidine 0.2%, a broad-spectrum antiseptic belonging to the biguanides class, has shown effectiveness against *Acanthamoeba*, bacteria, and fungi [296, 297]. Moreover, it has certain advantages, including the topical application, general availability, low costs, broad-spectrum activity, and fungicidal mechanism of action at relatively low concentrations [298]. Some evidence suggests it may serve as an early adjuvant in treating fungal keratitis, particularly when combined with other antifungal agents [298]. Interestingly, two RCTs reported that chlorhexidine 0.2% was more effective than natamycin in managing fungal keratitis [299, 300]. A Cochrane systematic review of treatments for fungal keratitis indicated a non-significant trend favoring chlorhexidine 0.2% over natamycin 5% in terms of "curing" the condition within 21 days when data from these two trials were combined [228]. Moreover, a recent non-inferiority trial comparing chlorhexidine 0.2% with natamycin 5% provided strong evidence that participants treated with natamycin had significantly better vision at 3 months compared to those treated with chlorhexidine. There was no difference in the rate of positive re-culture results between the two groups on day 7. While most patients treated with chlorhexidine did heal, the healing rate was lower compared to those treated with natamycin. Furthermore, patients in the natamycin group were less likely to experience perforation or require an emergency corneal graft [301, 302]. Results from this trial suggest that chlorhexidine is initially effective during the sterilization phase; however, extended treatment may lead to delayed re-epithelialization and increased scarring.

On the other hand, *in vitro* studies assessing the antimicrobial activity of hexamidine di-isethionate 0.05% (Keratosept®) and povidone-iodine 0.6% (IODIM®) found that both agents exhibit antimicrobial activity against *Candida* species [303].

7.10 Interventional and Surgical Therapy

Local antifungal injections. Severe and extensive fungal keratitis frequently requires the administration of larger doses and loads of antifungal agents in the form of subconjunctival, intrastromal, and intracameral injections, particularly when dense biofilms or compact infiltrates preclude the efficient delivery of medication via the topical route. The preparation, administration methodology, and doses of local antifungal injections are described in Table 7.4.

1. *Subconjunctival injections.* Subconjunctival injections permit the administration of antifungal medications directly into the subconjunctival space, creating a drug deposit near the site of infection. This delivery method can overcome some limitations associated with topical eye drops, such as inadequate corneal penetration and the requirement for frequent dosing. Fluconazole and amphotericin B are the most used antifungal agents delivered via this route [304, 305].

   The clinical applications of subconjunctival injections include: (1) Treating severe fungal keratitis, where the infection is present deep within the cornea and is not responding adequately to topical medications; (2) addressing non-compliant patients who struggle to use eye drops regularly; (3) serving as an adjunct to topical antifungal drops to enhance overall treatment efficacy; and (4) avoiding or delaying the need for surgical interventions, such as corneal transplantation [306].

   The potential benefits of this procedure include: (1) Direct drug delivery to the affected area, which may improve treatment effectiveness; (2) overcoming the challenge of poor drug penetration associated with topical treatments; and (3) reduced drug toxicity, such as with liposomal amphotericin B compared to its conventional form [305, 307]. However, there are potential risks associated with subconjunctival injections, including conjunctival necrosis (especially with amphotericin B), scleritis, scleral thinning, mild and temporary bleeding at the injection site, conjunctival chemosis, dilated conjunctival vessels, and a yellow appearance of the conjunctiva [239].

   In conclusion, subconjunctival injections can be a valuable tool in managing severe fungal keratitis. They offer a method to deliver antifungal medications near the cornea, potentially improving treatment outcomes, especially when topical medications are inadequate or when patient compliance poses a challenge.
2. *Intrastromal injections.* Since most topical antifungal agents are larger molecules that do not penetrate the stroma well, a direct drug delivery method, such as repeated intrastromal injections, may be suitable for managing dense and deep fungal stromal infiltrates often found in advanced cases of severe fungal keratitis [308]. However, the results of such therapeutic strategy are contradictory, while a RCT performed in corneas with moderate to severe filamentous fungal keratitis show no benefit of adding intrastromal voriconazole injections to topical natamycin, other similar design study exploring the benefits of voriconazole, amphotericin B, and natamycin intrastromal injections in recalcitrant fungal keratitis found them safe and effective adjunct to conventional therapy [230,

242, 309, 310]. Considering the current evidence, this should be a case-by-case strategy to be used based on the type of infection and clinical experience. Intrastromal injections should be performed under an operating microscope after administering topical or peribulbar anesthesia, along with basal sedation. It is essential to maintain full aseptic conditions throughout the procedure. The needle, with the bevel facing down, is inserted obliquely from an area of the cornea that is not affected, aiming to reach the abscess at the mid-stromal level, which is the targeted area for drug deposition. After inserting the needle, the medication is injected, using the degree of corneal hydration as a guide to assess the area covered by the drug. Once the desired amount of medication is delivered into the stroma, the plunger is pulled back slightly to disrupt the capillary column and prevent any back-leakage of the drug. Around five divided doses are administered around the abscess to create a drug deposit that encircles the lesion. This technique is performed in such a way that a centripetal wave of fluid appears to surround the abscess along each meridian. By employing circumferential injections, a barrier of intrastromal medication is established around the entire abscess [243]. Most studies indicate that a minimum of three injection sessions is necessary to achieve an optimal therapeutic response [309].

The advantages of intrastromal injection are: (1) Direct drug delivery to the target area, (2) injection into the corneal stroma effectively addresses the issue of poor drug penetration, (3) the intrastromal drug functions as a depot, allowing for a slow release of medication over time, and (4) it results in reduced epithelial toxicity [311].

However, intrastromal injection is not exempted from potential complications, and includes corneal edema, epithelial defects, neovascularization, corneal perforation, Descemet's membrane detachment, and even endophthalmitis [244]. Other complications reported with amphotericin b intrastromal injections include ocular surface and retinal toxicity [309].

3. *Intracameral injections* involve the direct administration of antifungal medications into the anterior chamber of the eye to treat severe fungal infections [234]. Although the evidence on the efficacy of delivering antifungal agents directly into the anterior segment is limited, this approach could be used for infections that affect the deep cornea or spread to the anterior chamber, posing a risk of endophthalmitis. It has been used when topical treatments are insufficient, allowing for higher concentrations of medication to be delivered directly to the site of infection [234]. We believe that intracameral injections should be used in certain instances, such as in "interface infections," during endothelial transplants, or as an adjunct to complete a therapeutic corneal transplantation. Antifungal medications used in this procedure include amphotericin B, voriconazole, fluconazole, and caspofungin [238, 312–314].

   The advantages of intracameral injections include the targeted delivery of antifungal medication at high concentrations to the site of infection, minimizing systemic side effects associated with oral antifungal treatments, and potentially reducing the need for more invasive procedures, such as TKP. However, in cases of severe and persistent infections, multiple injections may be required to fully eradicate the fungus [315, 316]. Finally, a combination of intrastromal and intracameral injections have proven efficacious for the management of certain cases of severe and recalcitrant fungal keratitis [212, 317].

Potential complications of intracameral antifungal injections can include sharp pain during and shortly after the procedure, intraocular inflammation, anterior chamber reactions, and transient hypopyon formation. More rarely, complications may include secondary infections due to paracentesis, bleeding from mechanical trauma to the iris, and the formation of anterior subcapsular cataracts if the needle inadvertently contacts the anterior lens capsule [318].

4. *Photo Activated Chromophore for Keratitis (PACK-CXL).* The mechanism behind PACK-CXL is rooted in the principles of corneal collagen crosslinking (CXL). This process involves irradiating the corneal stroma, which has been prepped with the photosensitizer riboflavin (vitamin B2), using ultraviolet-A (UV-A) light. This irradiation leads to the production of reactive oxygen species and singlet oxygen, enhancing corneal biomechanical stability by establishing covalent bonds between the collagen fibrils within the stroma. Schnitzler et al. (2000) were pioneers in demonstrating the efficacy of CXL for treating erosive and ulcerative corneal conditions, showing remarkable results [319]. Recently, there has been a growing interest in employing CXL as an adjunctive treatment for infective keratitis. The proposed mechanisms of action include: (1) An anti-inflammatory and antimicrobial effect by damaging the DNA/RNA of pathogens, (2) increased resistance of the tissue to enzymatic degradation by organisms, and (3) improved ocular penetration of antifungal agents facilitated by CXL [320, 321]. Experimental studies have demonstrated that CXL can serve as an effective adjunctive treatment in the management of fungal keratitis, particularly when combined with antifungal agents during the early stages of the disease [320–322]. It has also been suggested that extending the duration of irradiation and using a higher concentration of riboflavin may enhance the efficacy of the procedure [321, 323]. However, the role of CXL in treating fungal keratitis in humans remains controversial, with various studies yielding conflicting results [320, 323–328]. While some case reports and significant studies indicate that CXL can be a beneficial adjunctive therapy for managing fungal keratitis, the Cross-Linking Assisted Infection Reduction Trial (CLAIR trial)—a randomized controlled trial aimed at evaluating CXL's effectiveness—found no additional benefits. In fact, it suggested that CXL could lead to inferior visual outcomes compared to standard medical management [320].
5. *Photodynamic Therapy (PDT)* involves the generation of reactive oxygen species (ROS) from photosensitizers when activated by a radiation source. These ROS damage cellular structures, leading to cell death. PDT has been proposed as an alternative treatment for corneal infections, including Fusarium keratitis [209]. This therapy is promising due to several advantages: It exhibits negligible drug resistance, offers high spatiotemporal control, and has fewer side effects compared to existing topical medications (Fig. 7.7). The therapeutic protocol for PDT is like that of riboflavin, using UV-A light in cases of keratoconus. Experimental studies comparing rose Bengal and riboflavin PDT have shown

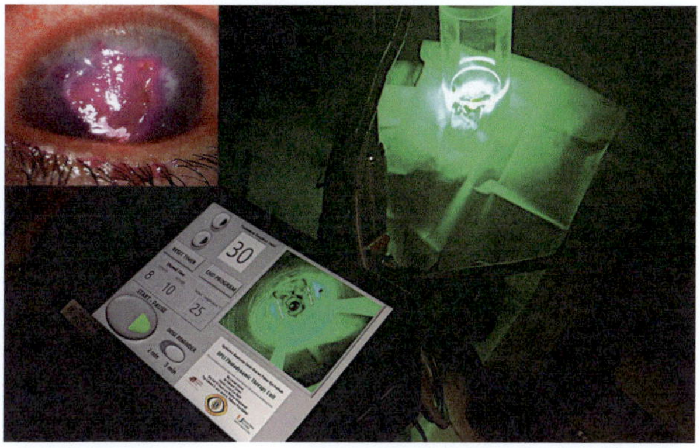

Fig. 7.7 Photodynamic therapy (PDT) with rose Bengal stain for the treatment of severe, recalcitrant filamentous fungal keratitis. The inset highlights the de-epithelialized cornea impregnated with rose Bengal stain. (Figures, courtesy of Bascom-Palmer Eye Institute photography department)

that rose Bengal PDT, when combined with green light (518 nm), is significantly effective *in vitro* against common fungal pathogens, including *Fusarium solani*, *Aspergillus fumigatus*, and *Candida albicans* [329]. The rose Bengal electromagnetic activation with green light for infection reduction (REAGIR) double-blinded, placebo-controlled RCT compared topical natamycin + rose Bengal PDT with topical natamycin + sham PDT found no overall benefit of RB-PDT vs sham. However, RB-PDT was beneficial in *Fusarium* keratitis, but not in other fungal species [330].

6. Recent innovative research has explored the use of mitochondrial-targeting luminogens with aggregation-induced emission characteristics (AIEgens) as photosensitizers instead of rose Bengal and riboflavin. These AIEgens selectively target fungal mitochondria, an organelle that has a lower likelihood of developing drug resistance [331]. This comparative study conducted in a rabbit model evaluated the efficacy and toxicity of these AIE agents—namely, IQTPE-2O, IQ-Cm, and IQ-TPA-assisted PDT—against rose Bengal PDT. The findings indicated that the AIE agents were less toxic and more effective [331].

7.11 Surgical Management

7.11.1 Therapeutic Keratoplasty (TPK)

Surgical intervention is a crucial modality in treating fungal keratitis, with a range of 15–55% of cases requiring therapeutic keratoplasty (TKP), indicating that medical treatment alone may not be sufficient for controlling the infection [218, 332] (Fig. 7.8a, b). A study found that 51.58% of severe and extensive filamentous fungal keratitis cases (43.33% *Aspergillus* and 60.86% *Fusarium*) and 100% of *Candida* cases needed TPK for the control of infection [170]. The most common indications for TPK include perforated ulcers, impending perforations, and recalcitrant keratitis that worsens despite medical management [207, 218]. A secondary analysis of the MUTT- II study which evaluated the predictors that could potentially indicate the need for a TPK in fungal keratitis found that hypopyon at baseline indicated 2.28

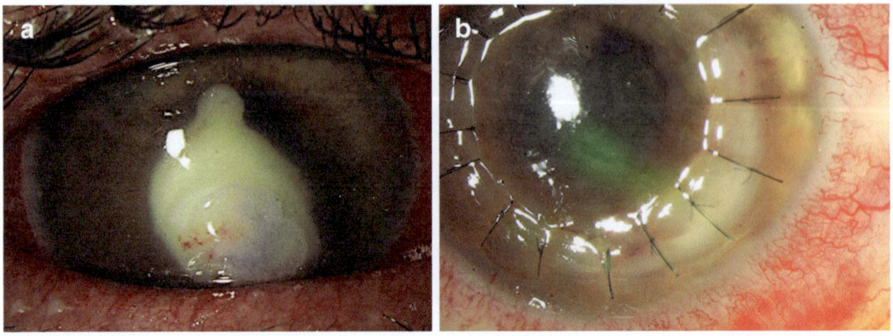

Fig. 7.8 Soft contact lens-associated fungal keratitis in a 33-year-old insulin-dependent diabetic patient. (**a**) Dense, large, and deep fungal infiltrate with significant central stromal melting. (**b**) Postoperative image after a few weeks of therapeutic penetrating keratoplasty (TPK) showing a clear donor button free of fungi and a quiet anterior chamber. (Figures, courtesy of Bascom-Palmer Eye Institute photography department)

times the odds of the patient developing corneal perforation and/or needing TPK (95% CI, 1.18–4.40; $P = 0.01$). Additionally, patients with a corneal infiltrate involving the posterior one-third of the stroma had a 71.4% risk of developing corneal perforation and/or needing TPK. For each 1-mm increase in the geometric mean of the infiltrate, there were 1.37 (95% CI, 1.12–1.67; $P = 0.002$) increased odds of developing perforation and/or needing TPK [333]. However, the survival rate of a corneal graft in an actively infected and inflamed eye is low with an increased chance of graft rejection, re-infection, and secondary glaucoma [207]. The rates of re-infection after keratoplasty procedures are a major concern in fungal keratitis with rates ranging from 6% to 16% [207, 218, 334]. Another important reason for rapid graft failure and poor outcomes is the limited availability of donor corneas with optimal endothelial cell counts in developing countries where non-optical grade tissue is used for TPK given the increased demand and paucity of donor corneal tissue. Furthermore, poorer surgical outcomes in fungal keratitis cases can occur due to the postoperative delayed use of corticosteroid drops due to the fear of re-infection, which hence an increase in inflammation and resultant graft decompensation and vascularization [207]. A study on the outcomes of TPK in fungal keratitis revealed that the probability of graft survival decreases over time after surgery, from 49% at 6 months to 29.5% at 1 year, 20.5% at 2 years, 13.7% at 3 years, and 10.6% at 4 years. The overall median graft survival rate was only 5.9 months. The risk factors for graft failure were categorized as follows: size of infiltrate (<6 mm, 6–8 mm, and > 8 mm), size of graft (8–9 mm, 9–11 mm, and > 11 mm), fungus species (*Acremonium, Aspergillus, Fusarium*, others), additional cataract surgery (presence/absence), and socio-economic status (higher/lower) [207, 335]. The univariate Cox proportional hazards regression analysis revealed that stromal infiltrate size (hazard ratio = 1.36; $P = 0.01$) and graft size (hazard ratio = 1.39; $P < 0.0001$) were the most significant risk factors for failure. The multivariate Cox proportional hazards regression analysis showed that the size of the stromal infiltrate is a significant risk factor for failure (hazard ratio = 1.37; $P = 0.0003$).

7.11.2 Lamellar Keratoplasty (LK) in Fungal Keratitis

Lamellar corneal surgery has emerged as a preferable surgical option for managing specific cases of fungal keratitis, primarily due to its advantages as a less risky and invasive technique compared to full-thickness TPK. A study involving 55 cases of fungal keratitis that were unresponsive to conventional treatments found that LK achieved a success rate of 92.7%, with only 7.3% experiencing a recurrence of infection. Positive visual and anatomical outcomes were noted during follow-up periods of 12–18 months [336]. Other research has indicated that early surgical intervention, such as deep anterior lamellar keratoplasty (DALK), can be a safe and effective approach for managing fungal keratitis [337, 338]. In a study involving 23 patients with fungal keratitis caused by various species, including *Fusarium*, *Aspergillus*, *Candida*, and *Curvularia*, early DALK was performed as an adjunctive therapy. Histopathological examination of the excised tissue showed no signs of fungal colonization in the deep stroma or peripheral lamellae. All grafts remained clear throughout the entire follow-up period (mean: 32 ± 10 months, range: 18–50 months; 95% CI, 27–36 months), with no recurrences of infection or episodes of graft rejection. Additionally, there was a significant improvement in best-corrected visual acuity (BCVA) ($p = 0.001$) [338]. A multicenter study analyzed 25 cases of fungal keratitis treated with DALK using cross-linked acellular porcine corneal stroma (APCS) along with topical tacrolimus. The results showed promising surgical and visual outcomes at the one-year follow-up. Only one patient experienced a fungal reinfection, and three patients had graft rejection [339].

7.11.3 Amniotic Membrane Transplantation (AMT)

AMT, either on its own or in combination with a partial conjunctival flap, has emerged as a viable option for delaying or preventing TPK due to fungal keratitis. Single or multi-layer cryopreserved and lyophilized amniotic membranes (AM) create a physical barrier that facilitates the migration of epithelial cells, promoting corneal re-epithelialization. Additionally, they possess several beneficial properties: they have anti-inflammatory effects by downregulating IL-1α and IL-1β in corneal epithelial cells, exhibit anti-angiogenic properties through the overexpression of thrombospondin-1, endostatin, and tissue inhibitors of metalloproteinases (TIMP-1, 2, 3, and 4), and demonstrate anti-fibrotic effects by suppressing TGFβ and its receptors. Furthermore, active components in the amniotic membrane, such as nerve growth factors, can also help reduce pain [340]. A study involving 23 patients with culture-proven acute fungal keratitis, who had non-healing corneal ulcers or were at risk of corneal perforation, was conducted to evaluate the effectiveness of AMT in promoting re-epithelialization and preventing TPK. AMT was performed during the active keratitis phase (with positive fungal cultures) for 16 patients (69.6%) and during the inactive phase (with negative fungal cultures) for 7 patients (30.4%). Complete epithelialization was achieved in 75% of the patients in the active group and 100% of the patients in the inactive group. In the active group, 25% of patients ultimately required TPK due to treatment failure. The final BCVA was greater than 20/400. It improved in 17 patients, remained unchanged in four, and worsened in two patients [341].

There is strong evidence from a systematic review and meta-analysis indicating that early adjuvant AMT leads to more rapid corneal healing and better visual outcomes for moderate to severe fungal keratitis [342]. The meta-analysis examined two RCTs and one non-randomized controlled study that compared AMT to standard antimicrobial treatment. The results showed that the AMT group experienced a faster time to complete corneal healing, averaging 6.90 days [342].

7.11.4 Partial Conjunctival Flaps and Gundersen Procedure

Partial conjunctival flaps are simple, cost-effective procedures that do not require donor tissue and have shown effectiveness in treating persistent fungal keratitis [343–345]. The rich network of blood and lymphatic vessels in the conjunctival flap enhances the cornea's resistance to fungal infections and collagen degradation [346, 347]. A partial flap, rather than the classic complete Gundersen procedure, is preferred for most cases, and particularly focal fungal intrastromal abscess, mainly because it permits direct visualization of the unaffected cornea during the infectious process, whereas the Gundersen flap impedes visualizing the anterior segment for potential infectious spread and endophthalmitis (Fig. 7.9a–g). A study involving 16 eyes investigated the use and effectiveness of a selective, partial, pedunculated

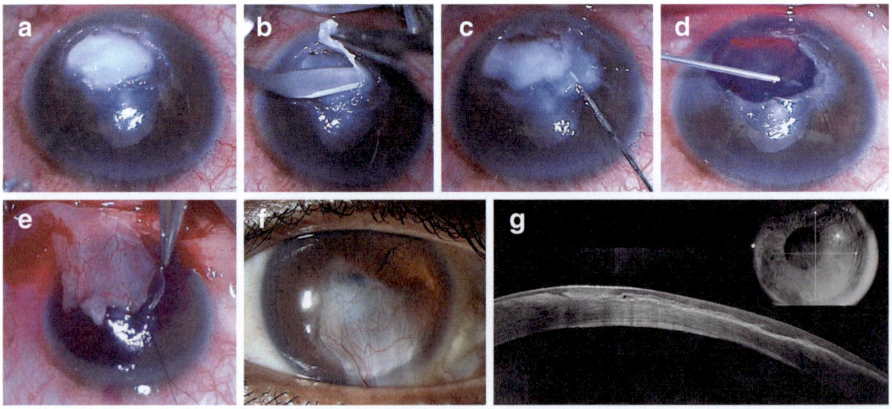

Fig. 7.9 Partial conjunctival flap in acute fungal keratitis. Intraoperative images: (**a**) De-epithelized fungal stromal infiltrate. (**b**) Manual superficial keratectomy with an angled crescent knife. (**c**) Voriconazole intrastromal injections around the infiltrate. (**d**) Rose Bengal lesion impregnation for photodynamic therapy (PDT). (**e**) Partial conjunctival flap advancement and sutured over the infiltrate. Postoperative images: (**f**) Partial conjunctival flap in place with resolved keratitis and a quiet eye at 6 months postoperative. (**g**) Transversal corneal AS-OCT image of the flap area showing a stable corneal stroma with adequate thickening. (Figures, courtesy of Bascom-Palmer Eye Institute photography department)

(tongue-shaped) conjunctival flap for treating refractory fungal keratitis, with or without perforation [344]. The results showed a favorable postoperative outcome for all patients, indicated by controlled eye infections and preservation of the eyeball. Postoperative visual acuity decreased in only 4 (25%) of the eyes, while it remained unchanged in 12 (75%). Three patients experienced post-surgical complications: one developed a corneal perforation, another showed uncontrolled spreading of purulent exudates (hypopyon) beyond the anterior chamber, and one patient presented with anterior chamber hypopyon [344]. A RCT comparing conjunctival flaps and AMT found no differences in re-epithelialization time, infection persistence, complications, and visual improvement [348]. Conjunctival flap reported complications include flap retraction and conjunctival buttonholes [349]. Hence, due to tectonic instability, conjunctival flaps used alone in cases of perforated fungal keratitis may lead to dissolution and recurrence of corneal perforation [350]. An oversized conjunctival flap with a partial Tenon's capsule placed over the cornea ensures abundant blood supply and prevents conjunctiva necrosis [350]. Furthermore, a combined technique utilizing AMT and partial conjunctival flap for treating corneal perforations due to fungal keratitis proved effective, with all 16 patients preserving their eyeballs. Over an average follow-up period of 11.0 ± 4.4 months (ranging from 6 to 18 months), none of the patients experienced a recurrence of fungal keratitis. Visual acuity improved in 93.8% of eyes, while one patient (6.3%) had no light perception at admission. This combined technique not only helps maintain the integrity of the eyeball but also prevents the recurrence of fungal keratitis, especially in circumstances where eye banks and fresh corneas are not available. Additionally, it provides a better opportunity for visual rehabilitation through future penetrating keratoplasty [350]. An alternative therapeutic approach involves a two-step surgical procedure that combines a conjunctival flap with a secondary DALK for patients with high-risk fungal keratitis [345]. In a study involving 10 subjects suffering from severe fungal keratitis, marked by hypopyon and endothelial plaques, there were no fungal recurrence or graft rejection. Additionally, all participants showed improvement in best-corrected visual acuity (BCVA). The study concluded that this two-step strategy is both safe and effective for treating high-risk fungal keratitis by converting a planned TPK during active infection into an optical DALK at a later stage [345]. This technique is also particularly useful in regions where access to fresh donor corneas and eye bank services is limited.

7.12 Prognosis and Visual Outcomes

The prognosis of fungal keratitis is influenced by several factors. These include the cause of the infection, such as trauma from plants or soil and contact lens usage; the time between the onset of symptoms and the first visit to an ophthalmologist, which reflects a delay in seeking attention; the immune status of the host, including factors like diabetes, immunosuppression, and prolonged use of topical corticosteroids; the amount of fungal inoculum present and the specific species of fungus involved, such as *Fusarium solani*; the fungus's sensitivity or resistance to available antifungal agents; the host's immune response to the infection; and the clinical progression and pathogenic characteristics of the infectious site, among other considerations [2, 9, 20, 25, 33, 115, 152, 274, 351].

The predictors of eye function, specifically regarding visual acuity outcomes after fungal keratitis, have been examined from various perspectives. Key predictors identified from the MUTT database include initial visual acuity, the size of the stromal infiltrate, male gender, older age, and the presence of a pigmented lesion [352]. It is reasonable to expect that poorer initial visual acuity is strongly associated with worse eventual vision. Similarly, a larger and deeper stromal infiltrate is likely to result in greater corneal damage, leading to a larger scar size and, thus, poorer visual outcomes [352]. Additionally, older age has been found to be a significant predictor of longer time to re-epithelialization and worse prognosis. This correlation may be attributed to reduced immunity in older adults or different risk factors that affect this population. Fungal keratitis is more common in men than in women. Male patients are often agricultural workers or engage in outdoor activities, which increases their risk of corneal trauma or injury [27]. There may also be differences in the types of fungi that infect men, as they might be exposed to more virulent strains [41]. Consequently, men could face a higher risk of poor outcomes due to these factors. The presence of pigmentation in corneal ulcers at the time of diagnosis provides valuable insights into predicting visual outcomes. Macroscopic pigmentation has been typically associated with dematiaceous fungi, such as *Curvularia* and *Bipolaris* species [353]. While several studies have proposed using macroscopic pigmentation as a diagnostic tool for fungal keratitis, they also suggest that pigmentation may indicate lower virulence and less severe inflammation, as well as the presence of fungal filaments on the anterior stroma [354]. However, an opposing view from the MUTT database analysis posits that the pigmentation of a corneal ulcer could serve as a prognostic indicator of worse visual outcomes. By the time pigmented hyphae become visible on the cornea, the infection may have been present for an extended period, leading to a more severe ulcer [352]. Some studies have examined the prognostic outcomes of fungal keratitis in relation to the etiopathogenic characteristics of the infection. They have identified several predictors of poor outcomes, including an infiltrated area greater than 16 mm^2, a hypopyon greater than 2 mm, the number of effective medications, *in vitro* resistance to those medications, and infections caused by *Fusarium* spp. or *Aspergillus* spp. [355].

7.13 Research Developments and Future Directions

7.13.1 Potential Immunologic Targets

A study has highlighted the role of the vitamin D receptor (VDR) in innate immunity, particularly its connection to the cathelicidin LL-37 antimicrobial peptide (CAMP). This may serve as a new treatment target for fungal keratitis [356]. Liposome-encapsulated mannan extracts from *Candida albicans* have been shown to stimulate the production of antibodies that provide protection against candidiasis [357]. Probiotics, such as *L. rhamnosus, L. acidophilus, L. pyogenes, L. casei,* and *Bifidobacterium*, have also been reported to offer protection against candidiasis by eliciting both immune and non-immune responses in mice. These experimental studies pave the way for further research focused on developing a vaccine for fungal keratitis and exploring the use of probiotics on ocular surfaces for disease prevention [358].

7.13.2 Antimicrobial Peptides

Antimicrobial peptides (AMPs) have significant potential for use as antimicrobial agents for ocular or other infections [359]. AMPs, also known as host defense peptides, are naturally produced, small, cationic, amphiphilic peptides ranging in length from 12 to 50 amino acids. They are present on the surfaces of the eyes and in tears. More than 500 AMPs have been reported, including large molecules (RNases and S100A proteins); small peptides α and β defensins in human cationic antibacterial protein (CAP) 18, and α 37 amino acids; proteins like lysozyme and peptidoglycan recognition protein with significant bactericidal activity. The cations carried by AMPs can bind to the anion surface of the bacterial plasma membrane, causing the perforation of cell membrane and subsequently microbial death. AMPs also prevent microbial adhesion to and access into host cells and cause digestion of fungal cell wall by lysozyme. *In vitro* studies have shown AMPs Pc-C and Pc-E reduced binding of Aspergillus fumigatus to cells; CAP37 inhibits candida infection by fungicidal activity [359, 360].

Wu et al. evaluated *in vivo* application of synthetic β-sheet forming peptide (IKIK) 2-NH2 and (IRIK) 2-NH2 for treatment of FK in comparison with amphotericin B. It was found that topical solutions of the designed peptides were safe, and as effective as the clinically used Amphotercin B. Many other AMPs such as Clavanin A, Chitinase 3-like 1, and CXCL 10 and S100 proteins may have role in prevention of infection [361].

7.13.3 Ocular Novel Drug Delivery Systems

Nanoparticles. Nanotechnology involves working with particles that range from 1 to 100 nm. In the field of ophthalmology, these technologies are being explored in various ways, particularly for developing novel drug delivery systems (NDDS) and gene delivery methods. Different types of nanoparticles, including nanosuspensions, liposomes, micelles, nanofibers, and nanotubes, are being utilized to deliver antifungal agents. The aim is to achieve better ocular penetration, increased retention, and improved bioavailability of these treatments [362].

Several *in vitro* and *in vivo* studies have shown promising results with these nanoformulations; however, further clinical studies are necessary to confirm their effectiveness in humans. For instance, a study on the liposomal formulation of the antifungal drug voriconazole demonstrated a sustained drug release profile and an eightfold increase in the amount of drug retained in the cornea after 1 h of exposure, compared to the conventional suspension formulation [363].

The microemulsion formulations of fluconazole demonstrated a controlled release profile, with 50–80% of the drug being released within 12 h. In contrast, the conventional drug solution released nearly the entire dose within the first 6 h [364]. These newer formulations may prove to be advantageous in the management of fungal keratitis in the future.

7.13.4 Impregnated Contact-Lens-Based Drug Delivery

Therapeutic contact lenses represent an innovative approach for treating infected corneas, considering they can continuously deliver medication while minimizing non-specific absorption and reducing drug loss due to tears. This method could significantly improve the management of infectious keratitis.

For patients with fungal keratitis, a contact lens drug delivery system offers a notable advantage, particularly because the challenging dosing regimens, combined with the limited availability of antifungal agents, often lead to poor treatment compliance. While some studies in this area show promise, there are currently no commercially available contact lens drug delivery systems specifically designed for fungal keratitis.

7.14 Conclusions

Given the widespread prevalence of fungal infections and the frequent failures of antifungal treatments, preventing corneal fungal infections and ensuring early diagnosis are essential. The severity of this condition, along with certain pathogenic factors such as fungal virulence, corneal defense mechanisms, and immune responses, significantly alter the outcome of the infection. Furthermore, delayed diagnosis, as well as untreated or mistreated fungal keratitis can result in a poor prognosis. When conventional diagnostic techniques, such as smear and culture, yield inconclusive results, IVCM becomes a game-changer in the definitive diagnosis of the disease, provided it is performed by a skilled technician and analyzed by an experienced viewer. Additionally, molecular diagnostic methods, like PCR, are becoming increasingly popular for enhancing diagnostic accuracy.

Recent advances in genomic, metagenomic, and tear proteomic methods have shown great promise for improving the diagnosis and management of fungal keratitis. Metagenomic sequencing enables rapid diagnosis and provides a more accurate assessment without the delays associated with fungal culture growth. Moreover, custom tear proteomic is becoming increasingly important for the diagnosis and management of fungal keratitis.

To improve treatment outcomes, rapid detection methods, such as multiplex PCR and antifungal susceptibility testing should become standard management protocols for fungal keratitis. Those, combined with the assessment of evident indications—such as perforated ulcers, impending perforations, and recalcitrant keratitis—along with known predictors like hypopyon and extensive and/or deep stromal infiltrates, are crucial for predicting outcomes and determining which cases require early TPK. Finally, recent antifungal medications and combination therapies have demonstrated greater efficacy in managing fungal keratitis compared to monotherapy.

References

1. Ung L, Acharya NR, Agarwal T, Alfonso EC, Bagga B, Bispo PJ, et al. Infectious corneal ulceration: a proposal for neglected tropical disease status. Bull World Heal Organ. 2019;97(12):854–6.
2. Song X, Xie L, Tan X, Wang Z, Yang Y, Yuan Y, et al. A multi-center, cross-sectional study on the burden of infectious keratitis in China. PLoS ONE. 2014;9(12):e113843.
3. Tran TM, Duong H, Bonnet C, Kashanchi A, Buckshey A, Aldave AJ. Corneal blindness in Asia: a systematic review and meta-analysis to identify challenges and opportunities. Cornea. 2020;39(9):1196–205.
4. Lakhundi S, Siddiqui R, Khan NA. Pathogenesis of microbial keratitis. Microb Pathog. 2017;104:97–109.
5. Ting DSJ, Settle C, Morgan SJ, Baylis O, Ghosh S. A 10-year analysis of microbiological profiles of microbial keratitis: the North East England study. Eye. 2018;32(8):1416–7.
6. Wong TY, Ng TP, Fong KS, Tan DT. Risk factors and clinical outcomes between fungal and bacterial keratitis: a comparative study. CLAO J: Off Publ Contact Lens Assoc Ophthalmol, Inc. 1997;23(4):275–81.
7. Stapleton F, Carnt N. Contact lens-related microbial keratitis: how have epidemiology and genetics helped us with pathogenesis and prophylaxis. Eye. 2012;26(2):185–93.
8. Thomas PA, Kaliamurthy J. Mycotic keratitis: epidemiology, diagnosis and management. Clin Microbiol Infect. 2013;19(3):210–20.
9. Leck AK, Thomas PA, Hagan M, Kaliamurthy J, Ackuaku E, John M, et al. Aetiology of suppurative corneal ulcers in Ghana and south India, and epidemiology of fungal keratitis. Br J Ophthalmol. 2002;86(11):1211.
10. Lan L, Wang FY, Zeng G. Staining with methylthioninium chloride for the diagnosis of fungal keratitis. Exp Ther Med. 2013;6(5):1229–32.
11. Rathi VM, Murthy SI, Mitra S, Yamjala B, Mohamed A, Sharma S. Masked comparison of trypan blue stain and potassium hydroxide with calcofluor white stain in the microscopic examination of corneal scrapings for the diagnosis of microbial keratitis. Indian J Ophthalmol. 2021;69(9):2457–60.
12. Mahmoudi S, Masoomi A, Ahmadikia K, Tabatabaei SA, Soleimani M, Rezaie S, et al. Fungal keratitis: an overview of clinical and laboratory aspects. Mycoses. 2018;61(12):916–30.
13. Ferrer C, Alió JL. Evaluation of molecular diagnosis in fungal keratitis. Ten years of experience. J Ophthalmic Inflamm Infect. 2011;1(1):15–22.
14. Kheirkhah A, Syed ZA, Satitpitakul V, Goyal S, Müller R, Tu EY, et al. Sensitivity and specificity of laser-scanning in vivo confocal microscopy for filamentous fungal keratitis: role of observer experience. Am J Ophthalmol. 2017;179:81–9.
15. Bakken IM, Jackson CJ, Utheim TP, Villani E, Hamrah P, Kheirkhah A, et al. The use of in vivo confocal microscopy in fungal keratitis – progress and challenges. Ocul Surf. 2022;24:103–18.
16. Manzouri B, Wyse RK, Vafidis GC. Pharmacotherapy of fungal eye infections. Expert Opin Pharmacother. 2001;2(11):1849–57.

17. Lakhani P, Patil A, Majumdar S. Challenges in the polyene- and azole-based pharmacotherapy of ocular fungal infections. J Ocul Pharmacol Ther. 2019;35(1):6–22.
18. McKay TB, Hutcheon AEK, Zieske JD. Biology of corneal fibrosis: soluble mediators, integrins, and extracellular vesicles. Eye. 2020;34(2):271–8.
19. Sharma N, Bagga B, Singhal D, Nagpal R, Kate A, Saluja G, et al. Fungal keratitis: a review of clinical presentations, treatment strategies and outcomes. Ocul Surf. 2022;24:22–30.
20. Bisen AC, Sanap SN, Agrawal S, Biswas A, Mishra A, Verma SK, et al. Etiopathology, epidemiology, diagnosis, and treatment of fungal keratitis. ACS Infect Dis. 2024;10(7):2356–80.
21. Prajna N, Lalitha P, Sharma S, de Freitas D, Höfling-Lima A, Varnado N, et al. A double-masked, sham-controlled trial of rose Bengal photodynamic therapy for the treatment of fungal and acanthamoeba keratitis: rose Bengal electromagnetic activation with green light for infection reduction (REAGIR) study. Trials. 2024;25(1):566.
22. Sourlis C, Seitz B, Roth M, Hamon L, Daas L. Outcomes of severe fungal keratitis using in vivo confocal microscopy and early therapeutic penetrating keratoplasty. Clin Ophthalmol (Auckl, NZ). 2022;16:2245–54.
23. Ibrahim YW, Boase DL, Cree IA. Epidemiological characteristics, predisposing factors and microbiological profiles of infectious corneal ulcers: the Portsmouth corneal ulcer study. Br J Ophthalmol. 2009;93(10):1319.
24. Brown L, Leck AK, Gichangi M, Burton MJ, Denning DW. The global incidence and diagnosis of fungal keratitis. Lancet Infect Dis. 2021;21(3):e49–57.
25. Keay LJ, Gower EW, Iovieno A, Oechsler RA, Alfonso EC, Matoba A, et al. Clinical and microbiological characteristics of fungal keratitis in the United States, 2001–2007: a multicenter study. Ophthalmology. 2011;118(5):920–6.
26. Tuft SJ, Tullo AB. Fungal keratitis in the United Kingdom 2003–2005. Eye. 2009;23(6):1308–13.
27. Gopinathan U, Sharma S, Garg P, Rao GN. Review of epidemiological features, microbiological diagnosis and treatment outcome of microbial keratitis: experience of over a decade. Indian J Ophthalmol. 2009;57(4):273–9.
28. Lalitha P, Prajna NV, Manoharan G, Srinivasan M, Mascarenhas J, Das M, et al. Trends in bacterial and fungal keratitis in south India, 2002–2012. Br J Ophthalmol. 2015;99(2):192.
29. Wang L, Sun S, Jing Y, Han L, Zhang H, Yue J. Spectrum of fungal keratitis in central China. Clin Exp Ophthalmol. 2009;37(8):763–71.
30. Wang L, Wang L, Han L, Yin W. Study of pathogens of fungal keratitis and the sensitivity of pathogenic fungi to therapeutic agents with the disk diffusion method. Curr Eye Res. 2015;40(11):1095–101.
31. Hoffman JJ, Burton MJ, Leck A. Mycotic keratitis—a global threat from the filamentous fungi. J Fungi. 2021;7(4):273.
32. Thomas PA, Leck AK, Myatt M. Characteristic clinical features as an aid to the diagnosis of suppurative keratitis caused by filamentous fungi. Br J Ophthalmol. 2005;89(12):1554.
33. Ong HS, Fung SSM, Macleod D, Dart JKG, Tuft SJ, Burton MJ. Altered patterns of fungal keratitis at a London ophthalmic referral hospital: an eight-year retrospective observational study. Am J Ophthalmol. 2016;168:227–36.
34. Jeng BH, Gritz DC, Kumar AB, Holsclaw DS, Porco TC, Smith SD, et al. Epidemiology of ulcerative keratitis in Northern California. Arch Ophthalmol. 2010;128(8):1022–8.
35. Mselle J. Fungal keratitis as an indicator of HIV infection in Africa. Trop Dr. 1999;29(3):133–5.
36. Koh YY, Sun CC, Hsiao CH. Epidemiology and the estimated burden of microbial keratitis on the health care system in Taiwan: a 14-year population-based study. Am J Ophthalmol. 2020;220:152–9.
37. Deorukhkar S, Katiyar R, Saini S. Epidemiological features and laboratory results of bacterial and fungal keratitis: a five-year study at a rural tertiary-care hospital in western Maharashtra. India. Singap Méd J. 2012;53(4):264–7.
38. Lamas-Francis D, Navarro D, Mansilla R, V d-R, Moreno C, Dios E, et al. Fungal keratitis in Northwestern Spain: epidemiology, risk factors and outcomes. J Fungi. 2024;10(10):689.

39. Köhler JR, Hube B, Puccia R, Casadevall A, Perfect JR. Fungi that infect humans. Microbiol Spectr. 2017;5(3) https://doi.org/10.1128/microbiolspec.FUNK-0014-2016.
40. Köhler JR, Casadevall A, Perfect J. The spectrum of fungi that infects humans. Cold Spring Harb Perspect Med. 2015;5(1):a019273.
41. Mills B, Radhakrishnan N, Rajapandian SGK, Rameshkumar G, Lalitha P, Prajna NV. The role of fungi in fungal keratitis. Exp Eye Res. 2021;202:108372.
42. O'Brien HE, Parrent JL, Jackson JA, Moncalvo JM, Vilgalys R. Fungal community analysis by large-scale sequencing of environmental samples. Appl Environ Microbiol. 2005;71(9):5544–50.
43. Thomas PA. Fungal infections of the cornea. Eye. 2003;17(8):852–62.
44. Weiss M, Molina R, Ofoegbuna C, Johnson DA, Kheirkhah A. A review of filamentary keratitis. Surv Ophthalmol. 2022;67(1):52–9.
45. Masterton S, Ahearne M. Mechanobiology of the corneal epithelium. Exp Eye Res. 2018;177:122–9.
46. Pflugfelder SC, Stern ME. Biological functions of tear film. Exp Eye Res. 2020;197:108115.
47. Prashanthi GS, Jayasudha R, Chakravarthy SK, Padakandla SR, SaiAbhilash CR, Sharma S, et al. Alterations in the ocular surface fungal microbiome in fungal keratitis patients. Microorganisms. 2019;7(9):309.
48. Mantelli F, Mauris J, Argüeso P. The ocular surface epithelial barrier and other mechanisms of mucosal protection. Curr Opin Allergy Clin Immunol. 2013;13(5):563–8.
49. Azkargorta M, Soria J, Acera A, Iloro I, Elortza F. Human tear proteomics and peptidomics in ophthalmology: toward the translation of proteomic biomarkers into clinical practice. J Proteom. 2017;150:359–67.
50. Kuo MT, Chen JL, Hsu SL, Chen A, You HL. An omics approach to diagnosing or investigating fungal keratitis. Int J Mol Sci. 2019;20(15):3631.
51. Hanstock HG, Edwards JP, Walsh NP. Tear lactoferrin and lysozyme as clinically relevant biomarkers of mucosal immune competence. Front Immunol. 2019;10:1178.
52. Farnaud S, Evans RW. Lactoferrin—a multifunctional protein with antimicrobial properties. Mol Immunol. 2003;40(7):395–405.
53. Fernandes KE, Carter DA. The antifungal activity of lactoferrin and its derived peptides: mechanisms of action and synergy with drugs against fungal Pathogens. Front Microbiol. 2017;8:2.
54. Leal SM, Roy S, Vareechon C, Carrion S d J, Clark H, Lopez-Berges MS, et al. Targeting iron acquisition blocks infection with the fungal pathogens Aspergillus Fumigatus and Fusarium oxysporum. PLoS Pathog. 2013;9(7):e1003436.
55. McDermott AM. Antimicrobial compounds in tears. Exp Eye Res. 2013;117:53–61.
56. Tsoni SV, Kerrigan AM, Marakalala MJ, Srinivasan N, Duffield M, Taylor PR, et al. Complement C3 plays an essential role in the control of opportunistic fungal infections. Infect Immun. 2009;77(9):3679–85.
57. Chairatana P, Chiang IL, Nolan EM. Human α-defensin 6 self-assembly prevents adhesion and suppresses virulence traits of candida albicans. Biochemistry. 2017;56(8):1033–41.
58. Swidergall M, Ernst JF. Interplay between Candida albicans and the antimicrobial peptide armory. Eukaryot Cell. 2014;13(8):950–7.
59. Brummer E, Stevens DA. Collectins and fungal pathogens: roles of surfactant proteins and mannose binding lectin in host resistance. Méd Mycol. 2010;48(1):16–28.
60. Zani M, Baranger K, Guyot N, Dallet-Choisy S, Moreau T. Protease inhibitors derived from Elafin and SLPI and engineered to have enhanced specificity towards neutrophil serine proteases. Protein Sci. 2009;18(3):579–94.
61. Baranger K, Zani M, Chandenier J, Dallet-Choisy S, Moreau T. The antibacterial and antifungal properties of trappin-2 (pre-Elafin) do not depend on its protease inhibitory function. FEBS J. 2008;275(9):2008–20.
62. Cabrera-Aguas M, Khoo P, Watson SL. Infectious keratitis: a review. Clin Exp Ophthalmol. 2022;50(5):543–62.

63. Niu L, Liu X, Ma Z, Yin Y, Sun L, Yang L, et al. Fungal keratitis: pathogenesis, diagnosis and prevention. Microb Pathog. 2020;138:103802.
64. Yang W, Zhang L. Association of tear film stability and corneal surface temperature in pudong patients. Curr Eye Res. 2017;42(5):655–60.
65. Hostetter MK. Adhesins and ligands involved in the interaction of Candida spp. with epithelial and endothelial surfaces. Clin Microbiol Rev. 1994;7(1):29–42.
66. Blango MG, Kniemeyer O, Brakhage AA. Conidial surface proteins at the interface of fungal infections. PLoS Pathog. 2019;15(9):e1007939.
67. Hardison SE, Brown GD. C-type lectin receptors orchestrate antifungal immunity. Nat Immunol. 2012;13(9):817–22.
68. Vila T, Romo JA, Pierce CG, McHardy SF, Saville SP, Lopez-Ribot JL. Targeting Candida albicans filamentation for antifungal drug development. Virulence. 2017;8(2):150–8.
69. Sheppard DC, Filler SG. Host cell invasion by medically important fungi. Cold Spring Harb Perspect Med. 2015;5(1):a019687.
70. Karthikeyan RS, Leal SM, Prajna NV, Dharmalingam K, Geiser DM, Pearlman E, et al. Expression of innate and adaptive immune mediators in human corneal tissue infected with Aspergillus or Fusarium. J Infect Dis. 2011;204(6):942–50.
71. Gao X, Zhao G, Li C, Lin J, Jiang N, Wang Q, et al. LOX-1 and TLR4 affect each other and regulate the generation of ROS in A. Fumigatus keratitis. Int Immunopharmacol. 2016;40:392–9.
72. Yuan K, Zhao G, Che C, Li C, Lin J, Zhu G, et al. Dectin-1 is essential for IL-1β production through JNK activation and apoptosis in Aspergillus Fumigatus keratitis. Int Immunopharmacol. 2017;52:168–75.
73. Muszkieta L, Carrion S d J, Robinet P, Beau R, Elbim C, Pearlman E, et al. The protein phosphatase PhzA of A. Fumigatus is involved in oxidative stress tolerance and fungal virulence. Fungal Genet Biol. 2014;66:79–85.
74. Vemuganti GK, Garg P, Gopinathan U, Naduvilath TJ, John RK, Buddi R, et al. Evaluation of agent and host factors in progression of mycotic keratitis a histologic and microbiologic study of 167 corneal buttons. Ophthalmology. 2002;109(8):1538–46.
75. Park M, Do E, Jung WH. Lipolytic enzymes involved in the virulence of human pathogenic fungi. Mycobiology. 2013;41(2):67–72.
76. Hohl TM, Feldmesser M. Aspergillus Fumigatus: principles of pathogenesis and host defense. Eukaryot Cell. 2007;6(11):1953–63.
77. Hedayati MT, Pasqualotto AC, Warn PA, Bowyer P, Denning DW. Aspergillus flavus: human pathogen, allergen and mycotoxin producer. Microbiology. 2007;153(6):1677–92.
78. Aboul-Nasr MB, Zohri ANA, Amer EM. Enzymatic and toxigenic ability of opportunistic fungi contaminating intensive care units and operation rooms at Assiut University Hospitals. Egypt. SpringerPlus. 2013;2(1):347.
79. Raza SK, Mallet AI, Howell SA, Thomas PA. An in-vitro study of the sterol content and toxin production of Fusarium isolates from mycotic keratitis. J Méd Microbiol. 1994;41(3):204–8.
80. Cusumano V, Costa GB, Seminara S. Effect of aflatoxins on rat peritoneal macrophages. Appl Environ Microbiol. 1990;56(11):3482–4.
81. Kupfahl C, Michalka A, Lass-Flörl C, Fischer G, Haase G, Ruppert T, et al. Gliotoxin production by clinical and environmental Aspergillus Fumigatus strains. Int J Méd Microbiol. 2008;298(3–4):319–27.
82. Ma JJK, Dohlman CH. Mechanisms of corneal ulceration. Ophthalmol Clin North Am. 2002;15(1):27–33.
83. Ballal S, Belur S, Laha P, Roy S, Swamy BM, Inamdar SR. Mitogenic lectins from Cephalosporium curvulum (CSL) and Aspergillus oryzae (AOL) mediate host–pathogen interactions leading to mycotic keratitis. Mol Cell Biochem. 2017;434(1–2):209–19.
84. Sangeetha AB, Abdel-hadi A, Hassan AS, Shobana CS, Suresh S, Abirami B, et al. Evaluation of in vitro activities of extracellular enzymes from Aspergillus species isolated from corneal ulcer/keratitis. Saudi J Biol Sci. 2020;27(2):701–5.

85. Monod M, Capoccia S, Léchenne B, Zaugg C, Holdom M, Jousson O. Secreted proteases from pathogenic fungi. Int J Méd Microbiol. 2002;292(5–6):405–19.
86. Yike I. Fungal proteases and their pathophysiological effects. Mycopathologia. 2011;171(5):299–323.
87. Zhu WS, Wojdyla K, Donlon K, Thomas PA, Eberle HI. Extracellular proteases of Aspergillus flavus: fungal keratitis, proteases, and pathogenesis. Diagn Microbiol Infect Dis. 1990;13(6):491–7.
88. Ibrahim-Granet O, Dubourdeau M, Latgé J, Ave P, Huerre M, Brakhage AA, et al. Methylcitrate synthase from Aspergillus Fumigatus is essential for manifestation of invasive Aspergillosis. Cell Microbiol. 2008;10(1):134–48.
89. Cassat JE, Skaar EP. Iron in infection and immunity. Cell Host Microbe. 2013;13(5):509–19.
90. Sandai D, Tabana YM, Ouweini AE, Ayodeji IO. Resistance of Candida albicans biofilms to drugs and the host immune system. Jundishapur J Microbiol. 2016;9(11):e37385.
91. Gulati M, Nobile CJ. Candida albicans biofilms: development, regulation, and molecular mechanisms. Microbes Infect. 2016;18(5):310–21.
92. Hirota K, Yumoto H, Sapaar B, Matsuo T, Ichikawa T, Miyake Y. Pathogenic factors in Candida biofilm-related infectious diseases. J Appl Microbiol. 2017;122(2):321–30.
93. Mukherjee PK, Chandra J. Candida biofilm resistance. Drug Resist Updat. 2004;7(4–5):301–9.
94. Ranjith K, Chakravarthy SK, Adicherla H, Sharma S, Shivaji S. Temporal expression of genes in biofilm-forming ocular Candida albicans isolated from patients with keratitis and orbital cellulitis. Investig Opthalmology Vis Sci. 2018;59(1):528.
95. Sardi JDCO, Pitangui NDS, Rodríguez-Arellanes G, Taylor ML, Fusco-Almeida AM, Mendes-Giannini MJS. Highlights in pathogenic fungal biofilms. Rev Iberoam Micol. 2014;31(1):22–9.
96. Al-Fattani MA, Douglas LJ. Biofilm matrix of Candida albicans and Candida tropicalis: chemical composition and role in drug resistance. J Méd Microbiol. 2006;55(8):999–1008.
97. Dongari-Bagtzoglou A, Kashleva H, Dwivedi P, Diaz P, Vasilakos J. Characterization of mucosal Candida albicans biofilms. PLoS ONE. 2009;4(11):e7967.
98. Silva S, Negri M, Henriques M, Oliveira R, Williams DW, Azeredo J. Adherence and biofilm formation of non-Candida albicans Candida species. Trends Microbiol. 2011;19(5):241–7.
99. Chang DC, Grant GB, O'Donnell K, Wannemuehler KA, Noble-Wang J, Rao CY, et al. Multistate outbreak of Fusarium keratitis associated with use of a contact lens solution. JAMA. 2006;296(8):953–63.
100. Leal SM, Pearlman E. The role of cytokines and pathogen recognition molecules in fungal keratitis – insights from human disease and animal models. Cytokine. 2012;58(1):107–11.
101. Sun Y, Abbondante S, Karmakar M, de Jesus Carrion S, Che C, Hise AG, et al. Neutrophil caspase-11 is required for cleavage of caspase-1 and secretion of IL-1β in aspergillus fumigatus infection. J Immunol. 2018;201(9):2767–75.
102. Theilgaard-Mönch K, Porse BT, Borregaard N. Systems biology of neutrophil differentiation and immune response. Curr Opin Immunol. 2006;18(1):54–60.
103. Sheshachalam A, Srivastava N, Mitchell T, Lacy P, Eitzen G. Granule protein processing and regulated secretion in neutrophils. Front Immunol. 2014;5:448.
104. Taylor PR, Roy S, Leal SM, Sun Y, Howell SJ, Cobb BA, et al. Activation of neutrophils by autocrine IL-17A–IL-17RC interactions during fungal infection is regulated by IL-6, IL-23, RORγt and dectin-2. Nat Immunol. 2014;15(2):143–51.
105. Roilides E, Antachopoulos C, Simitsopoulou M. Pathogenesis and host defence against mucorales: the role of cytokines and interaction with antifungal drugs. Mycoses. 2014;57(s3):40–7.
106. Acharya Y, Acharya B, Karki P. Fungal keratitis: study of increasing trend and common determinants. Nepal J Epidemiology. 2017;7(2):685–93.
107. Xie L, Zhong W, Shi W, Sun S. Spectrum of fungal keratitis in North China. Ophthalmology. 2006;113(11):1943–8.
108. Haseeb AA, Elhusseiny AM, Siddiqui MZ, Ahmad KT, Sallam AB. Fungal endophthalmitis: a comprehensive review. J Fungi. 2021;7(11):996.

109. Kernt M, Kampik A. Endophthalmitis: pathogenesis, clinical presentation, management, and perspectives. Clin Ophthalmol. 2010;4(0):121–35.
110. Klotz SA, Penn CC, Negvesky GJ, Butrus SI. Fungal and parasitic infections of the eye. Clin Microbiol Rev. 2000;13(4):662–85.
111. Kaminishi H, Miyaguchi H, Tamaki T, Suenaga N, Hisamatsu M, Mihashi I, et al. Degradation of humoral host defense by candida albicans proteinase. Infect Immun. 1995;63(3):984–8.
112. Leema G, Kaliamurthy J, Geraldine P, Thomas PA. Keratitis due to aspergillus flavus: clinical profile, molecular identification of fungal strains and detection of aflatoxin production. Mol Vis. 2010;16:843–54.
113. Griffiths JS, Thompson A, Stott M, Benny A, Lewis NA, Taylor PR, et al. Differential susceptibility of dectin-1 isoforms to functional inactivation by neutrophil and fungal proteases. FASEB J. 2018;32(6):3385–97.
114. Toumasis P, Tsantes AG, Tsiogka A, Samonis G, Vrioni G. From clinical suspicion to diagnosis: a review of diagnostic approaches and challenges in fungal keratitis. J Clin Med. 2024;13(1):286.
115. Atta S, Perera C, Kowalski RP, Jhanji V. Fungal keratitis: clinical features, risk factors, treatment, and outcomes. J Fungi. 2022;8(9):962.
116. Dahlgren MA, Lingappan A, Wilhelmus KR. The clinical diagnosis of microbial keratitis. Am J Ophthalmol. 2007;143(6):940–944.e1.
117. Ting DSJ, Galal M, Kulkarni B, Elalfy MS, Lake D, Hamada S, et al. Clinical characteristics and outcomes of fungal keratitis in the United Kingdom 2011–2020: a 10-year study. J Fungi. 2021;7(11):966.
118. Hagan M, Wright E, Newman M, Dolin P, Johnson G. Causes of suppurative keratitis in Ghana. Br J Ophthalmol. 1995;79(11):1024.
119. Furlanetto RL, Andreo EGV, Finotti LGA, Arcieri ES, Ferreira MA, Rocha FJ. Epidemiology and etiologic diagnosis of infectious keratitis in Uberlandia. Brazil. Eur J Ophthalmol. 2010;20(3):498–503.
120. Thomas PA. Current perspectives on ophthalmic mycoses. Clin Microbiol Rev. 2003;16(4):730–97.
121. Srinivasan M. Fungal keratitis. Curr Opin Ophthalmol. 2004;15(4):321–7.
122. Eleinen KGA, Mohalhal AA, Elmekawy HE, Abdulbaki AM, Sherif AM, El-Sherif RH, et al. Polymerase chain reaction-guided diagnosis of infective keratitis – a hospital based study. Curr Eye Res. 2012;37(11):1005–11.
123. Bharathi MJ, Ramakrishnan R, Meenakshi R, Mittal S, Shivakumar C, Srinivasan M. Microbiological diagnosis of infective keratitis: comparative evaluation of direct microscopy and culture results. Br J Ophthalmol. 2006;90(10):1271.
124. Ansari Z, Miller D, Galor A. Current thoughts in fungal keratitis: diagnosis and treatment. Curr Fungal Infect Rep. 2013;7(3):209–18.
125. Hudson J, Al-khersan H, Carletti P, Miller D, Dubovy SR, Amescua G. Role of corneal biopsy in the management of infectious keratitis. Curr Opin Ophthalmol. 2022;33(4):290–5.
126. Anthony PP. A guide to the histological identification of fungi in tissues. J Clin Pathol. 1973;26(11):828.
127. Grocott RG. A stain for fungi in tissue sections and smears. Am J Clin Pathol. 1955;25(8_ts):975–9.
128. Dadaci Z, Kılınç F, Ozer TT, Sahin GO, Acir NO, Borazan M. Periodic acid–Schiff staining demonstrates fungi in chronic anterior blepharitis. Eye. 2015;29(12):1522–7.
129. Gelder RNV. Applications of the polymerase chain reaction to diagnosis of ophthalmic disease. Surv Ophthalmol. 2001;46(3):248–58.
130. Itahashi M, Higaki S, Fukuda M, Shimomura Y. Detection and quantification of pathogenic bacteria and fungi using real-time polymerase chain reaction by cycling probe in patients with corneal ulcer. Arch Ophthalmol. 2010;128(5):535–40.
131. Nakayama T, Yamazaki T, Yo A, Tone K, Alshahni MM, Fujisaki R, et al. Detection of fungi from an indoor environment using loop-mediated isothermal amplification (LAMP) method. Biocontrol Sci. 2017;22(2):97–104.

132. Kuo MT, Chang HC, Cheng CK, Chien CC, Fang PC, Chang TC. A highly sensitive method for molecular diagnosis of fungal keratitis a dot hybridization assay. Ophthalmology. 2012;119(12):2434–42.
133. Zhao G, Zhai H, Yuan Q, Sun S, Liu T, Xie L. Rapid and sensitive diagnosis of fungal keratitis with direct PCR without template DNA extraction. Clin Microbiol Infect. 2014;20(10):O776–82.
134. Koay SY, Tuft S. False positive fungus results from investigation of microbial keratitis. Eye. 2023;37(3):574–5.
135. Kim E, Chidambaram JD, Srinivasan M, Lalitha P, Wee D, Lietman TM, et al. Prospective comparison of microbial culture and polymerase chain reaction in the diagnosis of corneal ulcer. Am J Ophthalmol. 2008;146(5):714–723.e1.
136. Lau A, Chen S, Sorrell T, Carter D, Malik R, Martin P, et al. Development and clinical application of a panfungal PCR assay to detect and identify fungal DNA in tissue specimens. J Clin Microbiol. 2006;45(2):380–5.
137. Sharma S, Silverberg M, Mehta P, Gopinathan U, Agrawal V, Naduvilath TJ. Early diagnosis of mycotic keratitis: predictive value of potassium hydroxide preparation. Indian J Ophthalmol. 1998;46(1):31–5.
138. Sabapathypillai SL, James HR, Lyerla RRL, Hassman L. The next generation of ocular pathogen detection. Asia-Pac J Ophthalmol. 2021;10(1):109–13.
139. Goldschmidt P, Degorge S, Benallaoua D, Semoun O, Borsali E, Bouter AL, et al. New strategy for rapid diagnosis and characterization of keratomycosis. Ophthalmology. 2012;119(5):945–50.
140. He D, Hao J, Gao S, Wan X, Wang W, Shan Q, et al. Etiological analysis of fungal keratitis and rapid identification of predominant fungal pathogens. Mycopathologia. 2016;181(1–2):75–82.
141. Bagyalakshmi R, Therese KL, Prasanna S, Madhavan HN. Newer emerging pathogens of ocular non-sporulating molds (NSM) identified by polymerase chain reaction (PCR)-based DNA sequencing technique targeting internal transcribed spacer (ITS) region. Curr Eye Res. 2008;33(2):139–47.
142. Manikandan P, Abdel-hadi A, Singh YRB, Revathi R, Anita R, Banawas S, et al. Fungal keratitis: epidemiology, rapid detection, and antifungal susceptibilities of fusarium and aspergillus isolates from corneal scrapings. BioMed Res Int. 2019;2019(1):6395840.
143. Hsiao CR, Huang L, Bouchara JP, Barton R, Li HC, Chang TC. Identification of medically important molds by an oligonucleotide array. J Clin Microbiol. 2005;43(8):3760–8.
144. Thomas PA, Teresa PA, Theodore J, Geraldine P. PCR for the molecular diagnosis of mycotic keratitis. Expert Rev Mol Diagn. 2012;12(7):703–18.
145. Vengayil S, Panda A, Satpathy G, Nayak N, Ghose S, Patanaik D, et al. Polymerase chain reaction-guided diagnosis of mycotic keratitis: a prospective evaluation of its efficacy and limitations. Investig Opthalmol Vis Sci. 2009;50(1):152.
146. Bu R, Sathiapalan RK, Ibrahim MM, Al-Mohsen I, Almodavar E, Gutierrez MI, et al. Monochrome LightCycler PCR assay for detection and quantification of five common species of Candida and Aspergillus. J Méd Microbiol. 2005;54(3):243–8.
147. Esposto MC, Cogliati M, Tortorano AM, Viviani MA. Determination of Cryptococcus neoformans var. neoformans mating type by multiplex PCR. Clin Microbiol Infect. 2004;10(12):1092–4.
148. Muraosa Y, Schreiber AZ, Trabasso P, Matsuzawa T, Taguchi H, Moretti ML, et al. Development of cycling probe-based real-time PCR system to detect Fusarium species and Fusarium solani species complex (FSSC). Int J Méd Microbiol. 2014;304(3–4):505–11.
149. Opathy C, Arastehfar A, Boekhout T, Butler G, Cesare GBD, Dolk E, et al. Recent trends in molecular diagnostics of yeast infections: from PCR to NGS. FEMS Microbiol Rev. 2019;43(5):517–47.
150. Souza M d, Matsuzawa T, Sakai K, Muraosa Y, Lyra L, Busso-Lopes AF, et al. Comparison of DNA microarray, loop-mediated isothermal amplification (LAMP) and real-time PCR with DNA sequencing for identification of Fusarium spp. Obtained from patients with hematologic malignancies. Mycopathologia. 2017;182(7–8):625–32.

151. Shigeyasu C, Yamada M, Aoki K, Ishii Y, Tateda K, Yaguchi T, et al. Metagenomic analysis for detecting Fusarium solani in a case of fungal keratitis. J Infect Chemother. 2018;24(8):664–8.
152. Kredics L, Narendran V, Shobana CS, Vágvölgyi C, Manikandan P, Group IFKW. Filamentous fungal infections of the cornea: a global overview of epidemiology and drug sensitivity. Mycoses. 2015;58(4):243–60.
153. Hassan AS, Al-Hatmi AMS, Shobana CS, van Diepeningen AD, Kredics L, Vágvölgyi C, et al. Antifungal susceptibility and phylogeny of opportunistic members of the genus Fusarium causing human Keratomycosis in South India. Sabouraudia. 2015;54(3):287–94.
154. Gaudin M, Desnues C. Hybrid capture-based next generation sequencing and its application to human infectious diseases. Front Microbiol. 2018;9:2924.
155. Turenne CY, Sanche SE, Hoban DJ, Karlowsky JA, Kabani AM. Rapid identification of fungi by using the ITS2 genetic region and an automated fluorescent capillary electrophoresis system. J Clin Microbiol. 1999;37(6):1846–51.
156. Jackson CJ, Barton RC, Evans EGV. Species identification and strain differentiation of dermatophyte fungi by analysis of ribosomal-DNA intergenic spacer regions. J Clin Microbiol. 1999;37(4):931–6.
157. Xia ZK, Yang RY, Wang WL, Ao JH, Wang CM, Zhu H. Significance of IGS1, ITS and D1/D2 regions in molecular identification of Trichosporon species and genotype of T. asahii in China. Zhonghua Yi Xue Za Zhi. 2008;88(44):3145–8.
158. Cantrell SA, Hanlin RT. Phylogenetic relationships in the family Hyaloscyphaceae inferred from sequences of ITS regions, 5.8S ribosomal DNA and morphological characters. Mycologia. 1997;89(5):745–55.
159. Sharma S, Balne PK, Motukupally SR, Das S, Garg P, Sahu SK, et al. Pythium insidiosum keratitis. Cornea. 2015;34(4):438–42.
160. Frau A, Kenny JG, Lenzi L, Campbell BJ, Ijaz UZ, Duckworth CA, et al. DNA extraction and amplicon production strategies deeply influence the outcome of gut mycobiome studies. Sci Rep. 2019;9(1):9328.
161. Wrent P, Rivas EM, Peinado JM, de Silóniz MI. Strain typing of Zygosaccharomyces yeast species using a single molecular method based on polymorphism of the intergenic spacer region (IGS). Int J Food Microbiol. 2010;142(1–2):89–96.
162. Ananthi S, Chitra T, Bini R, Prajna NV, Lalitha P, Dharmalingam K. Comparative analysis of the tear protein profile in mycotic keratitis patients. Mol Vis. 2008;14:500–7.
163. Ananthi S, Prajna NV, Lalitha P, Valarnila M, Dharmalingam K. Pathogen induced changes in the protein profile of human tears from Fusarium keratitis patients. PLoS ONE. 2013;8(1):e53018.
164. Kandhavelu J, Demonte NL, Namperumalsamy VP, Prajna L, Thangavel C, Jayapal JM, et al. Aspergillus flavus induced alterations in tear protein profile reveal pathogen-induced host response to fungal infection. J Proteom. 2017;152:13–21.
165. Kuo MT, Fang PC, Chao TL, Chen A, Lai YH, Huang YT, et al. Tear proteomics approach to monitoring sjögren syndrome or dry eye disease. Int J Mol Sci. 2019;20(8):1932.
166. Obayashi T, Yoshida M, Tamura H, Aketagawa J, Tanaka S, Kawai T. Determination of plasma (1 → 3)-β-d-glucan: a new diagnostic aid to deep mycosis. J Méd Vet Mycol. 1992;30(4):275–80.
167. Odabasi Z, Mattiuzzi G, Estey E, Kantarjian H, Saeki F, Ridge RJ, et al. β-d-glucan as a diagnostic adjunct for invasive fungal infections: validation, cutoff development, and performance in patients with acute myelogenous leukemia and myelodysplastic syndrome. Clin Infect Dis. 2004;39(2):199–205.
168. Kaji Y, Hiraoka T, Oshika T. Increased level of (1,3)-β-D-glucan in tear fluid of mycotic keratitis. Graefe's Arch Clin Exp Ophthalmol. 2009;247(7):989–92.
169. Kolomeyer AM, Murphy KM, Traband A, Frank I, Kim BJ. BETA-D-GLUCAN TESTING IN PATIENTS WITH FUNGAL ENDOPHTHALMITIS. Retina. 2018;38(4):650–9.
170. Awad R, Ghaith AA, Awad K, Saad MM, Elmassry AA. Fungal keratitis: diagnosis, management, and recent advances. Clin Ophthalmol. 2024;18(0):85–106.

171. Labbé A, Khammari C, Dupas B, Gabison E, Brasnu E, Labetoulle M, et al. Contribution of In vivo confocal microscopy to the diagnosis and management of infectious keratitis. Ocul Surf. 2009;7(1):41–52.
172. Chidambaram JD, Prajna NV, Larke N, Macleod D, Srikanthi P, Lanjewar S, et al. In vivo confocal microscopy appearance of Fusarium and Aspergillus species in fungal keratitis. Br J Ophthalmol. 2017;101(8):1119.
173. Aggarwal S, Yamaguchi T, Dana R, Hamrah P. Exophiala phaeomuriformis fungal keratitis. Eye Contact Lens: Sci Clin Pr. 2017;43(2):e4–6.
174. Mitani A, Shiraishi A, Uno T, Miyamoto H, Hara Y, Yamaguchi M, et al. In vivo and in vitro investigations of fungal keratitis caused by Colletotrichum gloeosporioides. J Ocul Pharmacol Ther. 2009;25(6):563–6.
175. Kumar RL, Cruzat A, Hamrah P. Current state of in vivo confocal microscopy in management of microbial keratitis. Semin Ophthalmol. 2010;25(5–6):166–70.
176. Kanavi MR, Javadi M, Yazdani S, Mirdehghanm S. Sensitivity and specificity of confocal scan in the diagnosis of infectious keratitis. Cornea. 2007;26(7):782–6.
177. Hau SC, Dart JKG, Vesaluoma M, Parmar DN, Claerhout I, Bibi K, et al. Diagnostic accuracy of microbial keratitis with in vivo scanning laser confocal microscopy. Br J Ophthalmol. 2010;94(8):982.
178. Chidambaram JD, Prajna NV, Larke NL, Palepu S, Lanjewar S, Shah M, et al. Prospective study of the diagnostic accuracy of the in vivo laser scanning confocal microscope for severe microbial keratitis. Ophthalmology. 2016;123(11):2285–93.
179. Wu X, Tao Y, Qiu Q, Wu X. Application of image recognition-based automatic hyphae detection in fungal keratitis. Australas Phys Eng Sci Med. 2018;41(1):95–103.
180. Ang M, Baskaran M, Werkmeister RM, Chua J, Schmidl D, Santos VAD, et al. Anterior segment optical coherence tomography. Prog Retin Eye Res. 2018;66:132–56.
181. Wang SB, Cornish EE, Grigg JR, McCluskey PJ. Anterior segment optical coherence tomography and its clinical applications. Clin Exp Optom. 2019;102(3):195–207.
182. Ramos JLB, Li Y, Huang D. Clinical and research applications of anterior segment optical coherence tomography – a review. Clin Exp Ophthalmol. 2009;37(1):81–9.
183. Wang J, Shousha MA, Perez VL, Karp CL, Yoo SH, Shen M, et al. Ultra-high resolution optical coherence tomography for imaging the anterior segment of the eye. Ophthalmic Surg Lasers Imaging Retin. 2011;42(4):S15–27.
184. Jin X, Jin H, Shi Y, Zhang N, Zhang H. Clinical observation of corneal endothelial plaques with fungal and bacterial keratitis by anterior segment optical coherence tomography and in vivo confocal microscopy. Cornea. 2022;41(11):1426–32.
185. Soliman W, Fathalla AM, El-Sebaity DM, Al-Hussaini AK. Spectral domain anterior segment optical coherence tomography in microbial keratitis. Graefe's Arch Clin Exp Ophthalmol. 2013;251(2):549–53.
186. D'Oria F, Galeone A, Pastore V, Cardascia N, Alessio G. Multi-drug resistant Enterococcus faecium in late-onset keratitis after deep anterior lamellar keratoplasty. Medicine. 2019;98(37):e17140.
187. Takezawa Y, Suzuki T, Shiraishi A. Observation of retrocorneal plaques in patients with infectious keratitis using anterior segment optical coherence tomography. Cornea. 2017;36(10):1237–42.
188. Abbouda A, Estrada AV, Rodriguez AE, Alió JL. Anterior segment optical coherence tomography in evaluation of severe fungal keratitis infections treated by corneal crosslinking. Eur J Ophthalmol. 2014;24(3):320–4.
189. Martone G, Pichierri P, Franceschini R, Moramarco A, Ciompi L, Tosi GM, et al. In vivo confocal microscopy and anterior segment optical coherence tomography in a case of Alternaria keratitis. Cornea. 2011;30(4):449–53.
190. Denk W, Strickler JH, Webb WW. Two-photon laser scanning fluorescence microscopy. Science. 1990;248(4951):73–6.

191. König K, So PTC, Mantulin WW, Tromberg BJ, Gratton E. Two-photon excited lifetime imaging of autofluorescence in cells during UVA and NIR photostress. J Microsc. 1996;183(3):197–204.
192. Gibson EA, Masihzadeh O, Lei TC, Ammar DA, Kahook MY. Multiphoton microscopy for ophthalmic imaging. J Ophthalmol. 2011;2011(1):870879.
193. Lee JH, Lee S, Gho YS, Song IS, Tchah H, Kim MJ, et al. Comparison of confocal microscopy and two-photon microscopy in mouse cornea in vivo. Exp Eye Res. 2015;132:101–8.
194. Lee JH, Le VH, Lee S, Park JH, Lee JA, Tchah H, et al. Two-photon microscopy of fungal keratitis-affected rabbit cornea ex vivo using moxifloxacin as a labeling agent. Exp Eye Res. 2018;174:51–8.
195. Viruni N, Zhang AY, Wang X, Handa JT, Liu TYA. Quantitative ocular ultrasound findings in microbial keratitis-associated endophthalmitis. Ophthalmol Retin. 2020;4(6):560–7.
196. Liu X, Lin TY, Lillehoj PB. Smartphones for cell and biomolecular detection. Ann Biomed Eng. 2014;42(11):2205–17.
197. Zhu H, Sikora U, Ozcan A. Quantum dot enabled detection of Escherichia coli using a cellphone. Analyst. 2012;137(11):2541–4.
198. Agarwal T, Bandivadekar P, Satpathy G, Sharma N, Titiyal JS. Detection of fungal hyphae using smartphone and pocket magnifier. Cornea. 2015;34(3):355–7.
199. Soleimani M, Esmaili K, Rahdar A, Aminizadeh M, Cheraqpour K, Tabatabaei SA, et al. From the diagnosis of infectious keratitis to discriminating fungal subtypes; a deep learning-based study. Sci Rep. 2023;13(1):22200.
200. Kalkanci A. Microbiological diagnosis of fungal keratitis. In: Mycotic keratitis.; 2019. p. 45–55.
201. Dalmon C, Porco TC, Lietman TM, Prajna NV, Prajna L, Das MR, et al. The clinical differentiation of bacterial and fungal keratitis: a photographic survey. Investig Opthalmology Vis Sci. 2012;53(4):1787.
202. Chatterjee S, Agrawal D, Gomase SN. Clinical differentiation of Pythium keratitis from fungal keratitis and development of a scoring system. Indian J Ophthalmol. 2022;70(10):3515–21.
203. Qi X, Liu T, Du M, Gao H. Endothelial plaques as sign of hyphae infiltration of Descemet's membrane in fungal keratitis. J Ophthalmol. 2020;2020(1):6083854.
204. Robbins N, Caplan T, Cowen LE. Molecular evolution of antifungal drug resistance. Annu Rev Microbiol. 2017;71(1):753–75.
205. Perlin DS, Rautemaa-Richardson R, Alastruey-Izquierdo A. The global problem of antifungal resistance: prevalence, mechanisms, and management. Lancet Infect Dis. 2017;17(12):e383–92.
206. Berkow EL, Lockhart SR, Ostrosky-Zeichner L. Antifungal susceptibility testing: current approaches. Clin Microbiol Rev. 2020;33(3) https://doi.org/10.1128/cmr.00069-19.
207. Mundra J, Dhakal R, Mohamed A, Jha G, Joseph J, Chaurasia S, et al. Outcomes of therapeutic penetrating keratoplasty in 198 eyes with fungal keratitis. Indian J Ophthalmol. 2019;67(10):1599–605.
208. Koçluk Y, Sukgen EA. Results of therapeutic penetrating keratoplasty for bacterial and fungal keratitis. Int Ophthalmol. 2017;37(5):1085–93.
209. Amescua G, Arboleda A, Nikpoor N, Durkee H, Relhan N, Aguilar MC, et al. Rose Bengal photodynamic antimicrobial therapy. Cornea. 2017;36(9):1141–4.
210. Prajna VN, Nirmalan PK, Saravanan S, Srinivasan M. Economic analysis of corneal ulcers in south India. Cornea. 2007;26(2):119–22.
211. Qiu S, Zhao GQ, Lin J, Wang X, Hu LT, Du ZD, et al. Natamycin in the treatment of fungal keratitis: a systematic review and meta-analysis. Int J Ophthalmol. 2015;8(3):597–602.
212. Hu J, Zhang J, Li Y, Han X, Zheng W, Yang J, et al. A combination of intrastromal and intracameral injections of amphotericin B in the treatment of severe fungal keratitis. J Ophthalmol. 2016;2016(1):3436415.
213. Ghenciu LA, Faur AC, Bolintineanu SL, Salavat MC, Maghiari AL. Recent advances in diagnosis and treatment approaches in fungal keratitis: a narrative review. Microorganisms. 2024;12(1):161.

214. FlorCruz NV, Peczon IV, Evans JR. Medical interventions for fungal keratitis. Cochrane Database Syst Rev. 2012;15(2):CD004241.
215. Knutsson KA, Iovieno A, Matuska S, Fontana L, Rama P. Topical corticosteroids and fungal keratitis: a review of the literature and case series. J Clin Med. 2021;10(6):1178.
216. Raj N, Vanathi M, Ahmed NH, Gupta N, Lomi N, Tandon R. Recent perspectives in the management of fungal keratitis. J Fungi. 2021;7(11):907.
217. Chander J, Sharma A. Prevalence of fungal corneal ulcers in Northern India. Infection. 1994;22(3):207–9.
218. Xie L, Dong X, Shi W. Treatment of fungal keratitis by penetrating keratoplasty. Br J Ophthalmol. 2001;85(9):1070.
219. Reference Method for Broth Dilution Antifungal Susceptibility Testing of Yeasts. Clinical and Laboratory Standards Institute; 2017. Report No.: M27.
220. Lalitha P, Prajna NV, Oldenburg CE, Srinivasan M, Krishnan T, Mascarenhas J, et al. Organism, minimum inhibitory concentration, and outcome in a fungal corneal ulcer clinical trial. Cornea. 2012;31(6):662–7.
221. Suman S, Jayangshu S, Debdulal B, Sunayana S, Archana K, Santi MM. Systemic evaluation on antifungal susceptibility of keratitis associated fungal pathogens in Eastern India. J Méd Microbiol Diagn. 2014;03(01):1.
222. Patil A, Lakhani P, Majumdar S. Current perspectives on natamycin in ocular fungal infections. J Drug Deliv Sci Technol. 2017;41:206–12.
223. Salvosa FAM, Cubillan LP, Nievera LF. In vitro evaluation of natamycin 5% suspension against Aspergillus flavus, Fusarium solani, and Candida parasilopsis. Philippine Journal of Ophthalmology. 2004;29(1):26–8.
224. Lalitha P, Vijaykumar R, Prajna NV, Fothergill AW. In vitro natamycin susceptibility of ocular isolates of Fusarium and Aspergillus species: comparison of commercially formulated natamycin eye drops to pharmaceutical-grade powder. J Clin Microbiol. 2008;46(10):3477–8.
225. Yildiz EH, Abdalla YF, Elsahn AF, Rapuano CJ, Hammersmith KM, Laibson PR, et al. Update on fungal keratitis from 1999 to 2008. Cornea. 2010;29(12):1406–11.
226. Prajna NV, Krishnan T, Mascarenhas J, Rajaraman R, Prajna L, Srinivasan M, et al. The mycotic ulcer treatment trial: a randomized trial comparing natamycin vs voriconazole. JAMA Ophthalmol. 2013;131(4):422–9.
227. Sharma S, Das S, Virdi A, Fernandes M, Sahu SK, Koday NK, et al. Re-appraisal of topical 1% voriconazole and 5% natamycin in the treatment of fungal keratitis in a randomised trial. Br J Ophthalmol. 2015;99(9):1190.
228. FlorCruz NV, Evans JR. Medical interventions for fungal keratitis. Cochrane Database Syst Rev. 2015;2015(4):CD004241.
229. Velpandian T, Nirmal J, Sharma HP, Sharma S, Sharma N, Halder N. Novel water soluble sterile natamycin formulation (Natasol) for fungal keratitis. Eur J Pharm Sci. 2021;163:105857.
230. Saluja G, Sharma N, Agarwal R, Sharma HP, Singhal D, Maharana PK, et al. Comparison of safety and efficacy of intrastromal injections of voriconazole, amphotericin B and natamycin in cases of recalcitrant fungal keratitis: a randomized controlled trial. Clin Ophthalmol. 2021;15:2437–46.
231. Nett JE, Andes DR. Antifungal agents spectrum of activity, pharmacology, and clinical indications. Infect Dis Clin North Am. 2016;30(1):51–83.
232. Saravolatz LD, Ostrosky-Zeichner L, Marr KA, Rex JH, Cohen SH. Amphotericin B: time for a new "gold standard.". Clin Infect Dis. 2003;37(3):415–25.
233. Qu L, Li L, Xie H. Corneal and aqueous humor concentrations of amphotericin B using three different routes of administration in a rabbit model. Ophthalmic Res. 2010;43(3):153–8.
234. Sharma N, Sankaran P, Agarwal T, Arora T, Chawla B, Titiyal JS, et al. Evaluation of intracameral amphotericin B in the management of fungal keratitis: randomized controlled trial. Ocul Immunol Inflamm. 2016;24(5):493–7.
235. Deswal J, Arya SK. Intracorneal amphotericin B injection in a case of indolent candidal keratitis. J Clin Diagn Res. 2017;11(5):ND01–2.

236. Bell RW, Ritchey JP. Subconjunctival nodules after amphotericin B injection: medical therapy for Aspergillus corneal ulcer. Arch Ophthalmol. 1973;90(5):402–4.
237. Aydin B, Cubuk MO, Ucgul A, Ertop M, Ozmen MC, Atalay T, et al. Combined intrastromal voriconazole and amphotericin B treatment for persistent fungal keratitis. Eye Contact Lens: Sci Clin Pr. 2020;46(5):269–73.
238. Yoon KC, Jeong IY, Im SK, Chae HJ, Yang SY. Therapeutic effect of intracameral amphotericin B injection in the treatment of fungal keratitis. Cornea. 2007;26(7):814–8.
239. Shu TH, Hussein A, Kursiah MR. Conjunctiva necrosis following subconjunctival amphotericin B injection in fungal keratitis. Cureus. 2019;11(9):e5580.
240. Arora R, Gupta D, Goyal J, Kaur R. Voriconazole versus natamycin as primary treatment in fungal corneal ulcers. Clin Exp Ophthalmol. 2011;39(5):434–40.
241. Dupuis A, Tournier N, Moal GL, Venisse N. Preparation and stability of voriconazole eye drop solution. Antimicrob Agents Chemother. 2008;53(2):798–9.
242. Narayana S, Krishnan T, Ramakrishnan S, Samantaray PP, Austin A, Pickel J, et al. Mycotic antimicrobial localized injection a randomized clinical trial evaluating intrastromal injection of voriconazole. Ophthalmology. 2019;126(8):1084–9.
243. Sharma N, Agarwal P, Sinha R, Titiyal JS, Velpandian T, Vajpayee RB. Evaluation of intrastromal voriconazole injection in recalcitrant deep fungal keratitis: case series. Br J Ophthalmol. 2011;95(12):1735.
244. Kalaiselvi G, Narayana S, Krishnan T, Sengupta S. Intrastromal voriconazole for deep recalcitrant fungal keratitis: a case series. Br J Ophthalmol. 2015;99(2):195.
245. Prajna NV, Krishnan T, Rajaraman R, Patel S, Srinivasan M, Das M, et al. Effect of oral voriconazole on fungal keratitis in the mycotic ulcer treatment trial ii (mutt ii): a randomized clinical trial. JAMA Ophthalmol. 2016;134(12):1365.
246. Prajna NV, Krishnan T, Rajaraman R, Patel S, Shah R, Srinivasan M, et al. Adjunctive oral voriconazole treatment of Fusarium keratitis: a secondary analysis from the mycotic ulcer treatment trial II. JAMA Ophthalmol. 2017;135(6):520.
247. Sharma N, Singhal D, Maharana PK, Sinha R, Agarwal T, Upadhyay AD, et al. Comparison of oral voriconazole versus oral ketoconazole as an adjunct to topical natamycin in severe fungal keratitis. Cornea. 2017;36(12):1521–7.
248. Chen D, Tan S, Zou W. Treating fungal keratitis with oral voriconazole only: a case series. Klin Monatsblätter für Augenheilkd. 2020;238(01):55–9.
249. Diekema DJ, Messer SA, Hollis RJ, Jones RN, Pfaller MA. Activities of caspofungin, itraconazole, posaconazole, ravuconazole, voriconazole, and amphotericin B against 448 recent clinical isolates of filamentous fungi. J Clin Microbiol. 2003;41(8):3623–6.
250. Al-Hatmi AMS, Meletiadis J, Curfs-Breuker I, Bonifaz A, Meis JF, Hoog GSD. In vitro combinations of natamycin with voriconazole, itraconazole and micafungin against clinical Fusarium strains causing keratitis. J Antimicrob Chemother. 2016;71(4):953–5.
251. Wagh VD, Deshmukh OJ. Itraconazole niosomes drug delivery system and its antimycotic activity against Candida albicans. Int Sch Res Not. 2012;2012(1):653465.
252. Lee EA, Balakrishnan P, Song CK, Choi JH, Noh GY, Park CG, et al. Microemulsion-based hydrogel formulation of itraconazole for topical delivery. J Pharm Investig. 2010;40(5):305–11.
253. Nakarani M, Misra AK, Patel JK, Vaghani SS. Itraconazole nanosuspension for oral delivery: formulation, characterization and in vitro comparison with marketed formulation. Daru: J Fac Pharm, Tehran Univ Méd Sci. 2010;18(2):84–90.
254. Mukherjee S, Ray S, Thakur RS. Solid lipid nanoparticles: a modern formulation approach in drug delivery system. Indian J Pharm Sci. 2009;71(4):349–58.
255. ElMeshad AN, Mohsen AM. Enhanced corneal permeation and antimycotic activity of itraconazole against Candida albicans via a novel nanosystem vesicle. Drug Deliv. 2016;23(7):2115–23.
256. Permana AD, Utami RN, Layadi P, Himawan A, Juniarti N, Anjani QK, et al. Thermosensitive and mucoadhesive in situ ocular gel for effective local delivery and antifungal activity of itraconazole nanocrystal in the treatment of fungal keratitis. Int J Pharm. 2021;602:120623.

257. Miller D, Alfonso EC. Management of fungal keratitis: topical or systemic therapy. Pan Am J Ophthalmol. 13(3):73–7.
258. Nagappan V, Deresinski S. Posaconazole: A broad-spectrum triazole antifungal agent. Clin Infect Dis. 2007;45(12):1610–7.
259. Arendrup MC, Cuenca-Estrella M, Donnelly JP, Hope W, Lass-Flörl C, Rodriguez-Tudela J-L, et al. EUCAST technical note on posaconazole. Clin Microbiol Infect. 2011;17(11):E16–7.
260. Sponsel WE, Graybill JR, Nevarez HL, Dang D. Ocular and systemic posaconazole (SCH-56592) treatment of invasive Fusarium solani keratitis and endophthalmitis. Br J Ophthalmol. 2002;86(7):829.
261. Guarascio AJ, Slain D. Review of the New Delayed-Release Oral Tablet and Intravenous Dosage Forms of Posaconazole. Pharmacother: J Hum Pharmacol Drug Ther. 2015;35(2):208–19.
262. Arnoldner MA, Kheirkhah A, Jakobiec FA, Durand ML, Hamrah P. Successful treatment of Paecilomyces lilacinus keratitis with oral posaconazole. Cornea. 2014;33(7):747–9.
263. Tu EY, McCartney DL, Beatty RF, Springer KL, Levy J, Edward D. Successful treatment of resistant ocular fusariosis with posaconazole (SCH-56592). Am J Ophthalmol. 2007;143(2):222–227.e1.
264. Altun A, Kurna SA, Sengor T, Altun G, Olcaysu OO, Aki SF, et al. Effectiveness of posaconazole in recalcitrant fungal keratitis resistant to conventional antifungal drugs. Case Rep Ophthalmol Med. 2014;2014(1):701653.
265. Tu EY, Park AJ. Recalcitrant Beauveria bassiana keratitis. Cornea. 2007;26(8):1008–10.
266. Durgun ME, Kahraman E, Hacıoğlu M, Güngör S, Özsoy Y. Posaconazole micelles for ocular delivery: in vitro permeation, ocular irritation and antifungal activity studies. Drug Deliv Transl Res. 2022;12(3):662–75.
267. Rao SK, Madhavan HN, Rao G, Padmanabhan P. Fluconazole in filamentous fungal keratitis. Cornea. 1997;16(6):700.
268. Sonego-Krone S, Martino DSD, Ayala-Lugo R, Torres-Alvariza G, Ta CN, Barbosa L, et al. Clinical results of topical fluconazole for the treatment of filamentous fungal keratitis. Graefe's Arch Clin Exp Ophthalmol. 2006;244(7):782–7.
269. Tanure MAG, Cohen EJ, Sudesh S, Rapuano CJ, Laibson PR. Spectrum of fungal keratitis at Wills Eye Hospital, Philadelphia, Pennsylvania. Cornea. 2000;19(3):307–12.
270. Dev S, Rajaraman R, Raghavan A. Severe fungal keratitis treated with subconjunctival fluconazole. Am J Ophthalmol. 2006;141(4):783.
271. Kaur IP, Rana C, Singh M, Bhushan S, Singh H, Kakkar S. Development and evaluation of novel surfactant-based elastic vesicular system for ocular delivery of fluconazole. J Ocul Pharmacol Ther. 2012;28(5):484–96.
272. Gupta AK, Foley KA, Versteeg SG. New antifungal agents and new formulations against dermatophytes. Mycopathologia. 2017;182(1–2):127–41.
273. Todokoro D, Suzuki T, Tamura T, Makimura K, Yamaguchi H, Inagaki K, et al. Efficacy of luliconazole against broad-range Filamentous fungi including Fusarium solani species complex causing fungal keratitis. Cornea. 2019;38(2):238–42.
274. Prajna NV, John RK, Nirmalan PK, Lalitha P, Srinivasan M. A randomised clinical trial comparing 2% econazole and 5% natamycin for the treatment of fungal keratitis. Br J Ophthalmol. 2003;87(10):1235.
275. Fernández-Ferreiro A, Barcia MG, Gil-Martínez M, Vieites-Prado A, Lema I, Argibay B, et al. In vitro and in vivo ocular safety and eye surface permanence determination by direct and magnetic resonance imaging of ion-sensitive hydrogels based on gellan gum and kappa-carrageenan. Eur J Pharm Biopharm. 2015;94:342–51.
276. Luaces-Rodríguez A, Díaz-Tomé V, González-Barcia M, Silva-Rodríguez J, Herranz M, Gil-Martínez M, et al. Cysteamine polysaccharide hydrogels: study of extended ocular delivery and biopermanence time by PET imaging. Int J Pharm. 2017;528(1–2):714–22.
277. Díaz-Tomé V, Luaces-Rodríguez A, Silva-Rodríguez J, Blanco-Dorado S, García-Quintanilla L, Llovo-Taboada J, et al. Ophthalmic econazole hydrogels for the treatment of fungal keratitis. J Pharm Sci. 2018;107(5):1342–51.

278. Mohanta P. Development of surfactant-based nanocarrier system for delivery of an antifungal drug. J Ocul Pharmacol Ther. 2017;11:1153–8.
279. Mselle J. Use of topical clotrimazole in human keratomycosis. Ophthalmologica. 2001;215(5):357–60.
280. Al-Shakarchi F. Use of clotrimazole eye suspension for fungal keratitis as monotherapy or sequentially with amphotercin-B. Mustansiriya Méd J. 2015;14(1):6.
281. Shobana CS, Mythili A, Homa M, Galgóczy L, Priya R, Singh YRB, et al. In vitro susceptibility of filamentous fungi from mycotic keratitis to azole drugs. J Mycol Médicale J Méd Mycol. 2015;25(1):44–9.
282. Patil A, Majumdar S. Echinocandins in ocular therapeutics. J Ocul Pharmacol Ther. 2017;33(5):340–52.
283. Gil-Lamaignere C, Salvenmoser S, Hess R, Müller FMC. Micafungin enhances neutrophil fungicidal functions against Candida pseudohyphae. Antimicrob Agents Chemother. 2004;48(7):2730–2.
284. Denning DW. Echinocandins: a new class of antifungal. J Antimicrob Chemother. 2002;49(6):889–91.
285. Revankar SG, Sobel JD. Are echinocandins better than azoles for invasive candidiasis? Curr Fungal Infect Rep. 2013;7(1):79–82.
286. Neoh CF, Daniell M, Chen SCA, Stewart K, Kong DCM. Clinical utility of caspofungin eye drops in fungal keratitis. Int J Antimicrob Agents. 2014;44(2):96–104.
287. Vorwerk CK, Tuchen S, Streit F, Binder L, Hofmüller W, Behrens-Baumann W. Aqueous humor concentrations of topically administered caspofungin in rabbits. Ophthalmic Res. 2009;41(2):102–5.
288. Neoh CF, Leung L, Misra A, Vajpayee RB, Davies GE, Fullinfaw RO, et al. Penetration of topically administered 0.5-percent caspofungin eye drops into human aqueous humor. Antimicrob Agents Chemother. 2011;55(4):1761–3.
289. Neoh CF, Leung L, Vajpayee RB, Stewart K, Kong DC. Treatment of alternaria keratitis with intrastromal and topical caspofungin in combination with intrastromal, topical, and oral voriconazole. Ann Pharmacother. 2011;45(5):681.
290. Tu EY. Alternaria keratitis: clinical presentation and resolution with topical fluconazole or intrastromal voriconazole and topical caspofungin. Cornea. 2009;28(1):116–9.
291. Hurtado-Sarrió M, Duch-Samper A, Cisneros-Lanuza A, Dı́iaz-Llopis M, Peman-Garcı́ia J, Vazquez-Polo A. Successful topical application of caspofungin in the treatment of fungal keratitis refractory to voriconazole. Arch Ophthalmol. 2010;128(7):941–2.
292. Gregory ME, Macdonald ECA, Lockington D, Ramaesh K. Recurrent fungal keratitis following penetrating keratoplasty: an unusual source of infection. Arch Ophthalmol. 2010;128(11):1490–1.
293. Matsumoto Y, Dogru M, Goto E, Fujishima H, Tsubota K. Successful topical application of a new antifungal agent, micafungin, in the treatment of refractory fungal corneal ulcers. Cornea. 2005;24(6):748–53.
294. Matsumoto Y, Murat D, Kojima T, Shimazaki J, Tsubota K. The comparison of solitary topical micafungin or fluconazole application in the treatment of Candida fungal keratitis. Br J Ophthalmol. 2011;95(10):1406–9.
295. Martin MJ, Rahman MR, Johnson GJ, Srinivasan M, Clayton YM. Mycotic keratitis: susceptibility to antiseptic agents. Int Ophthalmol. 1995;19(5):299–302.
296. Xu Y, He Y, Zhou L, Gao C, Sun S, Wang X, et al. Effects of contact lens solution disinfectants against filamentous fungi. Optom Vis Sci. 2014;91(12):1440–5.
297. Oliveira Dos Santos C, Kolwijck E, van der Lee HA, Tehupeiory-Kooreman MC, Al-Hatmi AMS, Matayan E, et al. In vitro activity of chlorhexidine compared with seven antifungal agents against 98 Fusarium isolates recovered from fungal keratitis patients. Antimicrob Agents Chemother. 2019;63(8) https://doi.org/10.1128/aac.02669-18.
298. Santos COD, Hanemaaijer NM, Ye J, van der Lee HAL, Verweij PE, Eggink CA. Chlorhexidine for the treatment of Fusarium keratitis: a case series and mini review. J Fungi. 2021;7(4):255.

299. Rahman MR, Minassian DC, Srinivasan M, Martin MJ, Johnson GJ. Trial of chlorhexidine gluconate for fungal corneal ulcers. Ophthalmic Epidemiol. 1997;4(3):141–9.
300. Rahman MR, Johnson GJ, Husain R, Howlader SA, Minassian DC. Randomised trial of 0.2% chlorhexidine gluconate and 2.5% natamycin for fungal keratitis in Bangladesh. Br J Ophthalmol. 1998;82(8):919.
301. Hoffman JJ, Yadav R, Sanyam SD, Chaudhary P, Roshan A, Singh SK, et al. Topical chlorhexidine 0.2% versus topical natamycin 5% for fungal keratitis in Nepal: rationale and design of a randomised controlled non-inferiority trial. BMJ Open. 2020;10(9):e038066.
302. Hoffman JJ, Yadav R, Sanyam SD, Chaudhary P, Roshan A, Singh SK, et al. Topical chlorhexidine 0.2% versus topical natamycin 5% for the treatment of fungal keratitis in Nepal a randomized controlled noninferiority trial. Ophthalmology. 2022;129(5):530–41.
303. Pinna A, Donadu MG, Usai D, Dore S, Boscia F, Zanetti S. In vitro antimicrobial activity of a new ophthalmic solution containing hexamidine diisethionate 0.05% (Keratosept). Cornea. 2020;39(11):1415–8.
304. Carrasco MA, Genesoni G. Treatment of severe fungal keratitis with subconjunctival amphotericin B. Cornea. 2011;30(5):608–11.
305. Tsai SH, Lin YC, Hsu HC, Chen YM. Subconjunctival injection of fluconazole in the treatment of fungal alternaria keratitis. Ocul Immunol Inflamm. 2016;24(1):103–6.
306. Yilmaz S, Maden A. Severe fungal keratitis treated with subconjunctival fluconazole. Am J Ophthalmol. 2005;140(3):454.e1–8.
307. Mahdy RA, Nada WM, Wageh MM. Topical amphotericin B and subconjunctival injection of fluconazole (combination therapy) versus topical amphotericin B (Monotherapy) in treatment of keratomycosis. J Ocul Pharmacol Ther. 2010;26(3):281–5.
308. Sharma N, Chacko J, Velpandian T, Titiyal JS, Sinha R, Satpathy G, et al. Comparative evaluation of topical versus intrastromal voriconazole as an adjunct to natamycin in recalcitrant fungal keratitis. Ophthalmology. 2013;120(4):677–81.
309. Maniam A, Yuen GS. Intrastromal antifungal injection as a successful modality of treatment for fungal keratitis: a case series. Int J Res Méd Sci. 2018;7(1):288–93.
310. Moramarco A, Grendele A, Iannetta D, Ottoboni S, Gregori G, Geronimo N d, et al. Efficacy of the combined intrastromal injection of voriconazole and amphotericin B in recalcitrant fungal keratitis. Microorganisms. 2024;12(5):922.
311. Konar P, Joshi S, Mandhare SJ, Thakur R, Deshpande M, Dayal A. Intrastromal voriconazole: an adjuvant approach for recalcitrant mycotic keratitis. Indian J Ophthalmol. 2020;68(1):35–8.
312. Shen YC, Wang CY, Tsai HY, Lee HN. Intracameral voriconazole injection in the treatment of fungal endophthalmitis resulting from keratitis. Am J Ophthalmol. 2010;149(6):916–21.
313. Indratno F, Vitresia H. The outcome of concurrent intracameral fluconazole injection with amniotic membrane transplantation for fungal keratitis in Dr. M. Djamil general hospital: a case series. Biosci Med J Biomed Transl Res. 2023;7(3):3204–9.
314. Nangia P, Gupta S, Lambat S, Nangia V. Role of intracameral Caspofungin in the management of Aspergillus keratitis: a case report. J Cornea Ocul Surf. 2023;1(2):134–6.
315. Dong LK, Krebs DB. An intracameral approach for recalcitrant fungal keratitis. Am J Ophthalmol Case Rep. 2022;25:101369.
316. Bezerra FM, Silva LNP, Aguiar LL, Yu MCZ, Rocha FJ, Sousa LB, et al. Intracameral voriconazole for severe fungal keratitis: a case series. Arq Bras Oftalmol. 2025;88(3):e2024–0207.
317. Dahiya M, Dua M, Rathi M, Sachdeva S, Dabas R. Intrastromal and intracameral voriconazole combination: an adjuvant therapy in intractable mycotic keratitis. Indian J Clin Exp Ophthalmol. 2023;9(1):45–8.
318. Kuriakose T, Kothari M, Paul P, Jacob P, Thomas R. Intracameral amphotericin B injection in the management of deep keratomycosis. Cornea. 2002;21(7):653–6.
319. Schnitzler E, Spörl E, Seiler T. Bestrahlung der Hornhaut mit UV-Licht und Riboflavingabe als neuer Behandlungsversuch bei einschmelzenden Hornhautprozessen, erste Ergebnisse bei vier Patienten1 2 3. Klin Monatsbl Augenheilkd. 2000;217(3):190–3.

320. Prajna NV, Radhakrishnan N, Lalitha P, Austin A, Ray KJ, Keenan JD, et al. Cross-linking–assisted infection reduction a randomized clinical trial evaluating the effect of adjuvant cross-linking on outcomes in fungal keratitis. Ophthalmology. 2020;127(2):159–66.
321. Wei A, Wang K, Wang Y, Gong L, Xu J, Shao T. Evaluation of corneal cross-linking as adjuvant therapy for the management of fungal keratitis. Graefe's Arch Clin Exp Ophthalmol. 2019;257(7):1443–52.
322. Alshehri JM, Caballero-Lima D, Hillarby MC, Shawcross SG, Brahma A, Carley F, et al. Evaluation of corneal cross-linking for treatment of fungal keratitis: using confocal laser scanning microscopy on an ex vivo human corneal model. Investig Opthalmology Vis Sci. 2016;57(14):6367.
323. Özdemir HB, Kalkancı A, Bilgihan K, Göçün PU, Öğüt B, Karakurt F, et al. Comparison of corneal collagen cross-linking (PACK-CXL) and voriconazole treatments in experimental fungal keratitis. Acta Ophthalmol. 2019;97(1):e91–6.
324. Zhu Z, Zhang H, Yue J, Liu S, Li Z, Wang L. Antimicrobial efficacy of corneal cross-linking in vitro and in vivo for Fusarium solani: a potential new treatment for fungal keratitis. BMC Ophthalmol. 2018;18(1):65.
325. Castellanos JCG, Osaba M, Reviglio V, Canchi MT, Arrigone MC, Reviglio VE. Early treatment of bilateral fungal keratitis with corneal cross-linking as adjuvant therapy. Oxf Méd Case Rep. 2020;2020(6):omaa032.
326. Mikropoulos DG, Kymionis GD, Voulgari N, Kaisari E, Nikolakopoulos KA, Katsanos A, et al. Intraoperative photoactivated chromophore for infectious keratitis–corneal cross-linking (PACK-CXL) during penetrating keratoplasty for the management of fungal keratitis in an immunocompromised patient. Ophthalmol Ther. 2019;8(3):491–5.
327. Mani VJ, Parthasarathy D, Padmanabhan P, Narayanan N, Lakshmipathy M, Pachayappan SK, et al. Therapeutic effect of corneal crosslinking on fungal keratitis: efficacy of corneal collagen crosslinking as an adjuvant therapy for fungal keratitis in a tertiary eye hospital in South India. Ocul Immunol Inflamm. 2021;29(7–8):1648–55.
328. Li M, Yu T, Gao X, Wu XY. Accelerated corneal collagen cross-linking in clinical management of infectious keratitis. J Int Méd Res. 2020;48(6):030006052092641l.
329. Arboleda A, Miller D, Cabot F, Taneja M, Aguilar MC, Alawa K, et al. Assessment of rose Bengal versus riboflavin photodynamic therapy for inhibition of fungal keratitis isolates. Am J Ophthalmol. 2014;158(1):64–70.e2.
330. Prajna V, Prajna L, Sharma S, de Freitas D, Höfling-Lima AL, Varnado N, et al. A double-masked, sham-controlled trial of rose bengal photodynamic therapy for the treatment of fungal and acanthameoba keratitis: Rose Bengal Electromagnetic Activation with Green Light for Infection Reduction (REAGIR) Study. Res Sq. 2024:rs.3.rs-4165312.
331. Zhou C, Peng C, Shi C, Jiang M, Chau JHC, Liu Z, et al. Mitochondria-specific aggregation-induced emission luminogens for selective photodynamic killing of fungi and efficacious treatment of keratitis. ACS Nano. 2021;15(7):12129–39.
332. Garg P, Roy A, Kalra P. Surgical management of fungal keratitis. Expert Rev Ophthalmol. 2018;13(6):351–9.
333. Prajna NV, Krishnan T, Rajaraman R, Patel S, Shah R, Srinivasan M, et al. Predictors of corneal perforation or need for therapeutic keratoplasty in severe fungal keratitis: a secondary analysis of the mycotic ulcer treatment trial II. JAMA Ophthalmol. 2017;135(9):987.
334. Xie L, Zhai H, Shi W. Penetrating keratoplasty for corneal perforations in fungal keratitis. Cornea. 2007;26(2):158–62.
335. Mohamed A, Chaurasia S, Murthy SI, Ramappa M, Vaddavalli PK, Taneja M, et al. Endothelial keratoplasty. Asia-Pac J Ophthalmol. 2014;3(4):207–10.
336. Xie L, Shi W, Liu Z, Li S. Lamellar keratoplasty for the treatment of fungal keratitis. Cornea. 2002;21(1):33–7.
337. Qu L-j, Xie L-x. Changing indications for lamellar keratoplasty in Shandong, 1993–2008. Chin Méd J. 2010;123(22):3268–71.

338. Sabatino F, Sarnicola E, Sarnicola C, Tosi GM, Perri P, Sarnicola V, et al. Early deep anterior lamellar keratoplasty for fungal keratitis poorly responsive to medical treatment. Eye. 2017;31(12):1639–46.
339. Zheng Q, Zhang Y, Ren Y, Zhao Z, Hua S, Li J, et al. Deep anterior lamellar keratoplasty with cross-linked acellular porcine corneal stroma to manage fungal keratitis. Xenotransplantation. 2021;28(2):e12655.
340. Sanders FWB, Huang J, del Barrio JLA, Hamada S, McAlinden C. Amniotic membrane transplantation: structural and biological properties, tissue preparation, application and clinical indications. Eye. 2024;38(4):668–79.
341. Chen HC, Tan HY, Hsiao CH, Huang SCM, Lin KK, Ma DHK. Amniotic membrane transplantation for persistent corneal ulcers and perforations in acute fungal keratitis. Cornea. 2006;25(5):564–72.
342. Ting DSJ, Henein C, Said DG, Dua HS. Amniotic membrane transplantation for infectious keratitis: a systematic review and meta-analysis. Sci Rep. 2021;11(1):13007.
343. Sun GH, Li SX, Gao H, Zhang WB, Zhang MA, Shi WY. Clinical observation of removal of the necrotic corneal tissue combined with conjunctival flap covering surgery under the guidance of the AS-OCT in treatment of fungal keratitis. Int J Ophthalmol. 5(1):88–91.
344. Nizeyimana H, Zhou DD, Liu XF, Pan XT, Liu C, Lu CW, et al. Clinical efficacy of conjunctival flap surgery in the treatment of refractory fungal keratitis. Exp Ther Med. 2017;14(2):1109–13.
345. Wang YC, Wang JS, Wang B, Peng X, Xie HT, Zhang MC. Two-step strategy-conjunctival flap covering surgery combined with secondary deep anterior lamellar keratoplasty for the treatment of high-risk fungal keratitis. Int J Ophthalmol. 2023;16(7):1065–70.
346. Lim LS, How AC, Ang LPK, Tan DTH. Gundersen flaps in the management of ocular surface disease in an Asian population. Cornea. 2009;28(7):747–51.
347. Zemba M, Stamate AC, Tataru CP, Branisteanu DC, Balta F. Conjunctival flap surgery in the management of ocular surface disease (review). Exp Ther Med. 2020;20(4):3412–6.
348. Abdulhalim BEH, Wagih MM, Gad AAM, Boghdadi G, Nagy RRS. Amniotic membrane graft to conjunctival flap in treatment of non-viral resistant infectious keratitis: a randomised clinical study. Br J Ophthalmol. 2015;99(1):59.
349. Alino AM, Perry HD, Kanellopoulos AJ, Donnenfeld ED, Rahn EK. Conjunctival flaps. Ophthalmology. 1998;105(6):1120–3.
350. Du YL, Wang JS, Geng W, Duan CY, Wang XH, Xie HT, et al. Amniotic membrane transplantation combined with conjunctival flap covering surgery for the treatment of corneal perforations in fungal keratitis. Heliyon. 2023;9(12):e22693.
351. Jin X, Feng J, Sun N, Jin H, Wang J, Song Z, et al. A 5-year retrospective analysis of the risk factors, treatment, and prognosis of patients with fungal keratitis in Heilongjiang, China. Am J Ophthalmol. 2022;244:48–57.
352. Prajna NV, Krishnan T, Mascarenhas J, Srinivasan M, Oldenburg CE, Toutain-Kidd CM, et al. Predictors of outcome in fungal keratitis. Eye. 2012;26(9):1226–31.
353. Berger ST, Katsev DA, Mondino BJ, Pettit TH. Macroscopic pigmentation in a dematiaceous fungal keratitis. Cornea. 1991;10(3):272–6.
354. Garg P, Vemuganti GK, Chatarjee S, Gopinathan U, Rao GN. Pigmented plaque presentation of dematiaceous fungal keratitis. Cornea. 2004;23(6):571–6.
355. Lulu WANG, Zhang Y, L Z, L W. Prognosis of clinical treatment for fungal keratitis and its influence factors. Chin J Exp Ophthalmol. 2016;34(8):734–8.
356. Cong L, Xia YP, Zhao GQ, Lin J, Xu Q, Hu LT, et al. Expression of vitamin D receptor and cathelicidin in human corneal epithelium cells during fusarium solani infection. Int J Ophthalmol. 2015;8(5):866–71.
357. Han Y, Ulrich MA, Cutler JE. Candida albicans mannan extract—protein conjugates induce a protective immune response against experimental candidiasis. J Infect Dis. 1999;179(6):1477–84.
358. Rossoni RD, de Barros PP, de Alvarenga JA, de Ribeiro F, Velloso MDS, Fuchs BB, et al. Antifungal activity of clinical Lactobacillus strains against Candida albicans biofilms:

identification of potential probiotic candidates to prevent oral candidiasis. Biofouling. 2018;34(2):212–25.
359. Brandt CR. Peptide therapeutics for treating ocular surface infections. J Ocul Pharmacol Ther. 2014;30(9):691–9.
360. Pereira HA, Tsyshevskaya-Hoover I, Hinsley H, Logan S, Nguyen M, Nguyen TT, et al. Candidacidal activity of synthetic peptides based on the antimicrobial domain of the neutrophil-derived protein, CAP37. Méd Mycol. 2009;48(2):1–11.
361. Wu H, Ong ZY, Liu S, Li Y, Wiradharma N, Yang YY, et al. Synthetic β-sheet forming peptide amphiphiles for treatment of fungal keratitis. Biomaterials. 2015;43:44–9.
362. de Sá FAP, Taveira SF, Gelfuso GM, Lima EM, Gratieri T. Liposomal voriconazole (VOR) formulation for improved ocular delivery. Colloids Surf B Biointerfaces. 2015;133:331–8.
363. Zhou W, Wang Y, Jian J, Song S. Self-aggregated nanoparticles based on amphiphilic poly(lactic acid)-grafted-chitosan copolymer for ocular delivery of amphotericin B. Int J Nanomed. 2013;8(0):3715–28.
364. Soliman OAEA, Mohamed EA, Khatera NAA. Enhanced ocular bioavailability of fluconazole from niosomal gels and microemulsions: formulation, optimization, and in vitro–in vivo evaluation. Pharm Dev Technol. 2019;24(1):48–62.
365. Cariello AJ, Passos RM, Yu MCZ, Hofling-Lima AL. Microbial keratitis at a referral center in Brazil. Int Ophthalmol. 2011;31(3):197.
366. Rautaraya B, Sharma S, Kar S, Das S, Sahu SK. Diagnosis and treatment outcome of mycotic keratitis at a tertiary eye care center in eastern India. BMC Ophthalmol. 2011;11(1):39.
367. Lin CC, Lalitha P, Srinivasan M, Prajna NV, McLeod SD, Acharya NR, et al. Seasonal trends of microbial keratitis in south India. Cornea. 2012;31(10):1123–7.
368. Marujo FI, Hirai FE, Yu MCZ, Hofling-Lima AL, de Freitas D, Sato EH. Distribuição das ceratites infecciosas em hospital terciário no Brasil. Arq Bras Oftalmol. 2013;76(6):370–3.
369. Kaliamurthy J, Kalavathy CM, Parmar P, Jesudasan CAN, Thomas PA. Spectrum of bacterial keratitis at a tertiary eye care centre in India. BioMed Res Int. 2013;2013(1):181564.
370. Hernandez-Camarena JC, Graue-Hernandez EO, Ortiz-Casas M, Ramirez-Miranda A, Navas A, Pedro-Aguilar L, et al. Trends in microbiological and antibiotic sensitivity patterns in infectious keratitis. Cornea. 2015;34(7):778–85.
371. Hsiao CH, Sun CC, Yeh LK, Ma DHK, Chen PYF, Lin HC, et al. Shifting trends in bacterial keratitis in Taiwan. Cornea. 2016;35(3):313–7.
372. Politis M, Wajnsztajn D, Rosin B, Block C, Solomon A. Trends of bacterial keratitis culture isolates in Jerusalem; a 13- years analysis. PLoS ONE. 2016;11(11):e0165223.
373. Tan SZ, Walkden A, Au L, Fullwood C, Hamilton A, Qamruddin A, et al. Twelve-year analysis of microbial keratitis trends at a UK tertiary hospital. Eye. 2017;31(8):1229–36.
374. Tam ALC, Côté E, Saldanha M, Lichtinger A, Slomovic AR. Bacterial keratitis in Toronto. Cornea. 2017;36(12):1528–34.
375. Khor WB, Prajna VN, Garg P, Mehta JS, Xie L, Liu Z, et al. The Asia Cornea Society infectious keratitis study: a prospective multicenter study of infectious keratitis in Asia. Am J Ophthalmol. 2018;195:161–70.
376. Tavassoli S, Nayar G, Darcy K, Grzeda M, Luck J, Williams OM, et al. An 11-year analysis of microbial keratitis in the South West of England using brain–heart infusion broth. Eye. 2019;33(10):1619–25.
377. Kowalski RP, Nayyar SV, Romanowski EG, Shanks RMQ, Mammen A, Dhaliwal DK, et al. The prevalence of bacteria, fungi, viruses, and acanthamoeba from 3,004 cases of keratitis, endophthalmitis, and conjunctivitis. Eye Contact Lens: Sci Clin Pr. 2020;46(5):265–8.
378. Lin L, Duan F, Yang Y, Lou B, Liang L, Lin X. Nine-year analysis of isolated pathogens and antibiotic susceptibilities of microbial keratitis from a large referral eye center in southern China. Infect Drug Resist. 2019;12(0):1295–302.
379. Green M, Carnt N, Apel A, Stapleton F. Queensland microbial keratitis database: 2005–2015. Br J Ophthalmol. 2019;103(10):1481.

380. Ting DSJ, Ho CS, Cairns J, Elsahn A, Al-Aqaba M, Boswell T, et al. 12-year analysis of incidence, microbiological profiles and in vitro antimicrobial susceptibility of infectious keratitis: the Nottingham Infectious Keratitis Study. Br J Ophthalmol. 2021;105(3):328–33.
381. Khoo P, Cabrera-Aguas MP, Nguyen V, Lahra MM, Watson SL. Microbial keratitis in Sydney, Australia: risk factors, patient outcomes, and seasonal variation. Graefe's Arch Clin Exp Ophthalmol. 2020;258(8):1745–55.
382. Bajracharya L, Bade AR, Gurung R, Dhakhwa K. Demography, risk factors, and clinical and microbiological features of microbial keratitis at a tertiary eye hospital in Nepal. Clin Ophthalmol. 2020;14:3219–26.
383. Soleimani M, Tabatabaei SA, Masoumi A, Mirshahi R, Ghahvechian H, Tayebi F, et al. Infectious keratitis: trends in microbiological and antibiotic sensitivity patterns. Eye. 2021;35(11):3110–5.
384. Hoffman JJ, Yadav R, Sanyam SD, Chaudhary P, Roshan A, Singh SK, et al. Microbial keratitis in Nepal: predicting the microbial aetiology from clinical features. J Fungi. 2022;8(2):201.
385. Shekhawat NS, Hall LN, Sulewski ME, Woreta F, Wang J, Smith K, et al. Corneal culture and antibiotic susceptibility results for microbial keratitis in the mid-Atlantic region of the United States, 2016 to 2020. Eye Contact Lens: Sci Clin Pr. 2023;49(7):267–74.
386. Kusumesh R, Ambastha A, Arya LK, Kumari A, Kumari N, Sinha BP, et al. Epidemiological and microbiological profiles of microbial keratitis in a tertiary eye center in Eastern India (Bihar). Indian J Ophthalmol. 2023;71(11):3506–12.
387. Kang L, Lu MC, Niziol LM, Greenwald MF, Mian SI, Thibodeau A, et al. Microbial keratitis isolates at a midwestern tertiary eye care center. Cornea. 2023;42(12):1488–96.
388. Ngarmsom R, Horatanaruang O. Epidemiology of microbial keratitis at a tertiary care hospital in Southern Thailand. Clin Ophthalmol. 2024;18(0):1267–75.
389. Kase C, Boppré YT, Rocchetti TT, Yu MCZ, Fernandes AG, Hofling-Lima AL. Microbial keratitis in Sao Paulo, Brazil: a 10-year review of laboratory results, epidemiological features, and risk factors. Arq Bras Oftalmol. 2023;87(6):e2022–00660.
390. Sharma P, Chipeta C, O'Kane K, Whiteman A, Francis B, Thornton R, et al. Five-year analysis of microbial keratitis incidence, isolates, and in vitro antimicrobial sensitivity in the South West of England: an epidemiological study. Microorganisms. 2025;13(7):1578.
391. Xu Y, Sun B, Shen Y, Xu H, Gu Y, Mao L, et al. Etiological characteristics of 3,691 cases of microbial keratitis: an 8-year longitudinal study. Microbiol Spectr. 2025;13(5):e02630–24.
392. Yamada N, Iwamoto N, Sakuma A, Sunada J, Aoki R, Mikuni M, et al. The temporal distribution and microbial spectrum in infectious keratitis: a comprehensive single-center study. J Clin Med. 2025;14(5):1613.
393. Ahmadikia K, Gharehbolagh SA, Fallah B, Eshkaleti MN, Malekifar P, Rahsepar S, et al. Distribution, prevalence, and causative agents of fungal keratitis: a systematic review and meta-analysis (1990 to 2020). Front Cell Infect Microbiol. 2021;11:698780.
394. Yue X, Wang A, Wang H, Li Q, Yue X. Evaluation of a new fluorescent reagent, fluorescent brightener 85, for the diagnosis of suspected onychomycosis compared with potassium hydroxide. Mycoses. 2018;61(4):279–82.
395. Shukla PK, Kumar M, Keshava GBS. Mycotic keratitis: an overview of diagnosis and therapy. Mycoses. 2008;51(3):183–99.
396. Younger JR, Johnson RD, Holland GN, Page JP, Nepomuceno RL, Glasgow BJ, et al. Microbiologic and histopathologic assessment of corneal biopsies in the evaluation of microbial keratitis. Am J Ophthalmol. 2012;154(3):512–519.e2.
397. Robaei D, Chan UT, Khoo P, Cherepanoff S, Li YC, Hanrahan J, et al. Corneal biopsy for diagnosis of recalcitrant microbial keratitis. Graefe's Arch Clin Exp Ophthalmol. 2018;256(8):1527–33.
398. Hwang DG. Lamellar flap corneal biopsy. Ophthalmic Surg. 1993;24(8):512–5.
399. Behera HS, Srigyan D. Evaluation of polymerase chain reaction over routine microbial diagnosis for the diagnosis of fungal keratitis. Optom Vis Sci. 2021;98(3):280–4.

400. Htun ZM, Rotchanapreeda T, Rujirawat T, Lohnoo T, Yingyong W, Kumsang Y, et al. Loop-mediated isothermal amplification (LAMP) for identification of pythium insidiosum. Int J Infect Dis. 2020;101:149–59.
401. Arbefeville S, Harris A, Ferrieri P. Comparison of sequencing the D2 region of the large subunit ribosomal RNA gene (MicroSEQ®) versus the internal transcribed spacer (ITS) regions using two public databases for identification of common and uncommon clinically relevant fungal species. J Microbiol Methods. 2017;140:40–6.
402. Kuo MT, Hsu SL, You HL, Kuo SF, Fang PC, Yu HJ, et al. Diagnosing fungal keratitis and simultaneously identifying fusarium and aspergillus keratitis with a dot hybridization array. J Fungi. 2022;8(1):64.
403. Doan T, Pinsky BA. Current and future molecular diagnostics for ocular infectious diseases. Curr Opin Ophthalmol. 2016;27(6):561–7.
404. Goodwin S, McPherson JD, McCombie WR. Coming of age: ten years of next-generation sequencing technologies. Nat Rev Genet. 2016;17(6):333–51.
405. Jayakumar M, Parthasarathy A. Isolated anterior-chamber fungal flocculosus in a healthy child with seeding through the trabecular meshwork. TNOA J Ophthalmic Sci Res. 2019;57(2):167.
406. Silverman RH. Focused ultrasound in ophthalmology. Clin Ophthalmol. 2016;10(0):1865–75.
407. Flynn HW, Batra NR, Schwartz SG, Iyer PG, Lytvynchuk L, Grzybowski A. Endophthalmitis in clinical practice. Clin Pr. 2023:45–60.
408. Konstantopoulos A, Kuo J, Anderson D, Hossain P. Assessment of the use of anterior segment optical coherence tomography in microbial keratitis. Am J Ophthalmol. 2008;146(4):534–542.e2.
409. Sharma N, Singhal D, Maharana PK, Agarwal T, Sinha R, Satpathy G, et al. Spectral domain anterior segment optical coherence tomography in fungal keratitis. Cornea. 2018;37(11):1388–94.
410. Ting DSJ, Gopal BP, Deshmukh R, Seitzman GD, Said DG, Dua HS. Diagnostic armamentarium of infectious keratitis: a comprehensive review. Ocul Surf. 2022;23:27–39.
411. Brasnu E, Bourcier T, Dupas B, Degorge S, Rodallec T, Laroche L, et al. In vivo confocal microscopy in fungal keratitis. Br J Ophthalmol. 2007;91(5):588.
412. Takezawa Y, Shiraishi A, Noda E, Hara Y, Yamaguchi M, Uno T, et al. Effectiveness of in vivo confocal microscopy in detecting filamentous fungi during clinical course of fungal keratitis. Cornea. 2010;29(12):1346–52.
413. Zemba M, Radu M, Istrate S, Dumitrescu OM, Ionescu MA, Vatafu A, et al. Intrastromal injections in the management of infectious keratitis. Pharmaceutics. 2023;15(4):1091.
414. Kalavathy CM, Parmar P, Kaliamurthy J, Philip VR, Ramalingam MDK, Jesudasan CAN, et al. Comparison of topical itraconazole 1% with topical natamycin 5% for the treatment of filamentous fungal keratitis. Cornea. 2005;24(4):449–52.
415. van der Wekken-Pas L, de Haas P, Wisse R, Rados M, van der Elst K. Candida keratitis and endopthalmitis after corneal transplantation; two case reports, a novel regimen and literature overview of therapeutic options. Eur J Ophthalmol. 2021;33(2):NP73–8.
416. Kernt M, Kampik A. Intraocular caspofungin: in vitro safety profile for human ocular cells. Mycoses. 2011;54(4):e110–21.
417. Liang Q-F, Jin X-Y, Wang X-L, Sun X-G. Effect of topical application of terbinafine on fungal keratitis. Chin Méd J. 2009;122(16):1884–8.

Fungal Endophthalmitis

8

Henry W. Zhou and Lucy H. Young

8.1 Introduction

Fungal endophthalmitis is a fungal infection of the intraocular contents. The recorded history of fungal ophthalmic infections begins with von Graefe's description of *Actinomyces* canaliculitis in 1854 [1]. The first two cases of intraocular fungal infection were described by Sorokin in 1881, and the first reported case of culture-positive fungal endophthalmitis was reported by Romer in 1902 in a case of *Aspergillus fumigatus* endophthalmitis secondary to penetrating eye trauma [2, 3]. Cavara compiled these early case reports, from which the exogenous causes were later organized into three distinct categories by Rychener in 1933: contiguous spread of external ocular infection, penetration from eye trauma, and iatrogenic from intraocular surgery [3]. The diagnosis and management of fungal endophthalmitis, in both its exogenous and endogenous forms, remain challenging. In this chapter, we provide an overview of the epidemiology, etiologies and pathogenesis, clinical presentation, diagnosis and differential diagnosis, treatment, and prognosis and complications of fungal endophthalmitis.

8.2 Epidemiology

Fungal endophthalmitis is relatively rare compared to bacterial endophthalmitis from all sources [4]. However, the incidence rate varies significantly when considering the etiologies of endophthalmitis. The overall incidence of fungal endophthalmitis post-keratoplasty is very low at 0.12–0.01% [5–7]. Incidence of fungal endophthalmitis postcataract extraction is even lower at 0.005–0.002% [8]. While a

H. W. Zhou · L. H. Young (✉)
Department of Ophthalmology, Mass Eye and Ear, Harvard Medical School, Boston, MA, USA
e-mail: hzhou22@meei.harvard.edu; Lucy_Young@meei.harvard.edu

M. C. Ramírez-Soto (ed.), *Fungal Eye Infections*,
https://doi.org/10.1007/978-3-032-19923-2_8

small minority of postsurgical exogenous endophthalmitis cases are fungal [5], significantly more cases of culture-proven endogenous endophthalmitis cases are of fungal origin (ranging from 18% to 62%) [9–11]. Certain regions may be more prone to fungal endophthalmitis, as one large multicenter review from India demonstrated that up to one in five cases of endophthalmitis might be of fungal origin [12]. Nevertheless, endophthalmitis remains relatively rare from a population-wide perspective, and fungal endophthalmitis is a yet-smaller proportion of overall endophthalmitis cases. However, in light of the current opioid crisis in the United States of America and other countries, and the corresponding increase in intravenous drug use, rates of endogenous fungal endophthalmitis have been on the rise [13, 14]. A corresponding shift in the demographics of such infections now includes higher numbers of young and otherwise healthy individuals with substance use disorders.

8.3 Etiologies and Pathogenesis

Fungal endophthalmitis is classified as either endogenous, originating from a systemic fungal infection that spreads through the blood to the eye, or exogenous, resulting from direct introduction of fungal organisms into the eye due to injury, surgery, or other external factors.

8.3.1 Exogenous Endophthalmitis

Exogenous sources of infection account for a majority of fungal endophthalmitis cases [4, 15]. Exogenous endophthalmitis may arise from a number of sources, namely from external ocular infection (e.g., keratitis), from penetrating eye trauma, or from intraocular surgery as originally outlined by Rychener [3]. Although modern advancements in ophthalmology further subdivide the postoperative group into more specific cohorts (postintravitreal injection fungal endophthalmitis being one such example).

Keratitis-associated endophthalmitis occurs when corneal infections spread posteriorly to involve the aqueous or vitreous humor [16]. Keratitis-associated fungal endophthalmitis is rare, but fungal infections of the cornea are more likely to cause endophthalmitis than bacterial infections of the cornea [17, 18]. Local environment, such as average temperature and humidity, may play a significant role in the variation seen between reported rates of keratitis-associated fungal endophthalmitis between different study sites, as overall rates of fungal keratitis appear to be lower in areas with more hostile climates (colder environments with less humidity) [19]. Unlike post-traumatic and postoperative associated cases, the most common etiology of keratitis-associated fungal endophthalmitis is *Fusarium*, followed by *Aspergillus* [15, 17, 20, 21].

Post-traumatic endophthalmitis is a rare complication of penetrating eye trauma [22]. Certain clinical features of open globe injuries are associated with a higher risk of endophthalmitis, such as delayed surgical repair beyond 24 to 36 hours and placement of primary IOL [22, 23]. Fungal endophthalmitis from penetrating eye injury is significantly less common than bacterial endophthalmitis, but some patients may develop mixed infections with both bacterial and fungal species [4, 24]. *Aspergillus* infection is more common than *Fusarium*, and yeast-form species such as *Candida* are also potential pathogens [24–26]. A vast number of organisms may be encountered in post-traumatic endophthalmitis, including *A. fumigatus*, *A. nidulans*, *A. niger*, *A. flavus*; *Fusarium solani*, *F. equiseti,* and *F. moniliforme*; *Bipolaris sorokiniana*; *Curvularia geniculata*; *Conidia*; and *Penicillium* [24]. *Sporothrix* has also been reported as an exceedingly rare cause of intraocular infections in the USA and Brazil [27].

Postsurgical endophthalmitis can encompass a wide range of intraocular surgeries and procedures with the potential to introduce infectious organisms into the intraocular space; these include but are not limited to cataract surgery, vitrectomy, penetrating keratoplasty, and intravitreal injection. Postcataract surgery endophthalmitis is the most well-studied postsurgical scenario, with the Endophthalmitis Vitrectomy Study providing standardized guidelines for the treatment of such cases [28]. However, the Endophthalmitis Vitrectomy Study excluded patients with a strong suspicion of fungal endophthalmitis, and postsurgical fungal endophthalmitis is generally less studied and less understood relative to its more common bacterial counterpart. Though postcataract surgery fungal endophthalmitis is considered far less common than bacterial etiologies [15, 29], this may not hold true in all climates/areas; studies from India and Jeju Island, as examples of regions with warmer climates and higher humidity, demonstrate generally higher rates of postcataract fungal endophthalmitis relative to studies from the West [30–32]. Postcataract surgery fungal endophthalmitis is most commonly caused by *Aspergillus* [17, 30, 31]. Like in cases of cataract surgery with primary intraocular lens (IOL) implantation, exogenous endophthalmitis is a rare complication of secondary IOL surgery. Similarly, the responsible pathogens are predominantly bacterial, with no reported cases of fungal endophthalmitis arising from secondary IOLs [33, 34]. Contaminated medical products and devices comprise another subgroup of patients with fungal endophthalmitis, as evidenced by one report from South Korea detailing a national outbreak of *Fusarium* endophthalmitis resulting from contaminated sodium hyaluronate (viscoelastic) [35]. Buchta and colleagues similarly described a series of 20 patients with *Fusarium oxysporum* endophthalmitis following cataract surgery. The cause of this outbreak was deemed most likely secondary to compromised viscoelasticity [36]. A cohort of patients in New York suffered from postintravitreal injection fungal endophthalmitis from *Bipolaris hawaiiensis* contamination from a single compounding pharmacy [37]. Finally, postsurgical fungal endophthalmitis is a rare but reported occurrence following corneal transplant surgeries such as penetrating keratoplasty (PK) and Descemet stripping automated endothelial keratoplasty (DSAEK) [5, 38]. *Candida* species comprised the vast majority of postcorneal surgery fungal endophthalmitis cases, with one reported case of *Aspergillus* endophthalmitis [5, 38, 39].

8.3.2 Endogenous Endophthalmitis

Endogenous endophthalmitis is a result of infectious organisms seeding ocular structures such as the choroid or vitreous via hematogenous spread. The most common cause of endogenous endophthalmitis is infection with *Candida* species, followed by *Aspergillus* [15]. Incidence of endogenous fungal endophthalmitis in patients with disseminated infection ranges from 2.5 to 45%, and recent practice of prophylaxis and prompt treatment of patients with positive fungal cultures have decreased the rate of ocular complications [40].

Patients afflicted with endogenous fungal endophthalmitis tend to have predisposing systemic risk factors resulting in immunosuppression, although cases occur in immunocompetent, otherwise healthy individuals [41]. Endogenous fungal endophthalmitis must also have a source of fungemia, including IV drug use, indwelling intravenous catheters, urinary tract infections, or prolonged hospital/ICU stays [4, 14]. Other risk factors for the development of endogenous fungal endophthalmitis include total parenteral nutrition, broad-spectrum antibiotics, recent abdominal surgery, neutropenia, glucocorticoid therapy, solid organ transplant, diabetes mellitus, chemotherapy, and chronic lung disease [15]. Endogenous fungal endophthalmitis cases caused by mold species (e.g., *Aspergillus*, *Fusarium*) are likely often missed while the patient is alive, due in part to high mortality rates within this very sick population and inability to report ophthalmic symptoms [42, 43].

Causative agents of endogenous fungal endophthalmitis include yeast forms such as *Candida albicans*, *Candida tropicalis*, *Cryptococcus neoformans*, and mold forms such as *Aspergillus fumigatus*, *Aspergillus glaucus*, *Fusarium oxysporum*, *Aspergillus terreus*, *Aspergillus niger*, and *Cladophialophora devriessi* [41]. The dimorphic fungus *Sporothrix schenkii* has also been identified in patients with endogenous endophthalmitis, and is more commonly seen in immunosuppressed patients from hyperendemic areas [27, 44, 45].

8.4 Clinical Presentation

The clinical presentation of fungal endophthalmitis differs based on the underlying etiology, as discussed previously. Although fungal endophthalmitis is generally more insidious than bacterial endophthalmitis, cases of exogenous fungal endophthalmitis tend to present more acutely than cases of endogenous fungal endophthalmitis, with more rapid progression of symptoms and exam findings, and may mimic bacterial endophthalmitis. A carefully collected clinical history is instrumental in the management of endophthalmitis with features concerning exogenous infection [17, 40].

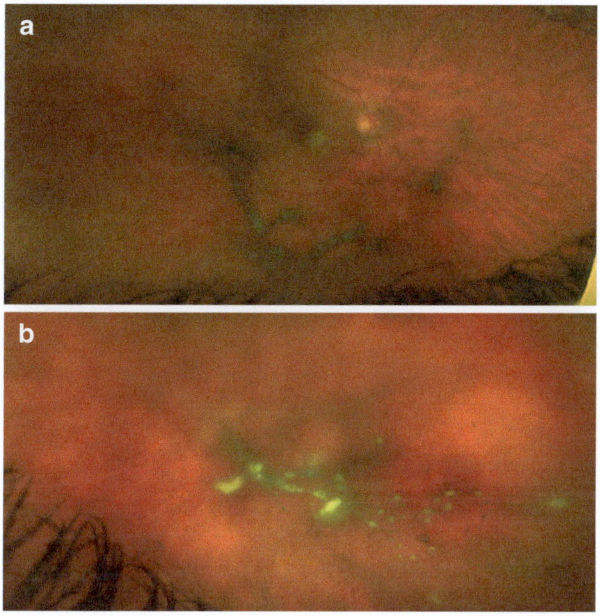

Fig. 8.1 String of pearls vitritis in fungal endophthalmitis. Widefield photographs of two separate patients, right eye/OD (**a**) and left eye/OS (**b**), demonstrating the classic "string of pearls" pattern of vitreous condensates secondary to *Candida* endophthalmitis. (Courtesy of Demetrios Vavvas, MD, PhD)

Patients with fungal endophthalmitis will typically report progressive vision loss and floaters that may progress over days to weeks. Other commonly reported symptoms include discomfort and pain, eye redness, and photophobia. The degree of vision loss can be strikingly debilitating in many cases, and many patients present with 20/200 vision or worse [46]. Patients with endogenous fungal endophthalmitis may also have accompanying systemic symptoms such as fever, chills, or weight loss, depending on the nature of the systemic infection.

On examination, the hallmark finding seen in fungal endophthalmitis is the presence of vitritis. Some specific patterns of vitritis and vitreous debris are associated with certain fungal infections, for example, the "string of pearls," "snowballs," or "fluff balls," often described in fungal endophthalmitis (Fig. 8.1) [16]. At an early stage, examination may reveal only chorioretinal lesions—often described as creamy-white, well-circumscribed lesions deep to the retina—without associated vitritis [40]. Patients with candidemia are more likely to have chorioretinitis without endophthalmitis [47].

Clinicians should try to distinguish between bacterial and fungal endophthalmitis for timely diagnosis and treatment. Features that typically help distinguish between bacterial and fungal endophthalmitis are displayed in Table 8.1.

Table 8.1 Clinical presentation of bacterial versus fungal endophthalmitis

	Bacterial endophthalmitis	*Fungal endophthalmitis*
Onset	Acute (hours to days)	Subacute to chronic (days to weeks), dependent on mechanism
Pain severity	Severe	Mild to moderate
Visual acuity loss	Rapid, profound loss	Gradual to rapid loss, dependent on the mechanism
Anterior chamber	Dense hypopyon, fibrin reaction	"Clumped" aggregates
Vitreous appearance	Diffuse vitritis	Vitritis with "string of pearls"
Retinal findings	Rapid retinal necrosis in some cases	Chorioretinal lesions, cotton-ball infiltrates
Intraocular pressure	Variable, often elevated at presentation	Normal to low

8.5 Diagnosis

Fungal endophthalmitis is a clinical diagnosis, though imaging and laboratory testing can provide significant supporting evidence in the appropriate clinical context.

8.5.1 Imaging

B-scan ultrasonography of the eye is often obtained when fungal endophthalmitis is suspected, particularly when the posterior segment is not amenable to direct examination. B-scan findings in fungal endophthalmitis may vary, but common features include chorioretinal masses and vitreous opacities or stranding [4].

8.5.2 Laboratory Diagnosis

Aqueous humor and/or vitreous samples are obtained in cases with high suspicion for endophthalmitis. Vitreous cultures are generally considered more appropriate than anterior chamber (AC) cultures for the diagnosis of fungal endophthalmitis [48], although both methods are hampered by relatively low sensitivity [49]. The acquisition of vitreous samples from vitrectomy demonstrates significantly higher rates of culture positivity [50]. Polymerase chain reaction (PCR) appears to have improved sensitivity for the detection of fungal infections, but the technology is limited by the number of pathogens that can be simultaneously targeted during an assay [51–53]. Vitreous galactomannan and 1–3 β-D-Glucan assays have been reported as useful biomarkers for insidious cases of fungal endophthalmitis, particularly culture-negative fungal endophthalmitis [54]. There are additional diagnostic tests with the potential for increased sensitivity, reduced testing costs, and faster turnaround time currently being developed: next-generation sequencing, such as nanopore sequencing [55], and CRISPR-CAS12a-based assays [56]. However, more data will be needed before these tests are viable for clinical use. Blood cultures should be obtained in cases where endogenous endophthalmitis is suspected, along with other ancillary testing such as an echocardiogram, liver ultrasound, or other testing/imaging in collaboration with internal medicine and infectious disease colleagues [15, 57]. Notably, negative blood cultures are possible in cases of endogenous fungal endophthalmitis, as fungemia may have been transient [15].

Standard microbiological evaluation for fungal organisms comprises direct microscopic examination using calcofluor white, Gram, and Giemsa stains, coupled with culture on blood agar, brain heart infusion, thioglycolate broth, potato dextrose agar, and Sabouraud's dextrose agar. A positive organism stain and culture is invaluable for accurate diagnosis and effective treatment of fungal endophthalmitis. However, culture media require incubation for a minimum of 14 days prior to reporting negative results. An extended incubation period is essential for the detection of slower-growing fungal organisms. Blood culture bottles have a higher fungal detection rate than other traditional forms of culture media, such as broth and solid media [58].

8.6 Differential Diagnosis

Accurate diagnosis of fungal endophthalmitis can be difficult even when several tests and assays are employed. The differential diagnosis for fungal endophthalmitis is broad and primarily includes infectious, inflammatory, and neoplastic etiologies. If misdiagnosed, the treatment of some masqueraders (such as noninfectious uveitis) can significantly worsen fungal endophthalmitis and lead to poor outcomes.

The most common misdiagnosis in cases of fungal endophthalmitis is noninfectious uveitis and other inflammatory etiologies [59]. Infectious etiologies include bacterial endophthalmitis, in addition to a variety of rarer etiologies. Lymphoma is a neoplastic process that commonly masquerades as other diseases, including fungal endophthalmitis. A detailed list of differential diagnoses is found in Table 8.2.

The ongoing opioid crisis accentuates the importance of establishing accurate accounts of prior/ongoing intravenous drug use. Many patients will not be forthcoming with their intravenous drug use history until asked directly, and some may not divulge the true extent of their substance use until they fully understand its

Table 8.2 Differential diagnosis for fungal endophthalmitis

Infectious	Noninfectious
Bacterial endophthalmitis	Lymphoma
Syphilis	Sarcoidosis
Toxoplasmosis	Intermediate/posterior uveitis
Tuberculosis	Vogt-Koyanagi-Harada disease
Herpes simplex virus	Sympathetic ophthalmia
Varicella zoster virus	Behcet's disease

necessity in accurate diagnosis and proper treatment. Moreover, these patients may not fall into the textbook cohort of endogenous endophthalmitis cases (i.e., frail, older, and/or sick-appearing). All cases of intraocular inflammation should prompt a high index of suspicion for infectious endophthalmitis, particularly in the setting of drug use [14].

8.7 Treatment

Medical management of fungal endophthalmitis may involve systemic and/or intravitreal antifungals. Systemic antifungals of choice include the azole-class medications, including voriconazole and fluconazole, which are particularly effective for *Candida* infection. However, growing resistance to this class of medications has become a point of increasing concern [60]. Beyond antimicrobial susceptibility, local therapeutic concentrations within ocular tissue must also be considered for each antifungal agent. Voriconazole's lipophilicity enhances penetration into ocular tissue relative to fluconazole [61]. Amphotericin B, while potent against many fungal species, suffers from relatively poor penetration given its large molecular weight and highly protein-bound structure [61]. To bypass the issue of ocular penetration, antifungal agents may also be delivered directly to ocular tissue via intravitreal injection. Agents of choice for intravitreal injection include voriconazole and amphotericin B [62, 63]. Culture samples should also be obtained at the time of intravitreal injection. An algorithm for the medical management of fungal endophthalmitis is shown in Fig. 8.2 and detailed in the following sections.

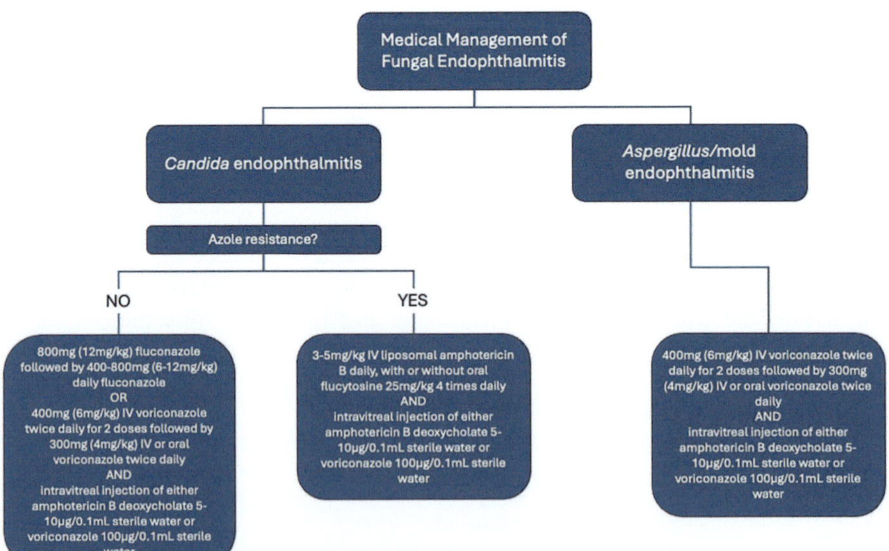

Fig. 8.2 Algorithm for the medical management of fungal endophthalmitis

8.7.1 Medical Management in *Candida* Endophthalmitis

Patients with *Candida* endophthalmitis, like many cases of endophthalmitis, are often managed in conjunction with colleagues in infectious diseases. For *Candida* isolates susceptible to fluconazole or voriconazole, a loading dose of 800 mg (12 mg/kg) fluconazole followed by 400–800 mg (6–12 mg/kg) daily fluconazole may be employed. Alternatively, a loading dose of 400 mg (6 mg/kg) IV voriconazole twice daily for two doses followed by 300 mg (4 mg/kg) IV or oral voriconazole twice daily is also appropriate. Voriconazole has a superior bioavailability profile relative to fluconazole [64]. For organisms resistant to fluconazole or voriconazole, liposomal amphotericin B 3–5 mg/kg IV daily, with or without oral flucytosine 25 mg/kg four times daily, is recommended. In addition to systemic therapy, intravitreal injection of either amphotericin B deoxycholate 5–10 μg/0.1 mL sterile water or voriconazole 100 μg/0.1 mL sterile water is recommended. Intravitreal amphotericin may be preferred given a longer half-life relative to intravitreal voriconazole (8.9 days vs. 2.5–6.5 h, respectively) [65]. Topical voriconazole, 1% solution applied every 1–2 h, demonstrates good penetration through the cornea and into the anterior chamber [66]. Treatment should last at least 4–6 weeks, with total duration of treatment pending clinical resolution [62].

8.7.2 Medical Management in *Aspergillus* Endophthalmitis

Similar to cases of *Candida* endophthalmitis, fungal endophthalmitis caused by *Aspergillus* should also be managed jointly with infectious disease physicians. Recommended therapy for all cases of *Aspergillus* endophthalmitis includes systemic oral or intravenous voriconazole (similar dosing as *Candida* regimens detailed above). In addition to systemic therapy, intravitreal injection of either amphotericin B deoxycholate or voriconazole (similar to *Candida* regimens) is recommended. Amphotericin B deoxycholate injected intravitreally appears to be particularly essential for adequate treatment of *Aspergillus* endophthalmitis [63]. However, other studies demonstrate that intravitreal voriconazole may provide the broadest spectrum of antifungal coverage and confer the least likelihood of resistance in cases of exogenous fungal endophthalmitis [67]. Echinocandins, such as micafungin and caspofungin, are generally not used for the treatment of fungal endophthalmitis due to poor bioavailability and penetration into the vitreous. However, there are reports of successful treatment with intravitreal caspofungin in cases of molds with high antifungal resistance [68].

8.7.3 Adverse Outcomes of Medical Therapy for Fungal Endophthalmitis

Antifungal agents employed in the treatment of fungal endophthalmitis are associated with a number of adverse effects. Within the azole class, fluconazole is generally better-tolerated compared to voriconazole, but all azole antifungals carry the risk of hepatic toxicity, cardiac arrhythmias, fever, and hypertension. Voriconazole serum concentrations are prone to more variability relative to fluconazole, as voriconazole follows nonlinear Michaelis-Menten pharmacokinetics while fluconazole adheres to linear pharmacokinetics [4]. Therefore, voriconazole trough levels must be carefully monitored to avoid adverse effects [69].

Amphotericin B is associated with the highest rate of systemic and ocular toxicities. Nephrotoxicity is the most prominent systemic adverse effect, particularly with conventional formulations; liposomal amphotericin B may reduce this risk and confer higher ocular penetration. Other adverse effects of amphotericin B include nausea, vomiting, rigors, fever, hypertension, hypotension, and hypoxia [4].

8.7.4 Surgical Management of Fungal Endophthalmitis

Surgical management of fungal endophthalmitis involves removal of the vitreous via pars plana vitrectomy (PPV). PPV serves both diagnostic and therapeutic roles in the management of fungal endophthalmitis, as culture yields from PPV are significantly higher than yields from needle vitreous tap alone [70]. PPV also mechanically reduces infection load and inflammatory mediators. However, there are risks of operating on an acutely inflamed eye. Current literature has not shown definitive evidence of long-term better visual acuity outcomes from PPV compared to medical management alone [46, 71]. For cases with intraocular foreign bodies causing fungal endophthalmitis, or cases of recalcitrant fungal endophthalmitis in eyes with intraocular lens (IOL) implants, surgery for explanation of a foreign body or an IOL may be necessary for complete resolution of infection [72]. Postoperative complications of PPV in eyes with fungal endophthalmitis include retinal detachment, cataract, hypotony, and choroidal effusions [73]. A case of fungal endophthalmitis managed successfully with surgical intervention is shown in Fig. 8.3.

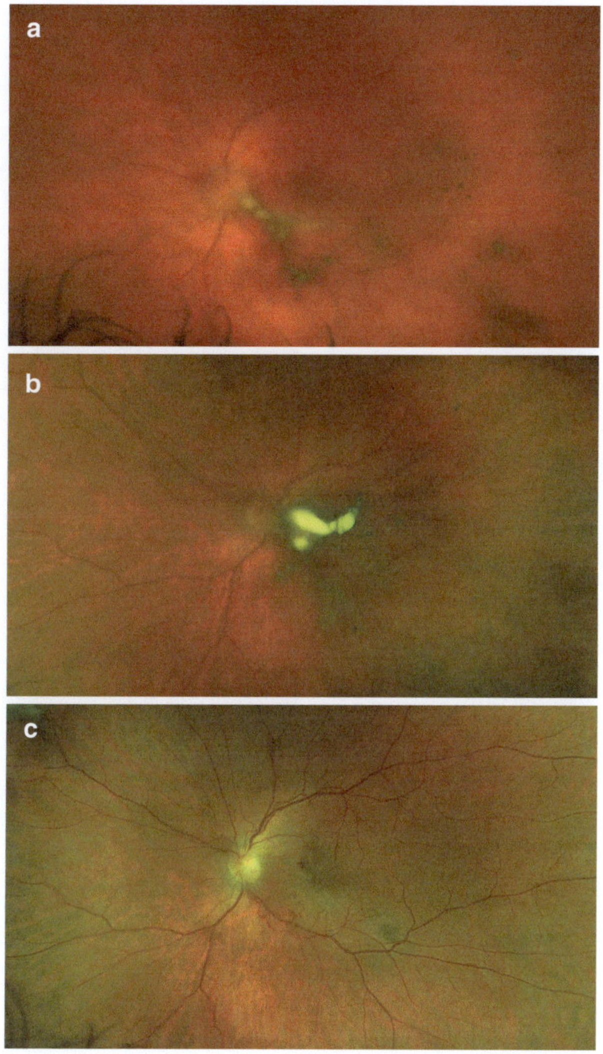

Fig. 8.3 Fungal endophthalmitis managed with surgery. (**a**) Widefield photograph of the patient's left eye demonstrating vitritis, vitreous clumps, and chorioretinal lesions. (**b**) 1 month later, and 1 week following vitreous tap and injection of voriconazole. Worsening preretinal/chorioretinal lesions, and with persistent vitritis. (**c**) 1 week later, now 5 days status post-pars plana vitrectomy, demonstrating good functional and anatomic outcomes. (Courtesy of Dean Eliott, MD)

8.8 Prognosis and Complications

Complications of fungal endophthalmitis include retinal detachment, cataract, hypotony, and phthisis [17, 71, 74]. Early vitrectomy in patients with fungal endophthalmitis may reduce the rate of retinal detachment (but notably, early vitrectomy does not improve visual acuity outcomes) [71, 75]. Patients with fungal endophthalmitis secondary to open globe injury have the worst visual outcomes and a high rate of enucleation [17]. Likewise, cases of fungal endophthalmitis secondary to molds (e.g., *Aspergillus* species) are more likely to undergo enucleation [41]. Patients with

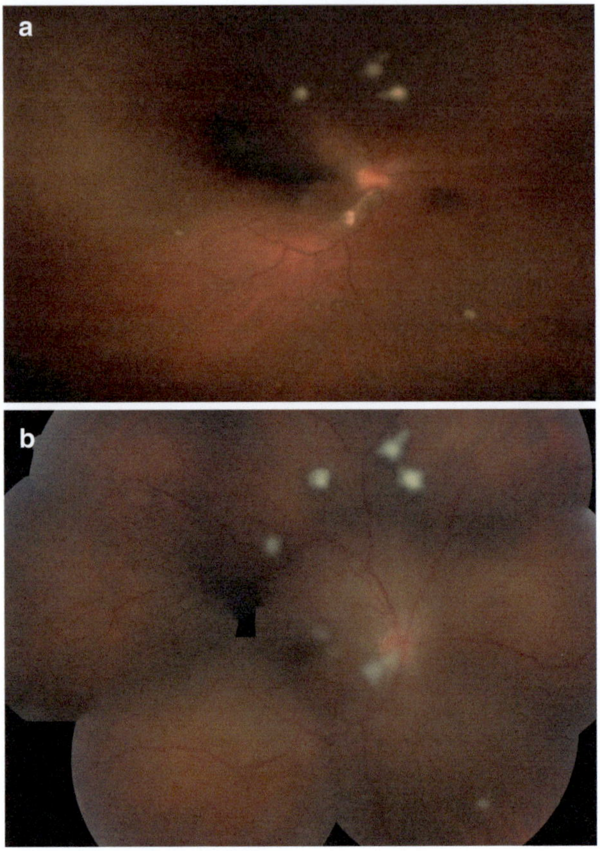

Fig. 8.4 Endogenous endophthalmitis managed with oral antifungals alone. (**a**) Widefield photograph of a patient with presumed endogenous endophthalmitis (patient deferred blood cultures and tap and inject) demonstrating several active chorioretinal lesions and vitritis. Inferior to the disc is an area of chronic fibrosis, likely from prior infection. (**b**) Composite color fundus photographs taken 2 months later after a course of oral fluconazole. Vitritis had resolved, and visual acuity remained good with foveal sparing

endogenous fungal endophthalmitis have high rates of overall mortality [74, 76]. Some cases of transient fungemia secondary to intravenous drug use and without active endovascular infection may have good outcomes with oral antifungals alone—one such case is demonstrated in Fig. 8.4. Nevertheless, patients with fungal endophthalmitis are at high risk of poor outcomes and may require urgent vitreoretinal intervention and multidisciplinary care.

References

1. von Graefe A. Koncretionen im unteren Thranenrohrchen durch Pilzbildung. Arch f Ophth. 1854;i:284.
2. Romer P. Eine intraoculare Schimmelpilz-Infection. Klin Monatsbl Augenheilkd. 1902:40;331–3.
3. Rychener RO. Intra-ocular mycosis. Trans Am Ophthalmol Soc. 1933;31:477–96.
4. Haseeb AA, Elhusseiny AM, Siddiqui MZ, Ahmad KT, Sallam AB. Fungal Endophthalmitis: a comprehensive review. J Fungi (Basel). 2021;7:996.
5. Keyhani K, Seedor JA, Shah MK, Terraciano AJ, Ritterband DC. The incidence of fungal keratitis and endophthalmitis following penetrating keratoplasty. Cornea. 2005;24:288–91.

6. Chen JY, Jones MN, Srinivasan S, Neal TJ, Armitage WJ, Kaye SB, et al. Endophthalmitis after penetrating keratoplasty. Ophthalmology. 2015;122:25–30.
7. Kloess PM, Stulting RD, Waring GO, Wilson LA. Bacterial and fungal endophthalmitis after penetrating keratoplasty. Am J Ophthalmol. 1993;115:309–16.
8. Du DT, Wagoner A, Barone SB, Zinderman CE, Kelman JA, MaCurdy TE, et al. Incidence of endophthalmitis after corneal transplant or cataract surgery in a medicare population. Ophthalmology. 2014;121:290–8.
9. Lim HW, Shin JW, Cho HY, Kim HK, Kang SW, Song SJ, et al. Endogenous endophthalmitis in the Korean population: a six-year retrospective study. Retina. 2014;34:592.
10. Binder MI, Chua J, Kaiser PK, Procop GW, Isada CM. Endogenous endophthalmitis: an 18-year review of culture-positive cases at a tertiary care center. Medicine (Baltimore). 2003;82:97–105.
11. Schiedler V, Scott IU, Flynn HW, Davis JL, Benz MS, Miller D. Culture-proven endogenous endophthalmitis: clinical features and visual acuity outcomes. Am J Ophthalmol. 2004;137:725–31.
12. Das T, Agarwal M, Anand AR, Behera UC, Bhende M, Das AV, et al. Fungal endophthalmitis: analysis of 730 consecutive eyes from 7 tertiary eye care centers in India. Ophthalmol Retina. 2022;6:243–51.
13. Luong PM, Tsui E, Batra N, Chapman CB, Zegans ME. Vision loss associated with the opioid epidemic. JAMA Ophthalmol. 2017;135:1449–51.
14. Mir TA, Papudesu C, Fang W, Hinkle DM. Incidence of drug use-related endogenous endophthalmitis hospitalizations in the United States, 2003 to 2016. JAMA Ophthalmol. 2021;139:18–26.
15. Durand ML. Bacterial and fungal endophthalmitis. Clin Microbiol Rev. 2017;30:597–613.
16. Durand ML. Endophthalmitis. Clin Microbiol Infect. 2013;19:227–34.
17. Wykoff CC, Flynn HW, Miller D, Scott IU, Alfonso EC. Exogenous fungal endophthalmitis: microbiology and clinical outcomes. Ophthalmology. 2008;115:1501–7, 1507.e1–2.
18. Henry CR, Flynn HW, Miller D, Forster RK, Alfonso EC. Infectious keratitis progressing to endophthalmitis: a 15-year study of microbiology, associated factors, and clinical outcomes. Ophthalmology. 2012;119:2443–9.
19. Malihi M, Li X, Patel S, Eck T, Chu DS, Zarbin MA, et al. Infectious keratitis-associated endophthalmitis: a 14-year study. Retina. 2017;37:662–6.
20. Shen Y-C, Wang C-Y, Tsai H-Y, Lee H-N. Intracameral voriconazole injection in the treatment of fungal endophthalmitis resulting from keratitis. Am J Ophthalmol. 2010;149:916–21.
21. Xie L, Zhong W, Shi W, Sun S. Spectrum of fungal keratitis in North China. Ophthalmology. 2006;113:1943–8.
22. Andreoli CM, Andreoli MT, Kloek CE, Ahuero AE, Vavvas D, Durand ML. Low rate of endophthalmitis in a large series of open globe injuries. Am J Ophthalmol. 2009;147:601–608.e2.
23. Tieger MG, Singh N, Bitar R, Makhoul K, Ashourizadeh H, Stryjewski TP, et al. Visual outcomes and risk of endophthalmitis in open globe injuries without intraocular foreign bodies with delayed repair. Ophthalmology. 2024;131:1398–402.
24. Long C, Liu B, Xu C, Jing Y, Yuan Z, Lin X. Causative organisms of post-traumatic endophthalmitis: a 20-year retrospective study. BMC Ophthalmol. 2014;14:34.
25. Jindal A, Moreker MR, Pathengay A, Khera M, Jalali S, Majji A, et al. Polymicrobial endophthalmitis: prevalence, causative organisms, and visual outcomes. J Ophthalmic Inflamm Infect. 2013;3:6.
26. Jindal A, Pathengay A, Mithal K, Jalali S, Mathai A, Pappuru RR, et al. Endophthalmitis after open globe injuries: changes in microbiological spectrum and isolate susceptibility patterns over 14 years. J Ophthalmic Inflamm Infect. 2014;4:5.
27. Ramírez-Soto MC, Tirado-Sánchez A, Bonifaz A. Ocular sporotrichosis. J Fungi. 2021;7:951.
28. Results of the endophthalmitis vitrectomy study: a randomized trial of immediate vitrectomy and of intravenous antibiotics for the treatment of postoperative bacterial endophthalmitis. Arch Ophthalmol 1995;113:1479–1496.

29. Mollan SP, Gao A, Lockwood A, Durrani OM, Butler L. Postcataract endophthalmitis: incidence and microbial isolates in a United Kingdom region from 1996 through 2004. J Cataract Refract Surg. 2007;33:265–8.
30. Gupta A, Gupta V, Gupta A, Dogra MR, Pandav SS, Ray P, et al. Spectrum and clinical profile of post cataract surgery endophthalmitis in North India. Indian J Ophthalmol. 2003;51:139–45.
31. Anand AR, Therese KL, Madhavan HN. Spectrum of aetiological agents of postoperative endophthalmitis and antibiotic susceptibility of bacterial isolates. Indian J Ophthalmol. 2000;48:123–8.
32. Park JH, Kim DY, Ha A, Ma DJ, Lee HJ, Jeong J, et al. Atypical microbiological feature of infectious endophthalmitis on Jeju Island: a 10-year study at a single tertiary referral center. J Ophthalmol. 2021;2021:6620926.
33. Scott IU, Flynn HW, Feuer W. Endophthalmitis after secondary intraocular lens implantation. A case-report study. Ophthalmology. 1995;102:1925–31.
34. Aaberg TM, Flynn HW, Schiffman J, Newton J. Nosocomial acute-onset postoperative endophthalmitis survey. A 10-year review of incidence and outcomes. Ophthalmology. 1998;105:1004–10.
35. Kim SW, Kim JH, Choi M, Lee SJ, Shin JP, Kim JG, et al. An outbreak of fungal endophthalmitis after cataract surgery in South Korea. JAMA Ophthalmol. 2023;141:226–33.
36. Buchta V, Feuermannová A, Váša M, Bašková L, Kutová R, Kubátová A, et al. Outbreak of fungal endophthalmitis due to Fusarium oxysporum following cataract surgery. Mycopathologia. 2014;177:115–21.
37. Sheyman AT, Cohen BZ, Friedman AH, Ackert JM. An outbreak of fungal endophthalmitis after intravitreal injection of compounded combined bevacizumab and triamcinolone. JAMA Ophthalmol. 2013;131:864–9.
38. Chew ACY, Mehta JS, Li L, Busmanis I, Tan DTH. Fungal endophthalmitis after descemet stripping automated endothelial keratoplasty—a case report. Cornea. 2010;29:346–9.
39. Mosca L, Guccione L, Toro ME, Scartozzi L, Fasciani R, Torelli R, et al. Non-pathogenic aspergillus oryzae acute exogenous endophthalmitis after penetrating keratoplasty: the first case report in the literature. Case Rep Ophthalmol. 2023;14:654–9.
40. Sallam A, Lynn W, McCluskey P, Lightman S. Endogenous Candida endophthalmitis. Expert Rev Anti-Infect Ther. 2006;4:675–85.
41. Sridhar J, Flynn HW, Kuriyan AE, Miller D, Albini T. Endogenous fungal endophthalmitis: risk factors, clinical features, and treatment outcomes in mold and yeast infections. J Ophthalmic Inflamm Infect. 2013;3:60.
42. Lamaris GA, Esmaeli B, Chamilos G, Desai A, Chemaly RF, Raad II, et al. Fungal endophthalmitis in a tertiary care cancer center: a review of 23 cases. Eur J Clin Microbiol Infect Dis. 2008;27:343–7.
43. Hunt KE, Glasgow BJ. Aspergillus endophthalmitis. An unrecognized endemic disease in orthotopic liver transplantation. Ophthalmology. 1996;103:757–67.
44. Ramírez Soto MC. Differences in clinical ocular outcomes between exogenous and endogenous endophthalmitis caused by Sporothrix: a systematic review of published literature. Br J Ophthalmol. 2018;102:977–82.
45. Chou B, McKay KM, Leveque TK. Thermal therapy for Sporothrix endogenous endophthalmitis of the anterior segment. Am J Ophthalmol Case Rep. 2022;25:101257.
46. Behera UC, Budhwani M, Das T, Basu S, Padhi TR, Barik MR, et al. Role of early vitrectomy in the treatment of fungal endophthalmitis. Retina. 2018;38:1385–92.
47. Oude Lashof AML, Rothova A, Sobel JD, Ruhnke M, Pappas PG, Viscoli C, et al. Ocular manifestations of candidemia. Clin Infect Dis. 2011;53:262–8.
48. Vilela RC, Vilela L, Vilela P, Vilela R, Motta R, Pôssa AP, et al. Etiological agents of fungal endophthalmitis: diagnosis and management. Int Ophthalmol. 2014;34:707–21.
49. Tanaka M, Kobayashi Y, Takebayashi H, Kiyokawa M, Qiu H. Analysis of predisposing clinical and laboratory findings for the development of endogenous fungal endophthalmitis. A retrospective 12-year study of 79 eyes of 46 patients. Retina. 2001;21:203–9.

50. Lingappan A, Wykoff CC, Albini TA, Miller D, Pathengay A, Davis JL, et al. Endogenous fungal endophthalmitis: causative organisms, management strategies, and visual acuity outcomes. Am J Ophthalmol. 2012;153:162–6.e1.
51. Hidalgo JA, Alangaden GJ, Eliott D, Akins RA, Puklin J, Abrams G, et al. Fungal endophthalmitis diagnosis by detection of Candida albicans DNA in intraocular fluid by use of a species-specific polymerase chain reaction assay. J Infect Dis. 2000;181:1198–201.
52. Danielescu C, Stanca HT, Iorga R-E, Darabus D-M, Potop V. The diagnosis and treatment of fungal endophthalmitis: an update. Diagnostics (Basel). 2022;12:679.
53. Sandhu HS, Hajrasouliha A, Kaplan HJ, Wang W. Diagnostic utility of quantitative polymerase chain reaction versus culture in endophthalmitis and uveitis. Ocul Immunol Inflamm. 2019;27:578–82.
54. Gandhi J, Gagan S, Mohamed A, Das T, Dave VP, Joseph J. Evaluation of vitreous galactomannan and (1, 3) β-D-glucan levels in the diagnosis of fungal endophthalmitis in southern India. Ocul Immunol Inflamm. 2023;31:734–40.
55. Jun KI, Oh B-L, Kim N, Shin JY, Moon J. Microbial diagnosis of endophthalmitis using nanopore amplicon sequencing. Int J Med Microbiol. 2021;311:151505.
56. Deivarajan HR, Prabhakara Sethupathy R, Elamurugan V, Akshayaa V, Reega P, Chelliah D, et al. Clinical evaluation of a novel CRISPR-Cas12a-based RID-MyC assay for the diagnosis of fungal endophthalmitis. Ophthalmol Retina. 2024;9(5):444–52. S2468-6530(24)00533-5.
57. Cho H, Shin YU, Siegel NH, Yu HG, Sobrin L, Patel A, et al. Endogenous endophthalmitis in the American and Korean population: an 8-year retrospective study. Ocul Immunol Inflamm. 2018;26:496–503.
58. Kehrmann J, Chapot V, Buer J, Rating P, Bornfeld N, Steinmann J. Diagnostic performance of blood culture bottles for vitreous culture compared to conventional microbiological cultures in patients with suspected endophthalmitis. Eur J Clin Microbiol Infect Dis. 2018;37:889–95.
59. Davis JL. Diagnostic dilemmas in retinitis and endophthalmitis. Eye (Lond). 2012;26:194–201.
60. Anderson MZ, Saha A, Haseeb A, Bennett RJ. A chromosome 4 trisomy contributes to increased fluconazole resistance in a clinical isolate of Candida albicans. Microbiology (Reading). 2017;163:856–65.
61. Khan FA, Slain D, Khakoo RA. Candida Endophthalmitis: focus on current and future antifungal treatment options. Pharmacotherapy. 2007;27:1711–21.
62. Pappas PG, Kauffman CA, Andes DR, Clancy CJ, Marr KA, Ostrosky-Zeichner L, et al. Clinical practice guideline for the management of candidiasis: 2016 update by the Infectious Diseases Society of America. Clin Infect Dis. 2016;62:e1–50.
63. Patterson TF, Thompson GR III, Denning DW, Fishman JA, Hadley S, Herbrecht R, et al. Practice guidelines for the diagnosis and management of aspergillosis: 2016 update by the Infectious Diseases Society of America. Clin Infect Dis. 2016;63:e1–60.
64. Hariprasad SM, Mieler WF, Lin TK, Sponsel WE, Graybill JR. Voriconazole in the treatment of fungal eye infections: a review of current literature. Br J Ophthalmol. 2008;92:871–8.
65. Patel TP, Zacks DN, Dedania VS. Antimicrobial guide to posterior segment infections. Graefes Arch Clin Exp Ophthalmol. 2021;259:2473–501.
66. Kauffman CA. Exogenous fungal endophthalmitis. In: Endophthalmitis [Internet]. Springer; 2016. p. 185–97. Available from: https://doi.org/10.1007/978-3-319-29231-1_11.
67. Silva RA, Sridhar J, Miller D, Wykoff CC, Flynn HW. Exogenous fungal endophthalmitis: an analysis of isolates and susceptibilities to antifungal agents over a 20-year period (1990–2010). Am J Ophthalmol. 2015;159:257–264.e1.
68. Danielescu C, Cantemir A, Chiselita D. Successful treatment of fungal endophthalmitis using intravitreal caspofungin. Arq Bras Oftalmol. 2017;80:196–8.
69. Hanai Y, Hamada Y, Kimura T, Matsumoto K, Takahashi Y, Fujii S, et al. Favorable effects of voriconazole trough concentrations exceeding 1 μg/mL on treatment success and all-cause mortality: a systematic review and meta-analysis. J Fungi (Basel). 2021;7:306.
70. Modjtahedi BS, Finn AP, Barb SM, MacLachlan MJ, van Zyl T, Papakostas TD, et al. Characteristics and outcomes of endogenous endophthalmitis: eight-year experience at a tertiary care center. Ophthalmol Retina. 2019;3:61–72.

71. Sallam A, Taylor SRJ, Khan A, McCluskey P, Lynn WA, Manku K, et al. Factors determining visual outcome in endogenous Candida endophthalmitis. Retina. 2012;32:1129–34.
72. Dave VP, Parmeshwarappa DC, Dogra A, Pappuru RR, Pathengay A, Joseph J, et al. Clinical presentations and comparative outcomes of delayed-onset low-grade endophthalmitis managed with or without intraocular lens explantation. Clin Ophthalmol. 2020;14:551–5.
73. Negretti GS, Chan W, Pavesio C, Muqit MMK. Vitrectomy for endophthalmitis: 5-year study of outcomes and complications. BMJ Open Ophthalmol. 2020;5:e000423.
74. Horn DL, Neofytos D, Anaissie EJ, Fishman JA, Steinbach WJ, Olyaei AJ, et al. Epidemiology and outcomes of candidemia in 2019 patients: data from the prospective antifungal therapy alliance registry. Clin Infect Dis. 2009;48:1695–703.
75. Zhang H, Liu Z. Endogenous endophthalmitis: a 10-year review of culture-positive cases in northern China. Ocul Immunol Inflamm. 2010;18:133–8.
76. Paulus YM, Cheng S, Karth PA, Leng T. Prospective trial of endogenous fungal endophthalmitis and chorioretinitis rates, clinical course, and outcomes in patients with fungemia. Retina. 2016;36:1357–63.

Fungal Choroiditis

9

Wijak Kongwattananon

9.1 Introduction

Fungal choroiditis is an inflammatory condition affecting the choroid, the vascular layer located between the retina and the sclera of the eye. This condition can be triggered by various fungi, with *Candida* and *Aspergillus* species among the most common causes [1]. The onset of fungal choroiditis typically occurs when fungi disseminate from other regions of the body, often via the bloodstream during systemic fungal infections, or through local spread from adjacent ocular structures. Patients may experience a range of symptoms, including blurred vision, floaters, photophobia, and ocular redness. A comprehensive eye examination is essential for diagnosing fungal choroiditis. Treatment protocols generally involve antifungal medications, which may be administered orally, intravenously (particularly in cases of systemic infection), or through direct injection into the eye (intravitreal injections). Given its potential severity, fungal choroiditis requires prompt diagnosis and intervention to mitigate the risk of vision loss and other complications. This chapter will discuss the primary diagnostic, prognostic, and therapeutic challenges associated with this serious infection.

W. Kongwattananon (✉)
Department of Ophthalmology, King Chulalongkorn Memorial Hospital, Thai Red Cross Society, Bangkok, Thailand

Center of Excellence in Retina, Department of Ophthalmology, Faculty of Medicine Chulalongkorn University and King Chulalongkorn Memorial Hospital, Thai Red Cross Society, Bangkok, Thailand
e-mail: wijak.k@chula.ac.th

M. C. Ramírez-Soto (ed.), *Fungal Eye Infections*,
https://doi.org/10.1007/978-3-032-19923-2_9

9.1.1 Epidemiology and Risk Factors

Fungal choroiditis is predominantly seen in patients with systemic immunosuppression, including those undergoing chemotherapy, organ transplant recipients, HIV/AIDS patients, and individuals with uncontrolled diabetes [2, 3]. It can occur due to endogenous hematogenous spread or direct ocular inoculation following trauma or surgery [4]. The prevalence varies geographically, with different fungal species being predominant in different regions. For example, histoplasmosis is endemic to certain parts of North America, whereas *Candida* and *Aspergillus* infections are more common worldwide in hospitalized, immunocompromised patients [2–4].

Recent epidemiological data indicate an increasing incidence of fungal choroiditis in patients receiving long-term immunosuppressive therapies, particularly in post-COVID-19 patients with prolonged corticosteroid use [5–7]. Additionally, climate change and increasing global travel have contributed to the spread of certain endemic fungi, altering regional distribution patterns [8].

9.1.2 Causative Fungal Organisms

Fungal choroiditis is primarily caused by opportunistic fungi that have the ability to invade ocular tissues, particularly in immunocompromised patients. The most commonly implicated fungi include *Candida*, *Aspergillus*, and *Cryptococcus* species, which have distinct pathogenic mechanisms and clinical manifestations. Additionally, less common fungal pathogens such as *Sporothrix brasiliensis* [9], dermatophytes like *Trichophyton* species, causing extensive tinea corporis [10, 11], *Pneumocystis jirovecii* [12], and *Coccidioides immitis* have also been reported to cause choroidal or retinochoroidal infections, particularly in immunosuppressed individuals [13]. The ability of these fungi to evade host immunity and establish intraocular infections makes their early detection and targeted treatment crucial. In this chapter, *Candida*, *Aspergillus*, and *Cryptococcus* are discussed in detail, highlighting their pathophysiology, clinical presentation, diagnosis, and treatment.

9.2 *Candida* Choroiditis

9.2.1 Pathogenesis

Candida choroiditis is typically caused by hematogenous dissemination of *Candida* species, most commonly *Candida albicans*. Other, less common *Candida* species causing choroiditis include *C. parapsilosis* [14, 15], *C. glabrata* [16], *C. tropicalis* [17], and *C. guilliermondii* [18]. It primarily occurs in patients with candidemia, which is often secondary to indwelling catheters, intravenous drug use, or systemic antibiotic therapy [19]. Candidemia can lead to chorioretinitis and endophthalmitis, with an incidence ranging from 9% to 37% [20].

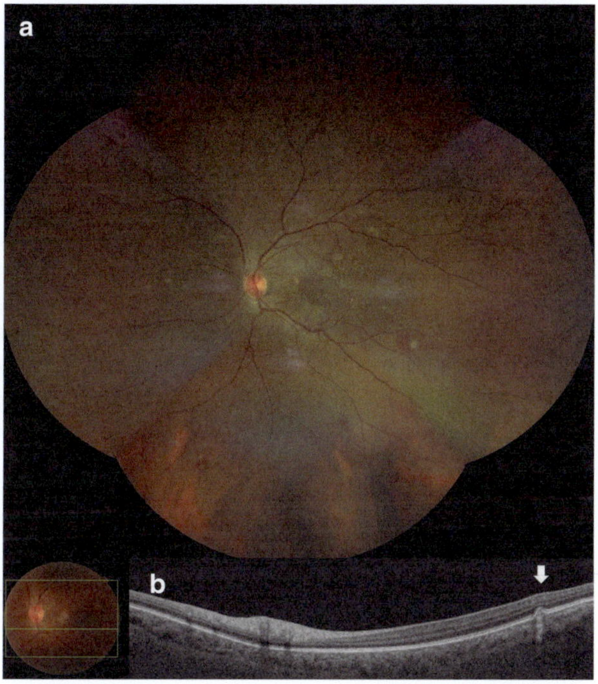

Fig. 9.1 Fundus photographs and optical coherence tomography (OCT) image in a patient with *Candida tropicalis* infection. (**a**) Fundus photograph shows multiple yellow-whitish chorioretinal infiltrates. (**b**) OCT image scanned along the green lines reveals a focal hyperreflective elevation of the retinal pigment epithelium (arrow), indicative of *Candida* chorioretinitis

9.2.2 Clinical Presentation

Candida choroiditis lesions initially localize in the choroid and/or retina (chorioretinitis) before extending into the well-circumscribed vitreous cavity. Early findings include multifocal white, infiltrative lesions (<1 mm) distributed throughout the postequatorial fundus, often with choroidal involvement and progressive inflammation (Fig. 9.1). These lesions may be accompanied by retinal hemorrhages surrounding small necrotic foci, resembling Roth spots, or perivascular sheathing. In some cases, occlusive retinal vasculitis may develop as a complication. Vitreous cellular inflammation is common, and vitreous exudates can take on a "string of pearls" or fluffy ball appearance [21]. In advanced stages, vitritis may obscure chorioretinal lesions, complicating clinical diagnosis.

If left untreated or inadequately managed, *Candida* chorioretinitis may progress to endogenous endophthalmitis, characterized by dense vitritis, marked vision loss, and panophthalmitis in severe cases [21, 22]. Complications of endophthalmitis can include retinal necrosis, tractional retinal detachment, optic atrophy, and irreversible vision loss [3, 23]. Chronic intraocular inflammation may also lead to secondary glaucoma or phthisis bulbi in advanced disease [1, 22].

9.2.3 Diagnosis

The diagnosis of *Candida* choroiditis typically relies on two key factors: the observation of characteristic fundus lesions and the presence of disseminated *Candida* infection or significant risk factors. Direct microscopic examination remains a critical first step. Gram staining can reveal yeast forms and pseudohyphae characteristic of *Candida* infection. If clinical suspicion for fungal infection is high, Calcofluor White staining can significantly improve detection sensitivity. Calcofluor binds to the chitin and cellulose in fungal cell walls, producing a bright fluorescent signal that enhances visualization of fungal elements, although caution is needed as cotton fibers and other chitin-containing materials may cause false-positive results [24].

Confirmation of *Candida* infection is often supported by culture of biological samples. *Candida* species can typically be recovered from blood cultures, vitreous specimens, or other sterile fluids. Positive blood cultures are highly indicative of systemic candidiasis, while isolation from nonsterile sites, such as urine or respiratory secretions, requires cautious interpretation due to possible colonization. Fungal cultures should be incubated for up to 4 weeks, particularly when clinical suspicion remains high, to ensure detection of slow-growing strains and to optimize diagnostic yield [24].

In cases with significant vitreous involvement, vitreous biopsy through pars plana vitrectomy (PPV) serves both diagnostic and therapeutic purposes. More recent diagnostic approaches include polymerase chain reaction (PCR) testing, which has demonstrated high specificity for fungal detection in vitreous samples [25]. Broad-range PCR targeting conserved fungal ribosomal regions (18S or 28S rDNA) can facilitate early detection, although species-level identification may not always be achieved [26].

Next-generation sequencing (NGS) technologies offer new possibilities for detecting *Candida* species directly from ocular samples in choroiditis cases. While not yet routine in clinical microbiology, NGS shows particular promise for fungal intraocular infections due to minimal background microbial DNA in these samples. NGS has successfully identified *Candida* species in choroidal lesions when conventional methods failed, proving valuable for diagnosing *Candida* choroiditis, especially in immunocompromised patients or those with disseminated infection [24].

Beta-D-glucan (BDG) is a polysaccharide component of the cell wall present in various fungal species, which is released into the bloodstream and bodily fluids of individuals with fungal infections. It is a promising biomarker for diagnosing **fungal chorioretinitis and endogenous endophthalmitis**, particularly in high-risk patients. The sensitivity of BDG testing in serum has been reported to be high, with levels frequently elevated before blood cultures turn positive [27]. Intraocular BDG testing has also been explored, showing significantly higher concentrations in patients with *Candida* endophthalmitis compared to controls, reinforcing its diagnostic utility [28]. However, BDG testing has limitations. **False positives** can result from **glucan contamination, dialysis, or bacterial infections,** while **false negatives** may occur if the fungal load is low [28]. Given its **high negative predictive value,** BDG testing in **vitreous fluid or blood** may help **rule out fungal involvement,** guiding clinical decisions and reducing unnecessary interventions.

The diagnosis of *Candida* choroiditis relies on multimodal ocular imaging techniques that provide valuable insights into the localization and progression of infection. **Fundus photography** is useful for documenting the presence of white, elevated, fluffy chorioretinal lesions, which are characteristic of *Candida* choroiditis. **Fluorescein angiography (FA)** reveals early hyperfluorescence with late staining, confirming the inflammatory nature of the lesion [29].

Spectral domain optical coherence tomography (SD-OCT) provides high-resolution cross-sectional images of the retina and choroid, allowing visualization of hyperreflective lesions at the vitreoretinal interface, loss of outer retinal layers, and disruption of the retinal pigment epithelium (RPE) [30]. In early stages, SD-OCT demonstrates an elevated lesion with poorly defined borders and obscured retinal structures. As the infection progresses, the lesion penetrates Bruch's membrane, leading to RPE atrophy and photoreceptor loss. In late stages, SD-OCT shows hyperreflective subretinal scar tissue with persistent outer retinal thinning and choroidal hyperreflectivity due to transmission defects [31–33].

Fundus autofluorescence (FAF) is another imaging modality that can highlight areas of RPE loss. Fundus autofluorescence reveals numerous scattered punctate hyperautofluorescent lesions, indicating early retinal pigment epithelium degeneration. Hypoautofluorescence corresponding to areas of atrophy indicates irreversible damage to the RPE. In advanced cases, FAF reveals a well-defined hypofluorescent scar at the fovea [34].

These imaging techniques allow for accurate diagnosis, monitoring of treatment response, and assessment of visual prognosis. Early identification of structural changes using SD-OCT and FAF is critical for guiding therapeutic interventions and preventing permanent vision loss.

9.2.4 Treatment

Candida chorioretinitis without vitritis requires prompt systemic antifungal therapy to prevent progression to endophthalmitis and preserve visual function. The 2016 Infectious Diseases Society of America (IDSA) guidelines recommend treatment with fluconazole (loading dose: 800 mg, then 400–800 mg daily) or voriconazole (loading dose: 400 mg IV twice daily for two doses, followed by 300 mg IV or oral twice daily) for isolates susceptible to these agents. In cases involving fluconazole-resistant *Candida*, the use of liposomal amphotericin B (3–5 mg/kg IV daily) with or without oral flucytosine is advised [35].

For cases with macular involvement, the IDSA recommends adjunctive intravitreal antifungal injections to enhance local drug concentrations. Options include amphotericin B deoxycholate (5–10 μg/0.1 mL) or voriconazole (100 μg/0.1 mL). The treatment duration is typically a minimum of 4–6 weeks, guided by clinical and ophthalmologic response. In patients with vitritis, systemic therapy must be supplemented with intravitreal antifungal agents to ensure adequate intraocular drug delivery and control of infection [35].

In contrast, the 2025 Global Guideline for Candidiasis, developed by the European Confederation of Medical Mycology (ECMM) in collaboration with ISHAM and ASM, provides updated pharmacokinetic-driven, weight-based recommendations [36]. For *Candida* chorioretinitis, fluconazole (200–400 mg daily), voriconazole (6 mg/kg IV twice a day for day 1, then 4 mg/kg twice a day from day 2), or liposomal amphotericin B (3–5 mg/kg IV once daily) may be used. The guideline tailors treatment duration based on disease severity:

- For patients with visual symptoms or macular involvement, systemic antifungal therapy should be continued for 4–6 weeks.
- For patients without visual symptoms or macular involvement, a shorter course of at least 2 weeks may be sufficient if clinical improvement is observed.

The 2025 guideline reinforces the importance of individualized treatment based on organism susceptibility, site of involvement, and host factors. Intravitreal antifungal therapy may still be considered in selected cases to achieve therapeutic drug levels within the eye, particularly when there is posterior segment involvement or limited systemic drug penetration [36]. A flowchart summarizing the treatment of *Candida* choroiditis is presented in Fig. 9.2.

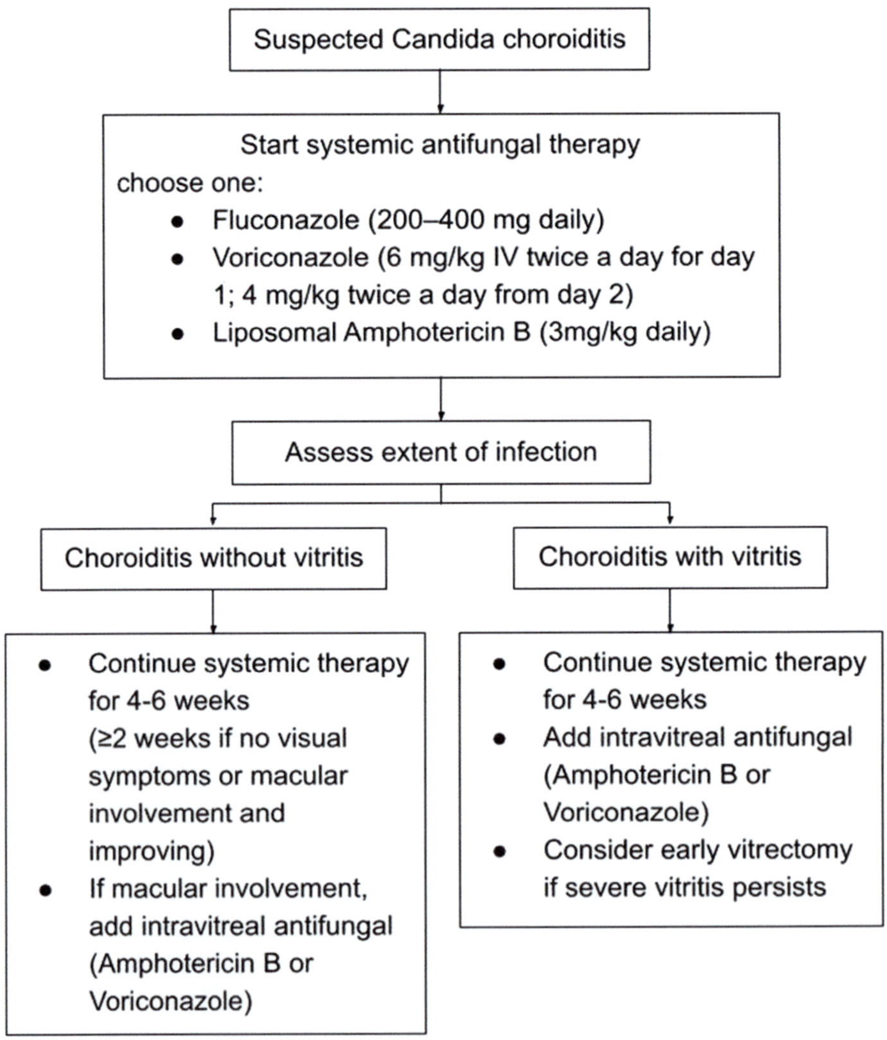

Fig. 9.2 A flowchart for the treatment of *Candida* choroiditis

In severe cases, vitrectomy is advised to reduce fungal burden and remove vitreous opacities [37]. Echinocandins (e.g., caspofungin, micafungin, anidulafungin) are not recommended due to their poor intraocular penetration, but may be considered in asymptomatic, well-localized chorioretinitis caused by echinocandin-susceptible isolates [36].

Prompt treatment with systemic antifungals, intravitreal injections, and surgical intervention, when needed, significantly improves visual outcomes and minimizes complications.

9.3 *Aspergillus* Choroiditis

9.3.1 Pathogenesis

Aspergillus species, particularly *Aspergillus fumigatus*, are angioinvasive fungi that can spread hematogenously, particularly in immunocompromised patients [38–41]. The lungs are the primary site of infection, with subsequent ocular involvement occurring through bloodstream dissemination [38, 41].

9.3.2 Clinical Presentation

Aspergillus choroiditis (Figs. 9.3 and 9.4) is characterized by rapidly progressive vision loss and yellow-white, confluent, deep infiltration lesions with ill-defined margins, typically located in the macula [38]. (Figs. 9.1 and 9.2). A large macular abscess and retinal pseudohypopyon formation are suggestive of the diagnosis [42]. Retinal involvement may range from subretinal or subhyaloid infiltrates to full-thickness retinal necrosis, sometimes associated with serous or exudative retinal detachment, intraretinal hemorrhages, choroidal or vitreous abscess, intravitreal granuloma, and posterior scleritis [43].

Aspergillus infections typically present with only one or two chorioretinitis lesions, unlike *Candida* infections, which often manifest as multiple lesions. *Aspergillus* tends to have more rapidly progressive and large macular lesions and is more hemorrhagic due to the angiocentric invasion of mold hyphae, leading to retinal and choroidal vessel occlusion and ischemia [22]. Vitreous involvement is also milder in Aspergillosis compared to *Candida* infections [44].

9.3.3 Diagnosis

The diagnosis of *Aspergillus* choroiditis presents significant challenges due to overlapping clinical presentations, low culture positivity rates, and the limitations of traditional diagnostic methods. Clinical suspicion should be particularly high in immunocompromised individuals, patients with hematologic malignancies,

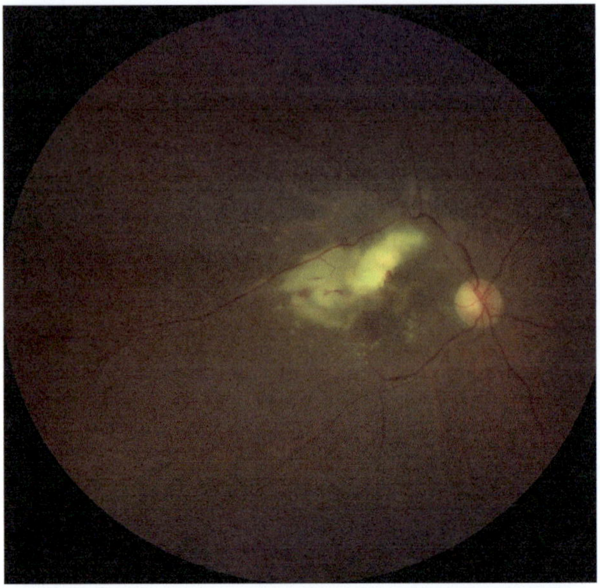

Fig. 9.3 Fundus photograph of a patient with *Aspergillus* chorioretinitis showing a yellow-whitish chorioretinal infiltrate, intraretinal hemorrhage, and associated retinal vasculitis

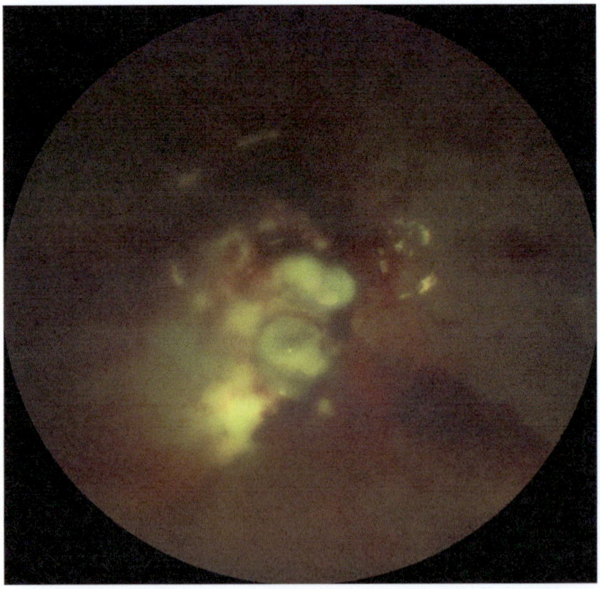

Fig. 9.4 Fundus photograph of a patient with *Aspergillus* fungemia, revealing diffuse intraretinal hemorrhages, along with a chorioretinal infiltrate and subhyaloid abscesses, indicative of chorioretinitis and endophthalmitis

intravenous drug users, or those with recent intraocular interventions [41]. Unlike *Candida*, *Aspergillus* choroiditis often demonstrates more extensive retinal and choroidal invasion, leading to vascular occlusion, increasing the risk of retinal detachment and irreversible vision loss.

The gold standard for diagnosing *Aspergillus* choroiditis remains direct fungal identification via culture or histopathology. However, *Aspergillus* is a fastidious organism with slow growth, and vitreous cultures have a sensitivity ranging from 30% to 70%, often delaying diagnosis and treatment [45]. Given these limitations, vitreous biopsy through PPV serves both a diagnostic and therapeutic role, particularly in cases with extensive vitreous involvement [25].

Molecular diagnostics have enhanced the detection of *Aspergillus* DNA in intraocular fluids, offering a faster and more sensitive alternative to culture. Broad-range real-time PCR targeting 18S rRNA has demonstrated high specificity, particularly for detecting *Aspergillus* in vitreous specimens [25]. Next-generation sequencing (NGS) has further improved diagnostic accuracy, allowing for comprehensive pathogen identification in intraocular infections [40]. Despite its promise, NGS remains costly and time-intensive, limiting its routine clinical applicability.

Galactomannan (GM) is a carbohydrate found in the cell wall, primarily specific to *Aspergillus* species, offering a rapid and highly specific alternative to culture-based methods. Research on intraocular GM levels in *Aspergillus* endophthalmitis found significantly higher levels compared to non-*Aspergillus* intraocular infections, including *Candida* [45]. GM testing at an optimal cutoff demonstrated perfect sensitivity and specificity for detecting *Aspergillus*, underscoring its potential as a highly accurate diagnostic tool [45].

Beta-D-glucan (BDG) has also been studied in *Aspergillus* choroiditis and endophthalmitis, particularly in exogenous cases following ocular trauma or surgery [46]. Studies have shown that BDG levels in intraocular fluid can be significantly elevated in *Aspergillus* endophthalmitis, providing a valuable adjunct to clinical suspicion and imaging findings [28]. The combination of BDG and GM testing has been proposed as a strategy to improve diagnostic accuracy, particularly in cases where conventional diagnostic methods are inconclusive [46].

Multimodal imaging plays an essential role in diagnosing *Aspergillus* choroiditis, distinguishing it from other infectious and inflammatory chorioretinal conditions. Fundus photography reveals deep-seated, fluffy, yellowish-white chorioretinal infiltrates, often accompanied by retinal hemorrhages and necrotic foci. FA further characterizes these lesions, showing early hypofluorescence due to vascular occlusion and late staining and leakage, indicative of an inflammatory process [47].

SD-OCT provides high-resolution cross-sectional imaging of *Aspergillus* choroiditis, revealing hallmark structural changes in retinal and choroidal tissues. Early findings include hyperreflective infiltrates at the vitreoretinal interface, with associated disruption of the outer retinal layers [48]. As the disease progresses, lesions penetrate Bruch's membrane, leading to retinal pigment epithelium (RPE) atrophy, photoreceptor loss, and choroidal hyperreflectivity. In late-stage *Aspergillus* choroiditis, SD-OCT reveals subretinal fibrosis, extensive outer retinal thinning, and hyperreflective scarring. The FAF findings are characterized by hypoautofluorescence in areas corresponding to RPE damage and hyperautofluorescence in regions of active inflammation [22].

9.3.4 Treatment

The management of *Aspergillus* choroiditis depends on the severity of intraocular involvement and the presence of vitritis. The following recommendations are based on the IDSA guidelines [49]. Systemic antifungal therapy with voriconazole (loading dose: 6 mg/kg IV every 12 h for two doses, then 4 mg/kg IV every 12 h or oral 200–300 mg twice daily) is the first-line treatment due to its superior ocular penetration and broad antifungal activity. Liposomal amphotericin B (3–5 mg/kg IV daily) is an alternative, particularly for patients in whom voriconazole is contraindicated. In cases with macular involvement, intravitreal antifungal injections of voriconazole (100 μg/0.1 mL) or amphotericin B deoxycholate (5–10 μg/0.1 mL) may be administered to enhance intraocular drug concentration.

For *Aspergillus* choroiditis with vitritis, systemic antifungal therapy should be supplemented with intravitreal antifungal injections to achieve effective intraocular penetration. PPV is recommended in cases with significant vitreous involvement or retinal detachment to reduce fungal burden and improve drug distribution. Echinocandins (e.g., caspofungin, micafungin), despite their limited vitreous penetration, may be considered in select cases of fungal choroiditis without vitritis or as an adjunctive salvage therapy. IDSA guidelines caution against corticosteroid use in fungal infections unless adequate antifungal coverage is ensured, as steroids may suppress immune responses and exacerbate infection.

Immunocompromised patients, including those undergoing chemotherapy or receiving organ transplants, require prolonged systemic therapy with therapeutic drug monitoring to prevent relapse. Despite aggressive treatment strategies, prognosis remains guarded, emphasizing the importance of early diagnosis and individualized management.

9.4 Cryptococcal Choroiditis

9.4.1 Pathogenesis

Cryptococcal choroiditis is a rare but significant manifestation of cryptococcal infection, primarily caused by *Cryptococcus neoformans* and *Cryptococcus gattii*. These encapsulated yeasts primarily affect immunocompromised individuals, particularly those with HIV/AIDS (especially with CD4 counts below 100 cells/μL), organ transplant recipients, and patients on prolonged corticosteroid or immunosuppressive therapy [50]. *Cryptococcus* is commonly found in soil contaminated with bird droppings, particularly pigeons, as well as fruit and plants [51]. The fungus gains entry into the human body through inhalation of airborne spores and disseminates hematogenously, most commonly to the brain, meninges, and spinal cord [52]. Intraocular cryptococcosis usually occurs through direct extension from the optic nerve sheath or hematogenous spread from the primary focus [51]. Direct ocular involvement by *Cryptococcus* is rare [52]. The main site of *Cryptococcus neoformans* involvement in the eyes is the choroid, with secondary spread to the retina or vitreous [50].

9.4.2 Clinical Presentation

Cryptococcal choroiditis often presents with blurred vision, floaters, and progressive visual impairment [53]. Patients may also exhibit signs of concurrent meningoencephalitis, including headaches, altered mental status, and neck stiffness [50]. Ophthalmoscopic examination may reveal multifocal yellow-white choroidal lesions, which can be bilateral and variably sized [52]. These lesions may coalesce, forming larger plaques [53]. Retinal involvement, including hemorrhages and vitritis, can sometimes accompany choroidal lesions, reflecting widespread fungal infiltration [54]. Chorioretinitis is characterized by discrete, multiple yellow-whitish lesions with slight elevation and is sometimes accompanied by retinal hemorrhage [51] (Fig. 9.5). Retinal necrosis, exudative retinal detachment, retinal vessel

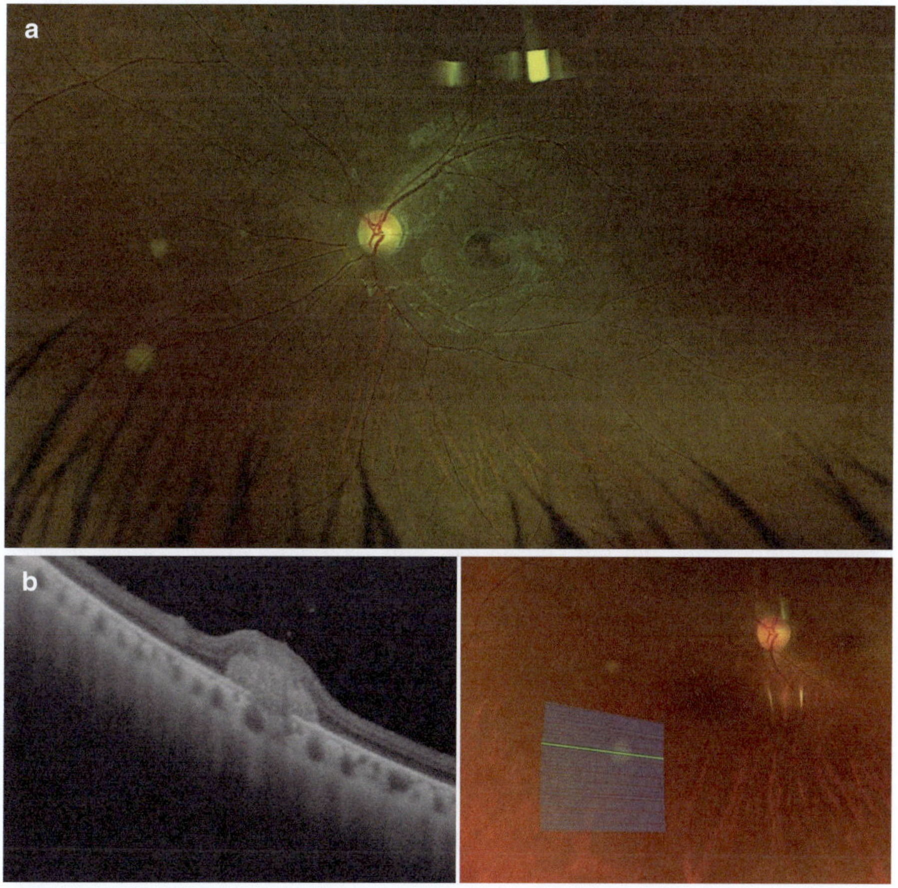

Fig. 9.5 Fundus photographs and optical coherence tomography (OCT) image in a patient with Cryptococcal choroiditis. (**a**) Fundus photograph shows a few whitish chorioretinal infiltrates. (**b**) OCT image scanned along the green lines reveals intraretinal hyperreflective infiltrates with overlying hyperreflective dots in the vitreous, consistent with focal vitritis

sheathing, optic disc edema, optic atrophy, and ophthalmoplegia may also occur [52]. Without treatment, the condition can progress to endophthalmitis, presenting as diffuse vitritis with haze, debris, and fluffy white vitreous exudates that progressively enlarge to involve the entire vitreous [50]. A mild inflammatory reaction is usually present in the anterior segment, and if left untreated, iris neovascularization and cataract formation may develop [51]. Visual outcomes are poor in most cases [52].

9.4.3 Diagnosis

The diagnosis of cryptococcal choroiditis is complicated by its frequent association with disseminated infection, particularly CNS involvement [55]. FA typically reveals hypofluorescent spots located under the neural retina without significant leakage in late stages [51]. Indocyanine green angiography (ICGA) reveals multifocal patterns and irregularly shaped hypofluorescent spots in the choroid, often appearing confluent and indicating active disease [51]. Lesions are often more numerous and distinct on ICGA compared to fundus examination and FA, and they tend to persist in late-phase ICGA imaging [56]. SD-OCT shows focal thickening of the choroid without disruption of the retinal pigment epithelium, supporting the localization of lesions at the inner choroid level [56]. If the causative organism is unknown, an early diagnostic vitreous tap or vitrectomy may be performed. Identification of the encapsulated organism in cerebrospinal fluid (CSF) stained with India ink is sufficient for making a presumptive diagnosis and initiating treatment pending culture results [53]. However, India ink preparations are negative in 50% of cases involving the CNS [52]. Therefore, serum cryptococcal antigen (CRAG) detection, which has high sensitivity, is often used in conjunction with CSF culture [56]. In suspected cases, urine, CSF, blood, and sputum should be cultured even in the absence of evidence suggesting genitourinary or pulmonary infection [50]. *Cryptococcus neoformans* grows well on both blood agar and Sabouraud medium, producing mucoid, cream, or pink colonies within 24–48 h [51]. Histological identification can be achieved using periodic acid-Schiff (PAS) or methenamine silver stains, while Mayer's mucicarmine stain highlights the polysaccharide capsule in red, distinguishing *Cryptococcus neoformans* from other organisms [52].

9.4.4 Management

The treatment of cryptococcal choroiditis aligns with systemic antifungal therapy for cryptococcosis. A flowchart for the treatment of cryptococcal choroiditis is presented in Fig. 9.6. According to the 2024 Global Guideline for Cryptococcosis [57],

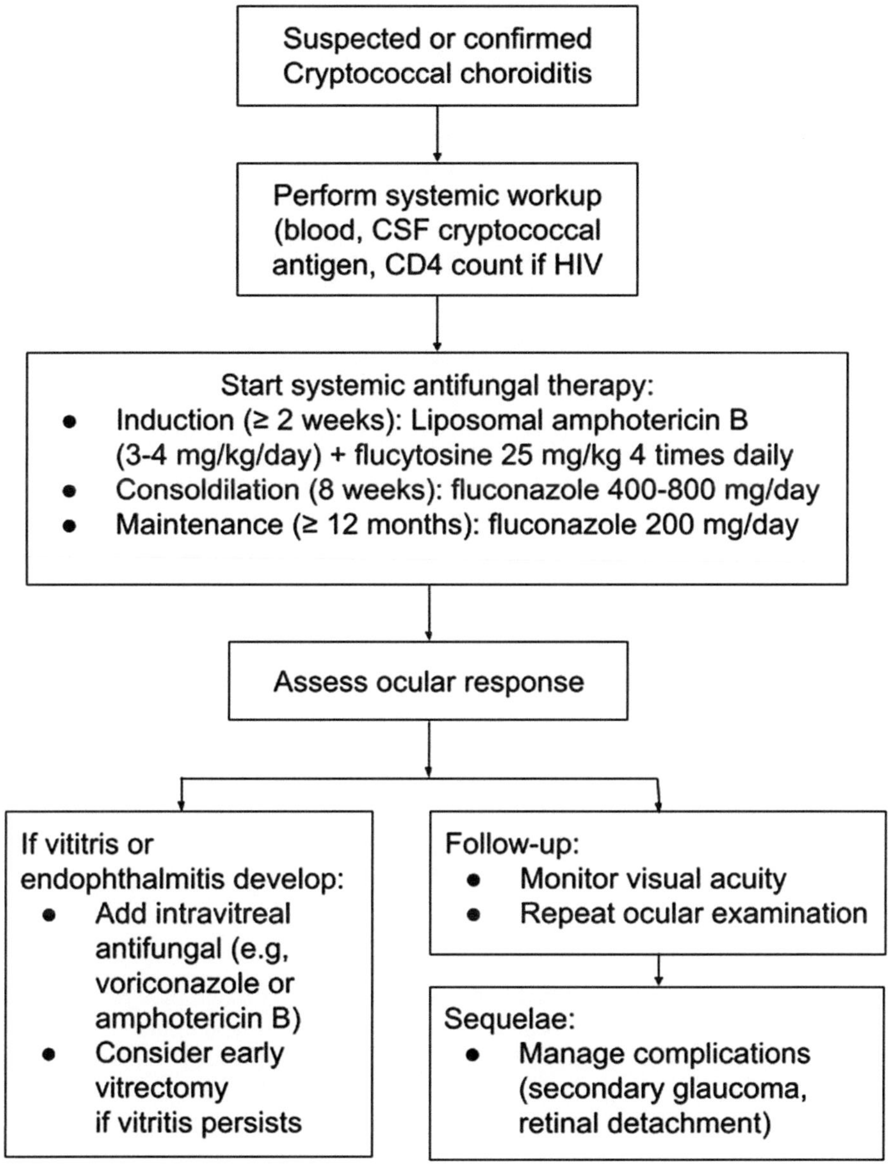

Fig. 9.6 A flowchart for the treatment of cryptococcal choroiditis

for disseminated cryptococcosis including ocular involvement, the preferred induction regimen is liposomal amphotericin B at 3–4 mg/kg daily plus flucytosine 25 mg/kg four times daily for at least 2 weeks. In low-resource settings, an alternative induction option includes a single dose of liposomal amphotericin B 10 mg/kg combined with 2 weeks of flucytosine and fluconazole 1200 mg daily, though this has only been studied in HIV-associated cryptococcosis.

Following induction, consolidation therapy with fluconazole 400–800 mg daily for 8 weeks is recommended, and maintenance therapy with fluconazole 200 mg daily should be continued for at least 12 months or until immune reconstitution [54, 57].

Therapeutic failure or relapse has been reported in approximately 33% of cases [53]. Voriconazole has a significantly broader spectrum of activity and the lowest minimum inhibitory concentration for *Cryptococcus neoformans* [55]. When administered systemically, voriconazole shows excellent bioavailability, penetrating well into the eye and reaching intravitreal concentrations of 1.0–1.5 mg/mL without significant toxicity [54]. Intravitreal voriconazole may therefore be a promising regimen for the treatment of cryptococcal choroiditis with endophthalmitis [51]. Early vitrectomy is recommended if severe vitritis fails to clear or worsens under antifungal therapy [52]. Enucleation is considered if the outcome is a blind, painful eye [50].

Despite antifungal therapy, cryptococcal choroiditis can lead to permanent visual impairment due to choroidal scarring, optic atrophy, or secondary complications such as retinal detachment [55]. Early recognition and prompt systemic therapy improve outcomes. In patients with underlying immunosuppression, recurrence remains a concern, necessitating prolonged antifungal prophylaxis [50]. Additionally, cases with neuro-ophthalmic involvement, such as optic nerve infiltration, may present with significant visual field defects [51].

9.5 Differential Diagnosis

The differential diagnosis of fungal choroiditis includes a range of infectious and noninfectious etiologies, which can present with similar clinical features. Table 9.1 **summarizes these conditions, highlighting key clinical clues and diagnostic considerations.**

Table 9.1 Differential diagnosis of fungal choroiditis and related conditions

Category	Disease/condition	Key clinical clues	Comments
Fungal infections	*Candida* chorioretinitis	Multifocal small white chorioretinal lesions; "string of pearls" vitreous exudates; systemic candidemia often present	Blood cultures, β-D-glucan positivity, PCR
	Cryptococcal choroiditis	Multifocal creamy-yellow choroidal lesions, usually bilateral; often associated with meningitis symptoms	Serum cryptococcal antigen positive
	Aspergillus choroiditis	Large, often hemorrhagic subretinal abscesses; profound vision loss	Blood cultures, PCR, galactomannan positivity
Bacterial infections	Tuberculous choroiditis	Solitary or multifocal yellow-white choroidal lesions; systemic TB signs	IGRA positive, PCR or culture confirmation
	Syphilitic chorioretinitis	Placoid chorioretinitis, retinal vasculitis, mild vitritis	Positive VDRL/FTA-ABS
	Bartonella neuroretinitis	Optic disc swelling with macular star; history of cat exposure	Bartonella serology positive
Viral infections	Cytomegalovirus (CMV) retinitis	Hemorrhagic necrotizing retinitis; brushfire margins; immunosuppressed patients	CMV PCR positive
	Herpes simplex/zoster necrotizing retinitis	Acute retinal necrosis: Peripheral necrotizing lesions, vasculitis, rapid progression	HSV/VZV PCR positive
Parasitic infections	Toxoplasmic retinochoroiditis	Focal necrotizing retinitis near old scars; dense vitritis ("headlight in fog")	Positive toxoplasma IgG/IgM, PCR
Chronic noninfectious diseases	Sarcoidosis	Multifocal choroidal granulomas; anterior uveitis; periphlebitis ("candle-wax drippings")	Chest CT, elevated ACE, biopsy
	Vogt-Koyanagi-Harada (VKH) disease	Bilateral serous retinal detachments, disc edema; systemic features (vitiligo, poliosis)	Clinical diagnosis
	Primary intraocular lymphoma	Subretinal infiltrates, vitreous cells, masquerading as chronic uveitis	Diagnostic vitrectomy for vitreous cytology

9.6 Conclusion

The diagnosis of fungal choroiditis requires a comprehensive approach that integrates clinical examination, microbiological testing, fungal biomarker assays, and advanced imaging techniques. While cultures remain the gold standard, their low sensitivity necessitates the use of complementary diagnostic tools, such as PCR-based molecular detection, galactomannan (GM) assays, and multimodal imaging. GM testing in vitreous fluid offers a rapid and highly specific diagnostic alternative, while beta-D-glucan

(BDG) assays improve diagnostic accuracy, particularly in culture-negative cases. Advanced imaging modalities, including FA, SD-OCT, and FAF, are indispensable for characterizing disease extent, monitoring progression, and guiding treatment decisions. Given the complexity of fungal choroiditis, a multidisciplinary collaboration between infectious disease specialists, ophthalmologists, and critical care teams is essential to optimize patient management and minimize complications.

References

1. Sharma S. Fungal infections of the eye. J Acad Clin Microbiol. 2021;23(1):1–8. https://doi.org/10.4103/jacm.jacm_53_21.
2. Chen KJ, Sun MH, Chen YP, Chen YH, Wang NK, Liu L, et al. Endogenous fungal endophthalmitis: causative organisms, treatments, and visual outcomes. J Fungi (Basel). 2022;8(6) https://doi.org/10.3390/jof8060641. Epub 2022/06/24. PubMed PMID: 35736124; PubMed Central PMCID: PMCPMC9225322
3. Lingappan A, Wykoff CC, Albini TA, Miller D, Pathengay A, Davis JL, et al. Endogenous fungal endophthalmitis: causative organisms, management strategies, and visual acuity outcomes. Am J Ophthalmol. 2012;153(1):162–6. https://doi.org/10.1016/j.ajo.2011.06.020. e1. Epub 2011/09/16. PubMed PMID: 21917234
4. Das T, Agarwal M, Anand AR, Behera UC, Bhende M, Das AV, et al. Fungal endophthalmitis: analysis of 730 consecutive eyes from 7 tertiary eye care centers in India. Ophthalmol Retina. 2022;6(3):243–51. Epub 2021/09/22. PubMed PMID: 34547530. https://doi.org/10.1016/j.oret.2021.09.006.
5. Markan A, Dogra M, Katoch D, Tomar M, Mittal H, Singh R. Endogenous endophthalmitis in COVID-19 patients: a case series and literature review. Ocul Immunol Inflamm. 2023;31(6):1191–7. Epub 2023/04/13. PubMed PMID: 37043623. https://doi.org/10.1080/09273948.2023.2192273.
6. Samanta R, Jayaraj S, Mittal SK, Kumari J, Naharwal A, Agrawal A. Post-COVID-19 endogenous endophthalmitis case series and review of literature. Indian J Ophthalmol. 2023;71(12):3677–83. https://doi.org/10.4103/IJO.IJO_3079_22. Epub 2023/11/22. PubMed PMID: 37991303; PubMed Central PMCID: PMCPMC10788740
7. Shroff D, Narula R, Atri N, Chakravarti A, Gandhi A, Sapra N, et al. Endogenous fungal endophthalmitis following intensive corticosteroid therapy in severe COVID-19 disease. Indian J Ophthalmol. 2021;69(7):1909–14. https://doi.org/10.4103/ijo.IJO_592_21. Epub 2021/06/20. PubMed PMID: 34146056; PubMed Central PMCID: PMCPMC8374784
8. Williams SL, Toda M, Chiller T, Brunkard JM, Litvintseva AP. Effects of climate change on fungal infections. PLoS Pathog. 2024;20(5):e1012219. https://doi.org/10.1371/journal.ppat.1012219. Epub 2024/05/30. PubMed PMID: 38814855; PubMed Central PMCID: PMCPMC11139277
9. Biancardi AL, Freitas DF, Valviesse VR, Andrade HB, de Oliveira MM, do Valle AC, et al. Multifocal choroiditis in disseminated sporotrichosis in patients with HIV/AIDS. Retin Cases Brief Rep. 2017;11(1):67–70. Epub 2016/03/12. PubMed PMID: 26967963. https://doi.org/10.1097/icb.0000000000000290.
10. Agarwal M, Gupta C, Gujral GS, Mittal M. Tinea corporis infection manifestating as retinochoroiditis-an unusual presentation. J Ophthalmic Inflamm Infect. 2019;9(1):8. https://doi.org/10.1186/s12348-019-0173-z. Epub 2019/05/28. PubMed PMID: 31131426; PubMed Central PMCID: PMCPMC6535422
11. Konana VK, Babu K. A rare case report of panuveitis with retinochoroidal involvement, retinitis, and retinal vasculitis due to extensive tinea corporis. Front Ophthalmol (Lausanne). 2023;3:1174414. https://doi.org/10.3389/fopht.2023.1174414. Epub 2023/06/09. PubMed PMID: 38983055; PubMed Central PMCID: PMCPMC11182326

12. Gupta A, Hustler A, Herieka E, Matthews BN. Pneumocystis choroiditis. Eye (Lond). 2010;24(1):178. Epub 2009/03/28. PubMed PMID: 19325571. https://doi.org/10.1038/eye.2009.52.
13. Reyes-Montes MDR, Leon-Garcia AA, Frias-De-Leon MG, Acosta-Altamirano G, Sanchez-Saavedra EP, Victoriano-Pastelin I, et al. Clinical cases of coccidioidomycosis in the Americas in the period 1950-2021: epidemiology data, diagnosis, and treatment. Life (Basel). 2023;13(11) https://doi.org/10.3390/life13112109. Epub 2023/11/25. PubMed PMID: 38004249; PubMed Central PMCID: PMCPMC10672650
14. Scartozzi R, Tom D, Liggett PE, Flynn HW Jr. Postoperative endophthalmitis caused by Candida parapsilosis: clinical features and treatment outcomes. Ophthalmic Surg Lasers Imaging. 2011;42 Online:e37–9. Epub 2011/03/18. PubMed PMID: 21410086. https://doi.org/10.3928/15428877-20110303-02.
15. Chen KJ. Atypical endogenous Candida parapsilosis Endophthalmitis. Ophthalmol Retina. 2018;2(3):200. Epub 2018/03/01. PubMed PMID: 31047586. https://doi.org/10.1016/j.oret.2017.12.008.
16. Chapman FM, Orr KE, Armitage WJ, Easty DL, Cottrell DG. Candida glabrata endophthalmitis following penetrating keratoplasty. Br J Ophthalmol. 1998;82(6):712–3. https://doi.org/10.1136/bjo.82.6.709c. Epub 1998/11/03. PubMed PMID: 9797681; PubMed Central PMCID: PMCPMC1722613
17. Shmuely H, Kremer I, Sagie A, Pitlik S. Candida tropicalis multifocal endophthalmitis as the only initial manifestation of pacemaker endocarditis. Am J Ophthalmol. 1997;123(4):559–60. Epub 1997/04/01. PubMed PMID: 9124260. https://doi.org/10.1016/s0002-9394(14)70189-8.
18. Tamura A, Kawamoto D, Minami K, Yasuda S, Tsujimoto H, Tsuda Y, et al. Candida guilliermondii-induced chorioretinitis in a patient with eating disorder. J Infect Chemother. 2021;27(4):642–6. Epub 2020/11/21. PubMed PMID: 33214072. https://doi.org/10.1016/j.jiac.2020.11.005.
19. Uppuluri A, Zarbin MA, Budoff G, Bhagat N. Risk factors for endogenous endophthalmitis in hospitalized patients with candida fungemia. Ophthalmol Retina. 2021;5(7):687–95. Epub 2020/10/20. PubMed PMID: 33075547. https://doi.org/10.1016/j.oret.2020.10.007.
20. Bae JH, Lee SC. Intravitreal liposomal amphotericin B for treatment of endogenous candida endophthalmitis. Jpn J Ophthalmol. 2015;59(5):346–52. Epub 2015/07/29. PubMed PMID: 26215152. https://doi.org/10.1007/s10384-015-0397-x.
21. Au L, Guduru K, Lipscomb G, Kelly SP. Candida endophthalmitis: a critical diagnosis in the critically ill. Clin Ophthalmol. 2007;1(4):551–4. Epub 2007/12/01. PubMed PMID: 19668535; PubMed Central PMCID: PMCPMC2704539
22. Haseeb AA, Elhusseiny AM, Siddiqui MZ, Ahmad KT, Sallam AB. Fungal endophthalmitis: a comprehensive review. J Fungi (Basel). 2021;7(11) https://doi.org/10.3390/jof7110996. Epub 2021/11/28. PubMed PMID: 34829283; PubMed Central PMCID: PMCPMC8623405
23. Sridhar J, Flynn HW Jr, Kuriyan AE, Miller D, Albini T. Endogenous fungal endophthalmitis: risk factors, clinical features, and treatment outcomes in mold and yeast infections. J Ophthalmic Inflamm Infect. 2013;3(1):–60. https://doi.org/10.1186/1869-5760-3-60. Epub 2013/09/24. PubMed PMID: 24053550; PubMed Central PMCID: PMCPMC3848556
24. Leal SM Jr, Rodino KG, Fowler WC, Gilligan PH. Practical guidance for clinical microbiology laboratories: diagnosis of ocular infections. Clin Microbiol Rev. 2021, e0007019;34(3) https://doi.org/10.1128/CMR.00070-19. Epub 2021/06/03. PubMed PMID: 34076493; PubMed Central PMCID: PMCPMC8262805
25. Sugita S, Kamoi K, Ogawa M, Watanabe K, Shimizu N, Mochizuki M. Detection of Candida and Aspergillus species DNA using broad-range real-time PCR for fungal endophthalmitis. Graefes Arch Clin Exp Ophthalmol. 2012;250(3):391–8. Epub 2011/09/29. PubMed PMID: 21947326. https://doi.org/10.1007/s00417-011-1819-1.
26. Ogawa M, Sugita S, Watanabe K, Shimizu N, Mochizuki M. Novel diagnosis of fungal endophthalmitis by broad-range real-time PCR detection of fungal 28S ribosomal DNA. Graefes Arch Clin Exp Ophthalmol. 2012;250(12):1877–83. Epub 2012/04/25. PubMed PMID: 22527320. https://doi.org/10.1007/s00417-012-2015-7.

27. Ammar MJ, Carroll R, Kolomeyer A, Ying GS, Whitehead G, Brucker AJ, et al. Clinical utility of Beta-D-Glucan testing for endogenous fungal chorioretinitis or endophthalmitis. Retina. 2021;41(2):431–7. Epub 2020/06/10. PubMed PMID: 32516224. https://doi.org/10.1097/iae.0000000000002861.
28. Kolomeyer AM, Murphy KM, Traband A, Frank I, Kim BJ. Beta-D-Glucan testing in patients with fungal endophthalmitis. Retina. 2018;38(4):650–9. Epub 2018/01/26. PubMed PMID: 29370030. https://doi.org/10.1097/iae.0000000000002049.
29. Lavine JA, Mititelu M. Multimodal imaging of refractory Candida chorioretinitis progressing to endogenous endophthalmitis. J Ophthalmic Inflamm Infect. 2015;5(1):54. https://doi.org/10.1186/s12348-015-0054-z. Epub 2015/08/09. PubMed PMID: 26253239; PubMed Central PMCID: PMCPMC4529431
30. Teixeira FHF, Santos NS, de Carvalho Mendes Paiva A, Carvalho EM, Biancardi AL, Curi ALL. Optical coherence tomography findings in fungal uveitis. Int Ophthalmol. 2023;43(8):3023–30. Epub 2023/04/03. PubMed PMID: 37004606. https://doi.org/10.1007/s10792-023-02696-0.
31. Kubicka-Trząska A, Bugara D, Żuber-Łaskawiec K, Pociej-Marciak W, Markiewicz A, Romanowska-Dixon B, et al. Use of optical coherence tomography and optical coherence tomography angiography in the diagnosis and follow-up of endogenous candida endophthalmitis: a case report. Medicina (Kaunas). 2024;60(2) https://doi.org/10.3390/medicina60020207. Epub 2024/02/24. PubMed PMID: 38399495; PubMed Central PMCID: PMCPMC10890289
32. Invernizzi A, Symes R, Miserocchi E, Cozzi M, Cereda M, Fogliato G, et al. Spectral domain optical coherence tomography findings in endogenous candida endophthalmitis and their clinical relevance. Retina. 2018;38(5):1011–8. Epub 2017/05/12. PubMed PMID: 28492430. https://doi.org/10.1097/iae.0000000000001630.
33. Zhuang H, Ding X, Gao F, Zhang T, Ni Y, Chang Q, et al. Optical coherence tomography features of retinal lesions in Chinese patients with endogenous Candida endophthalmitis. BMC Ophthalmol. 2020;20(1):52. https://doi.org/10.1186/s12886-020-01337-9. Epub 2020/02/16. PubMed PMID: 32059661; PubMed Central PMCID: PMCPMC7020574
34. Veronese C, Maiolo C, Gurreri A, Morara M, Ciardella AP, Yannuzzi LA. Multimodal imaging of multifocal chorioretinitis secondary to endogenous candida infection. Int Ophthalmol. 2019;39(9):2137–42. Epub 2018/10/08. PubMed PMID: 30293205. https://doi.org/10.1007/s10792-018-1025-9.
35. Pappas PG, Kauffman CA, Andes DR, Clancy CJ, Marr KA, Ostrosky-Zeichner L, et al. Clinical practice guideline for the management of candidiasis: 2016 update by the Infectious Diseases Society of America. Clin Infect Dis. 2016;62(4):e1–e50. https://doi.org/10.1093/cid/civ933. Epub 2015/12/19. PubMed PMID: 26679628; PubMed Central PMCID: PMCPMC4725385
36. Cornely OA, Sprute R, Bassetti M, Chen SC, Groll AH, Kurzai O, et al. Global guideline for the diagnosis and management of candidiasis: an initiative of the ECMM in cooperation with ISHAM and ASM. Lancet Infect Dis. 2025;25(5):e280–e93. Epub 2025/02/17. PubMed PMID: 39956121. https://doi.org/10.1016/S1473-3099(24)00749-7.
37. Chee YE, Eliott D. The role of vitrectomy in the management of fungal endophthalmitis. Semin Ophthalmol. 2017;32(1):29–35. Epub 2016/10/30. PubMed PMID: 27792412. https://doi.org/10.1080/08820538.2016.1228396.
38. Weishaar PD, Flynn HW Jr, Murray TG, Davis JL, Barr CC, Gross JG, et al. Endogenous Aspergillus endophthalmitis. Clinical features and treatment outcomes. Ophthalmology. 1998;105(1):57–65. Epub 1998/01/27. PubMed PMID: 9442779. https://doi.org/10.1016/s0161-6420(98)71225-3.
39. Li X, Chen Z, Zhang X, Zhou Z, Boost M, Huang T, et al. Fungal endophthalmitis: clinical characteristics, pathogens, and factors affecting visual outcome. Antibiotics (Basel). 2024;13(3) https://doi.org/10.3390/antibiotics13030199. Epub 2024/03/27. PubMed PMID: 38534634; PubMed Central PMCID: PMCPMC10967284
40. Danielescu C, Stanca HT, Iorga RE, Darabus DM, Potop V. The diagnosis and treatment of fungal endophthalmitis: an update. Diagnostics (Basel). 2022;12(3) https://doi.org/10.3390/diagnostics12030679. Epub 2022/03/26. PubMed PMID: 35328231; PubMed Central PMCID: PMCPMC8947249

41. Khambati A, Wright RE 3rd, Das S, Pasula S, Sepulveda A, Hernandez F, et al. Aspergillus endophthalmitis: epidemiology, pathobiology, and current treatments. J Fungi (Basel). 2022;8(7) https://doi.org/10.3390/jof8070656. Epub 2022/07/28. PubMed PMID: 35887412; PubMed Central PMCID: PMCPMC9318612
42. Sahu ES, Lahoti K, Bhargava A, Subhedar V, Sahu A. Subretinal aspergillus abscess in post COVID-19 recovered patients – an emerging problem. Ocul Immunol Inflamm. 2023;31(1):127–33. Epub 2021/11/17. PubMed PMID: 34784260. https://doi.org/10.1080/09273948.2021.1993271.
43. Spadea L, Giannico MI. Diagnostic and management strategies of aspergillus endophthalmitis: current insights. Clin Ophthalmol. 2019;13:2573–82. https://doi.org/10.2147/OPTH.S219264. Epub 2020/01/11. PubMed PMID: 31920280; PubMed Central PMCID: PMCPMC6939405
44. Hariprasad SM, Mieler WF, Holz ER, Gao H, Kim JE, Chi J, et al. Determination of vitreous, aqueous, and plasma concentration of orally administered voriconazole in humans. Arch Ophthalmol. 2004;122(1):42–7. Epub 2004/01/14. PubMed PMID: 14718293. https://doi.org/10.1001/archopht.122.1.42.
45. Yu T, Chen L, Qian Z, Tao Y. Examination of galactomannan levels in intraocular fluid to assist the diagnosis of aspergillus endophthalmitis. Retina. 2024;44(8):1449–55. Epub 2024/04/03. PubMed PMID: 38569210. https://doi.org/10.1097/iae.0000000000004119.
46. Chen L, Feng J, Hu X, Bao H, Luan F, Tao Y. Valuable application of thE β- d -glucan testing of intraocular fluid for the diagnosis of fungal endophthalmitis. Retina. 2022;42(8):1560–7. Epub 2022/07/26. PubMed PMID: 35877967. https://doi.org/10.1097/iae.0000000000003491.
47. Adam CR, Sigler EJ. Multimodal imaging findings in endogenous aspergillus endophthalmitis. Retina. 2014;34(9):1914–5. Epub 2014/04/04. PubMed PMID: 24695061. https://doi.org/10.1097/iae.0000000000000135.
48. Burton E, Reddy V, Venkat AG. Endogenous fungal endophthalmitis: a single-center retrospective study and review of the literature. Am J Ophthalmol. 2024;262:97–106. Epub 2024/01/28. PubMed PMID: 38280676. https://doi.org/10.1016/j.ajo.2024.01.018.
49. Patterson TF, Thompson GR 3rd, Denning DW, Fishman JA, Hadley S, Herbrecht R, et al. Practice guidelines for the diagnosis and management of aspergillosis: 2016 update by the Infectious Diseases Society of America. Clin Infect Dis. 2016;63(4):e1–e60. https://doi.org/10.1093/cid/ciw326. Epub 2016/07/02. PubMed PMID: 27365388; PubMed Central PMCID: PMCPMC4967602
50. Sanfilippo S, Docquier B, Schrooyen PL, Makhoul D, Le A. Bilateral cryptococcal choroiditis in a human immunodeficiency virus-infected patient: a case report. Case Rep Ophthalmol. 2024;15(1):157–62. https://doi.org/10.1159/000535151. Epub 2024/02/15. PubMed PMID: 38357214; PubMed Central PMCID: PMCPMC10866609
51. Baillif S, Delas J, Asrargis A, Gastaud P. Multimodal imaging of bilateral cryptococcal choroiditis. Retina. 2013;33(1):249–51. Epub 2012/11/30. PubMed PMID: 23190924. https://doi.org/10.1097/IAE.0b013e318271f290.
52. Canfield GS, Reingold S, Ho A, Thor AD, Pecen PE, DeSanto K, et al. AIDS-related Cryptococcus neoformans choroiditis. IDCases. 2020;22:e00931. https://doi.org/10.1016/j.idcr.2020.e00931. Epub 2020/09/05. PubMed PMID: 32884904; PubMed Central PMCID: PMCPMC7452429
53. Andreola C, Ribeiro MP, de Carli CR, Gouvea AL, Curi AL. Multifocal choroiditis in disseminated Cryptococcus neoformans infection. Am J Ophthalmol. 2006;142(2):346–8. Epub 2006/08/01. PubMed PMID: 16876530. https://doi.org/10.1016/j.ajo.2006.03.024.
54. Aderman CM, Gorovoy IR, Chao DL, Bloomer MM, Obeid A, Stewart JM. Cryptococcal choroiditis in advanced AIDS with clinicopathologic correlation. Am J Ophthalmol Case Rep. 2018;10:51–4. https://doi.org/10.1016/j.ajoc.2018.01.045. Epub 2018/05/22. PubMed PMID: 29780913; PubMed Central PMCID: PMCPMC5956675
55. Larochelle RD, Larochelle MB, Aung YY, Linn T, Heiden D, Vitale AT. Bilateral placoid choroiditis in an HIV-positive patient with cryptococcus neoformans meningitis and disseminated cryptococcal disease. J Vitreoretin Dis. 2020;4(6):530–3. https://doi.org/10.1177/2474126420936191. Epub 2020/07/21. PubMed PMID: 37007659; PubMed Central PMCID: PMCPMC9976065

56. Paiva A, Biancardi AL, Curi A. Clinical-laboratory outcome of cryptococcus sp. multifocal choroiditis in acquired immunodeficiency syndrome patients. Ocul Immunol Inflamm. 2024;32(10):2421–7. Epub 2024/09/09. PubMed PMID: 39250593. https://doi.org/10.1080/09273948.2024.2392201.
57. Chang CC, Harrison TS, Bicanic TA, Chayakulkeeree M, Sorrell TC, Warris A, et al. Global guideline for the diagnosis and management of cryptococcosis: an initiative of the ECMM and ISHAM in cooperation with the ASM. Lancet Infect Dis. 2024;24(8):e495–512. https://doi.org/10.1016/S1473-3099(23)00731-4. Epub 2024/02/13. PubMed PMID: 38346436; PubMed Central PMCID: PMCPMC11526416

10 Fungal Infections of the Orbit

Anjali Anil, Ayush Vasisth,
and Shivaprakash M. Rudramurthy

10.1 Introduction

Infections of the orbit are included under the term 'periocular infections', along with pre-septal infections. Although fungi are less common in orbital infections, they are associated with debilitating clinical progression that can result in poor visual outcomes and potential systemic consequences [1]. Commonly associated with coexisting sinusitis or dental infections, these infections may present with confusing ocular symptoms and signs [2, 3]. Owing to the associated vision loss and likely systemic involvement, including extension to the brain, ophthalmologists need to identify these infections and treat them at the earliest. In this chapter, we review the current epidemiology, pathogenesis, varying clinical features, diagnosis and present treatment modalities for fungal infections of the orbit.

10.2 Epidemiology

(a) Fungi Involved in Orbital Infections

Orbital infections (including cellulitis, subperiosteal abscess and orbital abscess) are most commonly caused by sinusitis-associated bacteria such as *Streptococcus pneumoniae* and *Haemophilus influenzae*. Other causative bacteria include *Staphylococcus aureus*, Group A *Streptococcus*, *Streptococcus anginosus* and, rarely, *Pseudomonas aeruginosa* and gram-negative anaerobes [4]. Fungal orbital infections are also typically linked with concurrent involvement of the paranasal sinuses and are potentially invasive, depending on the causative pathogen and the host's immune status. Consequently, they are most frequently associated with the

A. Anil · A. Vasisth · S. M. Rudramurthy (✉)
Department of Medical Microbiology, Post Graduate Institute of Medical Education and Research, Chandigarh, India

M. C. Ramírez-Soto (ed.), *Fungal Eye Infections*,
https://doi.org/10.1007/978-3-032-19923-2_10

condition known as fungal rhinosinusitis (FRS). Mucorales and *Aspergillus* species are the most common fungi involved in orbital infections.

One of the earliest population-based studies of invasive fungal infections in 1992–1993 in the USA reported the incidence of *Aspergillus* at 12.4/million/year and Mucorales at 1.7/million/year [5]. However, there is a rising incidence of invasive fungal infections due to the interplay of host, pathogen and environmental risk factors. In 2024, Denning DW stated that over 6.5 million people have a life-threatening fungal infection every year globally [6]. Among these, the true incidence of fungal orbital infections is difficult to estimate. Owing to their varying clinical presentation, patients are initially misdiagnosed with bacterial cellulitis, inflammatory disease, or neoplasms. A 2005–2019 study on orbital infections in India reported a steady trend of fungal orbital infections at 6–7% of all causes [7]. The prevalence of mucormycosis is significantly higher in India, estimated at 0.14 cases per 1000 population, which is approximately 80 times the global average [8]. During the second wave of the COVID-19 pandemic, there was a sharp rise in cases of rhino-orbito-cerebral mucormycosis (ROCM). Increased risk has been reported in association with natural disasters, as well as increased spore count in indoor environments due to air coolers and air-conditioning filters [9–12]. With the increase in immunocompromised and susceptible populations, invasive aspergillosis, as well as chronic non-invasive aspergillosis, is on the rise.

The order Mucorales, belonging to the subphylum Mucoromycotina, comprises a diverse group of around 55 genera, with 38 established human pathogenic species [13]. They are common inhabitants of wet and decaying organic matter, also known to cause plant rot and spoilage. Rhino-orbital/rhino-orbital-cerebral mucormycosis (ROCM) is the term used to refer to the invasive orbital infection caused by them. This clinical entity is more common in Asia, in comparison with the West. The most common pathogens include *Rhizopus* spp., *Lichtheimia* spp., *Rhizomucor* spp. and *Mucor* spp. Mucorales morphologically produce aseptate or pauci-septate hyphal forms in tissue, with septations produced at irregular distances if present [13].

Aspergillus species are also involved in acute and chronic forms of orbital infection, particularly associated with rhinosinusitis [14]. They belong to the order Eurotiales under the phylum Ascomycota, and are commonly associated with soil and decaying vegetation. The most common species implicated are *Aspergillus fumigatus* and *Aspergillus flavus*. However, in tropical and subtropical regions, *A. flavus* is reported predominantly, likely due to its ability to survive in warmer and drier conditions [7, 15]. Also, in such regions, the sino-orbital-cerebral form is significantly higher than in temperate areas [16].

Rare reports of *Scedosporium apiospermum* and *Lomentospora prolificans* in sinusitis and orbital apex syndrome have been described [17, 18]. Primary orbital infections by *Cryptococcus neoformans, Histoplasma capsulatum, Conidiobolus* spp. and *Blastomyces* spp. have also been reported [19–22]. However, these are uncommon, varying with local epidemiological patterns and the patient's immune status.

(b) **Underlying Risk Factors**

Primary fungal orbital infections without involvement of surrounding structures are quite rare. Like bacterial orbital infections, they occur most commonly due to pre-existing rhinosinusitis. Other risk factors include dental infection/procedure, direct inoculation via orbital trauma or surgery, lacrimal system infections, endophthalmitis and peribulbar anaesthesia for surgery [4, 23]. Rarely, fungi may cause orbital infections via the hematogenous route [3]. Both Mucorales and *Aspergillus* include species that are thermotolerant/thermophilic, hence favourable for invasive infections [24].

Rhino-Orbital-Cerebral Mucormycosis (ROCM) The established risk factors include:

- Diabetes mellitus with/without ketoacidosis [25]
- Solid organ transplant/haematopoietic stem cell transplant recipients on immunosuppressants
- Haematological malignancy/solid organ tumour, chemotherapy
- Corticosteroid therapy
- Neutropenia
- Iron overload, deferoxamine therapy

The presence of uncontrolled diabetes mellitus is significantly associated with the rhino-orbital form [26]. Regional differences in risk factors exist, with diabetes mellitus being most common in Asia, as compared with the West, with haematological malignancy and solid organ transplant being most common [27]. Accordingly, ROCM is the predominant form in India, Mexico, Iran and other parts of Asia. Type 2 diabetes mellitus disrupts both innate and adaptive immune pathways. It reduces polymorphonuclear lymphocyte activity, including their mobilisation and chemotaxis. Also, IL-10 activity is significantly reduced [28]. Additionally, in a hyperglycaemic state, there is increased expression of GRP-78 protein, expressed within the endoplasmic reticulum of mammalian cells. This binds to CotH3 protein, serving as its ligand, which is part of the spore coating protein family for *Rhizopus* spp. [29, 30].

Iron is vital for the survival and growth of Mucorales in a susceptible host. In a ketoacidosis state, iron is displaced from the iron-carrying proteins transferrin, ferritin and lactoferrin. The resulting serum-free iron is taken up by these organisms with the help of siderophores. It is also studied that in patients undergoing deferoxamine therapy, *Rhizopus delemar* utilises the iron-rich form of deferoxamine (ferrioxamine) for its growth as a siderophore [31, 32]. As a result, these organisms can produce a rapidly invasive infection.

The COVID-19 pandemic introduced a new entity, COVID-associated mucormycosis (CAM), particularly in India. The most common clinical form associated with CAM is the rhino-orbital-cerebral form, with the mean interval between COVID-19 and development of mucormycosis reported as 14.4 +/− 4.3 days [33]. Hyperglycaemia, increased usage of corticosteroids, endothelial injury and hyperferritinaemia were understood as causative factors [24, 34]. SARS-CoV-2 binds to angiotensin-converting enzyme receptors present in significant proportions in pancreatic islet cells, thereby causing their disruption of activity. This itself results in acute diabetes and consequent ketoacidosis [24]. The increased expression of GRP-78 levels in COVID-19 has also been studied, explaining its role in ROCM [35].

Orbital Aspergillosis Aspergillosis of the orbit can present as either invasive or non-invasive forms. Each of these can occur in acute, fulminant or chronic, indolent courses.

The acute invasive form is more common in the presence of an underlying phagocytic defect. However, the absence of risk factors should not negate invasive rhino-orbital aspergillosis as a differential diagnosis, particularly in endemic regions. The following are the risk factors associated with invasive aspergillosis [16, 36]:

- Neutrophil disorder/neutropenia (associated with neoplasms)
- Increased dose of corticosteroid therapy
- Diabetes mellitus
- Bone marrow and solid organ transplant
- HIV-AIDS (CD4 < 50 cells)
- Increased environmental exposure to conidia (demolition/construction nearby)
- Alcoholism
- Others include the presence of post-operative orbital dressing, prosthetic devices [36, 37]

The chronic invasive form results in gradual destruction of orbital tissue in non-atopic patients with a history of chronic sinusitis. Though *Aspergillus* is the most common genus involved, reports of dematiaceous fungi (*Bipolaris, Exserohilum, Curvularia* and *Alternaria* spp.) have also been described [38].

The non-invasive form of orbital involvement can occur either due to allergic sinusitis or as a result of chronic, non-destructive mycetoma or aspergilloma in non-atopic, immunocompetent individuals. The orbital involvement occurs in ~20% of cases of allergic fungal rhinosinusitis [38]. Multiple cases of orbital cellulitis and aspergilloma of the orbit in immunocompetent populations (or with subtle immunodeficiencies) have been reported previously [23, 36, 39, 40].

10.3 Pathophysiology

(a) **Anatomy of the Orbit**

The pathophysiology, as well as the resulting clinical features and complications of these infections, can be better understood by visualising the anatomical structures within and around the orbit. The conical orbit whose apex is shifted medially is surrounded by paranasal sinuses on most sides. This explains the contiguous manner of spread of infection from these sinuses to the orbit. Superiorly, the orbit is

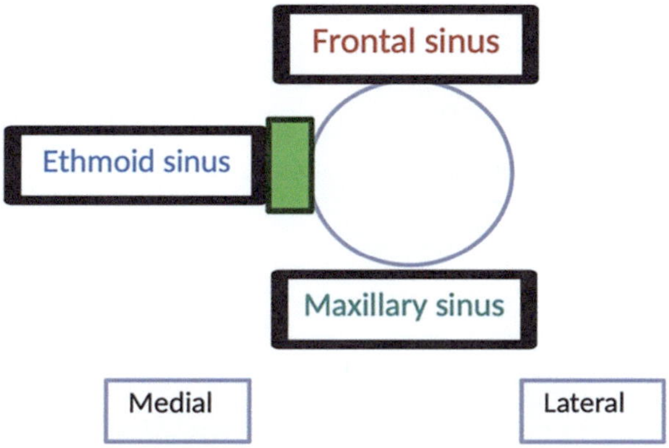

Fig. 10.1 Anterior view of orbit (created with Biorender.com)

bound by the frontal sinus, whose inferior wall forms the roof of the orbit, and inferiorly lies the maxillary sinus. Medially, the ethmoid sinus lies, separated by a thin lamina papyracea (indicated by the green box in Fig. 10.1). Through this lamina, multiple blood vessels and nerves pass. Hence, the ethmoid sinus is the most implicated in sinus-associated orbital infections [4].

The orbital apex is traversed by the optic nerve (second cranial nerve), as well as the IIIrd, IVth, VIth cranial nerves and the first division of cranial nerve V. The orbital apex syndrome associated with dysfunction of these nerves is commonly associated with mucormycosis, less commonly with invasive aspergillosis. The venous drainage of the paranasal sinuses is into the orbital veins, further draining into the pterygoid plexus inferiorly and the cavernous sinus posteriorly. Contiguous spread of infection to the brain can occur through the cribriform plate and the orbital apex [2]. The associated complications are explained later.

(b) **Mode of Infection and Pathogenesis**

Mucormycosis is an angio-invasive fungal infection, usually acquired by inhalation of propagative sporangiospores, and less commonly by traumatic inoculation. Mucorales produce spores of varying sizes (3–11 μm). As *Rhizopus* spp. produce larger spores, they tend to settle within the upper respiratory tract, including the sinuses, while the smaller spores of *Cunninghamella* spp. tend to travel to the lower respiratory tract. This explains their predominant involvement in ROCM and pulmonary mucormycosis, respectively [27]. However, previous literature has also reported that any of the genera can cause either of the manifestations [41].

Similar to mucormycosis, orbital aspergillosis is also commonly acquired via inhalation and concurrent paranasal sinus involvement. However, this entity could occur in immunocompromised or immunocompetent individuals. *Aspergillus flavus,* owing to its ability to survive in warm and arid environments, as well as larger spore size, is more likely to be associated with sinusitis and orbital aspergillosis.

Once these spores encounter a suitable environment, they sporulate and produce hyphae. In normal individuals, the nasal mucosa can mount an adequate local

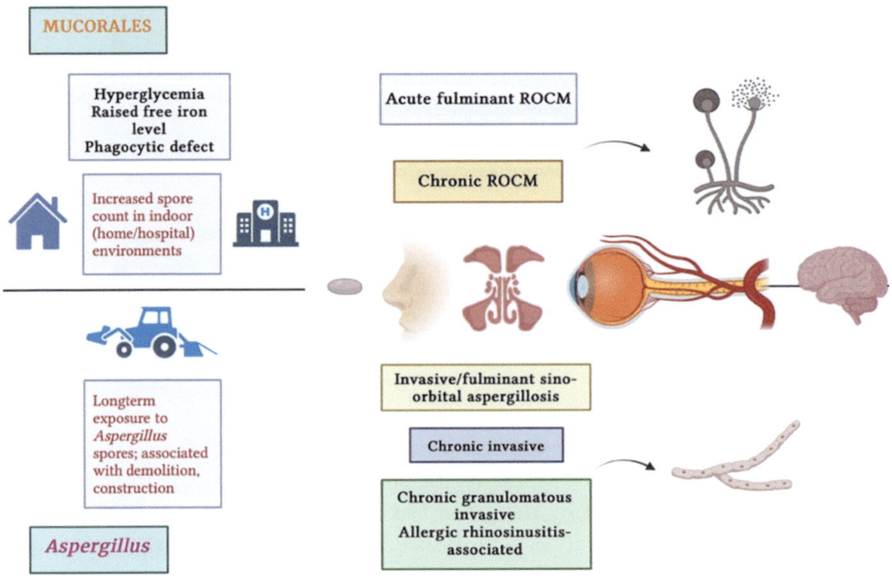

Fig. 10.2 Pathogenesis of orbital infections by Mucorales and *Aspergillus* (created in https://BioRender.com) [12, 43]

immune response, thereby preventing sporulation and spread of hyphae. In the presence of neutrophil dysfunction (in function or number), as commonly seen in the predisposing conditions mentioned previously, the hyphae are able to cause invasion of neurovascular structures and bone erosion. The spread occurs contiguously inferiorly to the hard palate, posteriorly to the sphenoid sinus and laterally to the orbit. Eventually, complications occur when the spread continues to the cavernous sinus or the brain [42]. The pathogenesis has been described in Fig. 10.2.

10.4 Clinical Presentation

Classically, orbital infections can be differentiated from their benign counterpart, pre-septal infections, by the presence of decreased vision, decreased extraocular movements and proptosis in the former entity [4]. Orbital infections, along with endogenous endophthalmitis and certain forms of uveitis, are particularly dangerous as they can cause systemic manifestations as well [44]. The presence of an underlying immune defect may suppress the local/systemic signs of infection, further confusing the clinician. The most common presenting features include: proptosis (>2 cm difference between either eye), diminution of vision (optic nerve involvement), pain and tearing and swelling of the periorbital region.

In rhino-orbital mucormycosis, the clinical features depend on the extent of involvement. The initial signs include facial/peri-orbital pain, nasal block and facial tenderness, with or without the presence of discharge. Nasal crusts and ulcers are

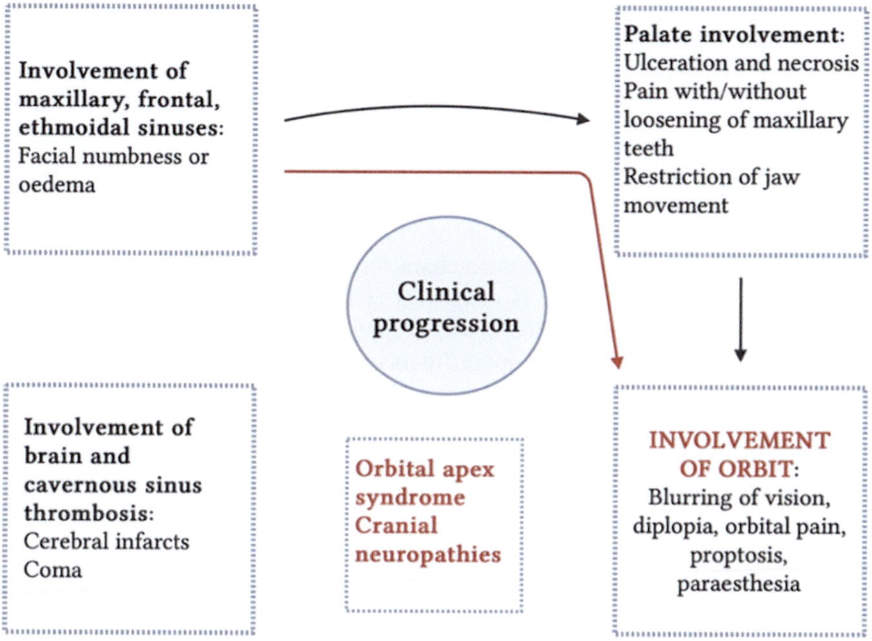

Fig. 10.3 Clinical progression of mucormycosis (created in https://BioRender.com)

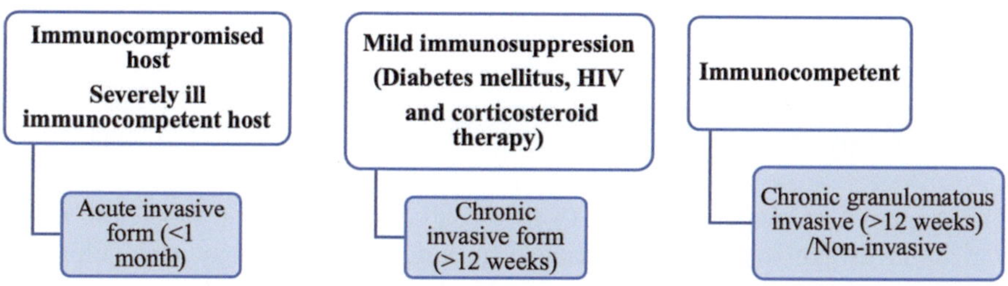

Fig. 10.4 Presentation of orbital aspergillosis depending on host status

also quite common [24, 43]. The presence of eschar on the hard palate is almost indicative of mucormycosis. However, it could be a late sign of orbital aspergillosis with spread to the hard palate. The clinical progression is explained in the Fig. 10.3.

Aspergillosis of the orbit can present either as an invasive (acute/chronic/chronic granulomatous) or a non-invasive form of infection. The presentation is dependent on the host's immune status (as described in Fig. 10.4) [15, 36, 45].

The non-invasive, indolent form of orbital aspergillosis can be either due to allergic fungal rhinosinusitis or fungal ball, with orbital or neuro-ophthalmic symptoms. When an allergic entity is present, the patient commonly presents with nasal obstruction, polyposis, chronic nasal discharge/crusting (greenish/black), not improving on antibiotics. Proptosis occurs due to secondary expansion of the orbit

[2, 46]. Orbital erosions have been reported in nearly 50% cases of AFRS in the paediatric population [46].

Invasive aspergillosis may present with varying clinical presentations, often confused with idiopathic orbital inflammatory disease, malignancy and temporal arteritis [36, 47–49]. The initial symptoms include headache, nasal congestion and facial pain. Occasionally, they develop severe retrobulbar pain due to sphenoidal involvement. Non-HIV immunocompromised patients typically present with acute proptosis, severe pain, and rapid diminution of vision. In contrast, patients with AIDS more often exhibit an insidious course characterised by headache, periorbital pain, and slowly progressive proptosis consistent with chronic invasive aspergillosis; diminution of vision is uncommon in this group [2].

Clinical diagnosis of orbital aspergillosis in immunocompetent hosts is rather challenging. As an adequate inflammatory response is mounted, these patients present with an acute onset of proptosis, severe headache, loss of vision and limitation of ocular movements. Being initially misdiagnosed as bacterial cellulitis, they go on to develop a chronic, untreated course [50]. The chronic granulomatous form of orbital aspergillosis could occur in immunocompetent individuals and is often associated with chronic rhinosinusitis, presenting with proptosis and occasionally headache [43]. They could present with bilateral orbital involvement and pansinusitis [2]. The differentiation between chronic invasive and chronic granulomatous invasive aspergillosis appears to be a dilemma. However, the two entities can be distinguished by host factors (AIDS, corticosteroid therapy, diabetes mellitus in chronic invasive), culture positivity (*Aspergillus fumigatus* in former (>50%), *Aspergillus flavus* in latter) and histopathological features [45].

10.5 Diagnosis

The diagnosis of fungal infections of the orbit combines clinical suspicion, radiological investigations and appropriate sampling for microscopy and culture in mycology, histopathology, as well as molecular diagnosis. The first step towards diagnosis is to identify the likelihood of an infectious process, as this would warrant urgent antifungal treatment with possible surgical intervention. Figure 10.5 illustrates the flowchart for the diagnosis of rhino-orbital mucormycosis.

10.5.1 Clinical History and Examination

When the patient presents to the clinician, a complete medical history should be obtained, detailing the onset, progression and appearance of symptoms and signs. Prior history of trauma, comorbidities, surgical procedures, drug intake and habits should be obtained. Also, the place of origin and occupation could point towards the likely cause of infection. A thorough examination should involve ophthalmic and

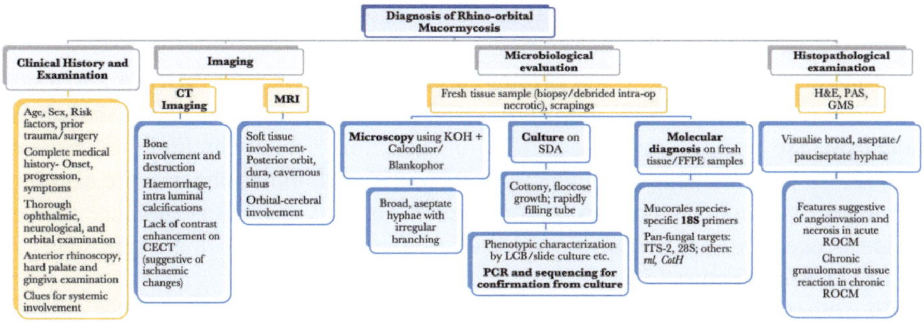

Fig. 10.5 Flowchart illustrating the diagnosis of Rhino-orbital Mucormycosis

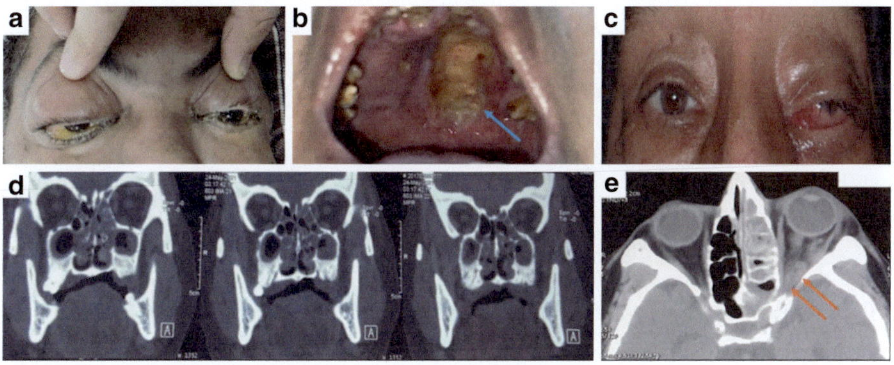

Fig. 10.6 Clinical and radiological features seen in fungal orbital infections. (**a**) Clinical presentation with cellulitis, periorbital oedema and conjunctival congestion. (**b**) Palatal eschar; a significant marker of rhino-orbital mucormycosis (blue arrow). (**c**) Patient with COVID-associated mucormycosis: mild proptosis, lid swelling and ptosis. (**d**) CT scan: coronal view: mass lesion & mucosal thickening in bilateral ethmoid, maxillary sinus and nasal cavity. (**e**) CT scan showing heterogenous opacity involving the entire left ethmoid sinus. Predominant left orbital apex involvement seen as a heterogenous hyperdensity at the apex, involving the medial rectus, the optic nerve sheath and surrounding fat (orange arrow). (Courtesy of Prof. Usha Singh, Department of Ophthalmology, Post Graduate Institute of Medical Education and Research, Chandigarh)

neuro-ophthalmic testing, orbital examination and testing for clues of systemic involvement. Anterior rhinoscopy, examination of the hard palate and gingiva, shall provide clues for upper respiratory or sinus involvement [2, 51] (Fig. 10.6).

10.5.2 Imaging

Imaging plays a significant role in understanding the anatomical involvement, particularly in aspergillosis. In mucormycosis, imaging also aids in preoperative planning. CT imaging provides an idea of bone involvement, as well as detecting the presence of haemorrhage and intraluminal calcifications. MRI highlights the soft tissue involvement, particularly that of the posterior orbit, dura mater close to paranasal sinuses and the cavernous sinus.

Bone destruction on CT and orbital-cerebral involvement on MRI in a diabetic patient with sinusitis, facial pain, proptosis, ophthalmoplegia or newly diagnosed amaurosis are highly suggestive of rhino-orbital/rhino-orbital-cerebral mucormycosis [52]. In patients with malignancy, thoracic and abdominal imaging are also recommended to understand the extent of disease. The lack of contrast enhancement of tissue is seen in ROCM due to ischaemic changes, owing to the angio-invasive nature of this infection [53].

In orbital aspergillosis, the findings can depict the invasiveness of the disease. CT scans are likely to depict soft tissue masses, with heterogenous enhancement post-contrast administration. This heterogeneous image may be due to the presence of iron, calcium or manganese in the fungal concretions. Calcification, when present, is highly suggestive of the chronic form of orbital aspergillosis [36]. Irregular, infiltrative soft tissue mass with extensive sinus involvement and bony destruction is more likely to be invasive aspergillosis. MRI demonstrates contrast-enhancing lesions that are hypointense on both T1- and T2-weighted sequences. This imaging profile contrasts with that of neoplasms and pyogenic infections, which generally exhibit T2 hyperintensity. In immunocompromised patients, despite extensive tissue involvement, the inflammatory signs may be minimal.

10.5.3 Microbiology and Histopathology

It is recommended that all patients undergo appropriate microbiological and histopathological sampling to establish the diagnosis of orbital fungal infections. The former helps to identify the causative pathogen, while the latter is important to check for the presence of invasive disease. The definitive diagnosis is based on culture of sterile site specimens or demonstration of hyphae on histopathology from the site. However, biopsy may not be tolerated in patients with rapidly progressive invasive mycosis [54]. Fine needle aspiration may be performed in patients who are unsuitable for surgery.

The general approach in microbiological diagnosis includes microscopy, culture, serology and, if required, molecular markers in culture-negative cases. Microscopy of tissue is performed by KOH mount, with enhancers such as calcofluor white or blankophor. Specimens of suspected mucormycosis should be processed with tissue teasing, and not grinding. The latter practice leads to the distortion of hyphae and a loss of culture positivity. Mucorales are visualised as broad, ribbon-like, aseptate hyphae with irregular branching on a KOH mount (Fig. 10.7). *Aspergillus* species are typically seen as septate hyphae with acute angle dichotomous branching. Culture of biopsy/aspirate is performed on Sabouraud dextrose agar and Brain Heart Infusion agar, preferably with added antibiotics. Mucorales are visualised as greyish, floccose growth that rapidly fills the tube or petri plate (Fig. 10.7). Further differentiation into genera can be done with the help of features such as the presence of rhizoids, the branching of sporangiophores, the shape of sporangia, the presence of apophyses and

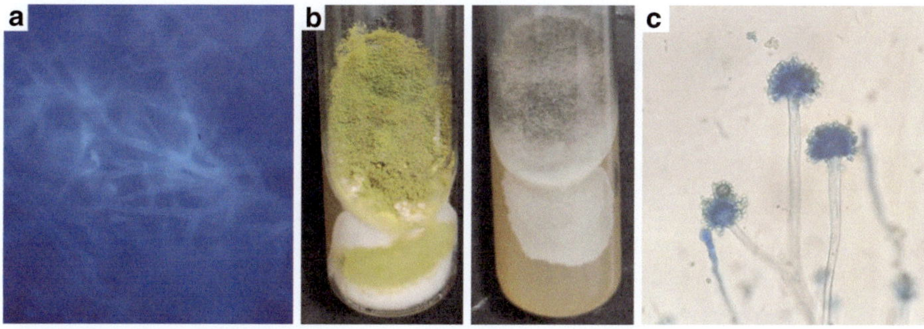

Fig. 10.7 Microscopy and culture findings of patients with suspected fungal orbital infections. (**a**) Palatal tissue—KOH-Calcofluor white preparation depicting broad, ribbon-like aseptate hyphae, with irregular branching. (**b**) Sabouraud dextrose agar (SDA) showing—left: yellow-green, granular growth of *Aspergillus flavus,* right: cottony, greyish growth of *Rhizopus arrhizus.* (**c**) Lactophenol cotton blue preparation showing hyaline, roughened conidiophore, conidial heads typically radiate, bearing biseriate/uniseriate phialides. Conidia are globose to sub-globose (3–6 μm in diameter), suggestive of *Aspergillus flavus*

the shape of the columella. Growth of *Aspergillus* species is initially white, and then turns into green, yellow, brown or black, depending on the species. Texture is usually velvety to powdery. *Aspergillus fumigatus* typically shows bluish green, powdery to velvety growth with a white border. *Aspergillus flavus* shows yellow-green to olive coloured growth, which is velvety to powdery in nature (Fig. 10.7).

In histopathological examination of tissue, stains utilised include haematoxylin and eosin, periodic acid-Schiff stain, Gomori's methenamine silver and Masson's Fontana stain (to highlight melanised fungi). Mucorales are generally visualised as broad non-septate/pauci-septate hyphae of width varying between 6 and 16 μm. False septations may be seen due to the folding over of hyphae during processing. Also, the angle of branching may be distorted due to the interstitial pressure of tissue. Hence, the width of fungal hyphae is a better indicator for histopathological diagnosis [52]. In acute lesions, thrombosing arteritis with invasion of vessels by fungal hyphae, with surrounding acute inflammatory infiltrate, is characteristic. Large areas of necrosis, accompanied by haemorrhage, can also be seen [2]. In chronic lesions, granulomatous inflammation is seen, with likely eosinophilic material surrounding fungal hyphae (Splendore-Hoeppli phenomenon) (Fig. 10.8).

In AFRS, the H&E section classically shows allergic mucin with variable staining, laminated accumulation of degenerating and intact eosinophils and Charcot-Leyden crystals [43, 55, 56]. The hyphae can be visualised as a negative image in nearly 67% cases [46]. Fungal ball/mycetoma typically shows tightly packed fungal hyphae, the morphology being better appreciated in the periphery. In invasive aspergillosis, a neutrophilic infiltrate (surrounding fungal elements) is classically seen. Granulomatous reaction, with a mixture of lymphocytes and giant cells, can be visualised in chronic lesions (Fig. 10.8) [43, 56].

Serodiagnosis can give an important clue for diagnosis where high suspicion is present on clinical and radiological features, but invasive sampling is not feasible.

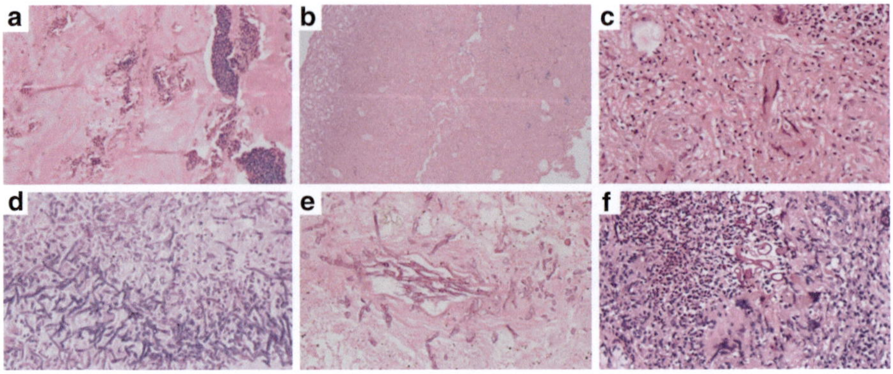

Fig. 10.8 Histopathological findings in fungal orbital infections. (**a**) H&E section in AFRS showing allergic mucin with variable intensity of staining, having folds and cracks and laminated accumulations of intact and degenerating eosinophils. (**b**) H&E section in fungal ball showing impacted fungal hyphae. (**c**) H&E section showing hyphal elements within a giant cell; chronic granulomatous lesion. (**d**) PAS highlighting septate hyphal elements in the case of acute invasive aspergillosis. (**e**) H&E section highlighting broad aseptate hyphal elements, with irregular branching in ROCM, (**f**) granulomatous response visualised on PAS in chronic rhino-orbital mucormycosis. (Courtesy of Prof. Amanjit Bal, Department of Pathology, Post Graduate Institute of Medical Education and Research, Chandigarh)

According to EORTC-MSG revised guidelines for diagnosis of invasive mould infections, galactomannan assay in serum/plasma is considered under the 'probable' category of invasive aspergillosis [57]. In allergic sinusitis associated with orbital complications, type I hypersensitivity to fungal antigens by the ImmunoCAP method can be demonstrated with good specificity and negative predictive value [58]. This helps to differentiate them from other causes of chronic rhinosinusitis. Also, the total IgE level is usually ≥1000 IU/ml [46]. There are no commercially available serodiagnostic tests for the diagnosis of mucormycosis. An in-house ELISA-based assay for the detection of antigens of *Rhizopus arrhizus* and *Rhizomucor* spp. has been described, with a sensitivity of 81% and a specificity of 94%. Also, lateral flow assays for the detection of γ-1,6-mannans and fucomannan antigen in Mucorales have been studied [54]. Choudhary H et al. evaluated an in-house indirect ELISA for antibody detection utilising secretory and mycelial antigens of *Rhizopus arrhizus*, showing better performance of IgG over IgM (84.6% vs. 69.2%) in diagnosing ROCM. When the tests were interpreted in combination, considering positivity for either IgG or IgM, the sensitivity for diagnosing ROCM increased to 94.9%, with a specificity of 80.0%. However, when both IgG and IgM had to be positive simultaneously, the sensitivity decreased to 60%, while the specificity increased to 95% [59].

PCR and sequencing techniques in tissue samples, including formalin-fixed paraffin-embedded (FFPE) samples, play a vital role in reducing the turnaround time. This helps to identify the pathogen up to genus or even species level. The targets include Mucorales-specific primers of the 18S gene, as well as pan-fungal targets including ITS-1/2 and 28S rRNA. Newer pan-Mucorales markers include *CotH* and *rnl* (encoding for spore coat protein and large subunit-ribosomal RNA, respectively) [60]. Fresh tissue samples are preferred over FFPE and have been noted to have more sensitivity (86–100% vs. 15–90%) [61]. Zaman K et al. have described a semi-nested PCR targeting Mucorales-specific primers of the 18S gene on fresh tissue samples. In comparison with (internal transcribed spacers) ITS primers (48% sensitivity), the Mucorales-specific primers were capable of detecting up to the species level in all samples [62]. However, the molecular diagnosis of mucormycosis in tissue faces several challenges, including a lack of standardisation, DNA degradation in FFPE samples and the risk of environmental contamination by Mucorales [54]. Also, performance on PCR in minimally contaminated BALF in pulmonary mucormycosis is considered superior to that in mucosal surfaces (nasal cavity and sinuses) [63]. Owing to the angio-invasive nature of this infection, several qPCR assays have been examined in serum for utility in high-risk patients. According to the MODIMUCOR multicentre prospective trial for multiplex qPCR assay targeting *Rhizopus*, *Mucor*, *Rhizomucor* and *Lichtheimia*, serum samples showed a sensitivity of 85.2% and a specificity of 89.8% in suspected invasive fungal disease. The PCR was able to detect invasive mucormycosis, 4 days prior to the mycological or histological examination and 1 day prior to the initial imaging results. Patients with consistently positive qPCR had a 100% mortality rate at 6 months despite antifungal treatment, while those with negative qPCR within 7 days of starting liposomal amphotericin B showed a markedly improved clinical outcome [64].

The EORTC-MSG guidelines for invasive fungal disease have classified *Aspergillus* PCR in blood and BALF under probable evidence for invasive aspergillosis. *Aspergillus* PCR can provide the benefits of identification of genetic markers of resistance and species-level differentiation, complementary to biomarker testing [63]. Previously studied assays are predominantly meant for the detection of invasive pulmonary aspergillosis. ITS1/ITS2, beta-tubulin and *Calmodulin*-based sequencing for *Aspergillus* have been performed.

10.6 Differential Diagnosis

Fungal infections of the orbit may be confused with other infectious causes (bacterial/parasitic), as well as neoplastic and non-infectious granulomatous processes. As a result, the patient may receive unwarranted corticosteroid therapy, which further potentiates the fungus. Also, as orbital infections could potentially cause a debilitating course, these infectious causes should be kept in mind when the patient presents to the ophthalmologist [36, 37] (Table 10.1).

Table 10.1 Differential diagnoses of fungal orbital infections

Type of disease	Aetiology
Infectious	*Bacterial*: Cellulitis, sub-periosteal abscess, *Mycobacterium tuberculosis,* non-tuberculous mycobacteria Syphilis: Gummatous involvement *Parasitic*: Toxoplasmosis, cysticercosis, hydatidosis, schistosomiasis
Inflammatory	Idiopathic orbital inflammatory disease Thyroid-associated ophthalmopathy Wegener's granulomatosis Sarcoidosis Polyarteritis nodosa Collagen vascular disorders
Neoplastic	Primary orbital neoplasm Metastasis, leukaemia, lymphoma, lacrimal gland neoplasm
Others	Drug-associated orbital inflammation Orbital foreign body, orbital haemorrhage Vascular involvement (fistula/thrombosis) Neuro-ophthalmic disorders (optic neuropathy/neuritis, cranial neuropathy)

10.7 Treatment

Management varies depending on the invasiveness, extent of involvement and pathogen involved. As *Mucorales* are angio-invasive, the resulting infection causes significant necrosis of the involved tissue. The Global Guideline for diagnosis and management of mucormycosis by ECMM-Mycoses Study Group Education and Research Consortium highlights that any suspected or confirmed case of mucormycosis warrants an urgent plan of action. A multipronged approach, including surgery, reversal of risk factors, wide surgical excision, systemic antifungal therapy and adequate sinus drainage, is required. For adequate drug delivery, the prime aspect of management is surgical debridement up to healthy margins [26]. The first-line antifungals include amphotericin B and isavuconazole. The recommended dose of amphotericin B is 5–10 mg/kg/day, which can be increased to 10 mg/kg/day in patients with CNS involvement. Both isavuconazole and posaconazole (delayed-release tablet/infusion therapy) are recommended as salvage therapy for mucormycosis. The duration of therapy depends on the reversal of inciting factors, the resolution of clinical signs and radiological improvement. Depending on the chronicity of the disease and the extent of orbital involvement, other treatment strategies include transcutaneous retrobulbar amphotericin B instillation and limited

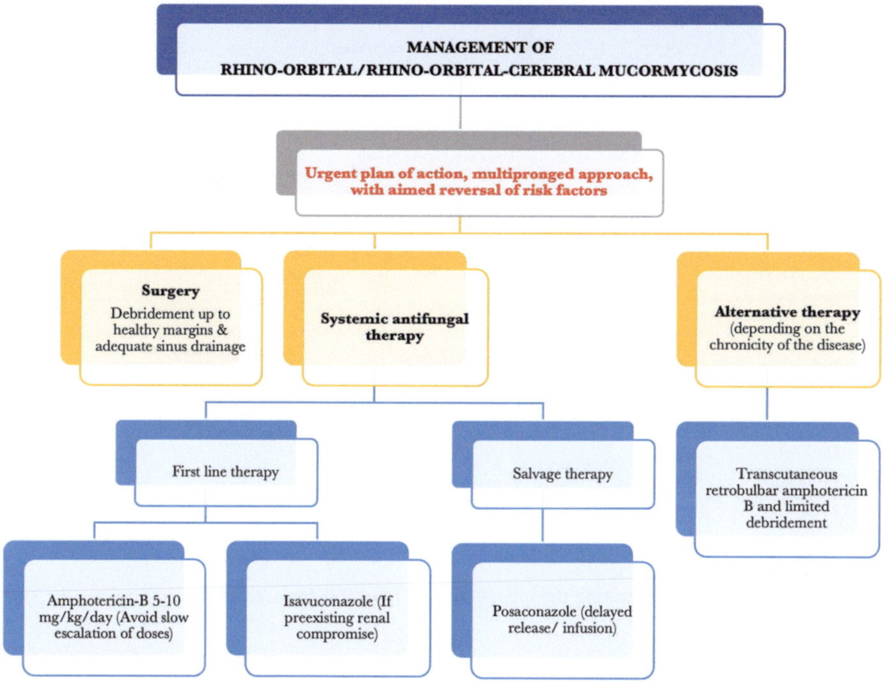

Fig. 10.9 Flowchart illustrating the management of Rhino-orbital Mucormycosis

debridement of infected tissue (Fig. 10.9) [1, 53]. Hyperbaric oxygen therapy (HBOT) has been shown to significantly inhibit the growth of Mucorales at the tissue level. Another therapeutic approach involves iron chelation with Deferasirox, which helps maintain iron homeostasis [60, 65].

In allergic *Aspergillus* rhinosinusitis and fungal ball, debridement of tissue along with aeration of the sinuses is required. Systemic antifungals are usually not warranted. Management of invasive aspergillosis depends on immunological status, early recognition and extent of disease [66]. While triazoles (particularly voriconazole and itraconazole) are the recommended first-line of antifungals, combination therapy of amphotericin B and itraconazole has also been given successfully [66, 67]. Oral isavuconazole is being investigated as a potential alternative to voriconazole, particularly in patients at increased risk of voriconazole-associated toxicity [68]. Surgical management depends on the extent of orbital involvement. Dhiwakar et al. reported that orbital exenteration is justified for posterior (retrobulbar, apical) disease, regardless of visual function, but is unnecessary for anterior (inferomedial) disease, where adequate debridement can preserve vision-critical structures [69].

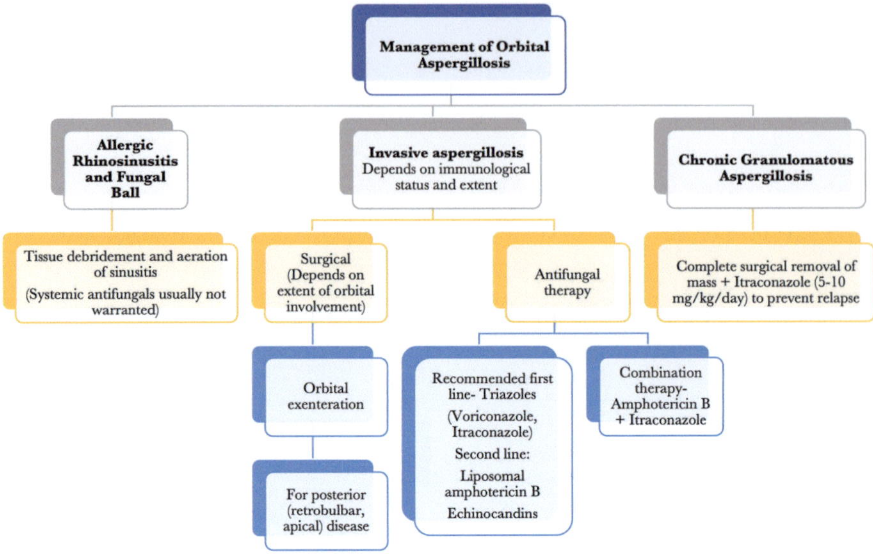

Fig. 10.10 Flowchart illustrating the management of Orbital Aspergillosis

However, controversy persists in terms of adequate surgical margins and drug delivery. In the chronic granulomatous form of aspergillosis, complete surgical removal of the mass is recommended. Itraconazole (5–10 mg/kg/day) is given in order to prevent relapse of the disease [43] (Fig. 10.10).

Newer antifungals and their formulations are being studied, owing to rising drug resistance, potential risk of systemic toxicity of the traditional drugs and poor compliance with drugs that require daily dosing [70]. Fosmanogepix (active moiety being Manogepix), a Gwt1 inhibitor, demonstrates activity against both *Aspergillus* and Mucorales, offering potential as a broad-spectrum agent. Cochleated amphotericin B, a lipid-crystal encapsulated oral formulation, allows targeted delivery with reduced toxicity, showing promise in treating invasive fungal diseases, including rhino-orbital mucormycosis, especially in patients unable to tolerate conventional amphotericin B. Opelconazole (PC945) is a novel triazole currently under investigation for the prophylaxis of invasive aspergillosis, delivered via the inhalational route in a micronised particulate formulation [70, 71]. Table 10.2 provides a summary of the drugs currently used in the management of fungal orbital infections.

Table 10.2 Summary of drugs required for management of fungal orbital infections

	Drug	Formulation	Dose	Remarks
Rhino-orbital/ rhino-orbital-cerebral mucormycosis (ROCM)	Liposomal amphotericin B	IV infusion	5–10 mg/kg/day	First-line. Higher doses (10 mg/kg) for CNS involvement. Monitoring of renal function.
	Isavuconazole	IV / oral (capsules)	Loading: 200 mg q8h × 6 doses (48 h), then 200 mg daily	First-line alternative to amphotericin. Less nephrotoxicity, once-daily dosing. Good oral bioavailability.
	Posaconazole	IV / oral (DR tablets/ susp.)	Loading: 300 mg BID day 1 → maintenance: 300 mg daily	Used as a step-down after amphotericin. DR tablets/IV preferred over suspension. TDM advised.
	Amphotericin B deoxycholate	IV infusion	0.7–1.0 mg/kg/ day	Used in resource-limited settings. Higher nephrotoxicity.
Invasive aspergillosis of the orbit	Voriconazole	IV / oral	Loading: 6 mg/kg IV q12h × 2 → maintenance: 4 mg/kg IV q12h OR 200–300 mg PO q12h	First-line. Requires TDM. Hepatotoxicity and neurotoxicity risk.
	Liposomal amphotericin B	IV infusion	3–5 mg/kg/day	Used if voriconazole contraindicated or resistance suspected.
	Posaconazole	IV / oral (DR tabs/ susp.)	Loading: 300 mg BID day 1 → maintenance: 300 mg daily	Step-down or salvage in azole failure. Monitoring required.
	Isavuconazole	IV / oral	Same as for ROCM	Useful in cases intolerant to voriconazole. Less QT prolongation risk.
Chronic granulomatous aspergillosis	Voriconazole/ itraconazole	IV/oral	5–10 mg/kg/day for itraconazole	Requires TDM.

10.8 Visual Prognosis and Complications

Fungal infections of the orbit are associated with a more debilitating course and serious sequelae, compared with bacterial cellulitis. As explained in earlier sections, the diagnosis and aggressive management are of utmost importance. As extensive surgical debridement is required in ROCM, the sequelae include significant facial disfigurement, exenteration and visual loss [26]. Rhino-orbital form of mucormycosis is, however, associated with better survival rates, as compared with its pulmonary counterpart. This is likely due to earlier presentation of the patient with facial and orbital signs, thereby leading to earlier diagnosis. Dissemination to the CNS, if present, is often associated with mortality rates of more than 80% [52]. A better survival rate is reported with infection by *Apophysomyces* species, and in the absence of neutropenia or haematological malignancy [72]. However, the visual outcome is generally poor.

Specific Complications:

- *Cavernous Sinus Thrombosis (CST):*

It is a rare yet life-threatening complication of fungal orbital infections. Once the infection reaches the cavernous sinus from the orbit, there is inflammation and thrombosis, potentially causing vision loss, seizures and could even be fatal. The management of this condition in the setting of fungal infections presents significant challenges. Treatment typically involves aggressive antifungal therapy and, in some instances, anticoagulation to address the risk of thrombosis. However, the use of anticoagulants in fungal CST remains controversial, as the combination of fungal invasion and anticoagulation therapy increases the risk of bleeding, and no clear consensus currently exists.

- *Intracranial Spread*:

Fungal invasion through the cribriform plate or superior orbital fissure can lead to brain abscess, cerebritis, stroke due to angioinvasion and vascular thrombosis. This requires aggressive management with liposomal amphotericin B and surgical debridement when feasible.

Other complications include systemic dissemination involving the lungs, skin and kidneys. Timely diagnosis is crucial to reduce morbidity and mortality, especially in high-risk patients such as those with uncontrolled diabetes mellitus and immunocompromised status.

10.9 Conclusion

Fungal orbital infections, particularly mucormycosis and aspergillosis, have emerged as significant threats to ocular and systemic health, especially in immunocompromised individuals. The COVID-19 pandemic notably contributed to a surge in cases, particularly in India, due to factors like uncontrolled diabetes and corticosteroid use. These infections are often aggressive, with high morbidity and mortality if not diagnosed and treated promptly. Early recognition and multidisciplinary management are critical to improving outcomes and reducing the risk of permanent vision loss or death.

Acknowledgements We would like to express our sincere gratitude to Prof. Usha Singh, Department of Ophthalmology, PGIMER Chandigarh, and Prof. Amanjit Bal, Department of Histopathology, PGIMER Chandigarh, for their generous contribution of images, which have significantly enhanced the understanding of this topic.

References

1. Chiou CA, Yoon MK. An update on fungal orbital infections. Int Ophthalmol Clin. 2022;62(2):55–69.
2. Mukherjee B, Raichura ND, Alam MS. Fungal infections of the orbit. Indian J Ophthalmol. 2016;64:337–45.
3. Kirszrot J, PAD R. Invasive fungal infections of the orbit. Int Ophthalmol Clin. 2007;47:117–32.
4. Durand L, Periocular M. Infections. In: Mandell, Douglas and Bennett's principles and practice of infectious diseases; 2020. p. 1541–7.
5. Rees JR, Pinner RW, Hajjeh RA, Brandt ME, Reingold AL. The epidemiological features of invasive mycotic infections in the San Francisco Bay area, 1992–1993: results of population-based laboratory active surveillance. Clin Infect Dis. 1998;27:1138–47.
6. Denning DW. Global incidence and mortality of severe fungal disease. Lancet Infect Dis. 2024;24:e428–38.
7. Joseph J, Karolia R, Sharma S, Choudhary H, Naik MN. Microbiological profile and antibiotic susceptibility trends in orbital cellulitis in India: an analysis over 15 years. Orbit. 2022;41:726–32.
8. Manuel RA, George A. Radiological findings of mucormycosis rhinosinusitis among Indian COVID-19 patients during the pandemic second wave. Egypt J Otolaryngol. 2023;39:94.
9. Benedict K, Park BJ. Invasive fungal infections after natural disasters. Emerg Infect Dis. 2014;20:349–55.
10. Davies BW, Smith JM, Hink EM, Durairaj VD. Increased incidence of rhino-orbital-cerebral mucormycosis after colorado flooding. Ophthalmic Plast Reconstr Surg. 2017;33:S148–51.
11. Caetano LA, Faria T, Springer J, Loeffler J, Viegas C. Antifungal-resistant Mucorales in different indoor environments. Mycology. 2019;10:75–83.
12. Ghosh AK, Singh R, Reddy S, Singh S, Rudramurthy SM, Kaur H, et al. Evaluation of environmental Mucorales contamination in and around the residence of COVID-19-associated mucormycosis patients. Front Cell Infect Microbiol. 2022;12:953750.
13. Walther G, Wagner L, Kurzai O. Updates on the taxonomy of Mucorales with an emphasis on clinically important taxa. J Fungi. 2019;5:106.
14. Green WR, Font RL, Zimmerman LE. Aspergillosis of the orbit: Report of Ten Cases and Review of the Literature. Arch Ophthalmol. 1969;82(3):302–313.
15. Rudramurthy SM, Paul RA, Chakrabarti A, Mouton JW, Meis JF. Invasive aspergillosis by *Aspergillus flavus*: epidemiology, diagnosis, antifungal resistance, and management. J Fungi. 2019;5 https://doi.org/10.3390/jof5030055.
16. Chakrabarti A, Chatterjee SS, Das A, Shivaprakash MR. Invasive aspergillosis in developing countries. Med Mycol. 2011;49:S35–47.
17. Sugiura Y, Sugimoto N, Takahashi T, Matsumoto T. Dual fungal infection with *Lomentospora prolificans* and *Aspergillus fumigatus*: a pathogenetic diagnosis elucidated after two decades by sequential examinations. Clin Case Rep. 2021;9:1383–6.
18. Jones J, Katz SE, Lubow M. *Scedosporium apiospermum* of the orbit. Arch Ophthalmol. 1999;117:272–3.
19. Vida L, Moel SA. Systemic North American blastomycosis with orbital involvement. Am J Ophthalmol. 1974;77:240–2.
20. Afkhamnejad ER, Turner C, Reynoso D. A case of orbital cryptococcosis. Am J Ophthalmol Case Rep. 2023;30:101821.
21. Pornpanich K, Uiprasertkul M, Luemsamran P, Jantharaworamet B, Vangveeravong S. Entomophthoramycosis: a rare fungal orbital infection presenting with dacryocystitis. Orbit. 2011;30:21–3.
22. Krakauer M, Prendes MA, Wilkes B, Lee HBH, Fraig M, Nunery WR. A case of orbital histoplasmosis. Ophthalmic Plast Reconstr Surg. 2016;32:e71–2.
23. Saini M, Singh U, Rudramurthy SM, Pokharel B. *Aspergillus terreus* panophthalmitis with orbital cellulitis. J Infect Chemother. 2025;31:102438.

24. Rudramurthy SM, Hoenigl M, Meis JF, Cornely OA, Muthu V, Gangneux JP, et al. ECMM/ISHAM recommendations for clinical management of COVID-19 associated mucormycosis in low- and middle-income countries. Mycoses. 2021;64:1028–37.
25. Jeong W, Keighley C, Wolfe R, Lee WL, Slavin MA, Kong DCM, et al. The epidemiology and clinical manifestations of mucormycosis: a systematic review and meta-analysis of case reports. Clin Microbiol Infect. 2019;25:26–34.
26. Morrissey CO, Kim HY, Garnham K, Dao A, Chakrabarti A, Perfect JR, et al. Mucorales: a systematic review to inform the World Health Organization priority list of fungal pathogens. Med Mycol. 2024;62:myad130.
27. Prakash H, Chakrabarti A. Global epidemiology of mucormycosis. J Fungi. 2019;5:26.
28. Morales-Franco B, Nava-Villalba M, Medina-Guerrero EO, Sánchez-Nuño YA, Davila-Villa P, Anaya-Ambriz EJ, et al. Host-pathogen molecular factors contribute to the pathogenesis of *Rhizopus* spp. in diabetes mellitus. Curr Trop Med Rep. 2021;8:6–17.
29. Gebremariam T, Liu M, Luo G, Bruno V, Phan QT, Waring AJ, et al. CotH3 mediates fungal invasion of host cells during mucormycosis. J Clin Invest. 2014;124:237–50.
30. Liu M, Spellberg B, Phan QT, Fu Y, Fu Y, Lee AS, et al. The endothelial cell receptor GRP78 is required for mucormycosis pathogenesis in diabetic mice. J Clin Invest. 2010;120:1914–24.
31. Ibrahim AS, Spellberg B, Walsh TJ, Kontoyiannis DP. Pathogenesis of mucormycosis. Clin Infect Dis. 2012;54(Suppl 1):S16–22.
32. Alqarihi A, Kontoyiannis DP, Ibrahim AS. Mucormycosis in 2023: an update on pathogenesis and management. Front Cell Infect Microbiol. 2023;13:1254919.
33. Bayram N, Ozsaygılı C, Sav H, Tekin Y, Gundogan M, Pangal E, et al. Susceptibility of severe COVID-19 patients to rhino-orbital mucormycosis fungal infection in different clinical manifestations. Jpn J Ophthalmol. 2021;65:515–25.
34. Chakrabarti A. The recent mucormycosis storm over Indian sky. Indian J Med Microbiol. 2021;39:269–70.
35. Sabirli R, Koseler A, Goren T, Turkcuer I, Kurt O. High GRP78 levels in covid-19 infection: a case-control study. Life Sci. 2021;265:118781.
36. Levin LA, Avery R, Shore JW, Woog JJ, Sullivan Baker A. The spectrum of orbital aspergillosis: a clinicopathological review. Surv Ophthalmol. 1996;41:142–54.
37. Lam Choi V, Yuen HunterKL, Biswas J, Yanoff M. Update in pathological diagnosis of orbital infections and inflammations. Middle East Afr J Ophthalmol. 2011;18:268.
38. Klapper SR, Lee AG, Patrinely JR, Stewart M, Alford EL. Orbital involvement in allergic fungal sinusitis. Ophthalmology. 1997;104:2094–100.
39. Lever M, Wilde B, Pförtner R, Deuschl C, Witzke O, Bertram S, et al. Orbital aspergillosis: a case report and review of the literature. BMC Ophthalmol. 2021;21:22.
40. Townes DE. Orbital aspergilloma. Surv Ophthalmol. 1967;12:337–43.
41. Rammaert B, Lanternier F, Zahar J-R, Dannaoui E, Bougnoux M-E, Lecuit M, et al. Healthcare-associated mucormycosis. Clin Infect Dis. 2012;54(Suppl 1):S44–54.
42. SMS H, Borghei P. Rhinocerebral mucormycosis: pathways of spread. Eur Arch Otorhinolaryngol. 2005;262:932–8.
43. Chakrabarti A, Das A, Panda NK. Overview of fungal rhinosinusitis. Indian J Otolaryngol Head Neck Surg. 2004;56:251–8.
44. M LD. Introduction to eye infections. In: Mandell, Douglas and Bennett's principles and practice of infectious diseases; 2020. p. 1493–6.
45. Chakrabarti A, Denning DW, Ferguson BJ, Ponikau J, Buzina W, Kita H, et al. Fungal rhinosinusitis: a categorization and definitional schema addressing current controversies. Laryngoscope. 2009;119:1809–18.
46. Chakrabarti A, Kaur H. Allergic aspergillus rhinosinusitis. J Fungi. 2016;2:32.
47. Mody KH, Ali MJ, Vemuganti GK, Nalamada S, Naik MN, Honavar SG. Orbital aspergillosis in immunocompetent patients. Br J Ophthalmol. 2014;98:1379–84.
48. Karakeçili F, Barkay O, Sümer B, Binay UD, Memiş KB, Yapıcıer Ö, et al. Invasive aspergillosis with cavernous sinus thrombosis following high-dose corticosteroid therapy: a challenging case of rhino-orbital-cerebral mycosis. J Fungi. 2024;10:788.

49. Zhang Y, He W. Orbital aspergillosis in an immunocompromised man with no history of trauma: a case report. J Int Med Res. 2024;52:03000605241239857.
50. Adulkar NG, Radhakrishnan S, Vidhya N, Kim U. Invasive sino-orbital fungal infections in immunocompetent patients: a clinico-pathological study. Eye (Basingstoke). 2019;33:988–94.
51. Johnson T. Fungal disease of the orbit. Ophthalmol Clin North Am. 2000;13:643–56.
52. Cornely OA, Alastruey-Izquierdo A, Arenz D, Chen SCA, Dannaoui E, Hochhegger B, et al. Global guideline for the diagnosis and management of mucormycosis: an initiative of the European confederation of medical mycology in cooperation with the mycoses study group education and research consortium. Lancet Infect Dis. 2019;19:e405–21.
53. Bhuskute GS, Keshri AK, Seduchidambaram M, Dubey A, Hameed N, Chidambaram K, et al. Changing spectrum of invasive fungal infections of the anterior skull base. J Neurol Surg B Skull Base. 2024;85:458–64.
54. Safiia J, Díaz MA, Alshaker H, Atallah CJ, Sakr P, Moshovitis DG, et al. Recent advances in diagnostic approaches for mucormycosis. J Fungi. 2024;10:727.
55. Schubert MS. Allergic fungal sinusitis: pathophysiology, diagnosis and management. Med Mycol. 2009;47:S324–30.
56. Das A, Bal A, Chakrabarti A, Panda N, Joshi K. Spectrum of fungal rhinosinusitis; histopathologist's perspective. Histopathology. 2009;54:854–9.
57. Donnelly JP, Chen SC, Kauffman CA, Steinbach WJ, Baddley JW, Verweij PE, et al. Revision and update of the consensus definitions of invasive fungal disease from the European organization for research and treatment of cancer and the mycoses study group education and research consortium. Clin Infect Dis. 2020;71:1367–76.
58. Calabria CW, Dietrich J, Hagan L. Comparison of serum-specific IgE (ImmunoCAP) and skin-prick test results for 53 inhalant allergens in patients with chronic rhinitis. Allergy Asthma Proc. 2009;30(4):386–96.
59. Choudhary H, Kaur H, Singh S, Singh R, Muthu V, Verma R, et al. A novel indirect ELISA for serodiagnosis of mucormycosis using antigens from *Rhizopus arrhizus*. Mycoses. 2024;67:e13730.
60. Lamoth F. Novel approaches in the management of mucormycosis. Curr Fungal Infect Rep. 2023; 17:98–107.
61. Gudisa R, Harchand R, Rudramurthy SM. Nucleic-acid-based molecular fungal diagnostics: a way to a better future. Diagnostics. 2024;14:520.
62. Zaman K, Rudramurthy SM, Das A, Panda N, Honnavar P, Kaur H, et al. Molecular diagnosis of rhino-orbito-cerebral mucormycosis from fresh tissue samples. J Med Microbiol. 2017;66:1124–9.
63. Brown L, Cruciani M, Morton CO, Alanio A, Barnes RA, Donnelly JP, et al. The molecular diagnosis of invasive fungal diseases with a focus on PCR. Diagnostics. 2025;15:1909.
64. Millon L, Caillot D, Berceanu A, Bretagne S, Lanternier F, Morio F, et al. Evaluation of serum mucorales Polymerase Chain Reaction (PCR) for the diagnosis of mucormycoses: the MODIMUCOR prospective trial. Clin Infect Dis. 2022;75:777–85.
65. John BV, Chamilos G, Kontoyiannis DP. Hyperbaric oxygen as an adjunctive treatment for zygomycosis. Clin Microbiol Infect. 2005;11:515–7.
66. Panda NK, Saravanan K, Chakrabarti A. Combination antifungal therapy for invasive aspergillosis: can it replace high-risk surgery at the skull base? Am J Otolaryngol. 2008;29:24–30.
67. Patterson TF, Thompson GR, Denning DW, Fishman JA, Hadley S, Herbrecht R, et al. Practice guidelines for the diagnosis and management of aspergillosis: 2016 update by the infectious diseases society of America. Clin Infect Dis. 2016;63:e1–e60.
68. Too A, Sowerby L, Bursztyn L, Rahimi R. Successful treatment of invasive aspergillus rhinosinusitis and orbital aspergillosis with oral isavuconazole in a patient with contraindications to conventional first- and second-line therapy. RPS Pharm Pharmacol Rep. 2025;4. https://doi.org/10.1093/rpsppr/rqae031.
69. Dhiwakar M, Thakar A, Bahadur S. Invasive sino-orbital aspergillosis: surgical decisions and dilemmas. J Laryngol Otol. 2003;117:280–5.

70. Lu X, Zhou J, Ming Y, Wang Y, He R, Li Y, et al. Next-generation antifungal drugs: mechanisms, efficacy, and clinical prospects. Acta Pharm Sin B. 2025; https://doi.org/10.1016/j.apsb.2025.06.013.
71. Kriegl L, Egger M, Boyer J, Hoenigl M, Krause R. New treatment options for critically important WHO fungal priority pathogens. Clin Microbiol Infect. 2025;31:922–30.
72. Lee AS, Lee PWY, Allworth A, Smith T, Sullivan TJ. Orbital mycoses in an adult subtropical population. Eye. 2020;34:1640–7.

Neuro-ophthalmological Manifestations of Fungal Infections

11

Jaeryung Kim and Kyung-Ah Park

11.1 Introduction

Fungal infections affecting the visual system and surrounding neural structures represent a significant clinical challenge with potentially devastating consequences. These infections have increased in prevalence over recent decades, largely due to the growing population of immunocompromised individuals, advances in diagnostic capabilities, and increased awareness among clinicians [1]. Fungi are ubiquitous in the environment, yet only a small subset causes human disease, with an even smaller number capable of invading the central nervous system (CNS) and visual pathways [2].

The neuro-ophthalmological manifestations of fungal infections are diverse and often represent advanced diseases with significant morbidity and mortality. These manifestations typically result from the direct invasion of neural structures, vascular compromise, inflammatory responses, or a combination of these mechanisms [3]. The clinical presentation may include visual loss, ophthalmoplegia, orbital pain, proptosis, and other cranial neuropathies, often in the setting of sinus disease or systemic fungal infection [4, 5].

Fungal infections affecting neuro-ophthalmological structures are often associated with high morbidity and mortality, particularly in immunocompromised or debilitated patients. Diagnosis can be challenging due to often nonspecific clinical presentations and imaging findings, and difficulty in identifying the organism from cerebrospinal fluid or non-biopsy samples. Nevertheless,

J. Kim · K.-A. Park (✉)
Subdivision of Neuro-ophthalmology, Department of Ophthalmology, Samsung Medical Center, Sungkyunkwan University School of Medicine, Seoul, South Korea
e-mail: kparkoph@skku.edu

M. C. Ramírez-Soto (ed.), *Fungal Eye Infections*,
https://doi.org/10.1007/978-3-032-19923-2_11

advances in antifungal agents combined with aggressive surgical approaches offer the prospect of improved outcomes [6]. Early recognition, prompt diagnostic evaluation (particularly, tissue biopsy where feasible), and timely initiation of aggressive medical and often surgical therapy are critical for survival and potential visual preservation [7].

The most common fungal pathogens causing neuro-ophthalmological disease include *Aspergillus* species and the *Mucorales* order (formerly classified as *Zygomycetes*), which includes *Rhizopus*, *Mucor*, and *Lichtheimia* species [8]. Other fungi, such as *Cryptococcus*, *Candida*, *Fusarium*, *Histoplasma*, and *Coccidioides*, may also cause neuro-ophthalmological manifestations, albeit less frequently [9].

The anatomical complexity of the orbit, paranasal sinuses, skull base, and intracranial compartments creates unique challenges in the diagnosis and management of these infections. The orbital apex, cavernous sinus, and adjacent neurovascular structures are particularly vulnerable to fungal invasion from the paranasal sinuses, creating distinctive clinical syndromes that require prompt recognition and intervention [10, 11].

This chapter will explore the pathophysiology, clinical presentations, diagnostic approaches, and management strategies for fungal infections manifesting with neuro-ophthalmological signs and symptoms, with particular emphasis on early recognition and appropriate intervention to optimize outcomes.

11.2 Epidemiology

Invasive fungal infections in the head and neck most commonly affect the sinonasal cavities. A study conducted at a large tertiary hospital over a 19-year period (2005–2024) found that among the 413 documented fungal head and neck infections, 77 were invasive. Of these invasive cases, the sinonasal cavities were the most frequent site, accounting for 58.4% (45 cases), followed by orbital involvement in 18.2% (14 cases) [1, 12]. This highlights the sinonasal region as a primary site for invasive fungal disease with a high potential for extension to adjacent neurovascular structures, including the orbit. While precise epidemiological data for fungal orbital apex syndrome (OAS) itself are scarce due to its rarity and its status as a complication of broader invasive fungal sinusitis, the prevalence of its underlying causes provides an indirect measure of risk.

Specifically, concerning invasive fungal sinusitis, which is a common precursor to neuro-ophthalmological complications like orbital apex syndrome, its incidence can vary. For instance, previous research reported an approximate incidence of 1.4% for invasive fungal disease affecting the sinuses, noting that its occurrence in immunocompetent individuals is even rarer [13, 14]. Despite its overall rarity, especially in those without underlying immune deficiencies, the severe consequences of invasive fungal sinusitis, including orbital apex syndrome and other neuro-ophthalmological sequelae, make it a critical diagnostic consideration [6, 9].

11.3 Etiologies and Pathogenesis

11.3.1 Mechanisms of Fungal Invasion and Spread

Fungal infections affecting the visual system and neural structures represent a complex interplay between pathogen virulence factors and host immune responses. Understanding the fundamental mechanisms by which these organisms invade and damage tissues is essential for appropriate clinical management and therapeutic intervention. Fungal pathogens employ multiple mechanisms to invade and spread through host tissues. Rather than operating in isolation, these processes often occur simultaneously, creating a cascade of pathological events that culminate in the clinical manifestations observed in affected patients.

11.3.1.1 Direct Invasion

Direct tissue invasion represents the primary mechanism by which fungi establish infection and spread to contiguous structures. This process frequently begins with the colonization of the nasal mucosa and paranasal sinuses, creating a reservoir from which fungi can invade deeper tissues. The close anatomical proximity between the paranasal sinuses, orbit, and intracranial compartments provides routes for fungal spread [15]. The pattern and speed of invasion vary by fungal species. *Aspergillus* species commonly demonstrate a more indolent pattern of invasion characterized by granulomatous inflammation and progressive bone erosion, particularly of the orbital walls and skull base [16]. This erosive process may evolve over weeks to months, creating a potential window for therapeutic intervention before irreversible damage occurs, while invasive Aspergillosis can progress rapidly, particularly in immunocompromised hosts [17]. In contrast, *Mucorales* typically exhibit a more aggressive, rapidly progressive pattern of invasion that can traverse tissue planes within days, often outpacing diagnostic and therapeutic efforts [18].

The orbital apex represents a critical anatomical junction where multiple cranial nerves (II, III, IV, VI, and V1) converge in a confined space. Direct fungal invasion of this region results in the characteristic orbital apex syndrome, manifesting as visual loss, ophthalmoplegia, and sensory deficits in the distribution of the ophthalmic division of the trigeminal nerve [6].

11.3.1.2 Angioinvasion and Thrombosis

Angioinvasion represents a particularly devastating mechanism of fungal pathogenesis, especially prominent in Mucormycosis. This process involves direct penetration of blood vessel walls by fungal hyphae, leading to endothelial damage, thrombosis, tissue ischemia, and ultimately necrosis [4]. The predilection of *Mucorales* for blood vessels explains the characteristic black eschar observed clinically and accounts for the fulminant course often associated with these infections. Vascular compromise may affect the ophthalmic artery and its branches, the central retinal artery, or the cavernous portion of the internal carotid artery. The resulting ischemia can cause optic neuropathy, retinal infarction, or cerebral infarction, depending on the specific vessels involved [19]. While angioinvasion is most characteristic of *Mucorales*, *Aspergillus* species may also invade blood vessels, albeit typically with less aggressive vascular tropism.

11.3.1.3 Inflammatory Response

The inflammatory response to fungal invasion contributes significantly to tissue damage and clinical manifestations. Host neutrophils, macrophages, and other immune cells respond to fungal antigens, producing cytokines and other inflammatory mediators that can cause collateral damage to surrounding tissues. Neutrophilic infiltration, granuloma formation, and edema may compress neural structures, exacerbating the direct effects of fungal invasion [4]. In some cases, particularly with more chronic or indolent infections, the inflammatory response may predominate over direct fungal invasion in producing clinical symptoms. The balance between protective immunity and immunopathology varies depending on the fungal species, host immune status, and anatomical location of infection.

11.3.1.4 Perineural Spread

Perineural spread represents an important and increasingly recognized mechanism of fungal dissemination and a key indicator of advanced disease. Fungi can use nerve sheaths as conduits for invasion, spreading along these structures to reach distant sites. This mechanism is particularly relevant for cranial nerves traversing the skull base, including the optic nerve, oculomotor nerve, trochlear nerve, abducens nerve, and trigeminal nerve [4]. Perineural dissemination provides a pathophysiological explanation for the apparent discontinuous distribution of infectious processes occasionally observed in clinical assessment and radiographic evaluation, whereby pathogens traverse neural pathways to establish secondary foci of infection at distal anatomical sites while sparing intervening tissues, and contribute to characteristic symptoms, such as pain.

11.3.2 Host Factors and Immunological Response

Host immune status profoundly influences the pathophysiology and clinical course of fungal infections. The integrity of host defense mechanisms, including innate and adaptive immune responses, determines whether exposure to fungal pathogens results in colonization, localized infection, or the aggressive proliferation and invasion characteristic of invasive disease [20]. Several specific host factors increase susceptibility to invasive fungal disease and shape its clinical presentation.

11.3.2.1 Diabetes Mellitus

Diabetes mellitus, particularly when poorly controlled or complicated by ketoacidosis, creates an environment highly conducive to fungal growth and invasion [21]. The pathophysiological basis for this association is multifactorial. The acidotic state impairs neutrophil function, including chemotaxis, phagocytosis, and oxidative killing mechanisms [22, 23]. Elevated serum glucose provides a nutrient-rich medium for fungal proliferation, while hyperglycemia-induced glycosylation of iron-sequestering proteins may increase free iron availability, enhancing fungal growth. Additionally, microangiopathy associated with diabetes may contribute to tissue ischemia and impaired delivery of immune cells and antifungal drugs to infected tissues [24]. These factors collectively explain the strong association between diabetic ketoacidosis and rhinocerebral mucormycosis, a relationship first recognized clinically and subsequently confirmed through experimental models.

11.3.2.2 Immunosuppression

Various forms of immunosuppression increase vulnerability to fungal infections through distinct mechanisms. Neutropenia, whether resulting from hematological malignancies, chemotherapy, or bone marrow failure, particularly predisposes to *Aspergillus* infections. Neutrophils represent the primary cellular defense against filamentous fungi, and their quantitative or qualitative deficiency permits uncontrolled fungal proliferation. Impaired phagocytic function in diabetic ketoacidosis increases the risk for Mucormycosis [4]. Corticosteroid therapy impairs macrophage function and T-cell responses, compromising granuloma formation and cell-mediated immunity against fungi. Solid organ or hematopoietic stem cell transplantation creates complex immune defects that evolve over time, with the specific risk of different fungal pathogens varying according to the type of transplant, degree of immunosuppression, and time post-transplantation. HIV/AIDS primarily affects cell-mediated immunity, increasing susceptibility to fungi like *Cryptococcus* and endemic mycoses, though advanced disease may also predispose to invasive mold infections.

11.3.2.3 Iron Metabolism

Iron metabolism plays a crucial and often underappreciated role in fungal pathogenesis, particularly of *Mucorales*. These organisms require iron for growth and virulence, and conditions that increase serum iron availability enhance their pathogenicity. Elevated serum iron, as seen in patients with diabetic ketoacidosis, hemochromatosis, or those receiving deferoxamine therapy (which paradoxically serves as a siderophore for *Mucorales*), promotes fungal growth and tissue invasion. Conversely, iron chelation with agents that do not supply iron to fungi (unlike deferoxamine) may have therapeutic potential by limiting fungal proliferation [4, 25], although a small clinical trial found an increased mortality rate in patients with Mucormycosis treated with deferasirox in combination with liposomal amphotericin B, particularly in those with hematologic malignancies [26]. The relationship between iron metabolism and fungal virulence represents an active area of research with promising therapeutic implications.

11.3.3 Specific Pathophysiological Mechanisms by Fungal Species

11.3.3.1 *Aspergillus* Species

Aspergillus species, particularly *A. fumigatus*, *A. flavus*, and *A. niger*, cause a spectrum of disease ranging from allergic manifestations to invasive infection. In the context of neuro-ophthalmological disease, invasive Aspergillosis typically follows a more indolent course compared to Mucormycosis, though exceptions occur, particularly in severely immunocompromised hosts [27]. The pathophysiology of invasive *Aspergillus* infections is characterized by granulomatous inflammation with variable tissue necrosis, a tendency for bone erosion (particularly of the orbital walls and skull base), and less pronounced angioinvasion compared to *Mucorales*. *Aspergillus* produces numerous virulence factors, including proteases, phospholipases, and mycotoxins, that facilitate tissue invasion and damage. The organism's small conidia (2–3 μm) can reach terminal airways when inhaled, establishing a pulmonary infection that may subsequently disseminate hematogenously in severely immunocompromised hosts. In the context of sinonasal disease with orbital extension, however, contiguous spread from the sinuses represents the primary route of invasion. The clinical course of *Aspergillus* infections varies from acute (less than a month) to chronic (months to years), depending on the specific form and host immune status, which can allow for a potential window of intervention before irreversible damage occurs, especially in chronic forms [3].

11.3.3.2 *Mucorales* (*Rhizopus, Mucor, Lichtheimia*)

Mucorales (including *Rhizopus*, *Mucor*, and *Lichtheimia* species) cause a distinctive and often devastating form of invasive fungal disease characterized by aggressive angioinvasion with thrombosis and tissue infarction. The pathophysiology of Mucormycosis is marked by rapid progression (often within days) from initial symptoms to severe disease, pronounced tissue necrosis with characteristic black eschar formation, and a predilection for diabetic, particularly ketoacidotic, patients [22]. *Mucorales* possess several virulence factors that contribute to their pathogenicity, including thermotolerance (allowing growth at human body temperature), rhizoid production (facilitating tissue adherence), and expression of various enzymes that degrade host tissues. Their pronounced resistance to host defense mechanisms, particularly in the setting of impaired phagocytosis, contributes to their virulence. The fulminant nature of Mucormycosis often results in a narrow window for therapeutic intervention before irreversible damage occurs [28], underscoring the importance of early diagnosis and aggressive management.

11.3.3.3 Other Fungal Pathogens

Other fungal pathogens may cause neuro-ophthalmological disease through various mechanisms, though less commonly than *Aspergillus* and *Mucorales*. *Cryptococcus neoformans* typically causes meningitis with secondary cranial neuropathies and may cause papilledema due to increased intracranial pressure [29]. Its polysaccharide capsule represents a key virulence factor, inhibiting phagocytosis and modulating host immune responses [30]. *Candida* species usually cause endogenous endophthalmitis via hematogenous spread and rarely invade orbital structures directly [31]. Their ability to form biofilms and transition between yeast and hyphal forms contribute to their pathogenicity [32]. *Fusarium* may cause keratitis with potential for intraocular spread but rarely causes primary orbital disease [33]. *Histoplasma* and *Coccidioides* primarily cause chorioretinal disease and rarely invade orbital or neural structures directly [34].

The complex pathophysiology of fungal infections affecting the visual system and neural structures reflects the interplay between fungal virulence factors and host immune responses. Understanding these mechanisms provides the foundation for appropriate diagnostic approaches and therapeutic interventions, which must be tailored to the specific fungal pathogen and host factors involved in each case. Early recognition of the characteristic patterns of disease associated with different fungi is essential for timely intervention and optimal outcomes.

11.4 Clinical Presentation

Fungal infections affecting the visual system and surrounding neural structures manifest through a diverse spectrum of clinical presentations, reflecting the complex interplay between pathogen virulence, host immune status, anatomical location, and the duration of infection [35]. Understanding these clinical manifestations in their full context is essential for early recognition and timely intervention, which remain the cornerstones of successful management.

The neuro-ophthalmological manifestations of fungal infections typically evolve along a continuum, beginning with subtle, non-specific symptoms that may progress to distinctive clinical syndromes as the infection advances. The tempo of this progression varies significantly between fungal pathogens and host conditions. Mucormycosis often demonstrates a fulminant and rapidly progressive course, with symptom onset to diagnosis/death often measured in days or weeks [5]. Aspergillosis, while frequently evolving more insidiously over weeks to months [36, 37], can also present with a fulminant and rapidly progressive course, particularly in severely immunocompromised hosts [17]. This temporal pattern provides valuable diagnostic clues when evaluating patients with suspected fungal infection.

11.4.1 Early Clinical Manifestations

The initial presentation of fungal infections with neuro-ophthalmological involvement is often characterized by non-specific symptoms that may be mistaken for more common conditions, such as bacterial sinusitis, orbital cellulitis, idiopathic orbital inflammatory disease, giant cell arteritis, or optic neuritis. Patients frequently report orbital or facial pain, which may be severe and poorly responsive to analgesics. This pain often precedes objective clinical findings and should prompt consideration of invasive fungal disease, particularly in at-risk populations. Nasal congestion, rhinorrhea, and facial pressure—symptoms commonly attributed to bacterial sinusitis—may represent early manifestations of invasive fungal sinusitis with potential for orbital extension [38].

Visual symptoms typically begin subtly, with patients reporting blurred vision, color desaturation, or visual field defects that may initially be attributed to more common conditions, such as optic neuritis. As the infection progresses, visual acuity deteriorates, often rapidly in Mucormycosis, with progression to severe vision loss or blindness within days if the infection remains untreated [39, 40]. This deterioration is often due to aggressive angioinvasion leading to thrombosis and infarction of blood vessels (e.g., central retinal artery, ophthalmic artery, internal carotid artery), direct invasion of the optic nerve, or compression from an orbital apex syndrome or cavernous sinus thrombosis [4, 15, 41]. This rapid visual deterioration represents a medical emergency requiring immediate intervention to preserve visual function.

Diplopia, often initially intermittent and position-dependent, signals involvement of the ocular motor nerves (cranial nerves III, IV, and VI) and may precede clinically apparent ophthalmoplegia. Patients may compensate for mild diplopia by adopting a head tilt or turn, which can be a subtle but important clinical sign in early disease. Facial numbness or paresthesia in the distribution of the ophthalmic division of the trigeminal nerve (V1) may indicate the perineural spread of infection along this important sensory pathway [42].

Systemic symptoms, including fever, malaise, and altered mental status, may be present but are often less prominent than local symptoms, particularly in immunocompromised hosts whose inflammatory response may be blunted. The absence of systemic symptoms should not dissuade clinicians from considering invasive fungal disease when other clinical features are suggestive.

11.4.2 Orbital Apex Syndrome

Orbital apex syndrome (OAS) represents a cardinal manifestation of advanced fungal infection affecting the visual system and surrounding neural structures. This distinctive clinical entity results from pathological processes involving the orbital apex—an anatomically confined space containing the optic nerve, superior orbital fissure (transmitting cranial nerves III, IV, VI, and V1), and adjacent structures. The syndrome's clinical significance extends beyond its diagnostic implications, as it often heralds impending intracranial spread with potentially catastrophic consequences.

11.4.2.1 Anatomical Considerations

OAS is characterized by visual loss due to optic neuropathy combined with ophthalmoplegia from dysfunction of cranial nerves III, IV, and VI, and sensory deficits in the distribution of the ophthalmic division of the trigeminal nerve (V1) [6].

The anatomical configuration of the orbital apex explains the characteristic constellation of clinical findings in OAS. The optic nerve traverses the apex via the optic canal, while the oculomotor, trochlear, and abducens nerves, along with the ophthalmic division of the trigeminal nerve, pass through the adjacent superior orbital fissure. This anatomical convergence creates a vulnerable region where pathological processes can simultaneously affect multiple cranial nerves within a limited space. Furthermore, the orbital apex's proximity to the cavernous sinus posterolaterally and the middle cranial fossa posteriorly creates potential pathways for the infection to spread beyond the orbit, explaining the frequent progression from orbital apex syndrome to cavernous sinus syndrome (CSS) and intracranial involvement in advanced fungal infections [10].

11.4.2.2 Clinical Features and Diagnostic Criteria

Clinically, OAS manifests as a triad of visual loss (due to optic neuropathy), ophthalmoplegia (due to involvement of oculomotor, trochlear, and abducens nerves), and sensory deficits in the distribution of the ophthalmic division of the trigeminal nerve [43, 44] (Fig. 11.1). Visual loss results from optic neuropathy, which may occur through several mechanisms in fungal infections, including direct invasion of the optic nerve, compression by inflammatory tissue, vascular compromise of the ophthalmic artery or its branches, or a combination of these processes. The pattern of visual loss varies according to the predominant mechanism, with vascular compromise typically producing sudden, profound visual loss, while direct invasion or compression may cause more gradual deterioration [45].

Ophthalmoplegia in OAS reflects the dysfunction of cranial nerves III, IV, and VI, which control extraocular muscle function. This dysfunction can arise from the direct fungal invasion of the nerves, compression by expanding inflammatory tissue or abscesses, or ischemic injury due to the angioinvasion and thrombosis of the blood vessels supplying these nerves and the surrounding orbital structures. Complete ophthalmoplegia manifests as ptosis (from oculomotor nerve involvement) and a fixed, divergent eye position. Partial ophthalmoplegia may present with more subtle limitations of eye movement, often beginning in the field of action of a particular extraocular muscle and progressing to involve multiple directions of gaze. The pattern of ophthalmoplegia may provide clues to the predominant site of neural involvement, with isolated abduction deficits suggesting early abducens nerve involvement, while combined ptosis, mydriasis, and limitation of adduction, elevation, and depression suggest oculomotor nerve dysfunction [43].

Sensory deficits in OAS involve the distribution of the ophthalmic division of the trigeminal nerve, manifesting as decreased sensation or paresthesia in the forehead, upper eyelid, and cornea [43]. Corneal hypoesthesia may be detected clinically using a cotton wisp or corneal esthesiometer and represents an important but often overlooked sign of trigeminal nerve involvement. This sensory deficit increases the risk of exposure keratopathy, particularly when combined with lagophthalmos from oculomotor nerve dysfunction.

The clinical presentation of OAS due to fungal infection is often accompanied by additional findings that reflect the underlying infectious process. Proptosis, though variable in degree, results from inflammatory tissue, edema, or hemorrhage within the orbit [24, 43]. In some cases, particularly early in the disease course, proptosis

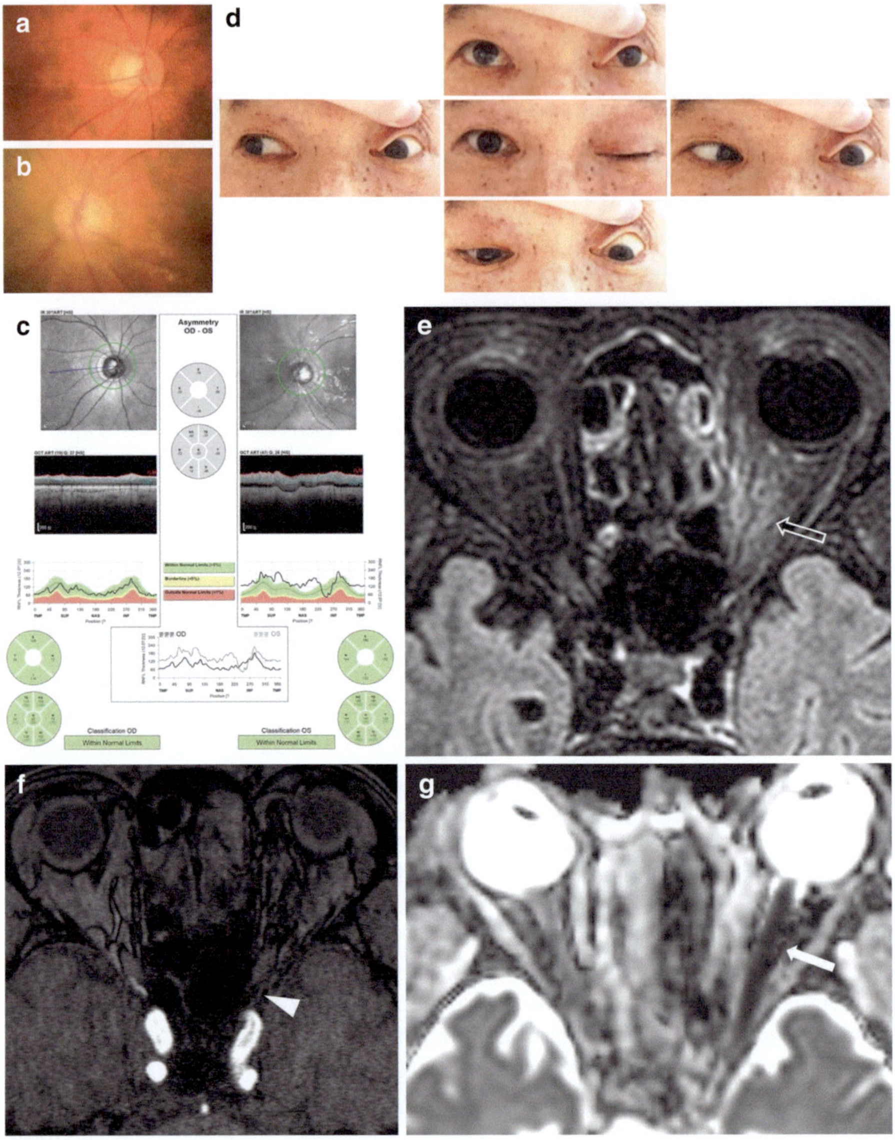
a
b
c
d
e
f
g
Asymmetry
OD - OS
Classification OD
Within Normal Limits
Classification OS
Within Normal Limits

Fig. 11.1 Orbital apex syndrome secondary to invasive fungal sinusitis in an immunocompromised patient with chronic lymphocytic leukemia. A 67-year-old male patient with chronic lymphocytic leukemia presented with an acute onset of visual loss in the left eye. The patient had a history of multiple chemotherapies for leukemia treatment. The patient developed rapid deterioration with left eye light perception vision, ptosis, optic disc swelling, extraocular movement limitation, and sensory loss in the distribution of the trigeminal nerve ophthalmic branch. Orbital magnetic resonance imaging (MRI) revealed infiltrative soft-tissue lesions involving the left orbital apex with involvement of the optic nerve and ophthalmic artery. Paranasal sinus biopsy confirmed invasive fungal infection with GMS (Grocott's methenamine silver) and PAS (Periodic acid-Schiff) stains demonstrating Mucormycosis. (**a**) Fundus photograph of the right eye showing normal optic disc appearance with sharp disc margins and normal retinal vasculature. (**b**) Fundus photograph of the left eye demonstrating severe optic disc swelling with blurred disc margins. (**c**) Peripapillary retinal nerve fiber layer (RNFL) optical coherence tomography (OCT) analysis showing normal thickness in the right eye within normal limits, while the left eye demonstrates optic disc swelling. (**d**) Ocular motility photographs showing left ptosis and limitation of extraocular movements in multiple directions, particularly affecting lateral, medial, and superior gaze, consistent with involvement of multiple ocular motor cranial nerves at the orbital apex. (**e–g**) Orbital MRI demonstrates an infiltrative lesion in the superior and medial orbit associated with sinonasal inflammation extending to the orbital apex to cause ophthalmic artery occlusion, resulting in optic nerve infarction. Post-contrast axial fluid-attenuated inversion recovery (FLAIR) image (**e**) with fat suppression demonstrates an infiltrative lesion in the superior and medial extraconal and intraconal orbit, reaching the orbital apex (*open white arrow*). Time-of-flight (TOF) MR angiography (**f**) demonstrates left ophthalmic artery occlusion (*solid white arrowhead*). A diffusion-weighted image (**g**) shows acute optic nerve infarction (*solid white arrow*)

may be minimal or absent despite significant neural involvement, a finding that should not dissuade clinicians from considering the diagnosis when other features are present. Chemosis and conjunctival injection reflect orbital inflammation and vascular congestion, while periorbital edema and erythema may signal the extension of the infectious process to the eyelids and periorbital tissues.

The tempo of symptom development in OAS provides important diagnostic clues regarding the underlying fungal pathogen. Mucormycosis typically presents with rapid progression over days, with patients often reporting dramatic worsening of symptoms within 24–48 h of onset. This fulminant course reflects the aggressive angioinvasive properties of *Mucorales* and the resulting tissue ischemia and necrosis. In contrast, while *Aspergillus* infections often evolve more gradually over weeks to months [10], they can also present with an acute or rapidly progressive course, particularly in severely immunocompromised hosts. The frequently non-specific initial symptoms of both Mucormycosis and Aspergillosis, coupled with their varied tempos, often lead to misdiagnosis and delayed treatment, which significantly worsens patient outcomes [10].

11.4.2.3 Prognostic Factors

Several factors influence the prognosis of OAS due to fungal infection, with the timing of intervention representing the most critical determinant of outcome. Early diagnosis and treatment significantly improve both visual and survival outcomes [46, 47], underscoring the importance of maintaining a high index of suspicion in at-risk populations. The causative organism also affects prognosis, with Mucormycosis generally carrying a worse prognosis than Aspergillosis due to its more aggressive course and greater resistance to antifungal therapy [48, 49]. Initial visual acuity provides an important prognostic indicator, with vision worse than 20/200 at presentation associated with poor prospects for visual recovery despite appropriate treatment [48]. The presence of cavernous sinus involvement, indicated by the extension of ophthalmoplegia to include the maxillary division of the trigeminal nerve (V2) or by radiographic evidence of cavernous sinus abnormalities, portends worse visual and survival outcomes [47–49]. Underlying host factors, including uncontrolled diabetes, profound immunosuppression, and advanced age, also adversely affect prognosis [47].

A recent retrospective study of 25 patients with OAS due to invasive fungal rhinosinusitis demonstrated the prognostic significance of initial visual acuity, with only 20% of patients presenting with vision worse than 20/200 recovering to better than 20/200 despite aggressive surgical and medical management [6]. This finding highlights the importance of early intervention before irreversible optic nerve damage occurs, as visual loss in these infections often becomes permanent [6].

11.4.2.4 Cavernous Sinus Syndrome

Cavernous sinus syndrome (CSS) represents an extension of the infectious process beyond the orbital apex into the cavernous sinus, with additional clinical manifestations reflecting the broader anatomical involvement. This progression signifies a critical deterioration in the patient's condition, as it indicates the extension of infection toward intracranial structures with increased risk of cerebral involvement and death.

11.4.2.5 Anatomical Considerations

The proximity of the cavernous sinus to the orbital apex and the valveless venous connections between these regions facilitate the spread of infection from the orbit to the cavernous sinus [15]. Additionally, the cavernous sinus receives venous drainage from the face and paranasal sinuses via the ophthalmic veins and pterygoid plexus, creating multiple potential routes for infectious spread. The absence of valves in these venous pathways allows bidirectional flow, explaining the occasional observation of bilateral cavernous sinus involvement via intercavernous connections, even when the primary infection appears unilateral.

11.4.2.6 Clinical Features

CSS due to fungal infection encompasses all the features of orbital apex syndrome with additional manifestations reflecting the broader anatomical involvement (Fig. 11.2). The most distinctive additional feature is involvement of the maxillary

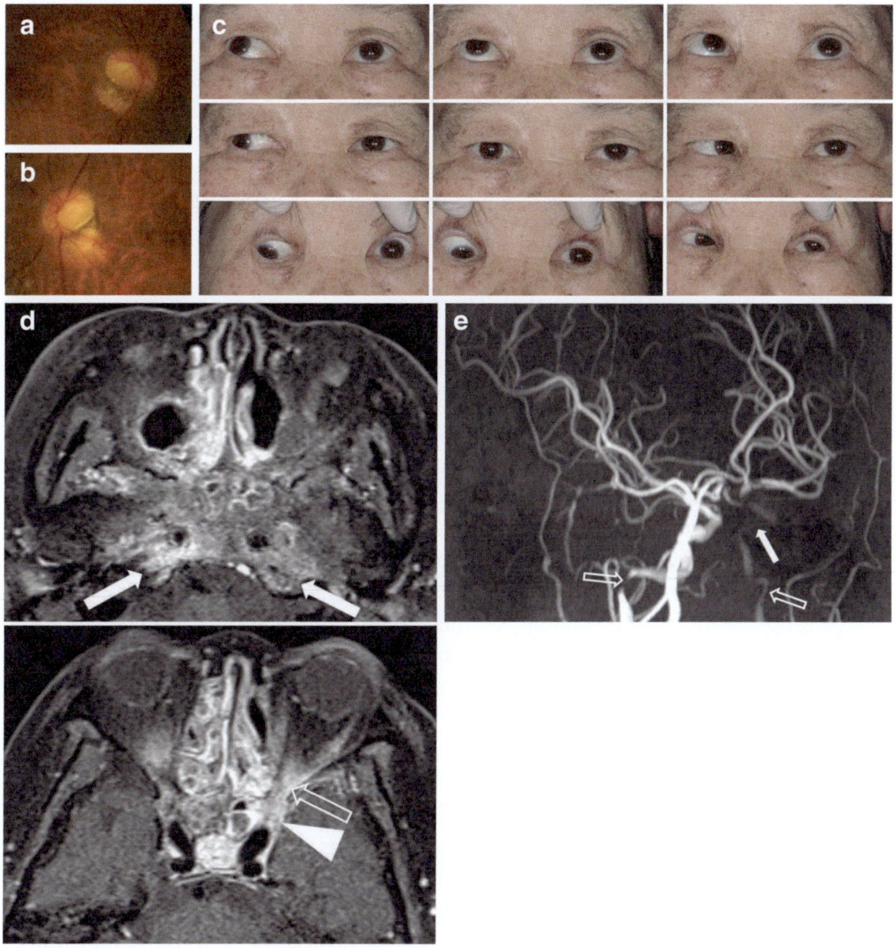

Fig. 11.2 Cavernous sinus syndrome secondary to invasive fungal sinusitis in a diabetic immunocompromised patient. A 66-year-old female patient with diabetes mellitus presented with visual loss in the left eye and extraocular movement limitation that had started two months prior to presentation. The patient had a history of diabetes mellitus for 20 years. One year prior to the visual symptoms, the patient presented with left cheek pain to another hospital, where an endoscopic biopsy was performed, revealing a fungal ball in the left maxillary sinus wall with Aspergillus confirmed by histopathological examination. She was treated with anti-fungal agents and showed improvement for approximately two months. However, the pain gradually worsened thereafter. Ophthalmologic examination revealed optic disc temporal pallor, with limitation of extraocular movements in all directions. Brain MRI and MRA revealed an infiltrative lesion of the skull base, with orbital apex, internal carotid artery, and cavernous sinus invasion. Endoscopic biopsy was performed, revealing sinusitis with marked edema and fibrosis. The patient was treated with amphotericin B, followed by voriconazole. (**a**) Fundus photograph of the right eye. (**b**) Fundus photograph of the left eye demonstrating temporal pallor of the optic disc. (**c**) Nine-gaze photographs showing severe extraocular movement limitation of the left eye in all directions. (**d**) On brain MRI, contrast-enhanced axial T1-weighted spin-echo images demonstrate infiltrative enhancing lesions involving the skull base (*solid white arrows*), orbital apex (*open white arrow*), and cavernous sinus (*solid white arrowhead*). (**e**) MR angiography shows occlusion of the left internal carotid artery (*solid white arrow*) and stenosis in both internal carotid arteries (*open white arrows*), secondary to a skull base infiltrative lesion

division of the trigeminal nerve (V2), manifesting as decreased sensation or paresthesias in the cheek, lower eyelid, lateral nose, and upper gum [50]. This finding helps distinguish CSS from isolated OAS and indicates the progression of the infectious process. The presence of CSS generally indicates advanced disease with higher morbidity and mortality compared to isolated OAS [10].

Horner syndrome, characterized by miosis, mild ptosis, and anhidrosis, may occur due to involvement of the sympathetic plexus surrounding the internal carotid artery within the cavernous sinus [51]. This finding may be difficult to appreciate in the setting of complete oculomotor nerve palsy with ptosis but becomes evident when the eyelid is manually elevated. The presence of Horner syndrome in a patient with ophthalmoplegia may suggest cavernous sinus involvement.

Internal carotid artery involvement represents a particularly ominous complication of cavernous sinus infection, potentially leading to thrombosis, stenosis, pseudoaneurysm formation, or rupture [52]. Carotid artery thrombosis may manifest as cerebral infarction in the corresponding vascular territory, with hemiparesis, hemisensory loss, aphasia (with dominant hemisphere involvement), or other focal neurological deficits [53]. Carotid pseudoaneurysm or rupture may cause catastrophic intracranial hemorrhage or carotid-cavernous fistula, the latter manifesting as pulsatile exophthalmos, orbital bruit, and severe chemosis [54].

The progression from orbital apex syndrome to cavernous sinus syndrome often occurs rapidly, particularly in Mucormycosis, with patients deteriorating clinically over hours to days [55]. This rapid progression underscores the need for frequent neurological and ophthalmological monitoring in patients with orbital apex syndrome and immediate intervention if signs of cavernous sinus involvement develop.

11.4.2.7 Isolated Cranial Neuropathies

While the orbital apex syndrome and cavernous sinus syndrome represent the most characteristic neuro-ophthalmological manifestations of fungal infections, isolated cranial neuropathies may occur as the predominant or initial presentation in some cases. These isolated deficits result from selective involvement of individual cranial nerves by the infectious process, often through perineural spread along nerve sheaths [56]. The pattern of cranial nerve involvement often reflects the anatomical pathway of infection spread.

Isolated optic neuropathy may present with visual loss in the absence of significant ophthalmoplegia or other cranial nerve deficits (Fig. 11.3). This pattern suggests selective involvement of the optic nerve, either through direct invasion, compression by inflammatory tissue, or vascular compromise of the ophthalmic artery or its branches. Visual outcomes are generally poor, particularly when initial visual acuity is worse than 20/200 or when treatment is delayed beyond 1–2 weeks from symptom onset [6].

Ocular motor cranial neuropathies (OMCNs) are common manifestations of fungal infections affecting the orbit and skull base, often occurring in characteristic patterns that provide diagnostic clues. Isolated OMCNs, particularly involving the abducens nerve (CN VI), may occur as an early manifestation of fungal infection [57] (Fig. 11.4). The abducens nerve's long intracranial course makes it particularly

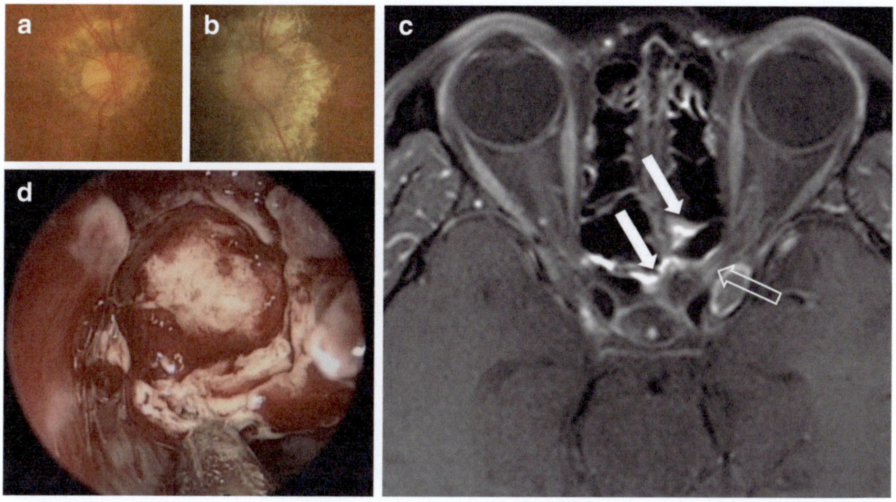

Fig. 11.3 Isolated optic neuropathy secondary to invasive fungal sinusitis in an immunocompromised patient with peripheral T-cell lymphoma. A 58-year-old male patient presented with a 5-month history of progressive left eye visual loss and headache following chemotherapy for peripheral T-cell lymphoma. Initial visual acuity was 20/50 in the left eye. Extraocular movements were normal and there was no diplopia. Orbit MRI revealed invasive inflammation involving the left posterior ethmoid sinus, sphenoid sinus, and anterior clinoid process with suspicious involvement of the adjacent optic nerve sheath and cavernous sinus, consistent with invasive sinus infection. Emergency endoscopic sinus surgery with biopsy was performed for definitive diagnosis, and post-operative tissue culture confirmed Aspergillus fumigatus. The patient was treated with voriconazole, and visual acuity improved to 20/30 at final follow-up. (**a**) Right optic disc appears normal with sharp disc margins. (**b**) Left optic disc shows mild swelling with blurred disc margins and a relative afferent pupillary defect positive. (**c**) On orbit MRI, T1-weighted fat-suppressed axial contrast-enhanced image demonstrates polypoid mucosal thickening in left posterior ethmoid and sphenoid sinuses (*solid white arrow*) with enhancement of optic nerve sheath and adjacent dura (*open white arrow*), consistent with invasive fungal sinusitis. (**d**) Endoscopic view during sinus surgery showing necrotic tissue and inflammatory changes consistent with invasive fungal sinus infection

vulnerable to various pathological processes, including fungal infection [58]. Isolated abduction deficit with horizontal diplopia should prompt consideration of fungal infection in at-risk populations, particularly when accompanied by severe, persistent pain or other suspicious features [57].

Isolated trigeminal neuropathy, manifesting as facial numbness or pain in the distribution of one or more divisions of the trigeminal nerve, may result from the perineural spread of fungi along trigeminal nerve branches. This pattern is more commonly associated with the perineural spread of malignancy but should prompt consideration of fungal infection in the appropriate clinical context, particularly when accompanied by other suspicious features or in immunocompromised hosts [59].

Facial nerve palsy may occur through an extension of infection from the middle ear or temporal bone, or through the direct invasion of the facial nerve within the

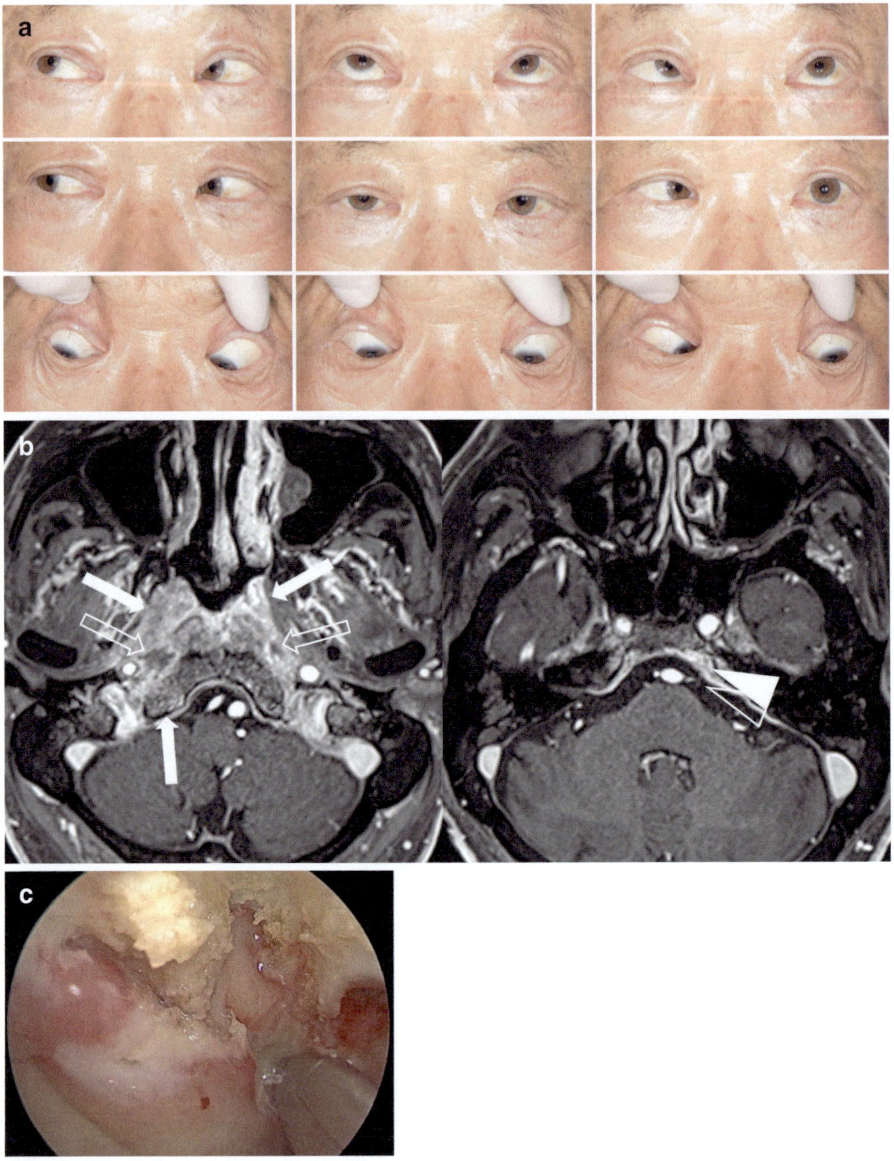
a
b
c

Fig. 11.4 Isolated abducens nerve palsy secondary to skull base osteomyelitis with otitis media complicated by invasive fungal sinusitis. A 67-year-old diabetic male patient with chronic alcoholism presented with progressive left eye abduction limitation and diplopia. The patient had a history of bilateral otitis media with tympanic membrane perforation and tube placement, which subsequently developed into skull base osteomyelitis. HbA1c was 8.6, indicating poor glycemic control with poorly controlled diabetes mellitus. Cranial nerve MRI revealed infiltrative enhancing lesions involving the central skull base and adjacent bilateral deep cervical spaces and probable abscess formation in the prevertebral space. Endoscopic transnasal biopsy of the clivus and nasopharyngeal mass confirmed invasive Aspergillosis. Pus drainage was performed during endoscopic surgery and sent for culture confirmation. The patient was treated with voriconazole. (**a**). Nine-gaze photograph demonstrating left abducens nerve palsy with limitation of left eye abduction and compensatory head turn to the left. (**b**) On cranial nerve MRI, contrast-enhanced axial T1-weighted fat-suppressed images show infiltrative enhancing soft-tissue lesions involving the central skull base and nasopharynx (*solid white arrows*) and abscesses in the prevertebral space (*open white arrows*). The infiltrative lesion probably involves the Dorello's canal portion of the left abducens nerve, so the Dorello's canal, which should normally appear as a filling defect, is not visible (*solid white arrowhead*). The cisternal segment of the abducens nerve shows subtle enhancement (*open white arrowhead*). (**c**) Endoscopic view during transnasal surgery showing necrotic tissue, with pus collected for culture confirmation of the causative organism

parotid gland. The combination of facial nerve palsy with ipsilateral ear pain or otorrhea should prompt consideration of fungal otomastoiditis, particularly in diabetic or immunocompromised patients [60].

Lower cranial nerve palsies (IX, X, XI, XII) may occur with fungal infections extending to the skull base, particularly those involving the jugular foramen or hypoglossal canal. These manifestations are less common than the neuro-ophthalmological presentations described above but should prompt consideration of fungal infection when occurring in at-risk populations or in conjunction with other suspicious features.

11.4.3 Other Neuro-ophthalmological Manifestations

Several additional neuro-ophthalmological manifestations may occur in the context of fungal infections, either as part of the syndromes described above or as distinct clinical entities.

Papilledema, reflecting increased intracranial pressure, may occur in fungal meningitis or with an intracranial extension of sinonasal fungal infections. This finding is particularly common in Cryptococcal meningitis, where communicating hydrocephalus from impaired cerebrospinal fluid reabsorption often leads to marked elevation of intracranial pressure [61]. Papilledema may also occur in invasive Aspergillosis or Mucormycosis with intracranial extension, reflecting mass effect from cerebral abscesses or infarction with associated edema [62].

Endophthalmitis, representing intraocular infection, may occur through hematogenous dissemination of fungi or through direct extension from adjacent structures. Endogenous fungal endophthalmitis typically presents with decreased vision, eye pain, and floaters, with examination revealing vitritis, chorioretinal lesions, and occasionally hypopyon. This manifestation is most common in patients with fungemia, with common predisposing factors including diabetes mellitus, recent hospitalization, central venous catheter use, intravenous drug use, and immunosuppression [9, 63]. Endophthalmitis represents a sight-threatening emergency requiring prompt diagnosis and intervention [9].

Rhino-orbital cerebral Mucormycosis (ROCM) represents a severe, rapidly progressive form of invasive fungal infection that begins in the nasal cavity or paranasal sinuses and extends to involve the orbit, cavernous sinus, and intracranial compartments. This entity encompasses many of the clinical manifestations described above but deserves special mention due to its fulminant course and high mortality rate [64]. ROCM typically begins with symptoms of sinusitis, including nasal congestion, facial pain, and rhinorrhea, often with characteristic black eschar visible in the nasal cavity or palate [65]. As the infection progresses, orbital involvement leads to orbital apex syndrome, followed by cavernous sinus syndrome and intracranial extension with altered mental status, focal neurological deficits, and seizures. The rapid progression from initial symptoms to death, often within days to weeks without treatment, underscores the importance of early recognition and aggressive intervention.

11.4.4 Clinical Variants by Host Factors

The clinical presentation of fungal infections with neuro-ophthalmological involvement varies significantly based on host factors, particularly immune status. Recognition of these variants is essential for appropriate clinical suspicion and timely diagnosis.

In diabetic patients, particularly those with ketoacidosis, Mucormycosis predominates with a characteristic fulminant course and prominent angioinvasion leading to tissue necrosis. The classic presentation includes rapid progression from sinusitis symptoms to the orbital apex syndrome, often with visible black eschar in the nasal cavity or palate reflecting tissue necrosis [66]. The combination of acute sinusitis, orbital pain, and cranial nerve deficits in a diabetic patient, particularly one with ketoacidosis, should prompt immediate consideration of Mucormycosis and urgent intervention.

In neutropenic patients, particularly those with hematological malignancies or hematopoietic stem cell transplantation, *Aspergillus* infections predominate [67]. While Mucormycosis is generally considered more aggressive, *Aspergillus* infections in this population are also rapidly progressive and severe [2, 67]. The presentation may be initially subtle and non-specific, with low-grade fever, mild orbital pain, and gradually progressive cranial nerve deficits. The absence of dramatic clinical findings should not dissuade clinicians from considering invasive fungal disease in these high-risk patients, as early intervention remains critical for favorable outcomes.

In solid organ transplant recipients, the clinical presentation varies based on the time post-transplantation and the degree of immunosuppression. Invasive fungal infections, including Aspergillosis, can occur both early (within the first month) and later (mean of approximately 184 days) post-transplantation, particularly in those requiring increased immunosuppression for rejection [68, 69]. The presentation may be modified by the immunosuppressive regimen, with corticosteroids potentially masking inflammatory signs and symptoms while permitting continued fungal invasion.

In HIV/AIDS patients, Cryptococcal meningitis represents the most common fungal infection with neuro-ophthalmological manifestations, typically presenting with headache, fever, and altered mental status, often with papilledema reflecting increased intracranial pressure [61]. Cranial neuropathies may occur but are less common than the diffuse meningeal signs. Other fungal pathogens, including *Histoplasma* and *Coccidioides*, may cause neuro-ophthalmological disease in endemic regions, particularly in patients with advanced immunosuppression [70].

In apparently immunocompetent hosts, fungal infections with neuro-ophthalmological involvement are rare but may occur, particularly in regions with high environmental exposure to pathogenic fungi. The presentation in these patients often includes more prominent inflammatory signs and symptoms compared to immunocompromised hosts, reflecting the intact immune response. Chronic invasive fungal sinusitis, typically caused by *Aspergillus* species, may present with gradually progressive proptosis, ophthalmoplegia, and visual loss over months to years, often mimicking orbital inflammatory disease or neoplasm [71].

The recognition of these clinical variants based on host factors allows clinicians to maintain appropriate suspicion for fungal infections in diverse patient populations and clinical scenarios, facilitating early diagnosis and intervention when these potentially devastating infections occur.

11.5 Diagnosis

The diagnosis of fungal infections with neuro-ophthalmological manifestations represents a complex clinical challenge requiring a multidisciplinary approach and integration of clinical, laboratory, and radiographic findings. Early and accurate diagnosis is paramount, as delays in recognition and treatment significantly impact visual and survival outcomes. The diagnostic approach must be systematic yet expeditious, balancing the need for definitive diagnosis with the urgency of initiating therapy before irreversible damage occurs.

11.5.1 Clinical Evaluation

The cornerstone of diagnosis begins with a comprehensive clinical evaluation, encompassing detailed history, thorough physical examination, and careful assessment of risk factors. This initial evaluation often provides the first indication of fungal infection and guides subsequent diagnostic investigations.

The history should focus on identifying predisposing conditions and exposures that increase susceptibility to invasive fungal disease. Diabetes mellitus, particularly when poorly controlled or complicated by ketoacidosis, represents a major risk factor for Mucormycosis and should prompt heightened suspicion when accompanied by compatible clinical features [72]. Other important risk factors include hematological malignancies, neutropenia, solid organ or hematopoietic stem cell transplantation, HIV/AIDS, prolonged corticosteroid therapy, and other forms of immunosuppression [72]. The temporal progression of symptoms provides valuable diagnostic clues, with Mucormycosis typically demonstrating a fulminant course measured in days, while Aspergillosis often evolves more insidiously over weeks to months [73]. The ophthalmological examination must be comprehensive, assessing both structural and functional aspects of the visual system. Findings such as ophthalmoplegia, proptosis, and optic neuropathy in an at-risk patient should trigger immediate further investigation [10].

Visual acuity testing provides an objective measure of visual function and establishes a baseline for monitoring disease progression and treatment response. Pupillary responses, particularly testing for relative afferent pupillary defect (RAPD), help localize pathology to the optic nerve or retina and may be present before clinically apparent visual loss. Ocular motility evaluation assesses the function of cranial nerves III, IV, and VI, with limitations in specific directions of gaze, providing clues to the pattern of neural involvement. Exophthalmometry quantifies proptosis, allowing objective monitoring of orbital disease progression, while slit-lamp examination may reveal anterior segment signs of orbital inflammation, including chemosis, conjunctival injection, and exposure keratopathy.

Dilated fundoscopic examination is essential for identifying optic nerve abnormalities, including optic disc edema, pallor, or atrophy, as well as retinal pathology, such as central retinal artery occlusion or chorioretinitis. Visual field testing, when the patient's condition permits, helps characterize the pattern of visual loss, with central scotomas suggesting direct optic nerve involvement, altitudinal defects suggesting vascular compromise, and progressive peripheral constriction suggesting compressive optic neuropathy. Color vision assessment provides a sensitive indicator of optic nerve dysfunction and may reveal abnormalities before significant visual acuity loss occurs.

The neurological examination complements the ophthalmological assessment, focusing on cranial nerve function, mental status, and evidence of intracranial involvement. Progression from orbital to neurological signs indicates advancing disease requiring urgent intervention [74]. Careful evaluation of trigeminal nerve function, including corneal sensation and facial sensibility in the distribution of V1 and V2, helps distinguish orbital apex syndrome from cavernous sinus syndrome and provides clues to the extent of neural involvement. Assessment of facial nerve function, lower cranial nerves, and long tract signs helps identify extension beyond the cavernous sinus to the cerebellopontine angle, skull base, or cerebral hemispheres. Signs of meningeal irritation, including nuchal rigidity and Kernig's or Brudzinski's signs, suggest meningeal involvement [75], while altered mental status, focal neurological deficits, or seizures indicate parenchymal disease requiring urgent intervention.

Nasal and oral examination represents a critical but often overlooked component of the clinical evaluation in suspected fungal infections. Careful inspection of the nasal cavity and palate may reveal the characteristic black eschar of Mucormycosis, representing necrotic tissue resulting from angioinvasion and infarction. This finding, when present, strongly supports the diagnosis of mucormycosis and indicates the need for immediate surgical and medical intervention [76].

The integration of clinical findings with the patient's risk profile often provides the first indication of fungal infection and guides the urgency and extent of subsequent diagnostic investigations. The presence of the orbital apex syndrome or cavernous sinus syndrome in a patient with diabetes, neutropenia, or other risk factors should trigger immediate consideration of invasive fungal disease and prompt expedited diagnostic evaluation and empiric therapy while awaiting definitive diagnosis.

11.5.2 Laboratory Investigations

Laboratory investigations play a crucial role in confirming the diagnosis of fungal infection, identifying the specific pathogen, and guiding targeted therapy. These investigations encompass microbiological studies, histopathological examination, serological tests, and molecular diagnostic techniques, each with specific advantages and limitations in the context of neuro-ophthalmological fungal disease.

Microbiological studies remain the gold standard for definitive diagnosis, providing direct evidence of fungal infection and allowing species identification and antifungal susceptibility testing. Direct microscopy of tissue samples using calcofluor white, potassium hydroxide (KOH), or other fungal stains permits rapid visualization of fungal elements, often within hours of sample collection. This approach provides immediate presumptive evidence of fungal infection and may guide initial therapy while awaiting culture results [1]. The morphological characteristics of fungal elements on direct microscopy may suggest the causative organism, with *Mucorales* demonstrating broad, ribbon-like, aseptate or pauciseptate hyphae with right-angle branching, while *Aspergillus* species typically show narrower, septate hyphae with acute-angle branching [77].

Fungal culture represents the definitive microbiological technique, allowing species identification and antifungal susceptibility testing. However, cultures may take days to weeks to yield results, and false negatives are common, particularly with prior antifungal therapy or inadequate sampling. The yield of cultures varies significantly based on the specimen type, with tissue biopsies providing higher sensitivity than swabs or aspirates [1]. Multiple media types, including Sabouraud dextrose agar, brain-heart infusion agar, and blood agar, should be inoculated to optimize the recovery of different fungal species [78]. Despite its limitations, culture remains essential for species identification and guiding targeted therapy, particularly in cases resistant to initial empiric treatment [79].

Histopathological examination of tissue specimens provides valuable diagnostic information [5], allowing visualization of fungal elements in the context of host tissue and inflammatory response. Special stains, including Gomori methenamine silver (GMS) and periodic acid-Schiff (PAS), enhance visualization of fungal elements within tissue sections [79]. Histopathology not only confirms the presence of fungi but also demonstrates tissue invasion, distinguishing colonization from invasive disease. The pattern of tissue invasion provides additional diagnostic clues, with *Nucorales* often demonstrating prominent angioinvasion and tissue necrosis [77], while *Aspergillus* typically shows more granulomatous inflammation with variable angioinvasion [80]. The integration of histopathological findings with clinical and radiographic features often provides the most comprehensive diagnostic picture.

Serological tests, including antigen and antibody detection, have variable utility and limitations in the diagnosis of invasive fungal infections with neuro-ophthalmological involvement. The galactomannan assay, which detects a cell wall component of *Aspergillus* species, may be useful in serum or bronchoalveolar lavage fluid but has limited sensitivity in localized sinonasal or orbital disease, with reduced performance noted in non-neutropenic or solid organ transplant recipients [81]. Similarly, the beta-D-glucan assay, which detects a cell wall component common to many fungi (except *Mucorales* and *Cryptococcus*), has variable sensitivity and specificity, with limitations in certain patient populations, such as non-hematological patients [81, 82]. Cryptococcal antigen testing in serum and cerebrospinal fluid has high sensitivity and specificity for Cryptococcal infection but is not relevant for the more common mold infections causing orbital and cranial nerve involvement [82]. False negatives are common with all serological tests, particularly in early disease or with concurrent antifungal therapy [5], limiting their utility as rule-out tests in suspected invasive fungal disease.

Molecular diagnostic techniques represent an evolving area with significant potential for improving the rapidity and accuracy of fungal diagnosis. Polymerase chain reaction (PCR) for fungal DNA offers greater sensitivity than culture and can provide results within hours rather than days [83]. Various PCR targets, including ribosomal DNA sequences and species-specific genes, allow broad fungal detection or focused testing for specific pathogens. Next-generation sequencing extends this capability, potentially identifying any fungal pathogen present in a clinical sample without prior knowledge of the likely organism. Matrix-assisted laser desorption/ionization time-of-flight mass spectrometry (MALDI-TOF MS) allows rapid identification of fungi from culture colonies, significantly reducing the time to species identification compared to traditional morphological methods [84].

Despite their potential advantages, molecular techniques face several limitations in clinical practice. Standardization remains challenging, with various in-house protocols limiting inter-laboratory comparability. Distinguishing colonization from invasion may be difficult with highly sensitive molecular methods, potentially leading to overdiagnosis. Additionally, these advanced techniques are not universally available, particularly in resource-limited settings where invasive fungal disease may be prevalent [84]. Nevertheless, molecular diagnostics represent a promising approach for improving the early diagnosis of fungal infections, particularly when combined with conventional microbiological and histopathological methods in a comprehensive diagnostic strategy.

11.5.3 Imaging Studies

Imaging studies play a crucial role in the diagnosis, staging, and management planning of fungal infections with neuro-ophthalmological involvement. Different imaging modalities offer complementary information, with computed tomography (CT) providing excellent bone detail and rapid assessment, while magnetic resonance imaging (MRI) offers superior soft tissue contrast and better evaluation of neural and vascular structures. The integration of radiographic findings with clinical and laboratory data provides the most comprehensive diagnostic picture and guides therapeutic interventions.

Computed tomography often serves as the initial imaging modality due to its widespread availability, rapid acquisition, and excellent visualization of bone structures. In the context of fungal infections, CT is particularly valuable for evaluating sinus opacification, bone erosion, and orbital involvement [85, 86]. Characteristic CT findings in invasive fungal sinusitis include unilateral or asymmetric sinus opacification with heterogeneous density, often with hyperdense foci representing fungal concretions or areas of hemorrhage. Bone erosion or destruction, particularly involving the orbital walls, skull base, or pterygopalatine fossa, suggests invasive disease and may be more prominent in Aspergillosis than Mucormycosis. Soft tissue infiltration of orbital fat, with obliteration of normal fat planes, indicates orbital extension, while air–fluid levels or hyperattenuating material with calcifications (often seen in Aspergillosis or fungus balls) within the sinuses may provide additional diagnostic clues [87].

The black turbinate sign, representing devitalized tissue due to vascular compromise, may be visible on contrast-enhanced T1-weighted MRI or CT as areas of non-enhancement within the nasal turbinates. This finding, when present, strongly suggests Mucormycosis and indicates the need for immediate surgical and medical intervention [88]. However, CT findings alone cannot reliably distinguish fungal from other causes of sinusitis or orbital disease, and the absence of characteristic findings does not exclude fungal infection, particularly in early disease or in immunocompromised hosts with attenuated inflammatory responses [4].

Magnetic resonance imaging provides superior soft tissue contrast and is invaluable for assessing orbital apex involvement, perineural spread, cavernous sinus invasion, and intracranial extension. The MRI characteristics of fungal infections reflect the paramagnetic properties of fungal elements, with T1 hypointensity and T2 hypointensity or heterogeneity of fungal concretions contrasting with the T2 hyperintensity typically seen in bacterial infections or inflammatory conditions [89, 90]. The "black turbinate" sign may be more conspicuous on T2-weighted MRI than on CT, appearing as areas of marked hypointensity within the nasal turbinates due to the combination of fungal elements, hemorrhage, and devitalized tissue. The presence of an infiltrative lesion in the cavernous sinus on MRI is associated with poor visual outcomes [6].

Post-contrast MRI sequences help distinguish fungal elements from surrounding inflammatory tissue, with fungal concretions typically demonstrating a lack of enhancement (e.g., "black turbinate sign") despite the avid enhancement of the surrounding inflammatory reaction [87]. For fungal abscesses, especially in Aspergillosis, a "target" appearance with peripheral enhancement and a non-enhancing necrotic core may be observed [91]. Perineural spread along cranial nerves appears as thickening and enhancement of the nerve and surrounding sheaths, often extending beyond the clinically apparent area of involvement [92]. Cavernous sinus involvement manifests as filling defects, abnormal enhancement, or expansion of the cavernous sinus, often with narrowing or occlusion of the internal carotid artery [93].

Diffusion-weighted imaging (DWI) provides additional diagnostic information, with fungal abscesses typically demonstrating restricted diffusion due to high viscosity and cellularity [94]. However, based solely on DWI, distinguishing pyogenic (bacterial) from fungal abscesses may not always be possible, as both can exhibit similar restricted diffusion patterns [95]. Susceptibility-weighted imaging (SWI) enhances detection of hemorrhage and fungal elements containing paramagnetic substances, potentially improving diagnostic sensitivity in early disease.

Vascular imaging, including CT angiography (CTA), MR angiography (MRA), or conventional angiography, plays an important role in evaluating vascular complications of fungal infections. These techniques allow the assessment of internal carotid artery involvement, including stenosis, occlusion, pseudoaneurysm formation, or cavernous-carotid fistula. Venous imaging may demonstrate cavernous sinus thrombosis or occlusion of other dural venous sinuses. The identification of vascular complications significantly impacts prognosis and management decisions, potentially necessitating neurovascular intervention in addition to antifungal therapy and surgical debridement.

The integration of multiple imaging modalities often provides the most comprehensive assessment of disease extent and complications. CT and MRI offer complementary information, with CT better demonstrating bone erosion and calcifications, while MRI provides superior evaluation of soft tissue, neural, and vascular structures. Serial imaging studies allow monitoring of disease progression and treatment response, guiding decisions regarding the need for additional surgical intervention or modification of medical therapy.

11.5.4 Diagnostic Sampling Procedures

Diagnostic procedures, particularly tissue sampling for microbiological and histopathological examination, represent a critical component of the diagnostic approach to suspected fungal infections. These procedures range from minimally invasive techniques, such as nasal endoscopy with targeted biopsy, to more extensive surgical exploration and debridement, with the choice of approach guided by the clinical presentation, radiographic findings, and the patient's overall condition.

Nasal endoscopy represents an essential diagnostic procedure in suspected sinonasal fungal infections, allowing direct visualization of the nasal cavity and paranasal sinuses. This approach permits the assessment of mucosal changes, identification of fungal debris or necrotic tissue, and targeted biopsy of suspicious areas. The characteristic finding of black eschar, when present, strongly suggests Mucormycosis and indicates the need for immediate surgical debridement [96]. Even in the absence of visible eschar, endoscopic examination may reveal subtle mucosal changes, including pale or violaceous discoloration, granulations, or ulcerations, that warrant biopsy and further evaluation [97].

Endoscopic biopsy provides tissue for microbiological and histopathological examination, often yielding the definitive diagnosis. Multiple, targeted biopsies should be obtained from areas of suspected invasion or necrosis, with specimens divided for various diagnostic studies, including direct microscopy, culture, histopathology, and molecular testing when available. The yield of endoscopic biopsy varies based on the extent and patchy nature of the disease, often requiring repeat biopsies if initial results are negative or clinical suspicion remains high.

Orbital biopsy may be necessary when sinonasal biopsies are non-diagnostic or when orbital disease appears primary rather than secondary to sinonasal infection. Various approaches exist, including anterior orbitotomy through a lid crease or conjunctival incision, endoscopic transnasal approaches to the medial orbit, and more extensive orbitotomy for lesions in the orbital apex or lateral compartments. The choice of approach depends on the location of the lesion, the patient's overall condition, and the surgeon's expertise. Orbital biopsy carries risks of vision loss, diplopia, and other complications, necessitating careful consideration of the risk–benefit ratio in each case [98].

Neurosurgical procedures, including craniotomy or endoscopic skull base approaches, may be required for the diagnosis and treatment of fungal infections with intracranial extension. These procedures allow access to the anterior and middle cranial fossae, cavernous sinus, and other intracranial compartments affected by fungal disease. The diagnostic yield of neurosurgical biopsy is generally high, but these procedures carry significant risks, including hemorrhage, stroke, and neurological deficits, necessitating careful patient selection and experienced surgical teams.

Fine-needle aspiration (FNA) represents a less invasive alternative for accessible lesions, particularly in the anterior orbit or periorbital tissues. This technique may provide diagnostic materials for cytological examination and culture while minimizing trauma to the surrounding structures. However, the limited sample volume obtained with FNA may reduce diagnostic yield, particularly for fungal infections, where abundant material is often necessary for definitive diagnosis [99].

Lumbar puncture for cerebrospinal fluid (CSF) analysis should be considered in patients with suspected meningeal involvement, particularly those with altered mental status, meningeal signs, or multiple cranial neuropathies. CSF findings in fungal meningitis vary by pathogen but may include pleocytosis (with varying cell predominance), elevated protein, decreased glucose, and positive fungal cultures or antigen tests [100]. CSF analysis is particularly valuable in Cryptococcal meningitis, where Cryptococcal antigen testing has high sensitivity and specificity [101]. However, lumbar puncture should be approached with caution in patients with mass lesions or elevated intracranial pressure, with neuroimaging recommended before the procedure to exclude contraindications.

The timing and extent of diagnostic procedures must balance the need for definitive diagnosis with the urgency of initiating therapy. In patients with high clinical suspicion of invasive fungal disease, particularly those with rapidly progressive symptoms or significant immunocompromise, empiric antifungal therapy should not be delayed while awaiting diagnostic results. Similarly, surgical debridement should proceed promptly when clinical and radiographic findings strongly suggest invasive fungal disease, even before microbiological confirmation, as delays in intervention significantly impact outcomes.

11.5.5 Diagnostic Challenges and Emerging Approaches

Despite advances in diagnostic techniques, the diagnosis of fungal infections with neuro-ophthalmological involvement remains challenging, with several persistent limitations and emerging approaches deserving consideration.

The non-specific nature of early clinical manifestations represents a significant diagnostic challenge, with symptoms such as headache, orbital pain, and sinusitis often attributed to more common conditions, delaying consideration of fungal infection. This challenge is particularly pronounced in immunocompromised patients, whose inflammatory response may be attenuated, masking classic signs and symptoms of infection. Maintaining a high index of suspicion in at-risk populations, even when presentations appear atypical, remains essential for early diagnosis.

The limitations of current diagnostic tests, including the low sensitivity of cultures, the time required for fungal growth, and the variable performance of serological assays, contribute to diagnostic uncertainty and potential delays in appropriate therapy. False negatives are common with all diagnostic modalities, necessitating a comprehensive approach that integrates clinical, laboratory, and radiographic findings rather than relying on any single test to exclude fungal infection.

The difficulty in distinguishing colonization from invasion represents another diagnostic challenge, particularly in the sinonasal region, where fungal colonization is common [102]. This distinction requires careful correlation of microbiological findings with histopathological evidence of tissue invasion and clinical signs of invasive disease. The presence of angioinvasion, tissue necrosis, or neural involvement on histopathology strongly supports invasive disease requiring aggressive intervention.

Emerging diagnostic approaches offer potential solutions to these challenges. Point-of-care diagnostic tests, including lateral flow assays for fungal antigens and rapid molecular tests, may provide results within minutes to hours rather than days, facilitating earlier diagnosis and intervention [103]. Metagenomic next-generation sequencing allows unbiased detection of all pathogens present in a clinical sample, potentially identifying unexpected or mixed fungal infections that might be missed with targeted testing [104]. Artificial intelligence algorithms applied to radiographic images may enhance the detection of subtle findings suggestive of fungal infection [105], potentially improving diagnostic sensitivity in early disease, though further research is needed to establish their clinical utility across different fungal infections.

Biomarkers of host response, including cytokine profiles [106], metabolomic signatures [107], and transcriptomic patterns [108], represent another promising approach for early diagnosis. These biomarkers may distinguish fungal from other infections based on the characteristic host response patterns they elicit, potentially allowing diagnosis before direct evidence of the pathogen is obtainable. While still investigational, these approaches may eventually complement traditional diagnostic methods, particularly in cases where conventional testing yields inconclusive results.

The integration of diagnostic information from multiple sources, facilitated by multidisciplinary teams including ophthalmologists, otolaryngologists, infectious disease specialists, radiologists, and pathologists, remains the most effective approach to diagnosing these complex infections. Regular communication among team members, with critical evaluation of all available data in the context of the individual patient's presentation and risk factors, provides the best opportunity for timely and accurate diagnosis, guiding appropriate intervention to optimize outcomes in these challenging cases.

11.6 Differential Diagnosis

The differential diagnosis of neuro-ophthalmological manifestations of fungal infections encompasses a diverse array of pathological processes that may mimic or coexist with fungal disease. Accurate differentiation is essential for appropriate management, as treatment approaches vary dramatically between fungal infections and their mimics. This differentiation requires careful integration of clinical features, laboratory findings, and radiographic characteristics, with consideration of the patient's risk factors and the temporal evolution of symptoms.

11.6.1 Neoplastic Processes

Neoplastic processes affecting the orbital apex, cavernous sinus, and adjacent structures can closely resemble fungal infections in their clinical presentation. Primary tumors, including meningiomas and sinonasal malignancies, may present with gradually progressive cranial neuropathies, proptosis, and visual loss, similar to the more indolent fungal infections such as Aspergillosis [43]. Metastatic lesions may also involve these regions, producing similar neuro-ophthalmological manifestations [109].

Several clinical features help distinguish neoplastic from fungal processes. Neoplastic lesions typically demonstrate a more indolent course measured in months rather than days or weeks, with gradually progressive symptoms rather than the rapid deterioration often seen in acute invasive fungal infections, such as Mucormycosis. However, chronic invasive fungal sinusitis may present with a more indolent course, sometimes mimicking malignancy. The absence of significant inflammatory signs, including pain, erythema, and edema, may also suggest neoplastic rather than infectious etiology, though this distinction becomes less reliable in immunocompromised hosts whose inflammatory response may be attenuated.

Radiographically, neoplastic processes often demonstrate more discrete margins and homogeneous enhancement compared to the infiltrative, heterogeneous appearance of fungal infections. Bone remodeling rather than frank destruction may be more characteristic of slow-growing neoplasms, while aggressive bone erosion may occur with both fungal infections and malignant tumors. The pattern of spread may provide additional clues, with perineural extension along specific cranial nerve pathways more characteristic of certain malignancies, particularly adenoid cystic carcinoma and squamous cell carcinoma, though fungal infections may also demonstrate perineural spread [110].

Ultimately, tissue diagnosis remains essential for definitive differentiation between neoplastic and fungal processes. Biopsy with appropriate microbiological and histopathological studies allows direct visualization of fungal elements or neoplastic cells, guiding appropriate management. In cases where clinical suspicion for fungal infection is high, particularly in immunocompromised hosts or those with diabetic ketoacidosis, empiric antifungal therapy may be initiated while awaiting definitive diagnosis, with modification of treatment based on biopsy results [111, 112].

11.6.2 Inflammatory Conditions

Inflammatory conditions affecting the orbit and cavernous sinus may closely mimic fungal infections, presenting with orbital pain, proptosis, ophthalmoplegia, and visual loss. These conditions include idiopathic orbital inflammation (formerly called orbital pseudotumor), Tolosa–Hunt syndrome, sarcoidosis, IgG4-related disease, and granulomatosis with polyangiitis (formerly Wegener's granulomatosis) [113].

Idiopathic orbital inflammation and Tolosa–Hunt syndrome, characterized by painful ophthalmoplegia due to non-specific inflammation of the orbital apex or cavernous sinus, respectively, can be particularly challenging to distinguish from fungal infections. Both conditions may present with an acute or subacute onset of pain, ophthalmoplegia, and variable visual loss, similar to fungal orbital apex syndrome. The dramatic response to corticosteroids often observed in these inflammatory conditions represents an important differentiating feature, though this response is not universal and may be seen to a lesser extent in some fungal infections, particularly when significant secondary inflammation is present [114].

Sarcoidosis, a multisystem granulomatous disorder of unknown etiology, may involve the orbit, cranial nerves, and meninges, producing neuro-ophthalmological manifestations that overlap with fungal infections. The presence of systemic manifestations, including pulmonary involvement, skin lesions, and lacrimal gland enlargement, may suggest sarcoidosis, though these findings are not universal. Elevated serum angiotensin-converting enzyme (ACE) and characteristic chest radiographic findings provide supportive evidence for sarcoidosis, though definitive diagnosis requires demonstration of non-caseating granulomas on biopsy with exclusion of infectious causes, including fungi.

IgG4-related disease, an immune-mediated fibroinflammatory condition, may involve the orbit, particularly the lacrimal gland, extraocular muscles, and orbital soft tissues. This condition can present with proptosis, diplopia, and orbital pain, potentially mimicking fungal orbital disease. The often bilateral and multifocal nature of IgG4-related disease, elevated serum IgG4 levels, and characteristic histopathological findings of lymphoplasmacytic infiltration with IgG4-positive plasma cells and storiform fibrosis help distinguish this entity from fungal infections [115].

Granulomatosis with polyangiitis may involve the orbit, paranasal sinuses, and upper respiratory tract, producing destructive lesions that can mimic invasive fungal disease. The presence of systemic vasculitis, particularly involving the kidneys and lungs, positive anti-neutrophil cytoplasmic antibodies (ANCA), and characteristic histopathological findings of necrotizing granulomatous vasculitis help distinguish this condition from fungal infections. However, limited forms of the disease may present with isolated sinonasal or orbital involvement, creating diagnostic challenges that require careful histopathological evaluation to exclude infectious etiologies.

Radiographically, the distinction between inflammatory conditions and fungal infections can be challenging due to overlapping features [95]. While fungal infections often involve bone destruction and demonstrate areas of necrosis, inflammatory conditions may also present with destructive changes or diffuse soft tissue involvement. These radiographic distinctions are not absolute, and tissue diagnosis remains essential for definitive differentiation.

The response to therapy provides important diagnostic information, with inflammatory conditions typically demonstrating rapid improvement with corticosteroid therapy, while fungal infections may worsen with immunosuppression. This differential response underscores the importance of excluding fungal infection before initiating corticosteroid therapy in patients with orbital inflammatory syndromes, particularly those with risk factors for fungal disease.

11.6.3 Other Infectious Causes

Various infectious processes beyond fungi may affect the orbit, cranial nerves, and adjacent structures, producing neuro-ophthalmological manifestations that mimic fungal infections. These include bacterial, viral, and parasitic infections, each with distinctive clinical and radiographic features that aid in differentiation.

Bacterial infections, including acute bacterial sinusitis with orbital complications, represent the most common infectious mimics of fungal orbital disease. Bacterial orbital cellulitis typically presents with acute onset of orbital pain, erythema, edema, proptosis, and variable ophthalmoplegia, often in the setting of preceding sinusitis or upper respiratory infection. The rapid onset and prominent inflammatory signs may resemble Mucormycosis, particularly in its early stages. However, bacterial infections can occur regardless of the patient's immune status, generally respond to appropriate antibiotic therapy, and show more homogeneous contrast enhancement on imaging, while characteristic T2-weighted imaging hypointensity or loss of mucosal enhancement (black turbinate sign), commonly observed in typical fungal elements, are absent.

Specific bacterial pathogens may produce distinctive clinical syndromes that enter the differential diagnosis of fungal neuro-ophthalmological disease. Tuberculosis may involve the orbit, skull base, and meninges, producing chronic granulomatous inflammation with cranial neuropathies and visual loss. The indolent course, presence of systemic tuberculosis, positive interferon-gamma release assays or tuberculin skin tests, and characteristic caseous granulomas on histopathology help distinguish tuberculosis from fungal infections. Actinomycosis, caused by filamentous bacteria of the *Actinomyces* genus, may produce chronic suppurative infections of the cervicofacial region with potential orbital extension. The presence of characteristic sulfur granules in purulent discharge and the filamentous, branching, gram-positive organisms on microscopy helps distinguish actinomycosis from fungal infections, though definitive differentiation may require culture or molecular testing.

Viral infections may produce focal orbital or cranial nerve involvement mimicking fungal disease but may cause meningoencephalitis with secondary cranial neuropathies. Herpes viruses, particularly herpes simplex virus (HSV) and varicella-zoster virus (VZV), may cause encephalitis or focal orbital and cranial nerve involvement with multiple cranial neuropathies [116]. The presence of characteristic vesicular skin lesions in VZV infection, cerebrospinal fluid pleocytosis with positive viral PCR, and response to antiviral therapy helps distinguish these conditions from fungal infections [117].

Parasitic infections, including toxoplasmosis, cysticercosis, and echinococcosis, may involve the orbit, brain, and cranial nerves, producing neuro-ophthalmological manifestations that enter the differential diagnosis of fungal disease. Toxoplasmosis typically causes chorioretinitis but may rarely involve the orbit or cause encephalitis with cranial neuropathies, particularly in immunocompromised hosts [118]. Positive serological tests for Toxoplasma gondii and response to specific anti-parasitic therapy help distinguish this entity from fungal infections. Cysticercosis, caused by the larval stage of Taenia Solium, may involve the extraocular muscles, orbital soft tissues, or intracranial structures, producing proptosis, ophthalmoplegia, or visual loss. The characteristic cystic lesions with eccentric scolex on imaging and positive serological tests help distinguish cysticercosis from fungal infections [119]. Echinococcosis, caused by *Echinococcus* species, may rarely involve the orbit, producing a slowly enlarging cystic mass with potential compression of adjacent structures [120]. The characteristic unilocular or multilocular cystic appearance on imaging and positive serological tests help distinguish echinococcosis from fungal infections [120].

The differentiation between fungal and other infectious causes often requires microbiological and histopathological examination of tissue specimens, with appropriate stains and cultures for bacteria, fungi, mycobacteria, and molecular tests for viruses and parasites. The integration of these findings with clinical features, radiographic characteristics, and response to empiric therapy guides appropriate management.

11.6.4 Vascular Conditions

Vascular conditions affecting the orbit, cavernous sinus, and adjacent structures may produce neuro-ophthalmological manifestations that mimic fungal infections. These conditions include cavernous sinus thrombosis, carotid-cavernous fistula, carotid artery aneurysm, and ischemic events affecting the ophthalmic or cerebral circulation.

Cavernous sinus thrombosis, often secondary to bacterial sinusitis or facial infections, presents with a rapid onset of orbital pain, proptosis, chemosis, ophthalmoplegia, and sensory deficits in the distribution of the ophthalmic and maxillary divisions of the trigeminal nerve [121]. This clinical presentation closely resembles fungal cavernous sinus syndrome, creating significant diagnostic challenges. The presence of high fever, marked leukocytosis, and rapid response to antibiotic therapy may suggest bacterial rather than fungal etiology, though these distinctions become less reliable in immunocompromised hosts. Imaging studies, particularly MR venography or CT venography, demonstrate filling defects within the cavernous sinus in thrombosis, while fungal invasion may show more infiltrative soft tissue abnormalities with potential vascular involvement [122]. Definitive differentiation often requires tissue sampling, with empiric coverage for both bacterial and fungal pathogens in high-risk cases while awaiting definitive diagnosis.

Carotid-cavernous fistula, representing abnormal communication between the carotid artery and cavernous sinus, may present with pulsatile proptosis, orbital bruit, chemosis, and ophthalmoplegia, potentially mimicking infectious or inflammatory conditions affecting the orbit and cavernous sinus. The characteristic orbital congestion with arterialized conjunctival vessels, often with a history of trauma or spontaneous onset in patients with connective tissue disorders, helps distinguish this entity from fungal infections. Definitive diagnosis relies on vascular imaging, including CT angiography, MR angiography, or conventional angiography, which demonstrates early venous filling from arterial supply.

A carotid artery aneurysm within the cavernous sinus may present with painful ophthalmoplegia, mimicking cavernous sinus syndrome due to fungal infection. The typically more indolent course, absence of inflammatory signs, and characteristic vascular abnormality on angiographic studies help distinguish a non-mycotic aneurysm from fungal infection. However, partially thrombosed aneurysms may present diagnostic challenges on routine imaging, necessitating dedicated vascular studies for definitive diagnosis [123].

Ischemic events affecting the ophthalmic or cerebral circulation may produce acute visual loss or focal neurological deficits that enter the differential diagnosis of neuro-ophthalmological manifestations of fungal infections. Central retinal artery occlusion presents with acute, painless visual loss and characteristic funduscopic findings of retinal whitening with a cherry-red spot at the fovea. Posterior cerebral artery occlusion may cause homonymous hemianopia, while middle cerebral artery occlusion may produce hemiparesis, hemisensory loss, or aphasia, depending on the hemisphere involved. The absence of orbital signs, including pain, proptosis, and ophthalmoplegia, helps distinguish primary vascular events from fungal infections, though fungal angioinvasion may itself cause vascular occlusion as a secondary phenomenon [124].

The differentiation between vascular conditions and fungal infections relies on careful clinical assessment, appropriate vascular imaging studies, and consideration of the patient's risk factors and the temporal evolution of symptoms. In cases where diagnostic uncertainty persists, empiric therapy for the most likely etiology based on clinical presentation and risk factors may be initiated while pursuing a definitive diagnosis.

11.6.5 Traumatic and Iatrogenic Causes

Traumatic and iatrogenic causes of the orbital apex syndrome or cavernous sinus syndrome may mimic the neuro-ophthalmological manifestations of fungal infections. These include orbital apex fractures, iatrogenic injury during sinus or orbital surgery, radiation-induced cranial neuropathies, and complications of local anesthetic injections.

Orbital apex fractures, particularly those involving the orbital roof or medial wall with extension to the optic canal or superior orbital fissure, may cause traumatic orbital apex syndrome with visual loss, ophthalmoplegia, and sensory deficits in the distribution of the ophthalmic division of the trigeminal nerve [125]. The history of trauma, characteristic fracture patterns on CT imaging, and absence of inflammatory or infectious signs help distinguish traumatic from fungal orbital apex syndrome [126]. However, secondary infection may complicate traumatic injuries, particularly those with communication to the paranasal sinuses, necessitating careful monitoring and a low threshold for antimicrobial therapy in high-risk cases [127].

Iatrogenic injury during sinus or orbital surgery may produce cranial neuropathies that mimic infectious processes. Direct injury to the optic nerve, ocular motor nerves, or trigeminal nerve branches may occur during endoscopic sinus surgery, orbital decompression, or skull base procedures [128]. The immediate onset of deficits following surgery, characteristic imaging findings of surgical changes without evidence of infection, and absence of progressive worsening help distinguish iatrogenic injury from fungal infection [129]. However, postoperative infections, including fungal infections, may complicate surgical procedures, particularly in immunocompromised hosts or those with pre-existing colonization, creating diagnostic challenges that require careful clinical and radiographic monitoring [130].

Radiation-induced cranial neuropathies may develop months to years after radiation therapy for head and neck malignancies, presenting with progressive ophthalmoplegia, visual loss, or facial sensory deficits that may mimic indolent fungal infections [131]. The history of radiation exposure, characteristic imaging findings of radiation-induced changes without evidence of infection or recurrent tumor, and absence of inflammatory signs help distinguish radiation injury from fungal infection [132]. However, radiation necrosis may create a favorable environment for opportunistic infections, including fungi, necessitating careful evaluation to exclude superimposed infection in patients with prior radiation therapy who develop new or progressive cranial neuropathies [133].

Complications of local anesthetic injections, particularly retrobulbar or peribulbar injections for ocular surgery, may cause direct nerve injury, vascular complications, or introduce infection, producing neuro-ophthalmological manifestations that may mimic fungal disease. The temporal relationship to the procedure, characteristic imaging findings, and clinical course help distinguish these iatrogenic complications from primary fungal infections.

The differentiation between traumatic or iatrogenic causes and fungal infections relies on careful history, appropriate imaging studies, and consideration of the temporal relationship between interventions and symptom onset. In cases where diagnostic uncertainty persists, particularly in immunocompromised hosts or those with other risk factors for fungal infection, empiric antifungal therapy should be considered while pursuing a definitive diagnosis.

11.6.6 Miscellaneous Conditions

Several additional conditions may enter the differential diagnosis of neuro-ophthalmological manifestations of fungal infections, including thyroid eye disease, orbital pseudotumor, amyloidosis, and various rheumatological disorders with orbital or cranial nerve involvement.

Thyroid eye disease, an autoimmune disorder associated with Graves' disease, may present with proptosis, eyelid retraction, chemosis, and variable ophthalmoplegia, potentially mimicking orbital inflammatory processes, including fungal infections. The typical bilateral involvement, characteristic enlargement of extraocular muscles with sparing of tendinous insertions on imaging, and associated systemic manifestations of thyroid dysfunction help distinguish thyroid eye disease from fungal infections [134]. However, asymmetric or unilateral presentations may occur, creating diagnostic challenges that require careful clinical and laboratory evaluation.

Orbital pseudotumor, representing idiopathic inflammation of orbital tissues, may present with orbital pain, proptosis, ophthalmoplegia, and variable visual loss, closely mimicking infectious orbital disease, including fungal infections. The absence of sinus disease, lack of bone destruction on imaging, and dramatic response to corticosteroid therapy help distinguish orbital pseudotumor from fungal infections [113]. However, these distinctions are not absolute, and tissue biopsy with appropriate microbiological studies may be necessary for definitive differentiation, particularly in immunocompromised hosts or those with risk factors for fungal infection.

Amyloidosis, characterized by extracellular deposition of insoluble fibrillar proteins, may involve the orbit, extraocular muscles, and cranial nerves, producing proptosis, ophthalmoplegia, and visual loss that may mimic chronic fungal infections. The typically indolent course, absence of inflammatory signs, and characteristic amorphous, eosinophilic deposits on histopathology with Congo red positivity and apple-green birefringence under polarized light help distinguish amyloidosis from fungal infections [135].

Various rheumatological disorders, including rheumatoid arthritis, systemic lupus erythematosus, and Sjögren's syndrome, may cause orbital inflammation or cranial neuropathies that enter the differential diagnosis of neuro-ophthalmological manifestations of fungal infections. The presence of characteristic systemic manifestations, positive serological markers, and absence of infectious signs on microbiological studies help distinguish these autoimmune conditions from fungal infections. However, patients with autoimmune disorders often receive immunosuppressive therapy, increasing their susceptibility to opportunistic infections, including fungi, creating complex diagnostic scenarios that require careful evaluation to distinguish disease flare from superimposed infection [136].

The differentiation between these miscellaneous conditions and fungal infections relies on careful clinical assessment, appropriate laboratory and imaging studies, and often tissue biopsy with comprehensive microbiological and histopathological evaluation. The integration of these findings with the patient's risk factors and the temporal evolution of symptoms guides appropriate management.

11.7 Management and Treatment

The management of fungal infections with neuro-ophthalmological manifestations represents one of the most challenging therapeutic scenarios in clinical medicine, requiring a coordinated multidisciplinary approach, rapid intervention, and careful balancing of aggressive infection control with preservation of function. The complexity of these infections stems from their occurrence in anatomically critical regions, rapid and severe progression patterns, and a tendency to affect patients with significant comorbidities, collectively complicating therapeutic decision-making [112]. Successful management requires integration of medical and surgical approaches, with individualized treatment plans that consider the specific pathogen, extent of disease, host factors, and available resources.

11.7.1 Principles of Management

The fundamental principles guiding the management of neuro-ophthalmological fungal infections emphasize early diagnosis, prompt intervention, multidisciplinary collaboration, and comprehensive care addressing both the infection and its underlying predisposing factors. These principles provide the framework for therapeutic decision-making across the spectrum of fungal pathogens and clinical presentations.

Early diagnosis and intervention represent the cornerstone of successful management, with previous research demonstrating significantly improved outcomes when treatment is initiated promptly [6]. In Mucormycosis, each day of delayed treatment has been associated with an approximately 1.5-fold increase in 30-day mortality, with delays beyond 6 days associated with a nearly two-fold increase in mortality compared to earlier intervention [137]. Similarly, in invasive Aspergillosis, delayed diagnosis and treatment correlate with increased mortality, particularly in immunocompromised hosts [69]. These observations underscore the critical importance of maintaining a high index of suspicion in at-risk populations, pursuing expedited diagnostic evaluation, and initiating empiric therapy when clinical suspicion is high, even before definitive diagnosis is established [111].

The multidisciplinary approach to management represents another fundamental principle, reflecting the complex nature of these infections and their involvement of multiple anatomical regions and organ systems. Effective management typically requires collaboration among ophthalmologists, otolaryngologists, infectious disease specialists, neurologists, neurosurgeons, radiologists, pathologists, and critical care specialists, with additional involvement of endocrinologists, hematologists, or transplant specialists depending on the patient's underlying conditions. This multidisciplinary team facilitates comprehensive assessment, coordinated intervention, and integrated care addressing both the infection and its complications. Regular communication among team members, with critical evaluation of clinical progress and therapeutic response, allows dynamic adjustment of the management plan as the clinical situation evolves.

Comprehensive care addressing both the infection and its underlying predisposing factors represents a third fundamental principle. In diabetic patients with Mucormycosis, aggressive management of hyperglycemia and ketoacidosis, with correction of metabolic derangements and optimization of glycemic control, plays a crucial role in improving host defense and enhancing treatment efficacy [138]. In neutropenic patients with invasive Aspergillosis, strategies to enhance neutrophil recovery, including growth factor support or reduction of myelosuppressive medications when possible, complement antifungal therapy in controlling infection [18, 139]. In transplant recipients, careful modulation of immunosuppressive regimens, balancing the risk of rejection against the need for improved immune function to combat infection, represents a critical aspect of comprehensive management [68, 140]. This holistic approach, addressing both the infection and its underlying predisposing factors, provides the best opportunity for successful outcomes in these complex cases.

The balance between aggressive infection control and preservation of function represents a fourth guiding principle, particularly relevant in the management of orbital and cranial involvement. The anatomical complexity of the orbital apex, cavernous sinus, and adjacent structures, with critical neurovascular elements in close proximity, creates significant challenges for surgical intervention. The decision regarding the extent of surgical debridement, particularly whether to pursue orbital exenteration, requires careful consideration of both infectious control and functional outcomes. Historical approaches often favored aggressive debridement, including orbital exenteration, to achieve infectious control, accepting significant functional and cosmetic morbidity as necessary consequences. Contemporary approaches increasingly emphasize tissue-sparing strategies when possible, with early medical intervention, targeted surgical debridement, and close monitoring potentially allowing preservation of the globe and some visual function in selected cases [36]. This evolution in approach reflects improved understanding of disease pathophysiology, advances in imaging and surgical techniques, and enhanced efficacy of modern antifungal agents, allowing more nuanced decision-making that considers both infectious control and quality of life.

The timing and sequence of interventions represent a fifth guiding principle, with optimal management typically involving concurrent medical and surgical approaches rather than sequential intervention. In invasive fungal sinusitis with orbital involvement, initial surgical debridement provides both diagnostic material and therapeutic benefit through removal of infected tissue, while immediate initiation of appropriate antifungal therapy addresses residual infection not amenable to surgical removal [36]. This concurrent approach, rather than waiting for surgical confirmation before starting medical therapy or delaying surgery until after a trial of medical therapy, provides the most rapid and effective control of infection, particularly in fulminant cases such as Mucormycosis [141]. The specific timing and sequence may require adjustment based on individual circumstances, including the patient's clinical stability, the extent and location of disease, and available resources, but the principle of prompt, coordinated intervention remains paramount.

11.7.2 Antifungal Therapy

Antifungal therapy represents the cornerstone of medical management for fungal infections with neuro-ophthalmological involvement, with the choice of agent, dose, route of administration, and duration guided by the specific pathogen, extent of disease, host factors, and therapeutic response. The major classes of antifungal agents include polyenes, azoles, and echinocandins, each with distinct mechanisms of action, spectra of activity, pharmacokinetic properties, and adverse effect profiles that influence their role in management.

Polyene antifungals, particularly amphotericin B and its lipid formulations, act by binding to ergosterol in the fungal cell membrane, creating pores that disrupt membrane integrity and lead to cell death [39]. These agents demonstrate broad-spectrum activity against most pathogenic fungi, including *Mucorales*, *Aspergillus* species, *Candida* species, and *Cryptococcus neoformans*, making them valuable for empiric therapy when the specific pathogen remains unidentified. Among the available formulations, liposomal amphotericin B is a preferred option for Mucormycosis and a key alternative for other invasive fungal infections, offering improved tissue penetration, enhanced efficacy, and reduced nephrotoxicity compared to conventional amphotericin B deoxycholate [111]. The standard dose of liposomal amphotericin B for invasive fungal infections is 3–5 mg/kg/day, with some experts advocating higher doses (7–10 mg/kg/day) for Mucormycosis, particularly in cases with central nervous system involvement or refractory disease [142]. The primary limitations of amphotericin B formulations include nephrotoxicity, infusion-related reactions, electrolyte disturbances (particularly, hypokalemia and hypomagnesemia), and the requirement for intravenous administration, necessitating careful monitoring and supportive care during therapy [143].

Azole antifungals, including voriconazole, posaconazole, isavuconazole, and itraconazole, inhibit fungal cytochrome P450-dependent enzymes, particularly lanosterol 14α-demethylase, disrupting ergosterol synthesis and leading to accumulation of toxic sterol precursors in the fungal cell membrane [144]. These agents vary in their spectrum of activity, with voriconazole demonstrating excellent activity against *Aspergillus* species but limited efficacy against *Mucorales*, while posaconazole and isavuconazole offer broader coverage, including activity against many *Mucorales* species [145]. Voriconazole represents the first-line agent for invasive Aspergillosis, with superior efficacy and improved survival compared to conventional amphotericin B demonstrated in randomized controlled trials [146]. The standard dose of voriconazole includes a loading dose of 6 mg/kg intravenously every 12 hours for two doses, followed by 4 mg/kg every 12 hours, with transition to oral therapy (typically 200–300 mg twice daily) when clinically appropriate [147]. Therapeutic drug monitoring is essential for voriconazole, with target trough concentrations of 2–5 μg/mL balancing efficacy against the risk of adverse effects, which increase significantly with higher levels [148].

Posaconazole and isavuconazole have emerged as important options for Mucormycosis, including as primary therapy (especially when amphotericin B is inappropriate), step-down therapy following initial amphotericin B, or as salvage therapy [5]. Posaconazole is available in both oral suspension and tablet formulations, with the delayed-release tablet offering improved bioavailability and more reliable serum concentrations [149]. The standard dose of posaconazole tablets is 300 mg twice daily on the first day, followed by 300 mg once daily, with therapeutic drug monitoring recommended to ensure adequate serum concentrations (target trough >1 μg/mL) [148]. Isavuconazole, the newest triazole antifungal, offers several advantages, including excellent bioavailability, predictable pharmacokinetics without requirement for therapeutic drug monitoring, and reduced drug interactions compared to other azoles [150]. The standard dose of isavuconazole includes a loading dose of 200 mg every 8 hours for six doses, followed by 200 mg once daily, with both intravenous and oral formulations available [151]. The primary limitations of azole antifungals include hepatotoxicity, QT interval prolongation (particularly with voriconazole), visual disturbances (with voriconazole), and numerous drug interactions mediated through cytochrome P450 enzymes, necessitating careful medication reconciliation and potential dose adjustments of concomitant medications [152].

Echinocandins, including caspofungin, micafungin, and anidulafungin, inhibit the synthesis of β-(1,3)-D-glucan, a critical component of the fungal cell wall, leading to osmotic instability and cell lysis. These agents demonstrate excellent activity against *Candida* species and variable activity against *Aspergillus* species, but minimal efficacy against *Mucorales* or *Cryptococcus neoformans* [153]. In the context of neuro-ophthalmological fungal infections, echinocandins play a limited role as primary therapy but may be valuable as part of combination regimens for invasive Aspergillosis or as initial therapy for invasive candidiasis. The standard doses include caspofungin (70 mg loading dose followed by 50 mg daily), micafungin (100–150 mg daily), or anidulafungin (200 mg loading dose followed by 100 mg daily), all administered intravenously [154]. The primary advantages of echinocandins include their excellent safety profile, with minimal nephrotoxicity, hepatotoxicity, or drug interactions, making them valuable options for critically ill patients or those with multiple comorbidities [155]. Their primary limitations include a lack of activity against *Mucorales*, poor central nervous system penetration, and the requirement for intravenous administration, restricting their utility for long-term therapy of neuro-ophthalmological fungal infections [156].

The selection of specific antifungal agents should be guided by the identified or suspected pathogen, with liposomal amphotericin B representing the first-line therapy for Mucormycosis, voriconazole for Aspergillosis, and tailored regimens for other fungal pathogens based on species identification and susceptibility testing when available. In cases where the specific pathogen remains unidentified, empiric therapy should provide coverage for the most likely pathogens based on the clinical presentation, host factors, and local epidemiology. In immunocompromised hosts with sinusitis and orbital involvement, empiric coverage for both *Aspergillus* species and *Mucorales* is often warranted, with liposomal amphotericin B representing the preferred initial agent due to its broad spectrum of activity [157]. The addition of voriconazole to provide enhanced coverage for *Aspergillus* species may be considered in selected cases, though potential antagonism between these agents has been suggested in some in vitro studies, creating uncertainty regarding the optimal approach to combination therapy [158].

The route of administration for antifungal therapy depends on the severity of infection, the specific agent selected, and the patient's clinical status. Intravenous therapy is generally preferred for the initial treatment of invasive fungal infections, particularly those with orbital or intracranial involvement, due to the reliability of drug delivery and the severity of these infections. Transition to oral therapy may be considered once clinical improvement is evident, particularly for agents with excellent bioavailability such as voriconazole, posaconazole tablets, or isavuconazole [159]. This transition facilitates long-term therapy and potential outpatient management, improving quality of life and reducing healthcare costs. The timing of transition to oral therapy should be individualized based on the patient's clinical response, the extent of residual disease, and host factors influencing immune recovery.

Local administration of antifungal agents, including irrigation of surgical cavities with amphotericin B solution during debridement procedures, represents an adjunctive approach that may enhance drug delivery to infected tissues [160]. This approach provides high local drug concentrations while minimizing systemic toxicity, potentially complementing systemic therapy in cases with extensive tissue involvement or anatomical barriers to drug penetration. However, evidence supporting the efficacy of local antifungal administration remains limited, and this approach should be considered complementary to, rather than a replacement for, systemic therapy [5].

The duration of antifungal therapy for neuro-ophthalmological fungal infections typically extends for months rather than weeks, reflecting the severity of these infections, their location in anatomically complex regions with potential barriers to drug penetration, and the immunocompromised status of affected patients. For invasive Aspergillosis, a minimum duration of 12 weeks is generally recommended, with longer courses for patients with persistent immunosuppression or extensive disease [69]. For Mucormycosis, treatment typically continues until resolution of all clinical and radiological evidence of active infection, often requiring longer than 6 months of therapy, particularly for cases with orbital or intracranial involvement [111]. The specific duration should be individualized based on the extent of initial disease, the completeness of surgical debridement, the response to therapy as assessed by serial clinical and radiographic evaluations, and host factors influencing immune recovery [161].

In patients with persistent immunosuppression that cannot be reversed, such as those requiring ongoing immunosuppressive therapy for organ transplantation or autoimmune disease, indefinite suppressive therapy may be necessary to prevent recurrence [162].

Monitoring during antifungal therapy should include regular assessment of therapeutic efficacy, drug toxicity, and potential complications. Clinical evaluation, including ophthalmological examination to assess visual function and ocular motility, should be performed regularly to document response to therapy and detect potential deterioration requiring modification of the treatment approach. Radiographic monitoring, with serial MRI or CT imaging at intervals determined by the severity and progression of disease, allows assessment of the extent of residual infection and detection of potential complications such as vascular involvement or intracranial extension. Laboratory monitoring should include regular assessment of renal function, hepatic function, and electrolytes, with specific parameters guided by the antifungal agent used. For voriconazole, therapeutic drug monitoring with trough levels is essential to ensure adequate drug exposure while minimizing toxicity [148]. For amphotericin B formulations, particular attention to renal function, electrolytes (especially potassium and magnesium), and markers of tubular injury is warranted [163]. Drug interactions represent another important consideration, particularly with azole antifungals, necessitating careful medication reconciliation and potential dose adjustments of concomitant medications metabolized through cytochrome P450 enzymes [152].

11.7.3 Surgical Interventions

Surgical intervention plays a crucial role in the management of fungal infections with neuro-ophthalmological involvement, serving both diagnostic and therapeutic purposes. The goals of surgery include obtaining tissue for diagnosis, debridement of infected and necrotic tissue, reducing fungal burden, improving drug penetration to infected areas, and addressing complications such as compressive optic neuropathy or intracranial extension. The specific surgical approach depends on the location and extent of disease, the patient's clinical status, and available surgical expertise, with options ranging from endoscopic techniques to open surgical approaches.

Endoscopic sinus surgery is a key surgical approach for invasive fungal sinusitis with orbital involvement, offering several advantages over traditional open techniques. These advantages include minimally invasive access to the paranasal sinuses and orbital apex, direct visualization of affected tissues with magnified views, preservation of normal anatomy, reduced morbidity compared to open approaches, and the potential for repeated procedures as needed for reassessment or additional debridement. The endoscopic approach typically begins with wide opening of the involved sinuses, including complete ethmoidectomy, middle meatal antrostomy, sphenoidotomy, and frontal sinusotomy as indicated by the extent of disease [164]. Removal of the lamina papyracea provides access to the medial orbit, while the endoscopic transpterygoid approach allows access to the lateral sphenoid recess, pterygopalatine fossa, and infratemporal fossa when these regions are involved [165]. The endoscopic transorbital approach, performed through various incisions including a superior eyelid crease incision, provides complementary access to the orbital apex and optic canal, potentially allowing decompression of the optic nerve in cases with compressive optic neuropathy [166].

During endoscopic surgery, careful assessment of tissue viability guides the extent of debridement, with removal of all necrotic and infected tissue while preserving vital structures when possible. The characteristic black eschar of Mucormycosis, when present, provides a visual marker for the extent of tissue necrosis, though the zone of invasion often extends beyond the visibly necrotic tissue [4]. Intraoperative frozen section analysis may help guide the extent of debridement, with examination of margins to assess for residual fungal elements. The use of angled endoscopes and specialized instruments allows access to difficult-to-reach areas, while navigation systems provide anatomical orientation in cases with distorted landmarks due to extensive disease or previous surgery [167]. At the conclusion of the procedure, the surgical cavity is typically irrigated with saline or dilute antimicrobial solutions, and local antifungal irrigation has also been used, with reported success [74, 168].

Open surgical approaches may be necessary in certain scenarios, including disease extending beyond endoscopic access, need for extensive debridement, failed endoscopic control, or anatomical variations limiting endoscopic access [169]. These approaches include external ethmoidectomy, providing access to the ethmoid sinuses and medial orbit through an incision along the medial orbital rim; maxillectomy, allowing wide exposure of the maxillary sinus and adjacent structures through a facial or transoral approach; and craniofacial resection [157], providing access to the anterior skull base and superior orbital regions through combined intracranial and extracranial approaches [170]. While these open techniques have largely been replaced by endoscopic approaches as the initial surgical intervention, they retain an important role in selected cases with extensive disease or complex anatomy [171]. The specific approach should be individualized based on the location and extent of disease, the patient's clinical status, and available surgical expertise, with the goal of achieving complete debridement while minimizing morbidity.

Orbital decompression represents a specific surgical intervention that may be indicated for compressive optic neuropathy, severe proptosis, orbital compartment syndrome with increased intraorbital pressure, or access to retrobulbar disease. This procedure involves removal of one or more orbital walls to expand the orbital volume, reducing pressure on intraorbital structures and potentially improving blood flow to the optic nerve and other tissues. Approaches include medial wall decompression, typically performed endoscopically through the ethmoid sinuses; lateral wall decompression, performed through a lateral orbitotomy approach; or combined approaches for maximal volume expansion [157, 172]. In the context of fungal infections, orbital decompression serves not only to relieve pressure but also to provide access for debridement of infected orbital tissues, particularly in the orbital apex region [157]. The decision regarding the extent and approach to orbital decompression should consider both the need for infectious control and the preservation of orbital function, with the specific technique individualized based on the location and extent of disease.

Orbital exenteration, involving removal of all orbital contents, including the globe, extraocular muscles, orbital fat, and periorbita, represents the most radical surgical intervention for orbital fungal infections. Historically considered necessary for the control of Mucormycosis with orbital involvement, this procedure results in significant functional and cosmetic morbidity, with profound impact on quality of life. Contemporary approaches increasingly question the necessity of exenteration in all cases, with several retrospective studies suggesting that orbital preservation may be possible in selected patients with limited orbital involvement, particularly when early diagnosis and aggressive medical therapy allow the control of infection before extensive orbital invasion occurs [160]. The decision regarding exenteration requires careful consideration of multiple factors, including the extent of orbital involvement, the specific fungal pathogen, the patient's immune status and potential for recovery, the response to initial medical therapy, and the availability of close monitoring and prompt intervention if clinical deterioration occurs. This decision should involve multidisciplinary discussion and careful communication with the patient and family regarding the potential risks and benefits of orbital preservation versus exenteration, with the understanding that delayed exenteration remains an option if initial conservative management fails to control infection.

Neurosurgical intervention may be necessary for fungal infections with intracranial extension, including involvement of the anterior cranial fossa, cavernous sinus, or brain parenchyma. These procedures may be performed through traditional craniotomy approaches or, increasingly, through endoscopic endonasal approaches to the skull base, depending on the location and extent of disease [173]. The goals of neurosurgical intervention include debridement of infected tissue, decompression of neural structures, management of vascular complications, such as aneurysm or thrombosis, and establishment of drainage for abscesses. The decision regarding neurosurgical intervention should consider both the potential benefits of direct access to infected areas and the significant risks associated with surgery in these critical regions, particularly in patients with multiple comorbidities or coagulopathy. Close collaboration between neurosurgeons, otolaryngologists, and infectious disease specialists is essential for optimal decision-making and coordinated care in these complex cases.

Postoperative care following surgical intervention for fungal infections includes continued antifungal therapy, regular debridement of the surgical cavity to remove debris and assess for residual or recurrent disease, and comprehensive monitoring for potential complications. Endoscopic examination of the sinonasal cavity should be performed regularly during the postoperative period, with removal of crusts and debris to maintain patency of sinus drainage pathways and allow assessment of mucosal healing. Any suspicious areas of necrosis or fungal debris should prompt biopsy and culture to assess for residual infection [174]. Radiographic monitoring with serial MRI or CT imaging allows assessment of the extent of residual disease and detection of potential complications, with the frequency of imaging guided by the severity and progression of disease. The duration of postoperative antifungal therapy should be individualized based on the extent of residual disease, the completeness of surgical debridement, and host factors influencing immune recovery, with regular reassessment to determine the appropriate endpoint of therapy.

11.7.4 Adjunctive Therapies

Adjunctive therapies for fungal infections with neuro-ophthalmological involvement encompass a diverse range of interventions beyond standard antifungal agents and surgical debridement, aimed at enhancing host defense, improving tissue oxygenation, modulating the inflammatory response, and addressing specific complications. While evidence supporting many of these interventions remains limited, they may provide valuable complementary approaches in selected cases, particularly those with refractory disease or significant complications [4].

Hyperbaric oxygen therapy (HBOT) represents one adjunctive approach that has generated considerable interest, particularly for Mucormycosis. This therapy involves breathing 100% oxygen at increased atmospheric pressure, typically 2.0–2.5 atmospheres absolute, in specialized chambers [175]. The proposed mechanisms of benefit include enhanced neutrophil function, direct fungistatic effects through increased tissue oxygen tension, improved tissue oxygenation in marginally perfused areas, and synergistic effects with antifungal agents [176]. Previous research has suggested the potential benefit of HBOT as an adjunct to standard therapy for Mucormycosis, with some patients demonstrating clinical improvement and survival despite extensive disease [177]. However, controlled studies are lacking, and the logistical challenges of HBOT, including the need for specialized facilities and the difficulty of transporting critically ill patients to these facilities, limit its widespread application. When available, HBOT may be considered as an adjunct to standard therapy for refractory Mucormycosis, particularly in cases with extensive tissue necrosis or vascular compromise, though it should not delay or replace standard surgical and medical interventions [5].

Immunomodulatory approaches represent another category of adjunctive therapy, aimed at enhancing host defense against fungal invasion. These approaches include cytokine therapy, such as interferon-gamma to enhance macrophage function or granulocyte-macrophage colony-stimulating factor (GM-CSF) to stimulate neutrophil production and function; granulocyte transfusions for neutropenic patients with refractory infection; reduction of immunosuppressive medications when possible in transplant recipients or those with autoimmune disorders; and correction of underlying immune defects through interventions such as iron chelation therapy for patients with iron overload, which may enhance neutrophil function and reduce fungal growth [26]. The specific immunomodulatory approach should be tailored to the individual patient's immune defect and clinical context, with careful consideration of potential risks, including exacerbation of underlying conditions such as graft-versus-host disease in hematopoietic stem cell transplant recipients or organ rejection in solid organ transplant recipients [178]. While evidence supporting these interventions remains largely anecdotal, they may provide valuable adjuncts to standard therapy in selected cases with refractory disease or profound immune dysfunction [179].

Corticosteroid use in the context of fungal infections presents a complex risk–benefit calculation, with potential to both exacerbate infection through immunosuppression and reduce inflammatory damage to adjacent structures. In general, corticosteroids are avoided in Mucormycosis due to their immunosuppressive effects and the association between corticosteroid therapy and increased risk of mucormycosis [180]. However, in Aspergillosis with significant inflammatory component, particularly allergic forms such as allergic bronchopulmonary Aspergillosis or allergic fungal sinusitis, corticosteroids may play a role in reducing inflammation and associated tissue damage [180]. Additionally, patients on chronic corticosteroid therapy for underlying conditions such as autoimmune disorders or graft-versus-host disease may require continued corticosteroid therapy, albeit at reduced doses when possible, to prevent exacerbation of these conditions [180]. The decision regarding corticosteroid use should consider the specific fungal pathogen, the extent of inflammatory component, the patient's underlying conditions, and the potential risks and benefits of corticosteroid therapy in the individual clinical context.

Anticoagulation represents another adjunctive therapy that may be considered for specific complications of fungal infections, particularly cavernous sinus thrombosis or cerebral venous sinus thrombosis [181]. These vascular complications, resulting from direct fungal invasion of vessel walls or secondary thrombosis due to adjacent inflammation, may contribute to tissue ischemia and neurological deficits beyond the direct effects of fungal invasion. Anticoagulation with heparin or low-molecular-weight heparin may prevent the propagation of thrombosis and potentially reduce ischemic complications, though the risk of hemorrhage must be carefully considered, particularly in the setting of tissue necrosis or potential vascular wall weakening due to fungal invasion [181, 182]. The decision regarding anticoagulation should involve multidisciplinary discussion, with careful consideration of the extent of thrombosis, the presence of ischemic complications, the risk of hemorrhage, and the patient's overall clinical status. When anticoagulation is initiated, close monitoring for both therapeutic efficacy and potential complications is essential, with regular reassessment of the risk–benefit balance as the clinical situation evolves.

11.8 Visual Prognosis and Complications

The visual and neurological outcomes of fungal infections with neuro-ophthalmological involvement represent a complex interplay between pathogen virulence, host factors, anatomical considerations, and therapeutic interventions. Understanding the prognostic factors and potential complications is essential for appropriate patient counseling, therapeutic decision-making, and rehabilitation planning. Despite advances in diagnosis and treatment, these infections continue to carry significant morbidity, with permanent visual loss and neurological deficits remaining common sequelae even with optimal management.

11.8.1 Visual Outcomes

Visual prognosis in fungal infections affecting the visual pathways is influenced by multiple factors, with the initial degree of visual impairment serving as one of the most significant predictors of final visual outcome. Patients presenting with severe visual loss, particularly those with visual acuity worse than 20/200, generally demonstrate poor recovery despite appropriate intervention. In a comprehensive review of invasive fungal rhinosinusitis cases, only approximately 20% of patients with initial visual acuity worse than 20/200 recovered to better than 20/200 despite aggressive medical and surgical management [6]. This limited recovery potential reflects the irreversible nature of optic nerve damage once significant visual loss has occurred, particularly with ischemic mechanisms of injury.

The duration of visual symptoms before therapeutic intervention represents another critical determinant of visual outcomes. The relationship between symptom duration and prognosis follows a relatively predictable pattern, with progressively diminishing recovery potential as the interval between symptom onset and treatment initiation increases [183]. This time-dependent relationship is particularly evident in Mucormycosis, where the rapidly progressive nature of the infection can lead to irreversible tissue damage within days. In Aspergillosis, while the progression may be more indolent, delayed diagnosis and treatment still correlate with poorer visual outcomes, emphasizing the critical importance of early recognition and intervention across the spectrum of fungal pathogens.

The specific mechanism of optic nerve injury significantly influences visual prognosis, with different pathophysiological processes carrying distinct implications for recovery potential [45]. Direct fungal invasion of the optic nerve typically results in poor visual outcomes, as the organism destroys neural tissue and disrupts axonal integrity, often beyond the capacity for meaningful regeneration [184]. Compressive optic neuropathy, resulting from orbital inflammation, abscess, or granuloma formation, may demonstrate better recovery potential if prompt decompression restores normal perfusion and axonal transport before irreversible damage occurs. Ischemic optic neuropathy, resulting from vascular compromise due to angioinvasion or thrombosis, generally carries the poorest prognosis, as the watershed vascular supply of the optic nerve renders it particularly vulnerable to irreversible damage from even brief periods of ischemia [45].

The presence of cavernous sinus involvement represents a particularly ominous prognostic factor for visual outcomes [184]. This anatomical region contains critical neurovascular structures, including the internal carotid artery, multiple cranial nerves, and venous drainage pathways for the orbit and brain. Fungal invasion of the cavernous sinus often leads to extensive vascular compromise, affecting both the ophthalmic artery and its branches and potentially the central retinal artery, resulting in profound ischemic damage to the retina and optic nerve [15]. Additionally, the complex anatomy and limited surgical accessibility of this region often preclude complete debridement, allowing persistent infection despite aggressive medical therapy [15]. The combination of vascular compromise and persistent infection typically results in poor visual outcomes, with permanent blindness being a common sequela of cavernous sinus involvement.

The causative organism also influences visual prognosis, with different fungal pathogens demonstrating distinct patterns of tissue invasion and damage. *Mucorales* species, with their predilection for angioinvasion and rapidly progressive course, generally carry a poorer visual prognosis than *Aspergillus* species [41], which typically demonstrates a more indolent, granulomatous pattern of inflammation. However, this generalization must be considered within the context of individual patient factors, including immune status, comorbidities, and the timing of intervention [185]. Even typically indolent pathogens can cause devastating visual loss if diagnosis is delayed or host defenses are severely compromised, while early intervention may preserve vision even in aggressive infections.

Host factors, particularly those influencing immune function and tissue perfusion, significantly impact visual outcomes. Diabetic patients, especially those with ketoacidosis or poor glycemic control, demonstrate poorer visual outcomes compared to non-diabetic patients with similar infections [41, 183]. This disparity reflects both the increased susceptibility to certain pathogens, particularly *Mucorales*, and the compromised tissue perfusion and wound healing associated with diabetic vasculopathy. Similarly, patients with profound neutropenia or defects in cell-mediated immunity demonstrate poorer visual outcomes, reflecting both increased susceptibility to infection and impaired tissue repair mechanisms [3]. The potential for immune recovery represents a critical prognostic factor, with patients experiencing transient immunosuppression (such as those recovering from chemotherapy) demonstrating better outcomes than those with permanent immune defects (such as advanced HIV disease or certain congenital immunodeficiencies) [186].

The extent and completeness of surgical debridement also influence visual outcomes, though this relationship is complex and sometimes paradoxical. While more extensive debridement may achieve better infectious control, it may also result in greater collateral damage to adjacent structures, including the optic nerve and its blood supply [168, 187]. The decision regarding the extent of debridement, particularly whether to pursue orbital exenteration, requires careful consideration of both infectious control and functional outcomes. In some cases, particularly with Mucormycosis and extensive orbital and intracranial involvement, aggressive debridement, including orbital exenteration, may be necessary for survival despite the certainty of permanent visual loss [188]. In other cases, particularly with more indolent infections or limited orbital involvement, tissue-sparing approaches may allow preservation of the globe and some visual function without compromising infectious control [187].

11.8.2 Neurological Outcomes and Cranial Nerve Function

The prognosis for neurological function, particularly cranial nerve recovery, demonstrates different patterns compared to visual outcomes. In general, cranial nerve function shows better recovery potential than vision, reflecting differences in pathophysiology and the greater regenerative capacity of peripheral nerves compared to central nervous system structures like the optic nerve [189]. Among the cranial nerves, those controlling ocular motility (cranial nerves III, IV, and VI) often show significant improvement, with complete or partial resolution of ophthalmoplegia occurring in approximately 50% to over 80% of survivors, depending on the specific pathogen and host factors [6, 190, 191].

The recovery of ocular motor function follows a relatively predictable time course, with initial improvement typically observed within a few weeks to months of successful infection control, followed by more gradual improvement over up to a year [192]. This recovery pattern reflects the sequential processes of resolution of inflammation, remyelination, and potential axonal regeneration. Patients with persistent ophthalmoplegia beyond 12 months have a low likelihood of further spontaneous improvement, suggesting permanent damage to the cranial nerves or their nuclear structures [192]. In such cases, strabismus surgery may be considered to address persistent diplopia, though the complexity of these procedures is increased by the unpredictable patterns of residual muscle function and potential for continued evolution of ocular alignment over time.

Sensory deficits, particularly those involving the trigeminal nerve, demonstrate more variable recovery patterns. Facial numbness may persist despite successful infection control, reflecting the extensive perineural spread of fungi along trigeminal branches and the limited regenerative capacity of sensory nerves compared to motor nerves [56]. The persistence of sensory deficits may have significant functional implications, particularly when involving the ophthalmic division of the trigeminal nerve. Decreased corneal sensation increases the risk of exposure keratopathy and neurotrophic keratitis, potentially threatening vision even after successful control of the primary infection. These complications necessitate vigilant monitoring and aggressive lubrication, with consideration of protective measures such as tarsorrhaphy in severe cases.

Cognitive and neurological sequelae are common in patients with cerebral involvement, reflecting both direct fungal invasion of brain parenchyma and secondary effects of vascular compromise, increased intracranial pressure, or inflammatory responses [193]. These sequelae may include memory deficits, executive dysfunction, focal neurological deficits corresponding to the areas of involvement, seizures, and various movement disorders [194]. The prognosis for cognitive recovery depends on the extent and location of cerebral involvement, the specific pathogen, the timing of intervention, and host factors influencing neural plasticity and recovery potential. In general, younger patients with limited, focal involvement and prompt intervention demonstrate better cognitive recovery than older patients with extensive, multifocal disease or delayed treatment [194].

As with visual outcomes, the duration of neurological deficits before intervention significantly influences recovery potential [6]. This time-dependent relationship reflects the progressive nature of neural damage with ongoing infection and the limited regenerative capacity of neural tissue once significant damage has occurred [2]. The window of opportunity for meaningful neurological recovery varies by specific deficit and mechanism of injury, but early intervention consistently correlates with improved outcomes across the spectrum of neurological manifestations [154]. This relationship underscores the critical importance of prompt recognition and aggressive management of fungal infections with neurological involvement, even when the initial deficits appear relatively minor.

11.9 Conclusion

Fungal infections with neuro-ophthalmological manifestations represent a significant clinical challenge requiring prompt recognition and aggressive intervention. The orbital apex and adjacent structures are particularly vulnerable to invasion from the paranasal sinuses, creating distinctive clinical syndromes that serve as important diagnostic clues.

The pathophysiology of these infections involves direct tissue invasion, angioinvasion with thrombosis, inflammatory responses, and perineural spread. Host factors, particularly immunosuppression and diabetes mellitus, profoundly influence susceptibility and clinical course. The complex interplay between fungal pathogenesis, host factors, and orbital anatomy creates unique diagnostic and therapeutic challenges that necessitate individualized approaches.

Clinical presentations vary by causative organism, with *Mucorales* species typically exhibiting a rapidly progressive, angioinvasive pattern, while *Aspergillus* can also be angioinvasive and aggressive, though some infections may present with a more indolent course. Orbital apex syndrome, cavernous sinus syndrome, optic neuropathy, and cranial nerve palsies represent the most common neuro-ophthalmological manifestations.

Diagnosis requires a high index of suspicion, comprehensive clinical evaluation, appropriate imaging, and tissue biopsy for definitive identification. Management involves a multidisciplinary approach combining surgical debridement, antifungal therapy, and adjunctive measures tailored to the specific pathogen and host factors.

Outcomes have improved with advances in diagnostic techniques, antifungal therapy, and surgical approaches. However, outcomes remain suboptimal, with significant morbidity and mortality even with optimal management. Visual prognosis is particularly poor once significant visual loss has occurred, reflecting the limited regenerative capacity of the optic nerve. Neurological outcomes show more variability, with better recovery potential for cranial nerve function than for vision.

Future improvements may come from several directions: advanced molecular diagnostic methods for rapid pathogen identification and monitoring, novel antifungal agents with enhanced efficacy and tissue penetration, refined surgical techniques, and targeted immunomodulatory approaches. However, early intervention remains the most critical determinant of outcomes, underscoring the importance of heightened awareness among clinicians across specialties.

The key to improving outcomes lies in heightened awareness among clinicians, prompt recognition of characteristic clinical patterns, and immediate implementation of a multidisciplinary approach with appropriate diagnostic and therapeutic measures. With this approach, the morbidity and mortality associated with these challenging infections can be significantly reduced.

References

1. Chakrabarti A, Denning DW, Ferguson BJ, Ponikau J, Buzina W, Kita H, et al. Fungal rhinosinusitis: a categorization and definitional schema addressing current controversies. Laryngoscope. 2009;119(9):1809–18.
2. Góralska K, Blaszkowska J, Dzikowiec M. Neuroinfections caused by fungi. Infection. 2018;46(4):443–59.
3. Levin LA, Avery R, Shore JW, Woog JJ, Baker AS. The spectrum of orbital aspergillosis: a clinicopathological review. Surv Ophthalmol. 1996;41(2):142–54.
4. Spellberg B, Edwards J Jr, Ibrahim A. Novel perspectives on mucormycosis: pathophysiology, presentation, and management. Clin Microbiol Rev. 2005;18(3):556–69.
5. Cornely OA, Alastruey-Izquierdo A, Arenz D, Chen SCA, Dannaoui E, Hochhegger B, et al. Global guideline for the diagnosis and management of mucormycosis: an initiative of the European Confederation of Medical Mycology in cooperation with the mycoses study group education and research consortium. Lancet Infect Dis. 2019;19(12):e405–e21.
6. Park M, Shin J, Lee E, Ryu G, Kang MC, Park KA, et al. Neuro-ophthalmologic outcomes of orbital apex syndrome caused by invasive fungal Rhinosinusitis. J Neurol Surg B Skull Base. 2025;86(1):66–75.
7. Raman SR. Fungal infections of the nervous system: current perspective and controversies in management. Int J Surg. 2010;8(8):591–601.
8. Jeong W, Keighley C, Wolfe R, Lee WL, Slavin MA, Kong DCM, et al. The epidemiology and clinical manifestations of mucormycosis: a systematic review and meta-analysis of case reports. Clin Microbiol Infect. 2019;25(1):26–34.
9. Klotz SA, Penn CC, Negvesky GJ, Butrus SI. Fungal and parasitic infections of the eye. Clin Microbiol Rev. 2000;13(4):662–85.

10. Thurtell MJ, Chiu AL, Goold LA, Akdal G, Crompton JL, Ahmed R, et al. Neuro-ophthalmology of invasive fungal sinusitis: 14 consecutive patients and a review of the literature. Clin Experiment Ophthalmol. 2013;41(6):567–76.
11. Middlebrooks EH, Frost CJ, De Jesus RO. Acute invasive fungal Rhinosinusitis: a comprehensive update of CT findings. AJNR Am J Neuroradiol. 2015;36(8):1529–35.
12. Hou T, Bell WR, Mesa H. Invasive fungal infections of the head and neck: a tertiary hospital experience. Pathogens. 2024;13(7)
13. Dabas Y, Xess I, Pandey M, Ahmed J, Sachdev J, Iram A, et al. Epidemiology and antifungal susceptibility patterns of invasive fungal infections (IFIs) in India: a prospective observational study. J Fungi (Basel). 2021;8(1)
14. Rehman A, Farooqi HA, Khan I, Akram F, Khan BA, Ihtesham A, et al. Unmasking Aspergillosis: a rare cause of facial palsy and vision loss in an immunocompetent patient-a case report and literature review. Clin Case Reports. 2025;13(2):e70152.
15. Coutel M, Duprez T, Huart C, Wacheul E, Boschi A. Invasive fungal sinusitis with ophthalmological complications: case series and review of the literature. Neuroophthalmology. 2021;45(3):193–204.
16. Sivak-Callcott JA, Livesley N, Nugent RA, Rasmussen SL, Saeed P, Rootman J. Localised invasive sino-orbital aspergillosis: characteristic features. Br J Ophthalmol. 2004;88(5):681–7.
17. Wiggins RE Jr. Invasive aspergillosis. A complication of treatment of temporal arteritis. J Neuroophthalmol. 1995;15(1):36–8.
18. Ibrahim AS, Spellberg B, Walsh TJ, Kontoyiannis DP. Pathogenesis of mucormycosis. Clin Infect Dis. 2012;54(Suppl 1):S16–22.
19. Kaushik KS, Ananthasivan R, Acharya UV, Rawat S, Patil UD, Shankar B, et al. Spectrum of intracranial complications of rhino-orbito-cerebral mucormycosis — resurgence in the era of COVID-19 pandemic: a pictorial essay. Emerg Radiol. 2021;28(6):1097–106.
20. Ghuman H, Voelz K. Innate and adaptive immunity to Mucorales. J Fungi (Basel). 2017;3(3):48.
21. Binder U, Maurer E, Lass-Flörl C. Mucormycosis – from the pathogens to the disease. Clin Microbiol Infect. 2014;20(Suppl 6):60–6.
22. Gebremariam T, Lin L, Liu M. Bicarbonate correction of ketoacidosis alters host-pathogen interactions and alleviates mucormycosis. J Clin Invest. 2016;126(6):2280–94.
23. Liu M, Spellberg B, Phan QT. The endothelial cell receptor GRP78 is required for mucormycosis pathogenesis in diabetic mice. J Clin Invest. 2010;120(6):1914–24.
24. Bhansali A, Bhadada S, Sharma A, Suresh V, Gupta A, Singh P, et al. Presentation and outcome of rhino-orbital-cerebral mucormycosis in patients with diabetes. Postgrad Med J. 2004;80(949):670–4.
25. Andrianaki AM, Kyrmizi I, Thanopoulou K. Iron restriction inside macrophages regulates pulmonary host defense against Rhizopus species. Nat Commun. 2018;9(1):3333.
26. Spellberg B, Ibrahim AS, Chin-Hong PV. The Deferasirox-AmBisome Therapy for Mucormycosis (DEFEAT Mucor) study: a randomized, double-blinded, placebo-controlled trial. J Antimicrob Chemother. 2012;67(3):715–22.
27. Dagenais TR, Keller NP. Pathogenesis of Aspergillus fumigatus in invasive Aspergillosis. Clin Microbiol Rev. 2009;22(3):447–65.
28. Sipsas NV, Gamaletsou MN, Anastasopoulou A, Kontoyiannis DP. Therapy of Mucormycosis. J Fungi (Basel). 2018;4(3)
29. Merkler AE, Gaines N, Baradaran H, Schuetz AN, Lavi E, Simpson SA, et al. Direct invasion of the optic nerves, chiasm, and tracts by Cryptococcus neoformans in an immunocompetent host. Neurohospitalist. 2015;5(4):217–22.
30. O'Meara TR, Alspaugh JA. The Cryptococcus neoformans capsule: a sword and a shield. Clin Microbiol Rev. 2012;25(3):387–408.
31. Sridhar J, Flynn HW Jr, Kuriyan AE, Miller D, Albini T. Endogenous fungal endophthalmitis: risk factors, clinical features, and treatment outcomes in mold and yeast infections. J Ophthalmic Inflamm Infect. 2013;3(1):60.

32. Nobile CJ, Johnson AD. Candida albicans biofilms and human disease. Ann Rev Microbiol. 2015;69:71–92.
33. Wykoff CC, Flynn HW Jr, Miller D, Scott IU, Alfonso EC. Exogenous fungal endophthalmitis: microbiology and clinical outcomes. Ophthalmology. 2008;115(9):1501–7. 7.e1–2
34. Cunningham ET Jr, Seiff SR, Berger TG, Lizotte PE, Howes EL Jr, Horton JC. Intraocular Coccidioidomycosis diagnosed by skin biopsy. Arch Ophthalmol. 1998;116(5):674–7.
35. Vaughan C, Bartolo A, Vallabh N, Leong SC. A meta-analysis of survival factors in rhino-orbital-cerebral mucormycosis-has anything changed in the past 20 years? Clin Otolaryngol. 2018;43(6):1454–64.
36. Kashkouli MB, Abdolalizadeh P, Oghazian M. Outcomes and factors affecting them in patients with rhino-orbito-cerebral mucormycosis. Br J Ophthalmol. 2019;103(10):1460–5.
37. Gamaletsou MN, Sipsas NV, Roilides E, Walsh TJ. Rhino-orbital-cerebral mucormycosis. Curr Infect Dis Rep. 2012;14(4):423–34.
38. Arora R, Goel R, Khanam S. Rhino-Orbito-cerebral Mucormycosis during the COVID-19 second wave in 2021 – a preliminary report from a single hospital. Clin Ophthalmol. 2021;15:3505–14.
39. Nithyanandam S, Jacob MS, Battu RR, Rhino-orbito-cerebral mucormycosis. A retrospective analysis of clinical features and treatment outcomes. Indian J Ophthalmol. 2003;51(3):231–6.
40. Talmi YP, Goldschmied-Reouven A, Bakon M. Rhino-orbital and rhino-orbito-cerebral mucormycosis. Otolaryngol Head Neck Surg. 2002;127(1):22–31.
41. Goel R, Arora R, Shah S, Chhabra M, Kumar J, Khurana N, et al. Clinico-radiological-pathological correlation of visual loss in COVID-associated rhino-orbito-cerebral Mucormycosis. Ophthalmic Plast Reconstr Surg. 2022;38(3):242–9.
42. Patel AK, Patel KK, Patel K. Mucormycosis at a tertiary care centre in Gujarat, India. Mycoses. 2017;60(6):407–11.
43. Badakere A, Patil-Chhablani P. Orbital apex syndrome: a review. Eye Brain. 2019;11:63–72.
44. Yeh S, Foroozan R. Orbital apex syndrome. Curr Opin Ophthalmol. 2004;15(6):490–8.
45. Kahloun R, Abroug N, Ksiaa I, Mahmoud A, Zeghidi H, Zaouali S, et al. Infectious optic neuropathies: a clinical update. Eye Brain. 2015;7:59–81.
46. Jiang N, Zhao G, Yang S, Lin J, Hu L, Che C, et al. A retrospective analysis of eleven cases of invasive rhino-orbito-cerebral mucormycosis presented with orbital apex syndrome initially. BMC Ophthalmol. 2016;16:10.
47. Mohankumar A, Gurnani B. Orbital apex syndrome. In: StatPearls. Treasure Island (FL): StatPearls; 2025.
48. Godinho G, Abreu I, Alves G, Vaz R, Leal V, Carvalho AC, et al. Orbital apex syndrome due to orbital Mucormycosis after teeth infection: a successful case report. Case Rep Ophthalmol. 2021;12(1):110–5.
49. Cullen GD, Davidson TM, Yetmar ZA, Pritt BS, DeSimone DC. Orbital apex syndrome due to invasive aspergillosis in an immunocompetent patient. IDCases. 2021;25:e01232.
50. Fernández S, Godino O, Martínez-Yélamos S, Mesa E, Arruga J, Ramón JM, et al. Cavernous sinus syndrome: a series of 126 patients. Medicine (Baltimore). 2007;86(5):278–81.
51. Lee JH, Lee HK, Lee DH, Choi CG, Kim SJ, Suh DC. Neuroimaging strategies for three types of Horner syndrome with emphasis on anatomic location. AJR Am J Roentgenol. 2007;188(1):W74–81.
52. Shen Y, Hu F, Wu L, Nie H. Concomitant rapidly growing aneurysm of intracavernous carotid artery and cavernous sinus thrombosis: case report and review of the literature. Medicine (Baltimore). 2024;103(30):e39022.
53. Ebright JR, Pace MT, Niazi AF. Septic thrombosis of the cavernous sinuses. Arch Intern Med. 2001;161(22):2671–6.
54. Liang W, Xiaofeng Y, Weiguo L, Wusi Q, Gang S, Xuesheng Z. Traumatic carotid cavernous fistula accompanying basilar skull fracture: a study on the incidence of traumatic carotid cavernous fistula in the patients with basilar skull fracture and the prognostic analysis about traumatic carotid cavernous fistula. J Trauma. 2007;63(5):1014–20. discussion 20

55. Honavar SG. Code Mucor: guidelines for the diagnosis, staging and management of rhino-orbito-cerebral Mucormycosis in the setting of COVID-19. Indian J Ophthalmol. 2021;69(6):1361–5.
56. Galletta K, Alafaci C, D'Alcontres FS, Maria ME, Cavallaro M, Ricciardello G, et al. Imaging features of perineural and perivascular spread in rapidly progressive rhino-orbital-cerebral mucormycosis: a case report and brief review of the literature. Surg Neurol Int. 2021;12:245.
57. Dubey S, Mukherjee D, Sarkar P, Mukhopadhyay P, Barman D, Bandopadhyay M, et al. COVID-19 associated rhino-orbital-cerebral mucormycosis: an observational study from eastern India, with special emphasis on neurological spectrum. Diabetes Metab Syndr. 2021;15(5):102267.
58. Alsaleh MA, Almomen AA. Abducens nerve palsy secondary to allergic fungal sinusitis. J Surg Case Rep. 2024;2024(11):rjae697
59. Razek AA, Castillo M. Imaging lesions of the cavernous sinus. AJNR Am J Neuroradiol. 2009;30(3):444–52.
60. Walton J, Coulson C. Fungal malignant otitis externa with facial nerve palsy: tissue biopsy AIDS diagnosis. Case Rep Otolaryngol. 2014;2014:192318.
61. Espino Barros Palau A, Morgan ML, Foroozan R, Lee AG. Neuro-ophthalmic presentations and treatment of Cryptococcal meningitis-related increased intracranial pressure. Can J Ophthalmol. 2014;49(5):473–7.
62. Sun G, Weiss A, Zhao J, Silver M, DeMaio M, Dehbashi S. Isolated cerebral Mucormycosis and Aspergillosis coinfection in an immunocompromised adult. BMJ Case Rep. 2023;16(8)
63. Chen KJ, Sun MH, Chen YP, Chen YH, Wang NK, Liu L, et al. Endogenous fungal Endophthalmitis: causative organisms, treatments, and visual outcomes. J Fungi (Basel). 2022;8(6)
64. Abdollahi A, Shokohi T, Amirrajab N, Poormosa R, Kasiri AM, Motahari SJ, et al. Clinical features, diagnosis, and outcomes of rhino-orbito-cerebral mucormycosis- a retrospective analysis. Curr Med Mycol. 2016;2(4):15–23.
65. Zia Z, Sajadi MJ, Bazrafshan H, Khademi B, Janipour M. Survival and prognostic factors in rhino-orbito-cerebral mucormycosis: a 3-year cohort study. Sci Rep. 2025;15(1):16088.
66. Boohaker L, Patel SM, Townsley E. Delay in the diagnosis of Osteoarticular Mucormycosis in diabetic ketoacidosis: a learning opportunity. Cureus. 2025;17(4):e82693.
67. Price EB, Dubey S, Sulaiman ZI, Samra H, Askar G. A silent threat unveiled: invasive fungal sinusitis in a high-risk hematologic malignancy patient. Cureus. 2024;16(5):e61232.
68. Shoham S, Marr KA. Invasive fungal infections in solid organ transplant recipients. Future Microbiol. 2012;7(5):639–55.
69. Patterson TF, Thompson GR III, Denning DW, Fishman JA, Hadley S, Herbrecht R, et al. Practice guidelines for the diagnosis and management of Aspergillosis: 2016 update by the Infectious Diseases Society of America. Clin Infect Dis. 2016;63(4):e1–e60.
70. Couppié P, Herceg K, Bourne-Watrin M, Thomas V, Blanchet D, Alsibai KD, et al. The broad clinical spectrum of disseminated histoplasmosis in HIV-infected patients: a 30 years' experience in French Guiana. Journal of Fungi. 2019;5(4):115.
71. Deshazo RD. Syndromes of invasive fungal sinusitis. Med Mycol. 2009;47(Supplement 1):S309–S14.
72. Jia G, Yang C, Feng Y. Diabetes-associated central nervous system mucormycosis with delayed diagnosis: a case report. Front Neurol. 2025;16:1596136.
73. Pushker N, Meel R, Kashyap S, Bajaj MS, Sen S. Invasive aspergillosis of orbit in immunocompetent patients: treatment and outcome. Ophthalmology. 2011;118(9):1886–91.
74. Siddiqui AA, Shah AA, Bashir SH. Craniocerebral aspergillosis of sinonasal origin in immunocompetent patients: clinical spectrum and outcome in 25 cases. Neurosurgery. 2004;55(3):602–11. discussion 11-3
75. Thomas KE, Hasbun R, Jekel J, Quagliarello VJ. The diagnostic accuracy of Kernig's sign, Brudzinski's sign, and nuchal rigidity in adults with suspected meningitis. Clin Infect Dis. 2002;35(1):46–52.

76. Sahota R, Gambhir R, Anand S, Dixit A. Rhinocerebral Mucormycosis: report of a rare case. Ethiop J Health Sci. 2017;27(1):85–90.
77. Sravani T, Uppin SG, Uppin MS, Sundaram C. Rhinocerebral mucormycosis: pathology revisited with emphasis on perineural spread. Neurol India. 2014;62(4):383–6.
78. Clinical, Laboratory Standards I. M54: principles and procedures for detection and culture of fungi in clinical specimens. 2nd ed. Wayne, PA: Clinical and Laboratory Standards Institute; 2021.
79. Guarner J, Brandt ME. Histopathologic diagnosis of fungal infections in the 21st century. Clin Microbiol Rev. 2011;24(2):247–80.
80. Challa S. Pathogenesis and pathology of invasive Aspergillosis. Curr Fungal Infect Rep. 2018;12:23–32.
81. Lamoth F. Galactomannan and 1,3-β-d-Glucan testing for the diagnosis of invasive Aspergillosis. J Fungi (Basel). 2016;2(3)
82. Theel ES, Doern CD. β-D-Glucan testing is important for diagnosis of invasive fungal infections. J Clin Microbiol. 2013;51(11):3478–83.
83. Millon L, Larosa F, Lepiller Q. Quantitative polymerase chain reaction detection of circulating DNA in serum for early diagnosis of mucormycosis in immunocompromised patients. Clin Infect Dis. 2013;56(10):e95–101.
84. Gabaldón T. Recent trends in molecular diagnostics of yeast infections: from PCR to NGS. FEMS Microbiol Rev. 2019;43(5):517–47.
85. Therakathu J, Prabhu S, Irodi A. Imaging features of rhinocerebral mucormycosis: a study of 43 patients. Egypt J Radiol Nucl Med. 2018;49(2):447–52.
86. Herrera DA, Dublin AB, Ormsby EL. Imaging findings of rhinocerebral mucormycosis. Skull Base. 2009;19(2):117–25.
87. Aribandi M, McCoy VA, Bazan C 3rd. Imaging features of invasive and noninvasive fungal sinusitis: a review. Radiographics. 2007;27(5):1283–96.
88. Joshi AR, Muthe MM, Patankar SH, Athawale A, Achhapalia Y. CT and MRI findings of invasive Mucormycosis in the setting of COVID-19: experience from a single center in India. Am J Roentgenol. 2021;217(6):1431–2.
89. Groppo ER, El-Sayed IH, Aiken AH, Glastonbury CM. Computed tomography and magnetic resonance imaging characteristics of acute invasive fungal sinusitis. Arch Otolaryngol Head Neck Surg. 2011;137(10):1005–10.
90. Sreshta K, Dave TV, Varma DR, Nair AG, Bothra N, Naik MN, et al. Magnetic resonance imaging in rhino-orbital-cerebral mucormycosis. Indian J Ophthalmol. 2021;69(7):1915–27.
91. Marzolf G, Sabou M, Lannes B, Cotton F, Meyronet D, Galanaud D, et al. Magnetic resonance imaging of cerebral Aspergillosis: imaging and pathological correlations. PLoS One. 2016;11(4):e0152475.
92. Parsi K, Itgampalli RK, Vittal R, Kumar A. Perineural spread of rhino-orbitocerebral mucormycosis caused by Apophysomyces elegans. Ann Indian Acad Neurol. 2013;16(3):414–7.
93. Chikley A, Ben-Ami R, Kontoyiannis DP. Mucormycosis of the central nervous system. J Fungi (Basel). 2019;5(3)
94. Dhande RP, Singhania A, Gupta A. Role of diffusion-weighted imaging in evaluation of intracranial infections. J Datta Meghe Inst Med Sci Univ. 2020;15(1):26–9.
95. Gabelmann A, Klein S, Kern W, Krüger S, Brambs HJ, Rieber-Brambs A, et al. Relevant imaging findings of cerebral aspergillosis on MRI: a retrospective case-based study in immunocompromised patients. Eur J Neurol. 2007;14(5):548–55.
96. Upadhayay P, Bansal K, Goyal A. Epidemiology, risk factors, diagnosis and treatment of Mucormycosis (black fungus): a review. Curr Pharm Biotechnol. 2023;24(13):1645–56.
97. Luo Y-t, Zhu C-r, He B, Yan A-h, Wei H-q. Diagnostic and therapeutic strategies of acute invasive fungal rhinosinusitis. Asian J Surg. 2023;46(1):58–65.
98. Ting DS, Perez-Lopez M, Chew NJ, Clarke L, Dickinson AJ, Neoh C. A 10-year review of orbital biopsy: the Newcastle eye centre study. Eye (Lond). 2015;29(9):1162–6.
99. Chew FS, Kline MJ. Diagnostic yield of CT-guided percutaneous aspiration procedures in suspected spontaneous infectious diskitis. Radiology. 2001;218(1):211–4.

100. Kauffman CA. Central nervous system infection with other endemic mycoses: rare manifestation of Blastomycosis, Paracoccidioidomycosis, Talaromycosis, and Sporotrichosis. J Fungi (Basel). 2019;5(3)
101. Temfack E, Rim JJB, Spijker R, Loyse A, Chiller T, Pappas PG, et al. Cryptococcal antigen in serum and cerebrospinal fluid for detecting Cryptococcal meningitis in adults living with human immunodeficiency virus: systematic review and meta-analysis of diagnostic test accuracy studies. Clin Infect Dis. 2021;72(7):1268–78.
102. Deutsch PG, Whittaker J, Prasad S. Invasive and non-invasive fungal Rhinosinusitis-a review and update of the evidence. Medicina (Kaunas). 2019;55(7).
103. Prattes J, Heldt S, Eigl S, Hoenigl M. Point of care testing for the diagnosis of fungal infections: are we there yet? Curr Fungal Infect Rep. 2016;10:43–50.
104. Benoit P, Brazer N, de Lorenzi-Tognon M, Kelly E, Servellita V, Oseguera M, et al. Seven-year performance of a clinical metagenomic next-generation sequencing test for diagnosis of central nervous system infections. Nat Med. 2024;30(12):3522–33.
105. Angelini E, Shah A. Using artificial intelligence in fungal lung disease: CPA CT imaging as an example. Mycopathologia. 2021;186(5):733–7.
106. Taj-Aldeen SJ, Mir FA, Sivaraman SK, AbdulWahab A. Serum cytokine profile in patients with Candidemia versus Bacteremia. Pathogens. 2021;10(10)
107. Brandt P, Garbe E, Vylkova S. Catch the wave: Metabolomic analyses in human pathogenic fungi. PLoS Pathog. 2020;16(8):e1008757.
108. Steinbrink JM, Zaas AK, Betancourt M, Modliszewski JL, Corcoran DL, McClain MT. A transcriptional signature accurately identifies Aspergillus infection across healthy and immunosuppressed states. Transl Res. 2020;219:1–12.
109. Janetos TM, Volpe NJ, Simon SS. Neuro-ophthalmic manifestations of cancer: a narrative review. Chin Clin Oncol. 2022;11(3):25.
110. Bonavolontà G, Strianese D, Grassi P. An analysis of 2,480 space-occupying lesions of the orbit from 1976 to 2011. Ophthalmic Plast Reconstr Surg. 2013;29(2):79–86.
111. Cornely OA, Arikan-Akdagli S, Dannaoui E. ESCMID and ECMM joint clinical guidelines for the diagnosis and management of mucormycosis 2013. Clin Microbiol Infect. 2014;20(Suppl 3):5–26.
112. Spellberg B, Walsh TJ, Kontoyiannis DP, Edwards J Jr, Ibrahim AS. Recent advances in the management of mucormycosis: from bench to bedside. Clin Infect Dis. 2009;48(12):1743–51.
113. Pakdaman MN, Sepahdari AR, Elkhamary SM. Orbital inflammatory disease: pictorial review and differential diagnosis. World J Radiol. 2014;6(4):106–15.
114. Colnaghi S, Versino M, Marchioni E. ICHD-II diagnostic criteria for Tolosa-hunt syndrome in idiopathic inflammatory syndromes of the orbit and/or the cavernous sinus. Cephalalgia. 2008;28(6):577–84.
115. Mulay K, Honavar SG. Orbital immunoglobulin G4–related disease: a systematic review. Asia-Pacific J Ophthalmol. 2014;3(5):322–5.
116. Stornaiuolo A, Iodice R, De Simone R, Russo C, Rubino M, Braca S, et al. Multiple cranial neuropathy due to varicella zoster virus reactivation without vesicular rash: a challenging diagnosis. Neurol Sci. 2023;44(10):3687–9.
117. Hesarur N, Seshagiri DV, Nagappa M, Rao S, Santosh V, Chandrashekar N, et al. Case report: chronic fungal meningitis masquerading as tubercular meningitis. Am J Trop Med Hyg. 2020;103(4):1473–9.
118. Butler NJ, Furtado JM, Winthrop KL, Smith JR. Ocular toxoplasmosis II: clinical features, pathology and management. Clin Experiment Ophthalmol. 2013;41(1):95–108.
119. Dhiman R, Devi S, Duraipandi K, Chandra P, Vanathi M, Tandon R, et al. Cysticercosis of the eye. Int J Ophthalmol. 2017;10(8):1319–24.
120. Alabed A, Alobaid B, Alhallak S, Alamawi S, Kadi Z. Orbital hydatid cyst from Echinococcus granulosus: a case report. J Surg Case Rep. 2025;2025(3):rjaf135.
121. Dowling E, Modzeski M, Choby G. Cavernous sinus thrombosis secondary to sphenoid sinus fungal ball. Ear Nose Throat J. 2019;98(9):540–2.

122. Digge P, Prakashini K, Bharath KV. Plain CT vs MR venography in acute cerebral venous sinus thrombosis: triumphant dark horse. Indian J Radiol Imaging. 2018;28(3):280–4.
123. Saposnik G, Barinagarrementeria F, Brown RD Jr, Bushnell CD, Cucchiara B, Cushman M, et al. Diagnosis and management of cerebral venous thrombosis: a statement for healthcare professionals from the American Heart Association/American Stroke Association. Stroke. 2011;42(4):1158–92.
124. Bawankar P, Lahane S, Pathak P, Gonde P, Singh A. Central retinal artery occlusion as the presenting manifestation of invasive rhino-orbital-cerebral mucormycosis. Taiwan J Ophthalmol. 2020;10(1):62–5.
125. Shokri T, Zacharia BE, Lighthall JG. Traumatic orbital apex syndrome: an uncommon sequela of facial trauma. Ear Nose Throat J. 2019;98(10):609–12.
126. Imaizumi A, Ishida K, Ishikawa Y, Nakayoshi I. Successful treatment of the traumatic orbital apex syndrome due to direct bone compression. Craniomaxillofac Trauma Reconstr. 2014;7(4):318–22.
127. Goormans F, Coropciuc R, Vercruysse M, Spriet I, Willaert R, Politis C. Systemic antibiotic prophylaxis in maxillofacial trauma: a scoping review and critical appraisal. Antibiotics (Basel). 2022;11(4)
128. Westfall E, Fridirici Z, El-Kouri N, McSpadden R, Loochtan M, Stankiewicz J. Diagnosis and management of orbital fat exposure during endoscopic sinus surgery. Ear Nose Throat J. 2023;102(9):573–9.
129. Illing E, Schlosser RJ, Palmer JN, Curé J, Fox N, Woodworth BA. Spontaneous sphenoid lateral recess cerebrospinal fluid leaks arise from intracranial hypertension, not Sternberg's canal. Int Forum Allergy Rhinol. 2014;4(3):246–50.
130. Roxbury CR, Smith DF, Higgins TS, Lee SE, Gallia GL, Ishii M, et al. Complete surgical resection and short-term survival in acute invasive fungal rhinosinusitis. Am J Rhinol Allergy. 2017;31(2):109–16.
131. Alhilali L, Reynolds AR, Fakhran S. Osteoradionecrosis after radiation therapy for head and neck cancer: differentiation from recurrent disease with CT and PET/CT imaging. AJNR Am J Neuroradiol. 2014;35(7):1405–11.
132. Glastonbury CM, Salzman KL. Pitfalls in the staging of cancer of nasopharyngeal carcinoma. Neuroimaging Clin N Am. 2013;23(1):9–25.
133. Pruitt AA. Central nervous system infections in immunocompromised patients. Curr Neurol Neurosci Rep. 2021;21(7):37.
134. Hoang JK, Branstetter BFT, Eastwood JD, Glastonbury CM. Multiplanar CT and MRI of collections in the retropharyngeal space: is it an abscess? AJR Am J Roentgenol. 2011;196(4):W426–32.
135. Mora-Horna ER, Rojas-Padilla R, López VG, Guzmán MJ, Ceriotto A, Salcedo G. Ocular adnexal and orbital amyloidosis: a case series and literature review. Int Ophthalmol. 2016;36(2):281–98.
136. Ramos-Casals M, Brito-Zerón P, Bombardieri S, Bootsma H, De Vita S, Dörner T, et al. EULAR recommendations for the management of Sjögren's syndrome with topical and systemic therapies. Ann Rheum Dis. 2020;79(1):3–18.
137. Chamilos G, Lewis RE, Kontoyiannis DP. Delaying amphotericin B-based frontline therapy significantly increases mortality among patients with hematologic malignancy who have zygomycosis. Clin Infect Dis. 2008;47(4):503–9.
138. Farmakiotis D, Kontoyiannis DP. Mucormycoses. Infect Dis Clin N Am. 2016;30(1):143–63.
139. Maertens JA, Raad II, Marr KA, Patterson TF, Kontoyiannis DP, Cornely OA, et al. Isavuconazole versus voriconazole for primary treatment of invasive mould disease caused by Aspergillus and other filamentous fungi (SECURE): a phase 3, randomised-controlled, non-inferiority trial. Lancet. 2016;387(10020):760–9.
140. Singh N, Husain S. Invasive aspergillosis in solid organ transplant recipients. Am J Transplant. 2009;9(Suppl 4):S180–91.
141. Spellberg B, Edwards Jr J, Ashraf I. Novel perspectives on mucormycosis: pathophysiology, presentation, and management. Clin Microbiol Rev. 2005;18(3):556–69.

142. Lanternier F, Poiree S, Elie C, Garcia-Hermoso D, Bakouboula P, Sitbon K, Herbrecht R, Wolff M, Ribaud P, Lortholary O; French Mycosis Study Group. Prospective pilot study of high-dose (10 mg/kg/day) liposomal amphotericin B (L-AMB) for the initial treatment of mucormycosis. J Antimicrob Chemother. 2015;70(11):3116–23.
143. Lestner JM, Howard SJ, Goodwin J, Gregson L, Majithiya J, Walsh TJ, et al. Pharmacokinetics and pharmacodynamics of amphotericin B deoxycholate, liposomal amphotericin B, and amphotericin B lipid complex in an in vitro model of invasive pulmonary aspergillosis. Antimicrob Agents Chemother. 2010;54(8):3432–41.
144. Odds FC, Brown AJ, Gow NA. Antifungal agents: mechanisms of action. Trends Microbiol. 2003;11(6):272–9.
145. Marty FM, Ostrosky-Zeichner L, Cornely OA, Mullane KM, Perfect JR, Thompson GR 3rd, et al. Isavuconazole treatment for mucormycosis: a single-arm open-label trial and case-control analysis. Lancet Infect Dis. 2016;16(7):828–37.
146. Herbrecht R, Denning DW, Patterson TF, Bennett JE, Greene RE, Oestmann JW, et al. Voriconazole versus amphotericin B for primary therapy of invasive aspergillosis. N Engl J Med. 2002;347(6):408–15.
147. Pascual A, Calandra T, Bolay S, Buclin T, Bille J, Marchetti O. Voriconazole therapeutic drug monitoring in patients with invasive mycoses improves efficacy and safety outcomes. Clin Infect Dis. 2008;46(2):201–11.
148. Ashbee HR, Barnes RA, Johnson EM, Richardson MD, Gorton R, Hope WW. Therapeutic drug monitoring (TDM) of antifungal agents: guidelines from the British Society for Medical Mycology. J Antimicrob Chemother. 2014;69(5):1162–76.
149. Krishna G, Ma L, Martinho M, Preston RA, O'Mara E. A new solid oral tablet formulation of posaconazole: a randomized clinical trial to investigate rising single- and multiple-dose pharmacokinetics and safety in healthy volunteers. J Antimicrob Chemother. 2012;67(11):2725–30.
150. Kovanda LL, Desai AV, Lu Q, Townsend RW, Akhtar S, Bonate P, et al. Isavuconazole population pharmacokinetic analysis using nonparametric estimation in patients with invasive fungal disease (results from the VITAL study). Antimicrob Agents Chemother. 2016;60(8):4568–76.
151. Maertens JA, Rahav G, Lee DG, Ponce-de-León A, Ramírez Sánchez IC, Klimko N, et al. Posaconazole versus voriconazole for primary treatment of invasive aspergillosis: a phase 3, randomised, controlled, non-inferiority trial. Lancet. 2021;397(10273):499–509.
152. Brüggemann RJ, Alffenaar JW, Blijlevens NM, Billaud EM, Kosterink JG, Verweij PE, et al. Clinical relevance of the pharmacokinetic interactions of azole antifungal drugs with other coadministered agents. Clin Infect Dis. 2009;48(10):1441–58.
153. Cappelletty D, Eiselstein-McKitrick K. The echinocandins. Pharmacotherapy. 2007;27(3):369–88.
154. Pappas PG, Kauffman CA, Andes DR, Clancy CJ, Marr KA, Ostrosky-Zeichner L, et al. Clinical practice guideline for the management of candidiasis: 2016 update by the Infectious Diseases Society of America. Clin Infect Dis. 2015;62(4):e1–e50.
155. Aguilar-Zapata D, Petraitiene R, Petraitis V. Echinocandins: the expanding antifungal armamentarium. Clin Infect Dis. 2015;61(Suppl 6):S604–11.
156. Felton T, Troke PF, Hope WW. Tissue penetration of antifungal agents. Clin Microbiol Rev. 2014;27(1):68–88.
157. Kalin-Hajdu E, Hirabayashi KE, Vagefi MR, Kersten RC. Invasive fungal sinusitis: treatment of the orbit. Curr Opin Ophthalmol. 2017;28(5):522–33.
158. Lewis RE, Kontoyiannis DP. Rationale for combination antifungal therapy. Pharmacotherapy. 2001;21(8 Pt 2):149s–64s.
159. Maertens JA, Girmenia C, Brüggemann RJ, Duarte RF, Kibbler CC, Ljungman P, et al. European guidelines for primary antifungal prophylaxis in adult haematology patients: summary of the updated recommendations from the European conference on infections in leukaemia. J Antimicrob Chemother. 2018;73(12):3221–30.

160. Hirabayashi KE, Kalin-Hajdu E, Brodie FL, Kersten RC, Russell MS, Vagefi MR. Retrobulbar injection of amphotericin B for orbital Mucormycosis. Ophthalmic Plast Reconstr Surg. 2017;33(4):e94–e7.
161. Skiada A, Lanternier F, Groll AH, Pagano L, Zimmerli S, Herbrecht R, et al. Diagnosis and treatment of mucormycosis in patients with hematological malignancies: guidelines from the 3rd European conference on infections in Leukemia (ECIL 3). Haematologica. 2013;98(4):492–504.
162. Kontoyiannis DP, Lewis RE. How I treat mucormycosis. Blood. 2011;118(5):1216–24.
163. Hamill RJ. Amphotericin B formulations: a comparative review of efficacy and toxicity. Drugs. 2013;73(9):919–34.
164. Nicolai P, Castelnuovo P, Lombardi D, Battaglia P, Bignami M, Pianta L, et al. Role of endoscopic surgery in the management of selected malignant epithelial neoplasms of the naso-ethmoidal complex. Head Neck. 2007;29(12):1075–82.
165. Falcon RT, Rivera-Serrano CM, Miranda JF, Prevedello DM, Snyderman CH, Kassam AB, et al. Endoscopic endonasal dissection of the infratemporal fossa: anatomic relationships and importance of eustachian tube in the endoscopic skull base surgery. Laryngoscope. 2011;121(1):31–41.
166. Balakrishnan K, Moe KS. Applications and outcomes of orbital and transorbital endoscopic surgery. Otolaryngol Head Neck Surg. 2011;144(5):815–20.
167. Citardi MJ, Batra PS. Intraoperative surgical navigation for endoscopic sinus surgery: rationale and indications. Curr Opin Otolaryngol Head Neck Surg. 2007;15(1):23–7.
168. Murthy R, Gote YS, Bagchi A. Localized surgical debridement for the management of orbital mucormycosis. Indian J Ophthalmol. 2022;70(2):649–52.
169. Kasapoglu F, Coskun H, Ozmen OA, Akalin H, Ener B. Acute invasive fungal rhinosinusitis: evaluation of 26 patients treated with endonasal or open surgical procedures. Otolaryngol Head Neck Surg. 2010;143(5):614–20.
170. Abu-Ghanem S, Fliss DM. Surgical approaches to resection of anterior skull base and paranasal sinuses tumors. Balkan Med J. 2013;30(2):136–41.
171. Nicolai P, Castelnuovo P, Bolzoni VA. Endoscopic resection of sinonasal malignancies. Curr Oncol Rep. 2011;13(2):138–44.
172. Leong SC, Karkos PD, Macewen CJ, White PS. A systematic review of outcomes following surgical decompression for dysthyroid orbitopathy. Laryngoscope. 2009;119(6):1106–15.
173. Kassam AB, Prevedello DM, Carrau RL, Snyderman CH, Thomas A, Gardner P, et al. Endoscopic endonasal skull base surgery: analysis of complications in the authors' initial 800 patients. J Neurosurg. 2011;114(6):1544–68.
174. Turner JH, Soudry E, Nayak JV, Hwang PH. Survival outcomes in acute invasive fungal sinusitis: a systematic review and quantitative synthesis of published evidence. Laryngoscope. 2013;123(5):1112–8.
175. Mathieu D, Marroni A, Kot J. Tenth European consensus conference on hyperbaric medicine: recommendations for accepted and non-accepted clinical indications and practice of hyperbaric oxygen treatment. Diving Hyperb Med. 2017;47(1):24–32.
176. John BV, Chamilos G, Kontoyiannis DP. Hyperbaric oxygen as an adjunctive treatment for zygomycosis. Clin Microbiol Infect. 2005;11(7):515–7.
177. Tragiannidis A, Groll AH. Hyperbaric oxygen therapy and other adjunctive treatments for zygomycosis. Clin Microbiol Infect. 2009;15(Suppl 5):82–6.
178. Kontoyiannis DP, Lewis RE, Alexander BD, Lortholary O, Dromer F, Gupta KL, et al. Calcineurin inhibitor agents interact synergistically with antifungal agents in vitro against Cryptococcus neoformans isolates: correlation with outcome in solid organ transplant recipients with cryptococcosis. Antimicrob Agents Chemother. 2008;52(2):735–8.
179. Wan L, Zhang Y, Lai Y, Jiang M, Song Y, Zhou J, et al. Effect of granulocyte-macrophage colony-stimulating factor on prevention and treatment of invasive fungal disease in recipients of allogeneic stem-cell transplantation: a prospective Multicenter randomized phase IV trial. J Clin Oncol. 2015;33(34):3999–4006.

180. Li Z, Denning DW. The impact of corticosteroids on the outcome of fungal disease: a systematic review and meta-analysis. Curr Fungal Infect Rep. 2023;17(1):54–70.
181. Amani K, Shahbazi M, Behkar A, Farahmand G, Ghafouri S, Heydari S, et al. Anticoagulation in the management of septic cavernous sinus thrombosis secondary to rhino-orbito-cerebral mucormycosis: a retrospective real-world experience. Curr J Neurol. 2024;23(1):44–58.
182. Karakeçili F, Barkay O, Sümer B, Binay UD, Memiş KB, Yapıcıer Ö, et al. Invasive Aspergillosis with cavernous sinus thrombosis following high-dose corticosteroid therapy: a challenging case of rhino-orbital-cerebral mycosis. J Fungi (Basel). 2024;10(11)
183. Aksoy M, Ozcan AA, Ulas B. Prognostic factors and clinical features of rhino-orbital-mucormycosis cases: an update for patient and visual survivals. Int J Ophthalmol. 2024;17(5):916–23.
184. Chen F, Shao Y, Huang Q, Chen Y, Yang B, Jiang L. Visual function loss in fungal sphenoid sinusitis: clinical characteristics and outcomes. Sci Rep. 2024;14(1):8649.
185. Adulkar NG, Radhakrishnan S, Vidhya N, Kim U. Invasive sino-orbital fungal infections in immunocompetent patients: a clinico-pathological study. Eye (Lond). 2019;33(6):988–94.
186. Son HJ, Kim MJ, Lee S, Choi S, Jung KH, Jung J, et al. Risk factors and outcomes of patients with ocular involvement of candidemia. PLoS One. 2019;14(9):e0222356.
187. Farooq S, Khan NA, Singh A, Khan A, Sharma P, Meena R, et al. Orbital Mucormycosis: understanding the deadly fungus sweeping the globe. Cureus. 2023;15(6):e41010.
188. Shah K, Dave V, Bradoo R, Shinde C, Prathibha M. Orbital exenteration in rhino-orbito-cerebral Mucormycosis: a prospective analytical study with scoring system. Indian J Otolaryngol Head Neck Surg. 2019;71(2):259–65.
189. Gupta N, Dembla S. Cranial nerve involvement in mucormycosis in post-COVID patients: a case series. Egypt J Radiol Nucl Med. 2022;53(1):28.
190. Al Saad M, Rimawi A, Saadeh A, Shehadeh A. Mucormycosis with extensive cranial nerve involvement as the first presentation of diabetes mellitus: a case report. Qatar Med J. 2021;2021(3):61.
191. Mehdi Z, Bhardwaj N, Aggarwal J, Kaur N, Singh B. Facial nerve palsy with Total Ophthalmoplegia; a novel presentation of fungal invasion. Arch Acad Emerg Med. 2021;9(1):e54.
192. Galtrey CM, Schon F, Nitkunan A. Microvascular non-Arteritic ocular motor nerve palsies-what we know and how should we treat? Neuroophthalmology. 2015;39(1):1–11.
193. Lange N, Wantia N, Jörger AK, Wagner A, Liesche F, Meyer B, et al. Fungal brain infection-no longer a death sentence. Neurosurg Rev. 2021;44(4):2239–44.
194. Schwartz S, Kontoyiannis DP, Harrison T, Ruhnke M. Advances in the diagnosis and treatment of fungal infections of the CNS. Lancet Neurol. 2018;17(4):362–72.

12 Artificial Intelligence in the Diagnosis and Management of Ocular Fungal Infections

William Rojas-Carabali, Carlos Cifuentes-González, Alejandra de-la-Torre, and Rupesh Agrawal

12.1 Introduction

Ocular fungal infections encompass infections of the cornea (fungal keratitis) and intraocular structures (fungal endophthalmitis). *Fungal keratitis* is a corneal infection often caused by filamentous fungi (e.g., *Fusarium*, *Aspergillus*) following plant-matter trauma, or yeast-like fungi (e.g., *Candida*), especially in eyes with surface disease [1]. It typically presents with corneal ulceration and characteristic clinical features such as a gray-white stromal infiltrate with feathery borders, satellite

W. Rojas-Carabali (✉)
Colombian Visual Science and Translational Eye Research Institute (CERI), Centre of Excellence in Ocular Inflammation, Bogotá, Colombia

Programme for Ocular Inflammation & Infection Translational Research, Department of Ophthalmology, National Healthcare Group Eye Institute, Tan Tock Seng Hospital, Singapore, Singapore

C. Cifuentes-González
Programme for Ocular Inflammation & Infection Translational Research, Department of Ophthalmology, National Healthcare Group Eye Institute, Tan Tock Seng Hospital, Singapore, Singapore

Lee Kong Chian School of Medicine, Nanyang Technological University, Singapore, Singapore

Ocular Immunology Department, Ophthalmology Research Center, SIGMA Clinic, Cali, Colombia

A. de-la-Torre
Neuroscience (NEUROS) Research Group, Neurovitae Research Center, Institute of Translational Medicine (IMT). Escuela de Medicina y Ciencias de la Salud, Universidad del Rosario, Bogotá, Colombia

M. C. Ramírez-Soto (ed.), *Fungal Eye Infections*,
https://doi.org/10.1007/978-3-032-19923-2_12

lesions, and often an immune ring or hypopyon (pus in the anterior chamber) [2]. *Fungal endophthalmitis*, in contrast, is a severe infection of the internal structures or fluids of the eye (aqueous and vitreous) that can occur exogenously (after surgery or trauma introducing fungi into the eye) or endogenously via hematogenous spread (e.g., yeast from a bloodstream infection seeding the eye) [3, 4]. These infections are less common than bacterial ocular infections but are often more challenging to eradicate and more vision-threatening.

Fungal keratitis is a major cause of corneal blindness, particularly in tropical and developing regions. It is estimated that over one million eyes are affected by fungal keratitis each year worldwide—likely around 1.4 million—leading to devastating outcomes if not promptly treated [2]. In high-incidence areas (South Asia, Africa, etc.), fungal pathogens may account for up to half of microbial keratitis cases [2]. Outcomes are often poor: approximately 10% of eyes with fungal keratitis suffer corneal perforation or require surgical removal, and around 60% are left blind in the affected eye despite treatment in low-income countries [2]. Fungal endophthalmitis is rarer but carries an equally grave prognosis, often resulting in severe vision loss or loss of the eye if diagnosis and therapy are delayed [3]. The global incidence of fungal endophthalmitis is not well quantified, but it commonly arises in immunocompromised patients or as postoperative infections, with *Candida albicans* being the most frequent culprit [3].

This review aims to evaluate the current and emerging applications of artificial intelligence in the diagnosis and management of ocular fungal infections, with a focus on imaging-based deep learning methods and their clinical implications (Fig. 12.1).

R. Agrawal
Programme for Ocular Inflammation & Infection Translational Research, Department of Ophthalmology, National Healthcare Group Eye Institute, Tan Tock Seng Hospital, Singapore, Singapore

Lee Kong Chian School of Medicine, Nanyang Technological University, Singapore, Singapore

National Healthcare Group Eye Institute, Tan Tock Seng Hospital, Singapore, Singapore

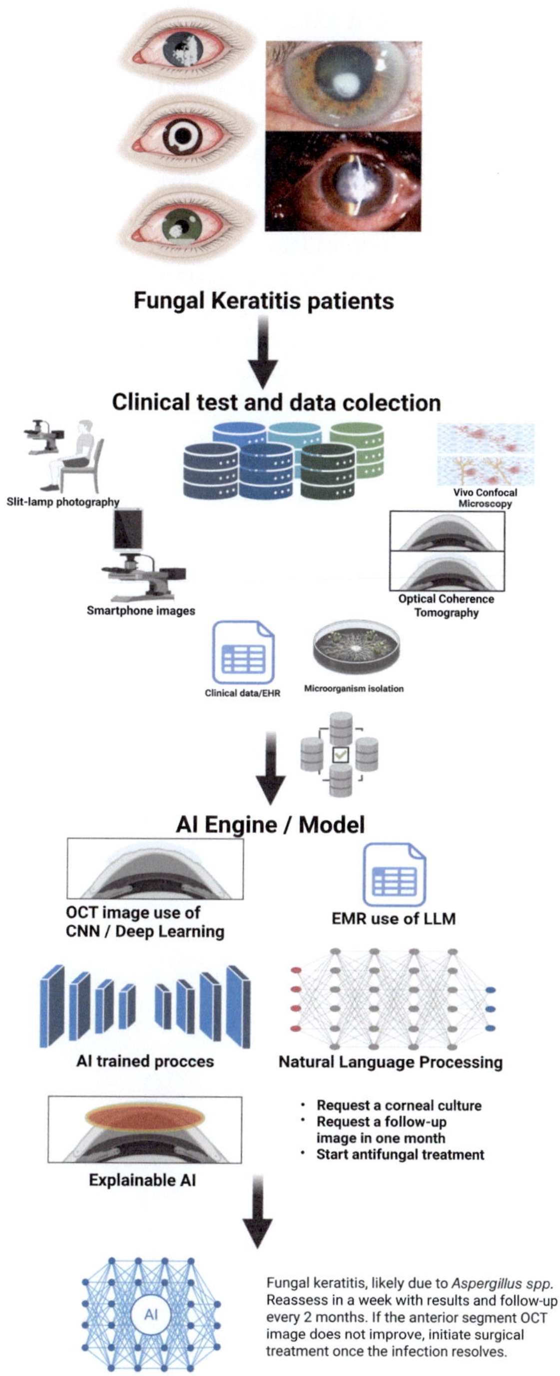

Fig. 12.1 Overall schematic diagram describing the practical application of AI in all common ophthalmic imaging modalities. Clinical data collection includes multimodal ophthalmic imaging—such as slit-lamp photography, smartphone images, in vivo confocal microscopy (IVCM), and anterior segment optical coherence tomography (OCT)—as well as laboratory data (microorganism isolation) and electronic medical records (EMR). These inputs are processed through a centralized AI engine comprising convolutional neural networks (CNN) for image analysis and large language models (LLM) for natural language processing of EMRs. AI outputs include diagnostic probabilities, explainable AI visualizations, and automated clinical decision support (e.g., treatment recommendation, follow-up scheduling). Finally, multimodal fusion enables the integration of imaging and textual data to improve diagnostic accuracy, identify antifungal resistance patterns, and support outcome prediction and individualized management plans

12.2 Current Challenges in Diagnosis and Management

Diagnosing ocular fungal infections accurately and rapidly remains challenging. Clinically, it is often difficult to distinguish fungal keratitis from other infections like bacterial keratitis based on the clinical examination alone—even expert cornea specialists misidentify the causative agent in a significant fraction of cases [3, 5]. Classic signs such as feathery-edged infiltrates or satellite lesions can suggest fungus, but there is considerable overlap with bacterial ulcers (Fig. 12.2) [2]. Definitive diagnosis requires laboratory tests (corneal scraping for microscopy and culture) or advanced imaging, which have limitations. Microscopy (e.g., KOH wet mount, Gram stain) and cultures are time-consuming (days to weeks for culture) and have relatively low sensitivity—many proven fungal cases are culture-negative due to prior treatment or difficult-to-grow organisms [5]. There is currently no point-of-care rapid diagnostic test for fungal keratitis, which is a major obstacle to early intervention [2]. In vivo confocal microscopy (IVCM) can visualize fungal filaments in the cornea and improve diagnostic yield, but it requires expensive equipment and specialized expertise [6, 7]. The net effect of these diagnostic challenges is that fungal infections are often diagnosed late or treated empirically as bacteria initially, contributing to worse outcomes.

Management of ocular fungal infections is also difficult. First-line therapy for fungal keratitis is topical antifungal medication (e.g., natamycin, voriconazole) [8, 9], but only a limited arsenal of antifungal eye drops exists, and many are not commercially available everywhere [10]. Fungal ulcers typically require longer treatment durations than bacterial ulcers, and even with appropriate therapy, they can progress, leading to corneal scarring or perforation [10]. If medical therapy fails or the cornea perforates, surgical intervention (such as therapeutic

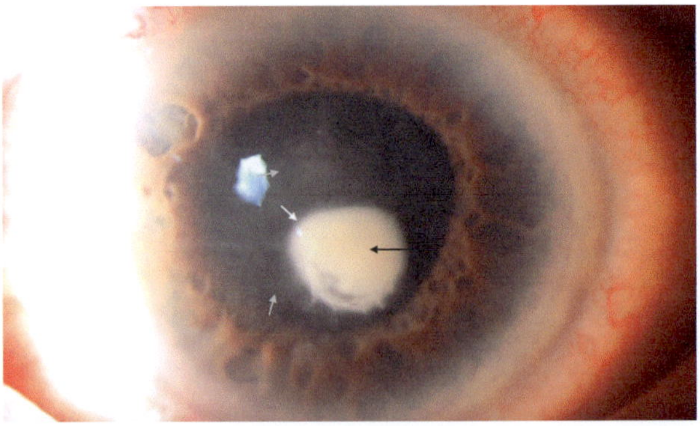

Fig. 12.2 Clinical features of fungal keratitis. Color slit-lamp image of a patient with fungal keratitis demonstrating a central dense stromal infiltrate with feathery margins (black arrow), satellite lesions (white arrows), and a small epithelial defect (gray arrow). These characteristic findings—particularly the branching borders and satellite lesions—are highly suggestive of filamentous fungal infection (e.g., *Fusarium* spp. or *Aspergillus* spp.). We acknowledge Dr. Carolina Mercado Acosta for providing the slit-lamp images used in this chapter

penetrating keratoplasty, i.e., corneal transplant) or even evisceration of the eye may be necessary [11]. In fungal endophthalmitis, treatment entails oral, intravitreal, and/or intravenous antifungal medications (e.g., fluconazole, amphotericin B, or voriconazole) and often vitrectomy surgery in addition to systemic antifungals [3, 12]. Despite aggressive treatment, outcomes are guarded, especially if the diagnosis is delayed. Thus, delays in diagnosis, limited therapeutic options, and the need for specialized care all pose significant challenges in managing these infections [2].

12.3 Overview of AI Technologies in Ophthalmology

Artificial intelligence (AI) has emerged as a promising tool to address gaps in healthcare, including ophthalmology. Machine learning (ML) refers to algorithms that learn patterns from data, encompassing a spectrum from traditional models (like support vector machines or random forests) to modern deep learning approaches [13]. In ophthalmology, deep learning—especially convolutional neural networks (CNNs)—has achieved remarkable image recognition performance, sometimes matching or exceeding experts in tasks such as detecting diabetic retinopathy in retinal photos and glaucoma in optic nerve images [14, 15]. These algorithms excel at analyzing complex imaging data: by training on large labeled datasets of medical images, CNNs can automatically extract features and classify diseases (for example, identifying hemorrhages and exudates in fundus photographs to detect diabetic retinopathy) [14]. AI systems like IDx-DR have even earned regulatory approval for autonomous retinal disease screening [16], underscoring the potential of AI in ophthalmic diagnosis.

Key AI technologies relevant to ophthalmology include: computer vision techniques (image processing algorithms to detect and classify features in images), deep neural networks for image classification and segmentation, and natural language processing (NLP) for analyzing textual data [17]. In the context of ocular infections, computer vision and deep learning are particularly pertinent, as diagnosis heavily relies on image-based findings (slit-lamp photos, microscopic images). For instance, AI models can be trained to distinguish subtle differences in lesion appearance that are not easily quantifiable by humans. Deep learning models are often criticized as "black boxes," but newer methods like explainable AI (XAI) attempt to highlight image regions driving the decision (e.g., heatmaps over an image to indicate detected fungal filaments) [18, 19]. NLP also has emerging roles—for example, algorithms have been developed to extract clinical descriptors of keratitis from electronic health records automatically [20]. Such AI-driven text mining can help gather epidemiological data or inform decision-support systems by integrating written clinical notes with image analysis [17]. Overall, AI technologies hold promise to improve diagnostic speed and consistency in ophthalmology, which is particularly relevant for time-sensitive conditions like ocular fungal infections.

12.4 AI Applications in Detecting Ocular Fungal Infections Using Imaging Modalities

12.4.1 AI for Ocular Imaging

Diagnosing fungal infections of the eye largely depends on recognizing patterns in clinical images—whether at the slit-lamp, under a microscope, or via ocular imaging devices. AI algorithms have been applied to a range of ophthalmic imaging modalities to assist in detecting fungal keratitis and endophthalmitis [21]. This section reviews how machine learning and deep learning models are being used with common modalities—slit-lamp photography, IVCM, and optical coherence tomography—as well as multimodal approaches. These AI applications aim to achieve faster and more accurate identification of fungal infections, aiding clinicians in situations where expertise or resources are limited (Fig. 12.1).

12.4.2 AI on Slit-Lamp Photography and External Eye Images

Slit-lamp photographs (or external eye images) of corneal ulcers are an accessible data source for AI. Several groups have trained deep learning models on clinical photographs to differentiate fungal keratitis from other causes of keratitis. Early work by Kuo et al. used a deep CNN (DenseNet architecture) on 288 clinical images of infectious keratitis (including fungal, bacterial, viral, and acanthamoeba cases) [22]. Their model achieved an average sensitivity of just above 70% for identifying fungal keratitis, with specificity slightly under 70% [22]. Notably, the AI's accuracy in that study was higher than that of general ophthalmologists but still lower than fellowship-trained cornea specialists—highlighting that while the AI could aid non-specialists, it did not yet surpass expert performance. Subsequent models have shown improving performance as larger image datasets became available. Koyama et al. trained a ResNet-50 CNN on over 4000 slit-lamp images to classify keratitis causes and reported an accuracy of about 83% in distinguishing fungal keratitis in their test set [22, 23]. Similarly, Ghosh et al. developed a deep learning model termed "DeepKeratitis" on a sizable image dataset; it achieved an area under the ROC curve (AUC) of ~0.90 for differentiating fungal versus bacterial ulcers [24], corresponding to substantial improvement over chance and approaching expert-level discrimination (Fig. 12.3).

Real-world deployment of these models is a key consideration. Some studies have tested AI using not only high-quality slit-lamp camera images but also photos taken with smartphones, which could enable telemedicine applications. Wang et al. (2021) evaluated a deep learning model on a set of keratitis images captured both via slit-lamp and smartphone cameras and found the AI could feasibly detect infectious keratitis features even in smartphone photos [25]. In that study, the system correctly identified the presence of infection in a majority of cases (with an estimated accuracy of around 77% for classifying fungal vs. bacterial) [25]. Another recent approach by Ueno et al. [26] in Japan involved a comprehensive deep

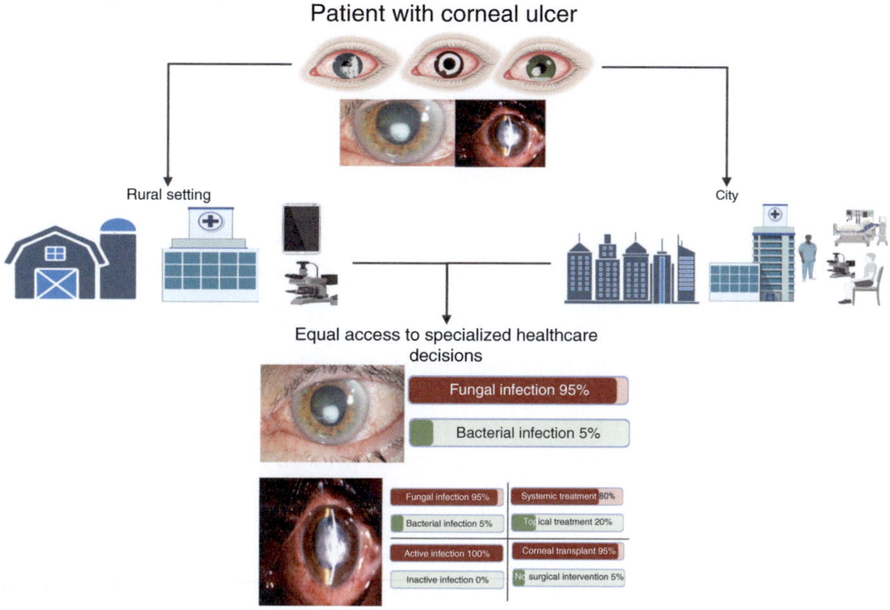

Fig. 12.3 AI-assisted decision support ensures equitable access to specialized care for patients with corneal ulcers. Patients presenting with corneal ulcers in either rural or urban settings undergo imaging (e.g., slit-lamp or smartphone photography), and the AI engine analyzes these inputs to deliver standardized diagnostic probabilities (e.g., 95% fungal, 5% bacterial infection). This system also supports individualized treatment recommendations, including the need for systemic or topical antifungal therapy, assessment of infection activity, and surgical intervention. Such AI-assisted tools democratize access to specialized care and help reduce disparities in outcomes for patients in remote or underserved areas

learning model for smartphone-based diagnosis of multiple corneal diseases, including infectious keratitis [26]. Such mobile AI solutions are particularly relevant for remote or resource-limited settings where an ophthalmologist may not be immediately available. Figure 12.2 shows a classic fungal ulcer; AI algorithms trained on thousands of such images can learn to recognize the telltale features (feathery infiltrates, etc.) and instantly flag an ulcer as "suspicious for fungus." In practice, this could guide clinicians to start antifungal therapy sooner rather than waiting days for lab results.

For example, researchers in India and the US collaborated on a multimodal AI system for keratitis diagnosis. They prospectively collected 599 patients' ulcer images in South India and compared three models: one using only clinical data, one using only the ulcer photograph (EfficientNet CNN), and one combining both [5]. The combined model outperformed the others, underscoring that while image-based AI is powerful, incorporating clinical context (e.g., lesion size, onset, prior therapy) can further boost accuracy. Indeed, clinical impression alone is unreliable in differentiating fungal versus bacterial keratitis [5], so an AI that integrates the image with clinical features or even lab results may provide the most robust decision support. The multimodal model in that study achieved a higher diagnostic accuracy than either the image or clinical model alone, demonstrating the synergistic value of combining data sources. Table 12.1 summarizes key AI studies that have applied deep learning to slit-lamp and external images for detecting fungal keratitis, showing the evolution from early models to more advanced, multi-input systems.

Mayya et al. proposed a novel two-stage DL framework for the early detection of fungal keratitis (FK) using slit-lamp images. Their method introduced a multi-scale convolutional neural network (MS-CNN) for precise segmentation of the corneal region, followed by a ResNeXt-based classifier to distinguish between fungal and nonfungal keratitis. Unlike previous studies that either required manual segmentation or operated on full-frame images, this approach automatically localized the region of interest (RoI), improving model focus and explainability. The segmentation model achieved a Dice coefficient of 96.42%, outperforming state-of-the-art methods like SLIT-Net and U^2-Net, while using significantly fewer parameters [27]. By isolating the corneal region prior to classification, the system enhanced diagnostic accuracy (88.96%) and offered visual explanations via Grad-CAM, reinforcing its clinical interpretability. The inclusion of attention mechanisms within the segmentation pipeline further ensured that key morphological features—often subtle and clinically relevant—were preserved. Importantly, their dataset incorporated publicly available, microbiologically confirmed images, enabling better generalizability [27].

Recent evidence from a comprehensive systematic review and meta-analysis by Ong et al. [28] reinforces the potential of DL in the diagnosis of infectious keratitis, including fungal keratitis. The review, encompassing 35 studies with over 136,000 corneal images, demonstrated that DL models achieved pooled sensitivity and specificity of 86.2% and 96.3%, respectively, in external validation, and 91.6% and 90.7%, respectively, in internal validation. Notably, DL performance was found to be comparable to that of ophthalmologists, highlighting its potential as a diagnostic adjunct, especially in settings with limited access to expert care [28].

However, several limitations in current research hinder widespread clinical deployment. Many studies included in the review exhibited a high risk of bias in the index test domain, primarily due to a lack of threshold prespecification and limited external validation. Furthermore, image-based analyses often failed to account for intrapatient correlation, potentially inflating diagnostic performance estimates. The authors advocate for future work to emphasize diverse, representative datasets, transparency in model development, and standardized evaluation metrics to enhance the reliability and generalizability of AI tools for IK diagnosis [28].

12.4.3 AI on In Vivo Confocal Microscopy Images

In vivo confocal microscopy is a specialized imaging technique that produces high-resolution, microscopic images of the living cornea. It can directly visualize fungal filaments in corneal tissue, essentially serving as a "virtual biopsy." Given its ability to reveal pathogen structures, IVCM has been a prime candidate for AI analysis

Table 12.1 Selected AI studies using slit-lamp or external photographs for diagnosing fungal keratitis

Study (year) [Ref]	Design	Data size	AI type	Task	Key findings
Kuo et al. (2020)[22]	Development and evaluation of a DL model	288 slit-lamp images	Deep CNN (DenseNet)	Multiclass mix of fungal, bacterial, and viral keratitis	Model sensitivity ~71%, specificity ~68% for fungal keratitis. Overall accuracy ~69%. Performed better than nonspecialist doctors but below cornea specialists.
Koyama et al. (2021) [23]	Development of a hybrid DL algorithm	4306 images	ResNet-50 CNN	Multiclass keratitis: fungal, bacterial, viral, acanthamoeba	Achieved ~83% accuracy in classifying FK in the test set. Demonstrated that deep learning can handle multiclass differentiation with reasonable accuracy.
Ghosh et al. (2022) [24]	Apply DL algorithms	2167 cornea images	Custom CNN ("DeepKeratitis"), VGG19, ResNet50, DenseNet121	Classification fungal vs. bacterial	AUC 0.90 + for distinguishing fungal vs. bacterial ulcers. Sensitivity and specificity were around 77% and 81%, respectively, indicating solid performance in a clinical dataset.
Wang et al. (2021) [25]	Apply DL algorithms	5673 slit-lamp photographs and 400 smartphone photographs	CNN, InceptionV3, ResNet50, DenseNet121	Classification of IK	Feasibility of smartphone imaging: model maintained accuracy ~77% on smartphone photos. Highlighted potential for tele-diagnosis with mobile devices.

(continued)

Table 12.1 (continued)

Study (year) [Ref]	Design	Data size	AI type	Task	Key findings
Wei et al. (2023) [7]	Development of a diagnostic model	Multicenter dataset (1916 images)	Ensemble ML with logistic regression and CNN	Detection of FK	High performance: ~90% accuracy for fungal keratitis detection, significantly outperforming earlier models (which had ~65–77% accuracy). Validated on external data with strong results (AUC > 0.90).
Prajna et al. (2024) [5]	Prospective study	599 patients	(EfficientNet) vs. combined	Compared the clinical data model vs. the image	Combined model (image + clinical features) was superior, illustrating that incorporating clinical context improves diagnostic accuracy. AI addressed cases where clinical impression was unreliable.
Ong et al. (2024) [28]	Systematic review and meta-analysis of 35 diagnostic accuracy studies	35 studies using 136,401 corneal images from over 56,011 patients	DL, predominantly CNNs	Diagnose IK from corneal images; subtasks include: Identifying IK presence Differentiating IK from healthy/non-IK eyes Identifying specific IK causes (bacterial, fungal, viral, Acanthamoeba)	DL showed good diagnostic accuracy: internal validation: 91.6% sensitivity, 90.7% specificity external validation: 86.2% sensitivity, 96.3% specificity DL and ophthalmologists had comparable accuracy IVCM-based DL models performed better than ASP-based models in cause differentiation Most studies had low bias, except for index test thresholding issues

Soleimani et al. (2023) [29]	Diagnostic development and evaluation study	9329 images from 977 patients (2505 healthy, 2008 FK, 4816 BK); subtypes: 1643 *Aspergillus/Fusarium* and 357 *Candida* images	DL using custom-designed CNNs, developed from scratch (not pretrained models)	Three-tier classification: **Model 1**—Differentiate healthy vs. keratitis **Model 2**—Differentiate FK vs. BK **Model 3**—Discriminate filamentous vs. yeast fungi	**Model 1:** 99.3% accuracy, 0.999 AUC **Model 2:** 84% accuracy, 0.96 AUC **Model 3:** 77.5% accuracy, 0.99 AUC CNNs outperformed or matched prior methods; first study to accurately subtype fungal keratitis
Hung et al. (2021) [30]	Model development and validation study	2685 images (from 1295 patients); 1175 BK, 918 FK, 592 healthy controls	Deep learning—multiple CNN architectures evaluated (e.g., InceptionV3, DenseNet121, ResNet50), with and without U^2-net segmentation preprocessing	Binary classification: FK vs. BK, with pre- and postsegmentation comparison	Without segmentation: best AUC = 0.853, accuracy ~70% With U^2-Net segmentation preprocessing: improved AUC to 0.887 and accuracy to ~80% Segmentation improved performance
Soleimani et al. (2025) [31]	Comparative study evaluating six DL models	13,557 slit-lamp images (training: 10,821; testing: 2,736) from 1,485 patients covering BK, FK, and healthy corneas	Deep learning—Four pretrained CNNs (ResNet50, MobileNetV2, EfficientNetB3, DenseNet121) and two custom CNN architectures (CNN1 and CNN2)	Multiclass classification of slit-lamp images into three categories: Healthy, BK, and FK	All models achieved high accuracy; CNN1 (custom) performed best with 94.5% accuracy, 0.987 AUC Pretrained models were close in performance Demonstrated potential for clinical deployment

(continued)

Table 12.1 (continued)

Study (year) [Ref]	Design	Data size	AI type	Task	Key findings
Li et al. (2024) [32]	Development and external validation of a DLS	23,055 slit-lamp images collected from 12 clinical centers nationwide in China	DenseNet121, InceptionResNetV2, Swin-Transformer, and DeepIK, a customized algorithm.	Multiclass classification: distinguishing BK, FK, AK, VK, and non-IK (healthy or other diseases)	External test AUCs: BK (0.88), FK (0.93), VK (0.90), AK (0.92), non-IK (0.899) Prospective validation AUCs: BK (0.92), FK (0.97), VK (0.89), AK (0.99), non-IK (0.87) Outperformed noncorneal specialists

Abbreviations: *AK,* amebic keratitis; *AUC,* area under the curve; *DL,* deep learning; *DLS,* deep learning system; *BK,* bacterial keratitis; *IK,* infectious keratitis; *FK,* fungal keratitis; *VK,* viral keratitis

[33]. Deep learning models have been developed to scan confocal images for the presence of fungal hyphae, aiming to assist or automate the diagnostic interpretation of these images [6]. One study by Lv et al. trained a CNN (ResNet) on confocal images to detect fungal keratitis; in an evaluation on 535 test images, the model correctly identified fungal presence in 515 of them (96.3% accuracy) [34]. This high performance suggests AI can effectively distinguish confocal images with fungal elements from those without. Other groups have reported similar results: Xu et al. (2021) developed an explainable deep learning system with an AUC of 0.983 and ~ 96% accuracy in classifying confocal images as fungal keratitis versus normal [18]. Impressively, their model's sensitivity (~93.6%) and specificity (~98.2%) were very high, and the addition of explanatory heatmaps (highlighting image regions corresponding to hyphae) improved less experienced clinicians' diagnostic accuracy when they used the tool (Fig. 12.3) [18].

Beyond simply detecting the presence of fungus, AI has also been used to identify fungal subtypes via confocal images. Tang et al. trained a model to classify pathogenic fungal genera on IVCM images [35]. Their algorithm could differentiate Fusarium versus Aspergillus hyphae with around 82% and 76% accuracy, respectively [6, 35]. This is a significant development because the optimal treatment can depend on the fungal species (for example, *Fusarium* is typically more responsive to natamycin). Another study by Essalat et al. included multiple classes (fungal vs. Acanthamoeba vs. other keratitis vs. normal cornea) using confocal images. It reported a sensitivity of ~97% and specificity of ~96% for identifying fungal keratitis [36], which is an outstanding diagnostic performance. These results underline that confocal imaging combined with AI can provide a rapid and highly reliable diagnosis, in many cases approaching the accuracy of culture or PCR without the time lag. Table 12.12.2 highlights several key studies of AI applied to confocal microscopy in fungal keratitis, showing consistently high accuracies. Confocal images of fungal keratitis typically show bright, branching filaments against the dark background of corneal stroma—AI models have learned to recognize these filamentous patterns, even when they are subtle or obscured by noise, with much greater speed than a human observer scanning hundreds of frames.

12.4.4 AI and Other Modalities (OCT, Ultrasound) and Multimodal Approaches

Other ophthalmic imaging techniques have comparatively smaller roles in fungal infection, but AI may still find its applications. Optical Coherence Tomography (OCT) of the anterior segment can visualize the cornea in cross section and measure lesion depth or thickness. Although OCT is not a primary diagnostic tool for keratitis etiology, researchers have considered using it to assess infection severity and monitor treatment response. In principle, a machine learning model could analyze corneal OCT scans to identify features suggestive of fungal versus nonfungal ulcers (such as deeper stromal involvement or hyper-reflective lines corresponding to hyphae). There is emerging work using OCT for corneal diseases—for instance,

Table 12.2 Selected AI studies using in vivo confocal microscopy (IVCM) for diagnosing fungal keratitis

Study (year) [Ref]	Design	Data size	AI type	Task	Key findings
Lv et al. (2020) [34]	Development of a DL algorithm	Confocal images from fungal keratitis patients (688 positive frames vs. 1400 negative)	Deep CNN (ResNet)	Detection of FK	~96% accuracy in identifying images with fungal hyphae. Only 20 of 535 test images were misclassified. Demonstrated automated confocal diagnosis is highly feasible.
Xu et al. (2021) [18]	Development of an XAI-based system	1089 IVCM images from a single center	Explainable AI with Grad-CAM heatmaps.	Detection of FK	Model AUC 0.983, accuracy 96.5% (sensitivity 93.6%, specificity 98.2%) for fungus detection. AI assistance significantly improved nonexperts' reading of confocal images without loss of speed .
Wu et al. (2021) [37]	Algorithm improvement	183 normal images and 195 abnormal images	Adaptive robust binary pattern	To classify normal cornea images with nerves and abnormal cornea images with hyphae, and to detect the hyphae	Near-perfect performance was reported (accuracy ~99.95%) using augmented data and image fusion. (indicates potential of AI, though such extreme accuracy may reflect limited test conditions).
Tang et al. (2023) [35]	Apply DL methods	3364 confocal images focusing on fungal genus identification (e.g., *Fusarium* vs. *Aspergillus*).	Machine learning, inception-ResNet V2, and a decision tree (DT) classifier	To identify pathogenic fungal genera	Achieved genus-level classification: ~82% accuracy for *Fusarium*, 76% for *Aspergillus*. It suggests that AI can provide organism-specific clues to guide therapy.

(continued)

Table 12.2 (continued)

Study (year) [Ref]	Design	Data size	AI type	Task	Key findings
Essalat et al. (2023) [36]	Development of multiple DL models	4001 confocal images of various keratitis (fungal, Acanthamoeba, other, normal)	Multiclass CNNs. Densenet161, Densenet121, Resnet152, Resnet101, Resnext101, Resnext50, Cspresnet50, Vgg19, Vgg16, and Vgg13	Classification of FK, acanthamoeba keratitis (AK), nonspecific keratitis (NSK), and healthy images	For fungal vs. others: sensitivity ~97%, specificity ~96%. High accuracy across multiple pathogens, with authors releasing a public confocal image dataset for further AI research.
Liang et al. (2023) [38]	Diagnostic model development and evaluation	7278 IVCM images from Zhongshan Ophthalmic Center (3862 with fungal hyphae, 3416 without)	DL—Structure-aware CNN (SACNN), combining GoogLeNet (main stream) and VGGNet (auxiliary stream for prior knowledge of hyphae structure)	Binary classification: presence vs. absence of fungal keratitis (based on hyphae detection in IVCM images)	Accuracy: 97.73%, sensitivity: 97.02%, specificity: 98.54%, F1-score: 97.84%, ROC-AUC: 0.993 Ablation study confirmed the benefit of integrating structural prior knowledge Outperformed previous methods like AlexNet+HMF and GoogLeNet+HMF

Abbreviations: *AI,* artificial intelligence; *DL,* deep learning; *CNN,* convolutional neural network; *IVCM,* in vivo confocal microscopy; *XIA,* explainable artificial intelligence

deep learning has been used to distinguish active infections from corneal scars on OCT or slit-lamp images [39]. In one study, a CNN: VGG16 could differentiate active keratitis versus healed scar with high accuracy (reporting over 90% accuracy in a test set) [39]. This sort of application could prevent the misdiagnosis of a quiescent scar as an active infection. For endophthalmitis, clinical imaging often involves an ultrasound B-scan (when the view to the retina is obscured by vitritis). In the future, AI image analysis might assist in detecting intraocular exudates or retinal lesions on ultrasound or fundus photos to raise suspicion for fungal endophthalmitis, though specific studies in this area are not yet prominent (Fig. 12.3).

Combining multiple data sources (multimodal AI) for decision support is an important trend. We saw an example of combining clinical data and photos. Some models integrate laboratory inputs as well—for instance, an AI could take as input the corneal image along with preliminary smear results or demographic risk factors. A multicenter study by Wei et al. (2023) developed a machine learning model for the early detection of fungal keratitis that incorporated images from different hospitals and potential laboratory parameters; it achieved a superior sensitivity (~90%) compared to earlier single-center models, which ranged around 65–77% [7]. By learning from a diverse dataset, such models become more generalizable. As another example, a natural language processing algorithm was devised to extract clinical morphological features of microbial keratitis (i.e., "feathery margin" or "satellite lesion") from clinical notes [20]. One can imagine a system that reads the clinic note and patient history, analyzes any available images, and then outputs a probability of fungal infection. This kind of holistic AI approach could function as an early warning system or a "second pair of eyes" for clinicians, ensuring subtle clues are not overlooked. While most current AI efforts focus on either image analysis or text analysis separately, future systems will likely merge these to mimic the comprehensive decision-making a seasoned clinician would perform.

While artificial intelligence has gained traction in fungal keratitis, its application is extending into other sight-threatening intraocular infections such as endophthalmitis and choroiditis. Demir et al. [40] evaluated the reliability of large language models (LLMs)—including ChatGPT-4.0 and a domain-specific tool, A-Eye Consult—in answering patient questions about endophthalmitis. The study found that A-Eye Consult provided the most accurate and detailed responses, scoring highest on both the DISCERN reliability scale and Likert accuracy ratings. These findings suggest that well-designed AI chatbots can serve as effective tools for patient education and potentially aid in early recognition of endophthalmitis symptoms, which is critical given the disease's rapid progression and high risk of vision loss.

Building on diagnostic support, Shaeri et al. [41] developed a smartphone-based clinical decision support system (CDSS) tailored for acute postoperative endophthalmitis. Using supervised machine learning models—such as Random Forest, SVM, and KNN—the application achieved 100% accuracy, sensitivity, and specificity in classifying cases. This user-centered tool not only assists physicians with early diagnosis and treatment but also empowers patients with symptom tracking and education. Meanwhile, Nezu et al. [42] demonstrated the value of AI in segmenting choroidal lesions using swept-source OCT in infectious choroiditis, marking a pivotal step toward AI-assisted disease monitoring and quantification in posterior segment infections.

12.5 AI in Therapeutic Decision-Making and Prognostication

Beyond diagnostics, AI can assist in treatment decisions and outcome prediction for ocular fungal infections. Once a fungal infection is identified, clinicians must decide on the optimal therapy (choice of antifungal agent, need for surgical intervention) and counsel patients on prognosis. AI models are being explored to aid these aspects. For instance, an algorithm could analyze initial presentation factors—ulcer size and depth (from images or OCT), organism type (from AI interpretation of confocal or culture data), and patient risk factors—to predict the risk of corneal perforation or the likelihood that medical therapy alone will succeed. In fungal keratitis, studies have shown that large, deep ulcers or certain fungal species (e.g., *Fusarium*) correlate with worse outcomes [2, 43]. A machine learning model trained on prior cases could quantitatively combine such factors to provide a prognostic risk score. This can help identify high-risk patients early; for example, an AI might flag that "this ulcer has an X% chance of requiring a transplant," prompting closer monitoring or earlier surgical referral (Fig. 12.3).

AI might also guide therapeutic decision-making by suggesting the most effective treatment. If an AI model can discern the likely fungal species (as demonstrated by Tang et al. for *Fusarium* vs. *Aspergillus*) [35], it could inform drug selection—natamycin is first-line for filamentous fungi like *Fusarium*, whereas voriconazole may be added or preferred for *Aspergillus* or yeasts. In the future, decision support systems could integrate diagnostic AI outputs with treatment protocols. For example, an AI system might automatically recommend topical natamycin and oral voriconazole if a filamentous fungal infection is detected in a deep ulcer in a patient from a region where *Fusarium* is common. Additionally, AI could aid in monitoring response to therapy. Image analysis algorithms can quantify changes in ulcer size or density over time from serial photos, providing objective measures of improvement or deterioration. This can complement the clinician's assessment in deciding whether to continue medical therapy or proceed to surgical management.

There is also interest in using AI for predicting visual outcomes. By learning from large cohorts, an AI model could estimate the likely final visual acuity given certain inputs (initial vision, organism, treatment delays). While currently such predictions are based on population statistics, AI could personalize them by recognizing patterns across multiple features. For example, a model might predict that a patient presenting 3 weeks after symptom onset, with a central 8 mm Fusarium ulcer and hypopyon, has a poor prognosis for recovering vision better than 20/200—alerting physicians and patients to brace for aggressive therapy and realistic expectations. Though these applications are still in the early stages, they represent a natural extension of diagnostic AI into the realm of treatment planning and prognostication.

12.6 Limitations, Ethical Considerations, and Implementation Challenges

Despite the promise of AI in ocular fungal infections, there are several limitations and ethical issues to address before such tools are widely implemented in clinical practice. Data quality and generalizability are primary concerns. Many AI models are trained on data from specific hospitals or regions; for example, a model developed on cases in South Asia might not perform as well on cases in Africa or Europe if fungal species and patient demographics differ. Ensuring diversity in training data is crucial so that the AI does not become overfit to a narrow population [14]. Likewise, image quality varies—photos taken with different cameras or under different lighting may affect AI performance. A model must be robust to such variability, and studies have shown that factors like image focus and illumination can impact algorithm accuracy [5, 44].

Another limitation is the "black box" nature of many deep learning models. Clinicians may be uncomfortable trusting an AI's output if they cannot understand the reasoning. This lack of transparency is an ethical and practical issue [45, 46]. Efforts like explainable AI (Grad-CAM heatmaps, etc.) are being used to provide visual explanation (e.g., highlighting the fungal filaments the model sees), which can increase clinician trust. Regulatory approval is also a hurdle—AI tools must be rigorously validated in clinical trials to ensure safety and efficacy [47]. There is a risk of algorithmic bias: if an AI is trained mostly on severe cases, it might overdiagnose fungus in mild cases (false positives), or vice versa. Continuous monitoring and periodic retraining with new data are needed to maintain calibration.

From an ethical perspective, important considerations include responsibility and liability. If an AI system misses a fungal infection or misclassifies a benign ulcer as fungal, leading to unnecessary treatment, who is accountable—the clinician or the AI developer? [45, 48] Clear guidelines are required for how clinicians should use (and not over-rely on) AI outputs. Many recommend that AI be an assistive tool, with final decisions made by physicians who consider the AI's suggestion in context. Patient privacy is another issue: AI development requires large datasets, so protecting patient data in images and records (via de-identification and secure data handling) is paramount. When deploying AI via cloud platforms or mobile apps, robust encryption and adherence to health data regulations are necessary to maintain confidentiality.

Practical implementation challenges also exist. Integrating AI into the clinical workflow means the system must provide results fast (ideally in real-time during an exam) and in an easily interpretable format. If an AI is too slow or gives cumbersome output, busy clinicians will not use it. There may be resource constraints in low-income areas—ironically, the same places that could benefit most from AI, due to a lack of specialists, might lack the hardware (good cameras, internet connectivity, computing power) to run advanced AI systems. Lightweight AI models deployable on smartphones offline are one solution to this. Training and acceptance: Clinicians need to be educated on the capabilities and limits of AI. Some clinicians may mistrust AI or fear it encroaching on their role; demonstrating that AI can reduce workload (e.g., quickly screening out nonfungal cases) and improve patient outcomes will be key to adoption. Finally, continuous evaluation is required after deployment—collecting feedback on AI errors and near-misses can help improve the system in a virtuous cycle.

12.7 Future Directions and Impact on Global Eye Health

The future of AI in ocular fungal infections is bright, with the potential to significantly improve global eye health if current hurdles are overcome. One central direction is the development of AI-assisted diagnostic platforms for remote and underserved areas. A smartphone-based AI tool could be revolutionary in rural clinics or developing countries, where specialist ophthalmologists and microbiology labs are scarce. A community health worker could take a corneal photograph of a patient with an ulcer and have an AI algorithm instantly classify it as likely fungal or not, guiding whether antifungal treatment should be started or if urgent referral is needed. This could reduce diagnostic delays dramatically. Given the heavy burden of fungal blindness in tropical regions [2, 49], such point-of-care AI diagnostics could help preserve sight for thousands of patients by enabling timely therapy. Global health organizations are interested in telementoring and diagnostic support networks—AI can function as a virtual "consultant" in places where human consultants are unavailable (Fig. 12.4).

In tertiary centers, the future may bring integrated AI diagnostics in ophthalmology EMR systems. For example, when an ulcer patient is seen, their information (images, exam findings, etc.) could automatically run through an AI, which provides a report: "80% probability fungal keratitis; predicted organism *Fusarium*; recommended actions: order natamycin drops, consider corneal scrape for culture." This report would accompany the clinician, who can then validate and act on it. Such systems would effectively raise the floor of care—helping less experienced doctors make sound decisions similar to an expert. Over time, as these systems accumulate more data (including outcomes), they might continuously learn to improve treatment recommendations and prognostic estimates.

Another future direction is the expansion of AI to new data modalities for fungal infections. Genomic and proteomic assays for pathogens are becoming faster; AI could potentially integrate genetic sequencing data of isolated organisms with clinical data to predict virulence or resistance patterns, customizing therapy. Furthermore, AI might assist in drug development. By analyzing large datasets of antifungal drug effects and fungal characteristics, machine learning could help identify patterns that lead to new therapeutic targets or optimize antifungal dosing regimens for better efficacy (Fig. 12.4).

On the technical side, future AI models will likely use multitask learning—a single unified model that can perform detection, classification, and outcome prediction simultaneously. For instance, one deep network might take an input image and output both a diagnosis (fungal vs. bacterial) and a risk assessment (chance of corneal perforation). This comprehensive approach can streamline workflows. Additionally, continual learning will be necessary: AI systems that update themselves as new cases are encountered (with appropriate oversight) to avoid obsolescence when pathogens evolve, or practice patterns change.

Ethically, the future will aim for transparent and human-compatible AI. Efforts will continue to make AI decisions more explainable so clinicians can trust and verify them. International guidelines and possibly regulatory frameworks will define standards for AI in ophthalmology (accuracy thresholds, required bias testing across populations, etc.). If these are implemented, clinicians and patients can be assured that an AI tool has been vetted much like a new diagnostic device or drug.

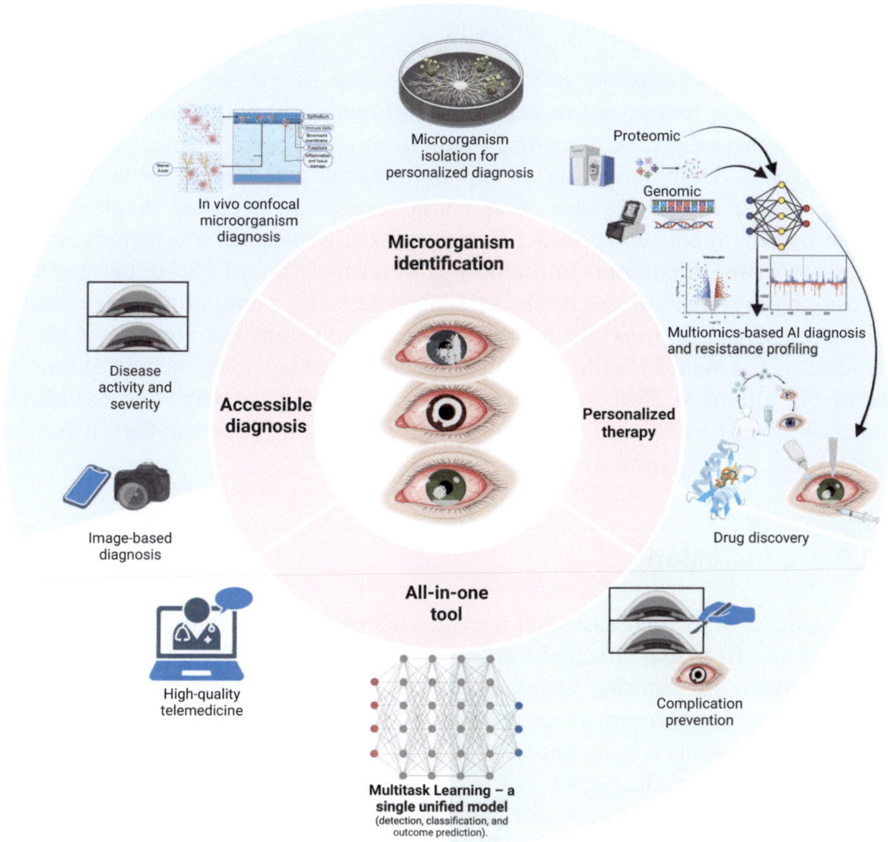

Fig. 12.4 Integrated artificial intelligence (AI) framework for accessible diagnosis, microorganism identification, and personalized therapy in fungal keratitis. The system combines image-based diagnostics (e.g., slit-lamp and smartphone photography, OCT) with in vivo confocal microscopy and telemedicine to enable accessible and equitable diagnosis. It incorporates microorganism isolation and multiomics profiling (genomics and proteomics) to support precise pathogen identification and resistance prediction. AI algorithms trained via multitask learning integrate clinical, imaging, and omics data for detection, classification, and outcome prediction. The tool enables therapeutic decision-making, drug discovery, and complication prevention, functioning as an all-in-one model to support precision care regardless of the healthcare setting

12.8 Global Impact

Ultimately, the widespread use of AI for ocular fungal infection could help reduce blindness and visual impairment worldwide. By overcoming the barrier of limited specialists, AI can bring expert-level diagnostic capability to any location. This democratization of expertise means a farmer in a low-resource setting with a fungal corneal ulcer could receive an accurate diagnosis and proper treatment plan early, rather than progressing to irreversible blindness due to late or wrong treatment. In public health terms, AI could be integrated into screening programs—for example, screening high-risk populations (agricultural workers with eye injuries) for early fungal infection signs via community health images. As the World Health Organization and other agencies push to eliminate avoidable blindness [50], such technology could be pivotal for corneal blindness, which has traditionally lagged behind other fields (like cataract or refractive error) in global initiatives (Fig. 12.4).

12.9 Conclusion

The use of AI in the diagnosis and management of ocular fungal infections is rapidly evolving from experimental studies to clinically applicable tools. While challenges remain in ensuring accuracy, ethics, and acceptance, the evidence so far—from high-performing image classifiers to improved clinical decisions with AI assistance—suggests a transformative potential. By augmenting ophthalmologists' capabilities and extending reach to where care is needed most, AI has the potential to markedly improve outcomes for patients with devastating fungal eye infections and, more broadly, to strengthen health systems' capacity to combat blindness on a global scale.

References

1. Centers for Disease Control and Prevention (2024) Fungal eye infections basics. Fungal Diseases.
2. Brown L, Leck AK, Gichangi M, Burton MJ, Denning DW. The global incidence and diagnosis of fungal keratitis. Lancet Infect Dis. 2021;21:e49–57.
3. Haseeb AA, Elhusseiny AM, Siddiqui MZ, Ahmad KT, Sallam AB. Fungal endophthalmitis: a comprehensive review. J Fungi (Basel). 2021;7:996.
4. Mishra C, Lalitha P, Rameshkumar G, Agrawal R, Balne PK, Iswarya M, Kannan NB, Ramasamy K. Incidence of endophthalmitis after intravitreal injections: risk factors, microbiology profile, and clinical outcomes. Ocul Immunol Inflamm. 2018;26:559–68.
5. Prajna NV, Assaf J, Acharya NR, Rose-Nussbaumer J, Lietman TM, Campbell JP, Keenan JD, Song X, Redd TK. Multimodal deep learning for differentiating bacterial and fungal keratitis using prospective representative data. Ophthalmol Sci. 2025;5:100665.
6. Soleimani M, Cheraqpour K, Sadeghi R, Pezeshgi S, Koganti R, Djalilian AR. Artificial intelligence and infectious keratitis: where are we now? Life. 2023;13:2117.

7. Wei Z, Wang S, Wang Z, et al. Development and multi-center validation of machine learning model for early detection of fungal keratitis. EBioMedicine. 2023;88:104438.
8. Qiu S, Zhao G-Q, Lin J, Wang X, Hu L-T, Du Z-D, Wang Q, Zhu C-C. Natamycin in the treatment of fungal keratitis: a systematic review and meta-analysis. Int J Ophthalmol. 2015;8:597–602.
9. McDonald EM, Ram FSF, Patel DV, McGhee CNJ. Effectiveness of topical antifungal drugs in the management of fungal keratitis: a systematic review and meta-analysis of randomized controlled trials. Asia-Pac J Ophthalmol. 2014;3:41–7.
10. Awad R, Ghaith AA, Awad K, Mamdouh Saad M, Elmassry AA. Fungal keratitis: diagnosis, management, and recent advances. Clin Ophthalmol. 2024;18:85–106.
11. Garg P, Roy A, Kalra P. Surgical management of fungal keratitis. Expert Rev Ophthalmol. 2018;13:351–9.
12. Xie CA, Singh J, Tyagi M, Androudi S, Dave VP, Arora A, Gupta V, Agrawal R, Mi H, Sen A. Endogenous endophthalmitis – a major review. Ocul Immunol Inflamm. 2023;31:1362–85.
13. Alzubi J, Nayyar A, Kumar A. Machine learning from theory to algorithms: an overview. J Phys Conf Ser. 2018;1142:012012.
14. Hashemian H, Peto T, Ambrósio R, Lengyel I, Kafieh R, Muhammed Noori A, Khorrami-Nejad M. Application of artificial intelligence in ophthalmology: an updated comprehensive review. J Ophthalmic Vis Res. 2024;19:354–67.
15. Li Z, Wang L, Wu X, Jiang J, Qiang W, Xie H, Zhou H, Wu S, Shao Y, Chen W. Artificial intelligence in ophthalmology: the path to the real-world clinic. Cell Rep Med. 2023;4:101095.
16. Abràmoff MD, Lavin PT, Birch M, Shah N, Folk JC. Pivotal trial of an autonomous AI-based diagnostic system for detection of diabetic retinopathy in primary care offices. npj Digital Med. 2018;1:39.
17. Rojas-Carabali W, Agrawal R, Gutierrez-Sinisterra L, et al. Natural language processing in medicine and ophthalmology: a review for the 21st-century clinician. Asia-Pac J Ophthalmol. 2024;13:100084.
18. Xu F, Jiang L, He W, et al. The clinical value of explainable deep learning for diagnosing fungal keratitis using in vivo confocal microscopy images. Front Med. 2021;8:797616.
19. Tan TF, Dai P, Zhang X, et al. Explainable artificial intelligence in ophthalmology. Curr Opin Ophthalmol. 2023;34:422–30.
20. Woodward MA, Maganti N, Niziol LM, Amin S, Hou A, Singh K. Development and validation of a natural language processing algorithm to extract descriptors of microbial keratitis from the electronic health record. Cornea. 2021;40:1548–53.
21. Sarayar R, Lestari YD, Setio AAA, Sitompul R. Accuracy of artificial intelligence model for infectious keratitis classification: a systematic review and meta-analysis. Front Public Health. 2023;11:1239231.
22. Kuo M-T, Hsu BW-Y, Yin Y-K, Fang P-C, Lai H-Y, Chen A, Yu M-S, Tseng VS. A deep learning approach in diagnosing fungal keratitis based on corneal photographs. Sci Rep. 2020;10:14424.
23. Koyama A, Miyazaki D, Nakagawa Y, Ayatsuka Y, Miyake H, Ehara F, Sasaki S, Shimizu Y, Inoue Y. Determination of probability of causative pathogen in infectious keratitis using deep learning algorithm of slit-lamp images. Sci Rep. 2021;11:22642.
24. Ghosh AK, Thammasudjarit R, Jongkhajornpong P, Attia J, Thakkinstian A. Deep learning for discrimination between fungal keratitis and bacterial keratitis: Deepkeratitis. Cornea. 2022;41:616–22.
25. Wang L, Chen K, Wen H, Zheng Q, Chen Y, Pu J, Chen W. Feasibility assessment of infectious keratitis depicted on slit-lamp and smartphone photographs using deep learning. Int J Med Inform. 2021;155:104583.
26. Ueno Y, Oda M, Yamaguchi T, et al. Deep learning model for extensive smartphone-based diagnosis and triage of cataracts and multiple corneal diseases. Br J Ophthalmol. 2024;108:1406–13.

27. Mayya V, Kamath Shevgoor S, Kulkarni U, Hazarika M, Barua PD, Acharya UR. Multi-scale convolutional neural network for accurate corneal segmentation in early detection of fungal keratitis. JoF. 2021;7:850.
28. Ong ZZ, Sadek Y, Qureshi R, et al. Diagnostic performance of deep learning for infectious keratitis: a systematic review and meta-analysis. EClinMed. 2024;77:102887.
29. Soleimani M, Esmaili K, Rahdar A, et al. From the diagnosis of infectious keratitis to discriminating fungal subtypes; a deep learning-based study. Sci Rep. 2023; https://doi.org/10.1038/s41598-023-49635-8.
30. Hung N, Shih AK-Y, Lin C, Kuo M-T, Hwang Y-S, Wu W-C, Kuo C-F, Kang EY-C, Hsiao C-H. Using slit-lamp images for deep learning-based identification of bacterial and fungal keratitis: model development and validation with different convolutional neural networks. Diagnostics. 2021;11:1246.
31. Soleimani M, Cheung AY, Rahdar A, et al. Diagnosis of microbial keratitis using smartphone-captured images; a deep-learning model. J Ophthalmol Inflamm Infect. 2025; https://doi.org/10.1186/s12348-025-00465-x.
32. Li Z, Xie H, Wang Z, et al. Deep learning for multi-type infectious keratitis diagnosis: a nationwide, cross-sectional, multicenter study. Npj Digit Med. 2024; https://doi.org/10.1038/s41746-024-01174-w.
33. Bakken IM, Jackson CJ, Utheim TP, Villani E, Hamrah P, Kheirkhah A, Nielsen E, Hau S, Lagali NS. The use of in vivo confocal microscopy in fungal keratitis – progress and challenges. Ocul Surf. 2022;24:103–18.
34. Lv J, Zhang K, Chen Q, et al. Deep learning-based automated diagnosis of fungal keratitis with in vivo confocal microscopy images. Ann Transl Med. 2020;8:706.
35. Tang N, Huang G, Lei D, et al. An artificial intelligence approach to classify pathogenic fungal genera of fungal keratitis using corneal confocal microscopy images. Int Ophthalmol. 2023;43:2203–14.
36. Essalat M, Abolhosseini M, Le TH, Moshtaghion SM, Kanavi MR. Interpretable deep learning for diagnosis of fungal and acanthamoeba keratitis using in vivo confocal microscopy images. Sci Rep. 2023;13:8953.
37. Wu X, Qiu Q, Liu Z, Zhao Y, Zhang B, Zhang Y, Wu X, Ren J. Hyphae detection in fungal keratitis images with adaptive robust binary pattern. IEEE Access. 2018;6:13449–60.
38. Liang S, Zhong J, Zeng H, Zhong P, Li S, Liu H, Yuan J. A structure-aware convolutional neural network for automatic diagnosis of fungal keratitis with in vivo confocal microscopy images. J Digit Imaging. 2023;36:1624–32.
39. Tiwari M, Piech C, Baitemirova M, et al. Differentiation of active corneal infections from healed scars using deep learning. Ophthalmology. 2022;129:139–46.
40. Demir S. Evaluation of the reliability and readability of answers given by chatbots to frequently asked questions about endophthalmitis: a cross-sectional study on chatbots. Health Informatics J. 2024; https://doi.org/10.1177/14604582241304679.
41. Shaeri M, Shoeibi N, Hosseini SM, Jeddi FR, Farrahi R, Nabovati E, Salehzadeh A. An intelligent decision support system for acute postoperative endophthalmitis: design, development and evaluation of a smartphone application. BMC Med Inform Decis Mak. 2023; https://doi.org/10.1186/s12911-023-02214-3.
42. Nezu N, Usui Y, Saito A, et al. Machine learning approach for intraocular disease prediction based on aqueous humor immune mediator profiles. Ophthalmology. 2021;128:1197–208.
43. Atta S, Perera C, Kowalski RP, Jhanji V. Fungal keratitis: clinical features, risk factors, treatment, and outcomes. J Fungi (Basel). 2022;8:962.
44. Hanif A, Prajna NV, Lalitha P, NaPier E, Parker M, Steinkamp P, Keenan JD, Campbell JP, Song X, Redd TK. Assessing the impact of image quality on deep learning classification of infectious keratitis. Ophthalmol Sci. 2023;3:100331.
45. Evans NG, Wenner DM, Cohen IG, Purves D, Chiang MF, Ting DSW, Lee AY. Emerging ethical considerations for the use of artificial intelligence in ophthalmology. Ophthalmol Sci. 2022;2:100141.

46. Floridi L, Cowls J, Beltrametti M, et al. AI4People—an ethical framework for a good AI society: opportunities, risks, principles, and recommendations. Minds Mach. 2018;28:689–707.
47. Han R, Acosta JN, Shakeri Z, Ioannidis JPA, Topol EJ, Rajpurkar P. Randomised controlled trials evaluating artificial intelligence in clinical practice: a scoping review. Lancet Digit Health. 2024;6:e367–73.
48. Jobin A, Ienca M, Vayena E. The global landscape of AI ethics guidelines. Nat Mach Intell. 2019;1:389–99.
49. Ahmadikia K, Aghaei Gharehbolagh S, Fallah B, Naeimi Eshkaleti M, Malekifar P, Rahsepar S, Getso MI, Sharma S, Mahmoudi S. Distribution, prevalence, and causative agents of fungal keratitis: a systematic review and meta-analysis (1990 to 2020). Front Cell Infect Microbiol. 2021;11:698780.
50. Pararajasegaram R. The global initiative for the elimination of avoidable blindness. Community Eye Health. 1998;11:29.

Correction to: Fungal Conjunctivitis

Andrés Tirado-Sánchez, Alexandro Bonifaz,
Jesús Heriberto Dávila-Alquisiras,
and Max Carlos Ramírez-Soto

Correction to:
Chapter 6 in: M. C. Ramírez-Soto (ed.), *Fungal Eye Infections*, https://doi.org/10.1007/978-3-032-19923-2_6

This title has been published recently. Figure 6.4 in Chapter 6 was inadvertently published with an incorrect detail–the following content in the flowchart "Mucopurulent or mucropurulent" should read only as "Mucopurulent". This correction chapter includes the updated figure.

The updated version of this chapter can be found at
https://doi.org/10.1007/978-3-032-19923-2_6

M. C. Ramírez-Soto (ed.), *Fungal Eye Infections*,
https://doi.org/10.1007/978-3-032-19923-2_13

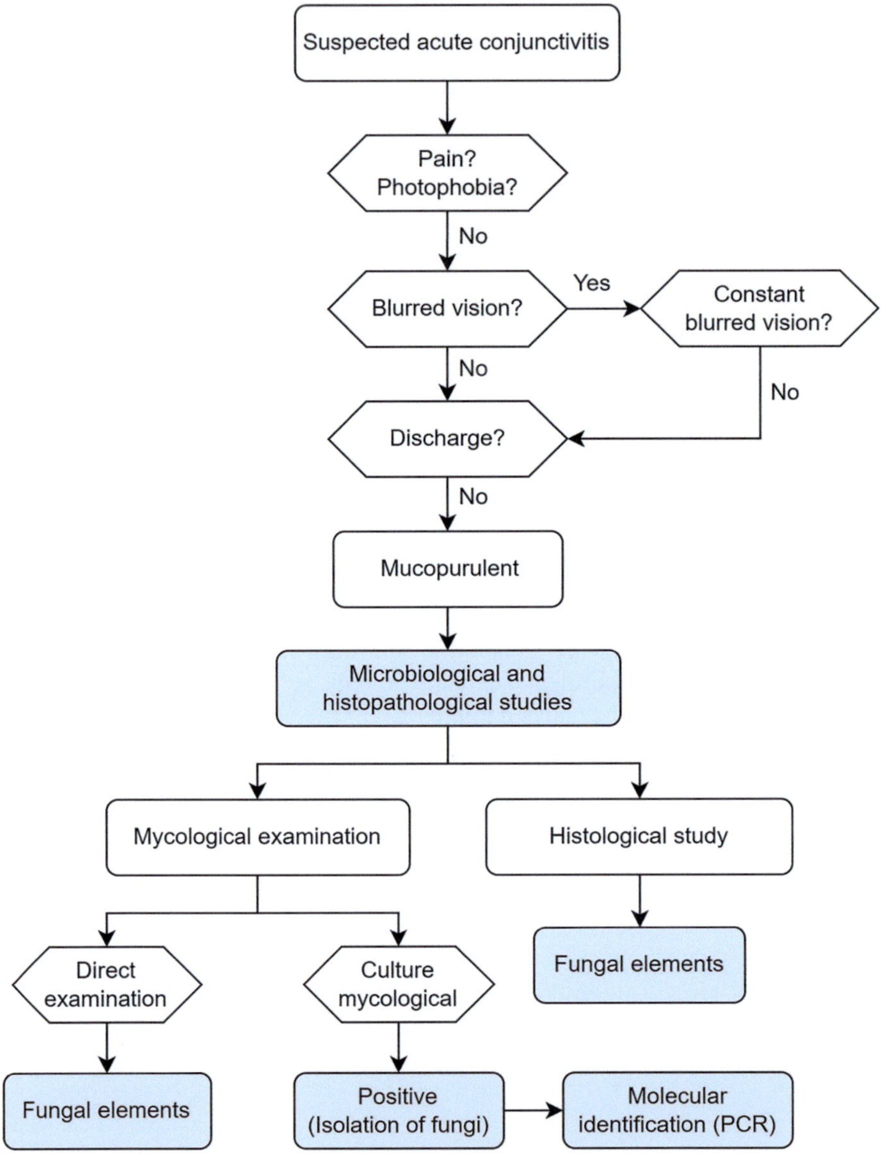

Fig. 6.4 Proposed algorithm for the diagnosis of fungal conjunctivitis

Index

M. C. Ramírez-Soto (ed.), *Fungal Eye Infections*,
https://doi.org/10.1007/978-3-032-19923-2

G

H

O

U

V

W

Y

Z

MIX
Papier aus verantwortungsvollen Quellen
Paper from responsible sources
FSC® C105338

If you have any concerns about our products,
you can contact us on
ProductSafety@springernature.com

In case Publisher is established outside the EU,
the EU authorized representative is:
Springer Nature Customer Service Center GmbH
Europaplatz 3, 69115 Heidelberg, Germany

Printed by Libri Plureos GmbH
in Hamburg, Germany